Liver/Biliary Cancer	Lung Cancer	Lymphoma (Hodgkin's)	Lymphoma (non-Hodgkin's)	Mouth and Throat Cancer	Multiple Myeloma	Ovarian Cancer	Pancreas Cancer	Prostate Cancer	Sarcomas: Bone, Cartilage and Soft-Tissue
Chapter 36 page 180	Chapter 22 page 132	Chapter 41 page 192	Chapter 41 page 192	Chapter 31 page 169	Chapter 43 page 200	Chapter 27 page 157	Chapter 35 page 178	Chapter 25 page 147	Chapter 39 page 187
M equal to F	M more than F	M more than F	M more than F	M more than F	M more than F	F	M more than F	M	M equal to F
over 65	55–65	20s, 70s	50–70	over 45	over 50	65–84	70–79	over 50	under 18
15,000	**155,000**	7,500	33,000	31,000	12,000	20,000	27,000	103,000	8,000
decreasing	increasing	constant	increasing	increasing	constant	constant	increasing	increasing	constant
clearly implicated; significant number of cases	somewhat implicated; some cases	not shown to be a factor	not shown to be a factor	slightly implicated; very few cases	not shown to be a factor	somewhat implicated; some cases	clearly implicated; significant number of cases	clearly implicated; significant number of cases	not shown to be a factor
not shown to be a factor	**strongly implicated; large number of cases**	not shown to be a factor	not shown to be a factor	**strongly implicated; large number of cases**	not shown to be a factor	not shown to be a factor	somewhat implicated; some cases	not shown to be a factor	not shown to be a factor
strongly implicated; large number of cases	slightly implicated; very few cases	clearly implicated; significant number of cases	clearly implicated; significant number of cases	not shown to be a factor	slightly implicated; very few cases	not shown to be a factor	not shown to be a factor	slightly implicated; very few cases	slightly implicated; very few cases
somewhat implicated; some cases	clearly implicated; significant number of cases	slightly implicated; very few cases	slightly implicated; very few cases	slightly implicated; very few cases	somewhat implicated; some cases	slightly implicated; very few cases	somewhat implicated; some cases	slightly implicated; very few cases	somewhat implicated; some cases
strongly implicated; large number of cases	not shown to be a factor	not shown to be a factor	not shown to be a factor	**strongly implicated; large number of cases**	not shown to be a factor	not shown to be a factor	somewhat implicated; some cases	not shown to be a factor	not shown to be a factor
slightly implicated; very few cases	somewhat implicated; some cases	slightly implicated; very few cases	slightly implicated; very few cases	slightly implicated; very few cases	somewhat implicated; some cases	slightly implicated; very few cases	slightly implicated; very few cases	not shown to be a factor	clearly implicated; significant number of cases
slightly implicated; very few cases	slightly implicated; very few cases	slightly implicated; very few cases	slightly implicated; very few cases	not shown to be a factor	slightly implicated; very few cases	slightly implicated; very few cases	slightly implicated; very few cases	slightly implicated; very few cases	somewhat implicated; some cases
gallstones	second-hand smoke	rich	immunity	poor	blacks	no children	poor	blacks	congenital
very good chance of prevention	**excellent chance of prevention**	hard to prevent	hard to prevent	**excellent chance of prevention**	hard to prevent	hard to prevent	very good chance of prevention	limited chance of prevention	hard to prevent
hard to detect early	hard to detect early	hard to detect early	hard to detect early	**excellent chance of early detection**	hard to detect early	hard to detect early	hard to detect early	limited chance of early detection	hard to detect early
surgery radiation therapy ? chemotherapy ?	surgery radiation therapy chemotherapy immunotherapy ?	radiation therapy chemotherapy	radiation therapy chemotherapy immunotherapy	surgery radiation therapy chemotherapy	chemotherapy radiation therapy immunotherapy ?	surgery chemotherapy radiation therapy	surgery radiation therapy ? chemotherapy ?	surgery chemotherapy radiation therapy	surgery radiation therapy chemotherapy
rarely curable 5%	rarely curable 13%	**fairly curable 70%**	possibly curable 50%	possibly curable 50%	possibly curable 25%	rarely curable 35%	rarely curable 3%	**fairly curable 70%**	**fairly curable 50%**

	Skin Cancer (Melanoma) Chapter 21 page 123	Skin Cancer (non-Melanoma) Chapter 21 page 123	Stomach Cancer Chapter 34 page 176	Testicular Cancer Chapter 29 page 163	Thyroid Cancer Chapter 38 page 184	Uterine-Cervical Cancer Chapter 26 page 150	Uterine-Endometrial Cancer Chapter 26 page 150	Vaginal Cancer Chapter 28 page 160
Epidemiology								
Sex (M: male, F: female)	M more or equal to F	M more than F	M more than F	M	F more than M	F	F	F
Age (range of peak incidence)	over 20	45 to 75	50–59	15–35	25–65	25–55	55–65	over 40
Cases Annually (approximately)	27,000	**500,000 +**	20,000	6,000	11,500	13,000	34,000	21,000
Incidence	increasing	increasing	increasing	increasing	increasing	increasing	increasing	increasing

Causes/Risk Factors

Strength of evidence for the listed factor as a cause of that type of cancer, and the approximate number of cases attributable to that factor.

	Skin Cancer (Melanoma)	Skin Cancer (non-Melanoma)	Stomach Cancer	Testicular Cancer	Thyroid Cancer	Uterine-Cervical Cancer	Uterine-Endometrial Cancer	Vaginal Cancer
Diet (causative, rather than preventive)	not shown to be a factor	not shown to be a factor	**strongly implicated; large number of cases**	not shown to be a factor	slightly implicated; very few cases	slightly implicated; very few cases	**strongly implicated; large number of cases**	somewhat implicated; some cases
Tobacco (smoked and smokeless)	not shown to be a factor	not shown to be a factor	somewhat implicated; some cases	not shown to be a factor	not shown to be a factor	somewhat implicated; some cases	different studies have shown both positive and negative effects	not shown to be a factor
Infection (primarily viruses, but also parasites)	not shown to be a factor	not shown to be a factor	not shown to be a factor	somewhat implicated; some cases	not shown to be a factor	clearly implicated; significant number of cases	slightly implicated; very few cases	slightly implicated; very few cases
Occupation (exposure at work, primarily chemical)	slightly implicated; very few cases	slightly implicated; very few cases	slightly implicated; very few cases	slightly implicated; very few cases	slightly implicated; very few cases	not shown to be a factor	not shown to be a factor	not shown to be a factor
Alcohol (alcohol alone or with smoking)	not shown to be a factor	not shown to be a factor	slightly implicated; very few cases	not shown to be a factor	not shown to be a factor	not shown to be a factor	not shown to be a factor	not shown to be a factor
Radiation (ionizing/medical, or non-ionizing/sun)	**strongly implicated; large number of cases**	**strongly implicated; large number of cases**	slightly implicated; very few cases	somewhat implicated; some cases	clearly implicated; significant number of cases	not shown to be a factor	not shown to be a factor	somewhat implicated; some cases
Genetics/Heredity (inherited risk, family history)	somewhat implicated; some cases	clearly implicated; significant number of cases	somewhat implicated; some cases	slightly implicated; very few cases	somewhat implicated; some cases	not shown to be a factor	somewhat implicated; some cases	not shown to be a factor
Unique causative factors	whites	whites	Japanese	undescended testes	Hawaiians	sex	estrogens	DES

Prevention/Early Detection

	Skin Cancer (Melanoma)	Skin Cancer (non-Melanoma)	Stomach Cancer	Testicular Cancer	Thyroid Cancer	Uterine-Cervical Cancer	Uterine-Endometrial Cancer	Vaginal Cancer
Primary prevention (prevent from beginning)	**excellent chance of prevention**	**excellent chance of prevention**	very good chance of prevention	very good chance of prevention	limited chance of prevention	**excellent chance of prevention**	very good chance of prevention	limited chance of prevention
Secondary prevention (early detection)	very good chance of early detection	**excellent chance of early detection**	limited chance of early detection	very good chance of early detection	limited chance of early detection	**excellent chance of early detection**	very good chance of early detection	very good chance of early detection

Treatment/Prognosis

	Skin Cancer (Melanoma)	Skin Cancer (non-Melanoma)	Stomach Cancer	Testicular Cancer	Thyroid Cancer	Uterine-Cervical Cancer	Uterine-Endometrial Cancer	Vaginal Cancer
Treatments used (? indicates that treatment is experimental, but may be effective)	surgery chemotherapy radiation therapy immunotherapy	surgery chemotherapy radiation therapy	surgery radiation therapy ? chemotherapy ?	surgery chemotherapy radiation therapy	surgery radiation therapy chemotherapy	surgery radiation therapy chemotherapy immunotherapy ?	surgery radiation therapy chemotherapy	surgery radiation therapy
Overall cure rate (percent free of cancer five years after treatment)	**fairly curable 80%**	**highly curable 95%**	rarely curable 10%	**highly curable 90%**	fairly curable 95%	fairly curable 65%	fairly curable 80%	fairly curable 30%

understanding cancer

Completely Revised Third Edition

Mark Renneker, M.D.

**Based on the premise
that education is our
most powerful weapon
against cancer.**

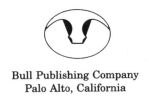

Bull Publishing Company
Palo Alto, California

Dedication

*To those who have struggled
to understand and combat
this dreadful disease.*

Copyright © 1988 Bull Publishing Company

Bull Publishing Company
P.O. Box 208
Palo Alto, CA 94302-0208
(415) 322-2855

ISBN 0-915950-86-3

First Edition: March 1977
Second Edition: June 1979, Updated 1984
Third Edition: September 1988, Updated 1989

Cover and interior design: Detta Penna
Production Manager: Helen O'Donnell

Library of Congress Cataloging-in-Publication Data
Understanding cancer / [edited by] Mark Renneker.
— 3rd ed.
        p. cm.
    Includes bibliographical references and index.
    ISBN 0-915950-86-3 : $24.95
    1. Cancer. I. Renneker, Mark, 1952-.
RC261.U44 1988
616.99'4—dc19   87-33804
                                                CIP

**A percentage of profits from this book will be
used to establish a Summer Fellowship
program for students interested in cancer
education.**

Table of Contents

Acknowledgements   v
Foreword   viii
Preface   ix
How to use this book   xi

Part 1   Orientation—*Renneker*   **1**

---

1. Introduction to Cancer   2
2. Principles of Cancer Prevention   5
3. The History of Cancer   8
4. The Cancer Field   13
5. Cancer Pathology–Terms and Concepts   17

Part 2   Biologic Aspects of Cancer   **25**

---

6. The Biology of Cancer—*Garrett*   26
7. Immunology—*Asimov/Clark*   52
8. Viruses and Cancer—*Starr*   61
9. Evolution and Cancer—*Dawe*   72

Part 3   Causes of Cancer   **77**

---

10. Overview–Everything Does Not Cause Cancer—*Renneker*   78
11. Diet and Cancer—*DiSogra*   81

12. Tobacco as a Cause of Cancer and Death—*Wilson/Renneker*   85
13. Parasites, Bacteria, and Cancer—*Renneker*   90
14. Reproductive and Sexual Behavior as a Cause of Cancer—*Doll/Peto*   93
15. Occupational Carcinogenesis—*Page/Asire*   95
16. Radiation and Cancer—*Renneker/Coggle/Walters*   100
17. Solar Radiation—*Page/Asire*   108
18. Iatrogenesis and Cancer—*Page/Asire*   110
19. Air and Water Pollution—*Page/Asire*   114

Part 4   Major Sites of Cancer—*Renneker*   **117**

---

20. Cancer Review   118
21. Skin Cancer (including Melanoma)   123
22. Lung Cancer   132
23. Cancer of the Colon and Rectum (and Anus)   135
24. Breast Cancer   139
25. Prostate Cancer   147
26. Uterine Cancer–Cervical and Endometrial   150
27. Cancer of the Ovary   157
28. Vagina, Vulvar, and Less Common Gynecological Cancers   160
29. Testicular and Male Genitalia Cancers   163
30. Urinary Tract Cancers–Kidney and Bladder   166
31. Cancer of the Mouth and Throat   169
32. Cancer of the Larynx   172
33. Cancer of the Esophagus   174

34. Cancer of the Stomach 176
35. Cancer of the Pancreas 178
36. Cancer of the Liver (and Gall Bladder) 180
37. Brain and Central Nervous System Tumors 182
38. Thyroid and Other Endocrine Gland Cancers 184
39. Sarcomas: Bone, Cartilage, and Soft-tissue Cancers 187
40. Introduction to Blood and Lymphoid Tissue Cancers 189
41. Lymphomas (including Hodgkin's Disease) 192
42. Leukemias 196
43. Multiple Myeloma 200
44. Childhood Cancers 202

Part 5   The Treatment of Cancer   207

45. Treatment Overview—*Renneker* 208
46. Principles of Cancer Surgery—*Renneker* 209
47. Radiation Oncology: Principles and Practice—*Odell* 213
48. Chemotherapy, Immunotherapy, and Biological Treatments—*McWaters/Renneker* 220
49. Spontaneous Regression of Cancer—*Cole* 233
50. What Is a Tumor Board?—*Renneker* 236
51. Cancer Registries—*Zippin* 238
52. Rights of the Cancer Patient—*Krant* 240
53. Cancer Quackery—*ACS* 243

Part 6   Understanding Cancer—For the Patient   251

54. Persons Who Have Had Cancer—*Bray* 252
55. Everything You Ever Wanted to Ask or Tell Your Physician But Were Afraid to, Lying on Your Back in a Hospital Bed, Tied to an IV Pole, Feeling Helpless, Vulnerable, and Dependent—*Leib* 255
56. Understanding Cancer: Personal, Interpersonal and Social Considerations—*Nathan* 257
57. For You, The Patient—*Rosenbaum* 263
58. The Will to Live—*Rosenbaum* 266
59. Nutrition for the Cancer Patient—*Rosenbaum* 271

60. Rehabilitation Exercises for the Cancer Patient—*Rosenbaum* 274
61. Sexuality and Cancer—*Rosenbaum* 276
62. Stress and Cancer—*Doolittle* 279
63. What is an Ostomy?—*Mullen/McGinn* 285
64. Job Discrimination—*ACS* 290
65. Death and Dying—Mortuis Vivos Docent—*White* 292
66. Questions and Answers on Death and Dying—*Kübler-Ross* 301
67. Hospice Care—*Larschan* 305
68. Living Wills—*Larschan* 308

Part 7   Cancer Prevention and Early Detection   313

69. Practicing Cancer Prevention—*Renneker* 314
70. Self-Examination for Cancer—*Renneker* 318
71. Breast Cancer Detection—Mammography and Other Methods—*McGinn* 330
72. Flexible Sigmoidoscopy 338
73. Diet and Cancer Prevention—*DiSogra* 343
74. Understanding Smoking—*Wilson* 358
75. Sputum Cytology: A Method to Assess Respiratory Health—*Sorenson* 367
76. Avoiding Unnecessary X-Rays—*Laws* 371
77. Environmental Cancer Issues Into the 1990s—*Raymond* 374
78. Cancer in the Economically Disadvantaged—*American Cancer Society* 380

Part 8   Understanding AIDS—*Eberle/Renneker*   385

79. History of the AIDS Epidemic 387
80. Cancer and AIDS 394
81. Clinical Spectrum of HIV Infection 399
82. Treatment for HIV Infection 403
83. Research and AIDS 407
84. The Prevention of AIDS 409
85. The Psychosocial Aspects of AIDS 416
86. The Future—Spread or Control? 419
87. Resources for Information and Support 421

Glossary 425
Appendix 435
Index 461

Acknowledgements

In three editions, extending over a decade, there have been many who deserve thanks and acknowledgement. In gratitude, then:

— to Steve Leib, for starting the Biology of Cancer;

— to the student coordinators, faculty sponsors, and guest speakers who volunteered their time and energy to the Biology of Cancer classes;

— to the members, then and now, of the Public Education Committee of the California Division of the American Cancer Society, for their continued support of the Biology of Cancer;

— to the valuable, behind-the-scenes assistance of an unsung legion, the staff of the American Cancer Society;

— for being friends along the way: Helene Brown, Jordan Wilbur, Marilyn Young, Debbie Rodgers, Charles Daniel, Henry Hilgard, Glenn Hildebrand, George Saunders, Barry Humphrey, Berkeley Mathews, Jennie Cook, Kent Sorenson, Lester and Devra Breslow, Sid Saltzstein, Bill Clark, Don Casperson, Laurens White, Anne Marie Daze, Lee Hilborne, Harold Harper, Carroll Pfrommer, Diane McCay, Eric Schmidt, Sylvia Davis, Leonardo Da Vinci, Del Paden (and friends), Jan Kirsch, Pat Rhyner, Gale Granger, Steve Trevor, Dick Ingraham, Denise Presotto, Melanie Wolf, Ric Loya, Laura Nathan, Nancy Evans, Ernie Rosenbaum, David McWaters, Micaela Thompson, Ron Goldschmidt, Laura Keranen, Gary Wilson, Craig Wilson, Steve Tillis, Shelly Bechtloff, Cathy Coleman, Joan Hall, Peggy Montagne, Arlyss Anderson, Robert Schweitzer, Davis Leino-Mills, May Sung, and Linda Cushman;

— to the following environments for the good eats and intense brainstorming they provided: Bill's Place, Mago's Famous Hamburgers, Lady Ester's, Everett and Jones BBQ, Ananda-Fuara, and Nepenthe;

— for love and support, from the Leib, Dunne, and Renneker families;

— to James Watson, for sharing in this project;

— to Helen O'Donnell and Pat Anderson of Bull Publishing, for their patience and professionalism;

— to Dave Bull, unwavering in his support and enthusiasm.

Understanding Cancer
Third Edition

Editor: Mark Renneker, M.D., A.B.F.P. (Diplomate, American Board of Family Practice). Assistant Clinical Professor, Department of Family and Community Medicine, University of California—San Francisco. Attending physician, the Cancer Education and Prevention Center, Merritt Hospital, Oakland, California (counseling, teaching, and examining patients); South of Market Health Center, San Francisco, California (inner-city family practice); Family Practice Residency Program, San Francisco General Hospital (teaching clinical preventive medicine and flexible sigmoidoscopy); and Laguna Honda Hospital (caring for the elderly). Fourteen-year-volunteer with the American Cancer Society, California Division, as a member of the Board of Directors and Public Education Committee (founding chair of the Biology of Cancer Sub-Committee, AIDS Work Group, and Aging Work Group). Member, the American Teachers of Preventive Medicine, the American Association of Cancer Education, the Surfer's Medical Association (founder and president). Founder of "Second Opinions"—a San Francisco/Oakland based consulting service devoted to finding new options for people in difficult medical situations.

Editors of Previous Editions: Mark Renneker and Steven Leib

Contributors to the Third Edition:

Adela Augsburger *Exam Questions*
Coordinator, 1986-88 Biology of Cancer
University of California, Irvine

Steven Bray, M.A. *Psychosocial Aspects*
Writer in residence
Olympia, Washington

William R. Clark, Ph.D. *Immunology*
Professor of Immunology
University of California, Los Angeles

Charles DiSogra, M.P.H., Ph.D. and
Lorelei DiSogra, Ed.D., R.D. *Diet and Cancer*
State Department of Public Health
Sacramento, California

Scott Eberle, M.D. *AIDS*
Family Practice Resident
Santa Rosa Community Hospital
Santa Rosa, California

Laurie Garrett *Biology of Cancer*
Broadcast Journalist
Berkeley, California

Steven Leib, M.D., A.B.F.P.
Private Practice, Family Medicine
Felton, California

David McWaters, Pharm. D. *Chemotherapy*
Assistant Professor
University of the Pacific, School of Pharmacy
(Stockton)
San Francisco, California

Laura E. Nathan, Ph.D. *Social Aspects*
Associate Professor of Sociology
Mills College
Oakland, California

Rollin Odell, M.D. *Radiation Oncology*
Chief, Radiation Oncology
Merritt Hospital
Oakland, California

Greg Raymond, M.S. *Environmental Aspects*
Industrial Hygienist
San Francisco, California

Ernest H. Rosenbaum, M.D. *Rehabilitation*
Medical Director
San Francisco Regional Cancer Foundation
San Francisco, California

Kent Sorenson *Sputum Cytology*
LungCheck
Cupertino, California

Karin Spears *Exam Questions*
Coordinator, 1986-87 Biology of Cancer
University of California, Irvine

Kevin Starr *Viruses*
4th Year Medical Student
University of California, San Francisco

Jeanette Wagner *Exam Questions*
Coordinator, 1986-87 Biology of Cancer
University of California, Irvine

Craig Wilson, M.D., M.P.H. *Smoking*
San Francisco Department of Public Health
San Francisco, California

Including Works by:
Isaac Asimov *Immunology*
Ardyce J. Asire *Causes of Cancer*
Judith Bray, O.T.R. *Rehabilitation*
David G. Bullard, Ph.D. *Sexuality*
Arthur Z. Cerf, M.D. *Rehabilitation*
J. E. Coggle, M.D. *Radiation*
Warren H. Cole, M.D. *Spontaneous Regression*
Clyde J. Dawe, M.D. *Comparative Neoplasia*
Sir Richard Doll, F.R.S. *Causes of Cancer*
Mark J. Doolittle, Ph.D. *Stress and Cancer*
Harry Drasin, M.D. *Nutrition*
Howard Franklin, M.D., M.P.H. *Occupational*
Melvin J. Krant, M.D. *Rights of Cancer Patients*
Elizabeth Kübler-Ross, M.D. *Death and Dying*
Edward J. Larschan, J.D., Ph.D. *Psychosocial*
Richard J. Larshcan, Ph.D. *Psychosocial*
Priscilla W. Laws *Radiation*
Francine Manuel, R.P.T. *Rehabilitation*
Kerry Anne McGinn, R.N. *Breast Cancer Detection*
Barbara Dorr Mullen *Ostomy*
Harriet S. Page *Causes of Cancer*
Richard Peto, M.D. *Causes of Cancer*
Stanley L. Robbins, M.D. *Pathology of Cancer*
Isadora R. Rosenbaum *Rehabilitation*
Carol A. Stitt, R.D. *Nutrition*
Jean M. Stoklosa, R.N., M.S.N. *Sexuality*
J. Walter, M.D. *Radiation*
Laurens P. White, M.D. *Death and Dying*
Calvin Zippin, Sc.D. *Cancer Registries*

Foreword

From the first edition

When I was in college in the mid 1940s, cancer was not a dominating factor in the public arena. We knew little about its fundamental nature, and there was no reason to believe that we should soon have any deep revelations, much less come up with some miracle cures. That being so, it probably made sense to ignore it as much as possible. Uncontrolled public discussion would probably generate more fear than hope, and broadcasting impotence reassures no one.

Today the situation could hardly be more different. It is almost impossible to read several issues of a major newspaper without coming across some new potential cause of cancer or of a new research lead that might help us cure it. The net effect of all this information flow, however, has not necessarily been more rational public behavior. Instead, I fear that all too many indigestible facts may make us even less able to prevent new cancers or find more inspired ways to fight already existing ones. So many things have been called cancer-causing agents, that there is an increasing tendency to lump all agents together, ignoring say, the fact that a mild reduction in tobacco consumption is likely to have far greater beneficial effects than the banning of all known food additives. And so many research leads have been overplayed for their curative consequences, that our words as scientists are often quickly dismissed by an ever desperate population that is increasingly tempted by worthless hoaxes like Laetrile.

There is no way, however, that we can return to the days when it made sense to keep cancer out of the public discussion. To try to do so would be a tragic response. We now know enough to be able to state with confidence that already much cancer could be prevented if we used preexisting knowledge. And there do exist some cancers which with proper medicine can be beaten. Unfortunately, many major forms are still effectively incurable, and we can only hope that someday new research kowledge will let us defeat them. Here it is important for the public to realize the great gaps which still exist in our fundamental knowledge, and the fact that many, many decades of high quality research may be necessary before we really know what to do.

A rational public response, however, requires an educated electorate, and I greatly applaud the student directed efforts which have led many colleges and universities to a series of courses aimed at presenting the current state of the cancer problem. No good text yet exists, and so they have put together this collection of the articles and essays. It provides many of the key facts that we should all know, and is to be especially commended for its broad overview that goes from pure science to the real social problems that cancer causes.

I thus hope it soon reaches a very wide audience.

James D. Watson
Cold Spring Harbor Laboratory

September 28, 1978

Preface

Understanding Cancer was first developed in 1976, in response to the textbook needs of students participating in the American Cancer Society "Biology of Cancer" courses.

The Biology of Cancer was first given at the University of California, Santa Cruz, in 1973. An accredited undergraduate biology course, it was conceived, designed, and coordinated entirely by Steven Leib, an undergraduate in his senior year of pre-medical studies. The class was sponsored by the American Cancer Society, and taught by a series of guest lecturers from all over California. Lectures ranged from the strictly biological aspects of cancer (cells, genetics, viruses, immunology) to the clinical and psychosocial aspects (diagnosis, treatment, prevention, quackery, death and dying). The class was an outstanding success: in a school of only 4,500 students, over 500 completed the course. I was one of those students.

That Biology of Cancer class was an exciting, spontaneous phenomenon that showed how hungry college students are to learn about cancer. Though many of the students were science majors or pre-medical students—such as myself—fifty percent were non-science majors and members of the community. For most, the reason for taking the class was personal: cancer strikes three out of four families. That, too, was my reason: my father had recently been diagnosed with a tumor (though it fortunately turned out to be benign).

Since 1973, I, along with many other students who were turned on by taking a Biology of Cancer class, have been starting and coordinating new courses throughout California. Variously titled "Biology of Cancer" or "Understanding Cancer," there have been over 100 such courses given, at virtually every college and university in California. Courses have been started in other states, too.

For the first several years, a good textbook for the class couldn't be found—a fact borne out by the student evaluations of the various books that were tried. These were found to be either too narrow in scope, too simplistic, or devastatingly scientific. And so, we, as students, decided to prepare our own textbook—*Understanding Cancer*.

The first edition, in 1976, was a purely grassroots effort. Steve Leib and I, both medical students at the University of California, San Francisco, made a book by cutting, pasting, and xeroxing the best of many cancer articles and books. We called it "stringing together pearls." The students loved it—we sold as many as we could print.

The second edition, in 1979, involved refining the rough cut "pearls" and having student coordinators research and write various chapters. Tired of sneaking into the university after hours to xerox yet more copies of the book, we found Dave Bull, of Bull Publishing, who, somewhat to our surprise, was happy to publish it. Dave quickly found that working with students was no easy task, as he began supplying books to up to twenty Biology of Cancer courses a year. He also introduced James Watson to the project.

Dave Bull took to heart James Watson's hope that the book would reach a very wide audience, and determined that a wide range of people were interested in the book—from the general public in local bookstores, to cancer patients and their families, to nurses using the book in home study continuing education courses.

Other cancer books have come on the market, some good, some not so good. Each has been tried by at least one of the Biology of Cancer classes, but they return to *Understanding Cancer*. Sales pitch aside, this is the book for the Biology of Cancer—student-developed, it's homegrown, it's The Original.

By 1982-83, enough had changed in the cancer field to merit a new edition. But with Steve Leib off at UCLA, finishing family practice residency and preparing to start a practice near Santa Cruz, and with my starting family practice residency at UCSF, the book had to wait. And then the AIDS epidemic hit.

I was particularly reluctant to put out a new edition in the light of AIDS' impact on the cancer field, to say nothing of the rest of science and medicine, and society. To have written then about AIDS would have ensured being out-of-date within weeks—things were changing that fast. Here was a totally mysterious, rapidly spreading, sometimes cancer-causing disease that seemed to be an encapsulation of everything that had already happened in cancer—the fear and hysteria, the seeming incurability, the stigmata of having it, the community organizations springing up, the need for education and service to patients, the accelerated and exciting research. In fact, AIDS was taking cancer's place as the most feared—and fascinating—of all diseases.

By 1986, the AIDS picture was becoming clear enough to write about—and include in this book. I think you'll see it as a true addition.

Steve Leib is happily ensconced in his family practice now, having created a comprehensive cancer prevention and screening center in his office, and wasn't able to help edit this time around.

In this edition, there are many new chapters and new contributors. Some of the past student coordinators are now health professionals and professors. I hope we haven't forgotten what it's like to *not* know the language and concepts of medicine and science, and that we can still speak (and write) in plain English. You be the judge.

Mark Renneker, M.D.
San Francisco, California

How to Use This Book

A primary goal of this book is to make you into an avid cancer preventionist. The first step in that process is to gain a broad understanding of cancer—what it is, what causes it, and how it affects people. Only then can you really begin to take steps, for yourself and the people close to you, to prevent cancer, or detect it early.

This book should be useful to a wide audience—college students from all disciplines, health professionals, patients and those close to them, anyone who is concerned about cancer. Whether directly or indirectly, cancer affects each of us. Though a purpose of this book is to serve as a textbook for courses in cancer,* it provides more than just fodder for the academic cannons. It provides ammunition for now (and the future) to understand cancer in your life.

ALL READERS

The minimum that all readers of this book—students, health professionals, patients, and the concerned public—should read:

- chapters 1 through 5 (Orientation);

- chapter 10 (Overview—Everything Does Not Cause Cancer);

*For anyone (student, faculty, American Cancer Society staff or volunteer) interested in starting a Biology of Cancer/Understanding Cancer class, a guide for starting such course is available from Bull Publishing—*The Biology of Cancer Sourcebook,* by Mark Renneker and Denise Presotto. The book is modeled after the "complete idiots' how-to-fix a Volkswagon" guide. Check it out!

- chapters 69 and 70 (Practicing Cancer Prevention and Self-Examination for Cancer);

- chapters on cancer that personally affect you—your own cancer (if any), a cancer in your family, or a cancer that you particularly worry about (see chapters 21–44, on each type of cancer).

STUDENTS

College and university students taking a cancer course, such as The Biology of Cancer, will almost certainly need to master the material in chapters 6, 7, and 8 (The Biology of Cancer, Immunology, and Viruses). Biology and science majors will have a headstart on these subjects; non-science majors may find it takes some work. Unfortunately, there may not be more than one or two lectures in your course on these subjects, and you probably will be tested on the material.

Check yourself out with Part 9, Testing Your Understanding of Cancer." This section is separately bound, but accompanies each book that will be used for a cancer course. It consists of the best exam questions from the many cancer courses given in recent years. (This isn't provided with all copies of the book, since it serves such a specialized function, i.e., cramming!)

Unlike some books you'll use in college, this book will be worth keeping—as a reference for the future. Someone you know will develop cancer, and you'll want to refer to it. I guarantee it.

Medical, nursing, and pharmacy students should pay special attention to the chapters on the major sites of cancer and on treatment (chapters 20 to 53). Though you may expect that during your health professional training you will be taught about cancer medicine, it is rarely done in a comprehensive manner.

HEALTH PROFESSIONALS

Understanding Cancer can be prescribed for patients and their families. Also, home-study, continuing education courses have been structured around this book. Write the publisher for additional information.

PATIENTS, FAMILIES, AND FRIENDS

If you are a patient, use this book to understand your own cancer; if you are a family member or a friend of a patient, use it to better understand what they are going through, and to help provide information to them.

You will undoubtedly want to first read the chapter on the type of cancer you are facing. Don't be surprised if you come away with more questions that you started with. That's the time to back up, and read Part 1 (Orientation) focussing on Chapter 1—Introduction to Cancer, and Chapter 5—Cancer Pathology—Terms and Concepts.

The most practical information will come from Part 6 (Understanding Cancer—for the Patient). It may expose you to a greater range of options than were presented to you by the cancer treatment team. Don't be afraid to act on them.

—*M.R.*

1

Orientation

1

Introduction to Cancer

Mark Renneker, M.D.

"What do you fear most?" asked a public opinion poll a few years ago. The list of possible answers included all forms of calamities and maladies, ranging from earthquakes and atomic war, to heart attacks and cancer. Ninety percent of people picked cancer. Why? What is it about cancer that makes us so fearful?

Tuberculosis was the feared disease earlier in this century, smallpox and plague before that. Cancer is the most feared disease of our age—despite the fact that it accounts for only about 20% of deaths in our country. More than twice as many people die from heart attacks and strokes (cardiovascular disease), our number one killer. Ask yourself, would you be as interested to read this book if it were on heart attacks and strokes? Not likely.

Some people have a cancerophobia, a constant anxiety about cancer. For others, the thought of cancer may occur only during fleeting moments—in wondering, for instance, why a cold or a pain is taking so long to go away.

All physicians have seen patients with an obviously simple problem, such as a rash or stomach ache, who, upon questioning, admit they'd come in because they were afraid it might be cancer. The routine physical or checkup is sought by many largely as a reassurance of not having cancer.

Practically everyone—you and me alike—has worried at one time or another, even if only for a moment, that we might have cancer.

UNDERSTANDING CANCER

The immediate goal of this book is to replace fear with understanding. Only then can the task of practicing early detection and prevention be effectively addressed. Fear paralyzes; understanding facilitates.

Ask yourself, "Do you believe that cancer can be cured?" For many people, usually because someone close to them died from cancer, the answer is NO. If you don't believe that cancer can be cured, then the concept of early detection will make no sense whatsoever. You may reason, what difference does it make to find it early if you're going to die from it anyway?

TEN CONCEPTS ESSENTIAL TO UNDERSTANDING CANCER

1. Cancer is not a single disease, it is a GROUP OF DISEASES. There are at least one hundred different types of cancer, differing as to their cause, type of cell or organ affected, and treatment. For instance, breast cancers are quite different from skin cancers, and brain cancers are different from bone cancers. That's why it's less meaningful to speak of finding the "cure" for cancer than to say "cures for cancers." There will probably never be a single "cure" for cancer, but there will be—as there already have been—cures for specific cancers.

2. What all cancers have in common is UNCONTROLLED GROWTH AND ABNORMAL SPREAD OF CELLS. That is the definition of cancer. Cancer is called LOCALIZED, if it hasn't spread beyond the tissue or organ it is growing in, and METASTATIC if it has spread to other parts of the body. But when most of us think of cancer, it isn't abnormal cells or diseased organs we picture, it's the faces of people we've known who have had cancer. That's the meaning of cancer.

3. Cancer affects all forms of life. Dinosaurs had it, plants get it, insects get it, fish, reptiles, cats, dogs—all mammals, ALL LIVING THINGS CAN GET CANCER.

4. MOST CANCERS ARE SLOW TO START AND TAKE UPWARDS OF TEN TO TWENTY, TO FORTY YEARS TO GROW. If they go undetected or if their growth is not stopped, they will kill the person. This is called the "natural history of cancer." How cancers start is thought to be a multi-step process, starting with an initiating event (INITIATOR) that is then promoted (PROMOTER).

For instance, an initiator would be a chemical or radiation that changed a gene, and the promoter could be diet or an infection that set the cancer to growing. It is reasoned that all of us have probably had cancer many times during our lifetime, but that our immune system mops it up before it has a chance to grow.

5. CANCER IS CURABLE. In the early 1900s, few cancer patients had any hope of long-term survival. In the 1930s, less than one-in-five in the U.S. were alive five years after treatment. In the 1950s that number had improved to one-in-four. By the 1970s, it was one-in-three. And now, in the late 1980s, the number is one-in-two. It depends on what type of cancer a person has as to when he or she can be considered "cured." For children with leukemia, they can be considered cured just three years after treatment. For women with breast cancer, five years is too early to speak of cure—and so is, perhaps, ten years. This is an example of how cancers differ, and underscores the importance of thinking of each cancer as a separate disease.

6. 75% OF CANCERS WOULD BE CURED in the U.S. if the early detection tests and self-examination methods that are presently known were put into practice.

7. Though 50% of cancers are now being cured, THE TOTAL NUMBER OF CANCERS IS INCREASING in the United States. This is almost entirely due to smoking. We may be winning the war against treating cancers, but not in preventing them. That will remain true until there is a drop in the total number of new cancer cases.

8. ONE-IN-THREE PEOPLE IN THE U.S. WILL GET CANCER. The fact that one-in-three people will get cancer means that CANCER WILL STRIKE THREE OUT OF FOUR FAMILIES. Think about an average-sized family, including grandparents, and you are looking at a group of at least nine or ten people—three of which can be expected to get cancer. It's the rare family that doesn't have a history of cancer.

9. POOR PEOPLE HAVE MORE CANCERS. Cancer incidence and survival is related to socio-economic factors—such as education and the availability of health services. In our country, poor people have more cancers—and worse survival rates. For instance, blacks have more cancers than whites, particularly of the lung, colon-rectum, prostate, esophagus, and uterus. And blacks have

an overall five-year cancer survival rate of only 38% compared to 50% in whites.

10.   CLOSE TO 90% OF CANCERS ARE PRE-VENTABLE. Only a small percentage of cancers are genetic or likely because of heredity, the rest are a result of what happens to you as you go through life.

CANCER STATISTICS

There is a sea of statistics in the cancer field, and to understand the basic concepts—as outlined above—you are already swimming in numbers. The numbers only have importance in appreciating the magnitude of the problem, and in deciding which areas deserve priority. The following numbers are worth knowing.

1.   The world population is about 4 billion. THE WORLD CANCER DEATH RATE IS ABOUT 4 MILLION PER YEAR. The number one cancer in the world is stomach cancer. Until the 1950s, stomach cancer was also the number one cancer in our country.

2.   There are approximately 1,000,000 NEW CASES OF CANCER A YEAR in the United States, divided almost equally between men and women. This does not include an additional 500,000 cases of non-melanoma skin cancer and 50,000 cases of the highly localized—confined to a small area in which it began—"carcinoma in situ" of the cervix and breast. They are so rarely fatal that they aren't considered in the overall statistics.

3.   In our country, THE NUMBER ONE CANCER IS LUNG CANCER. For men, lung cancer is number one in cancer incidence and deaths. For women, breast cancer is number one in cancer incidence, but lung cancer causes almost as many deaths as breast cancer. Of the over 150,000 people diagnosed with lung cancer each year, 135,000 or more will die. That means the cure rate is less than one-in-ten.

4.   In our country, THE NUMBER TWO CANCER IS COLON-RECTAL CANCER (cancer of the large bowel—the colon and rectum). It affects men and women almost equally, but many people erroneously think that women don't get it. It was the number one cancer in this country in the late 1970s, but lung cancer passed it up. Of the almost 150,000 people diagnosed with colon-rectal cancer each year, only about 40% are presently being cured.

5.   In our country, BREAST CANCER IS THE NUMBER THREE CANCER. There are about 130,000 cases a year, and 40,000 deaths—meaning that the overall survival rate is about 70%. For every 100 cases in women, there is one in a man.

2

Principles of Cancer Prevention

Mark Renneker, M.D.

The orientation of this book is decidedly towards prevention. In the field of preventive medicine is a conceptual framework called the "levels" of prevention: primary, secondary, and tertiary. It is suggested that the same framework be used to think about cancer.

THE LEVELS OF PREVENTION

1. Primary prevention is the absence of disease. It's the steps taken to prevent a disease from ever developing. Childhood vaccinations against polio is a good general example. With cancer it would be not to smoke cigarettes. There are numerous other examples of primary prevention with cancer, and you should learn them all. That will be a major focus of this book—to teach you how to prevent cancer. Primary prevention is health and wellness.

2. Secondary prevention is early detection or screening for asymptomatic disease (where the disease is present, but not yet causing symptoms). Skin testing for tuberculosis is an example, or, with cancer, getting a Pap test to find early cervical cancer. Again, there are many other methods of screening for cancer—and you will be taught them.

3. Tertiary prevention is the level where, at present, most medical care is rendered—when a disease has gone too far and it is symptomatic (called "acute care"). The difference in viewing it from the perspective of prevention is that the goal of treatment is to prevent recurrence, but also to prevent the harmful effects of treatment—for instance, choosing a method of breast cancer surgery that has the best chance for cure, but is the least disfiguring. Tertiary prevention also includes the idea that if a disease is incurable, as in a terminal cancer, that pain and suffering will be ameliorated. Hospice care is an example of this.

PREVENTION IN THE CONTEXT OF THE NATURAL HISTORY OF CANCER

Think of primary, secondary, and tertiary prevention as occurring in a continuum, and overlay that continuum with the natural history of cancer [see Figure 2-1.]. The cutoff between the levels is somewhat arbitrary—health or disease is not an absolute. Secondary prevention would be the largest level: few of us are completely healthy, but most of us don't have active cancers.

At the top of Figure 2-1 is a normal cell whose DNA (genes) is altered by exposure to a carcinogen (cancer-causing agent), such as radiation, chemicals, or viruses. Cancer begins when that altered cell next divides, producing cancer cells. First there will be two cancer cells, then four, then eight, and so on. The natural history of cancer is that it will continue to grow until it kills the host. The time it takes to

Figure 2-1 The Levels of Prevention and the Natural History of Cancer. Illustration by Ken Miller.

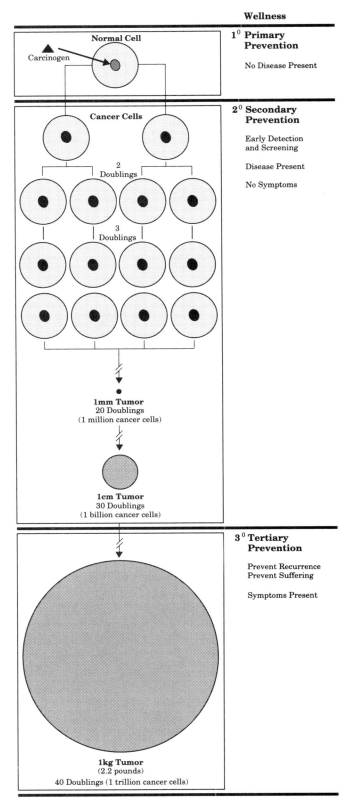

double the number of cancer cells is called the "doubling time."

The duration for doubling varies from tumor to tumor. Most people have an image of cancer as an explosive growth, rapid and frantic like a machine out-of-control. Bear in mind, though, that cancer cells sometimes duplicate more slowly than normal cells. For instance, a normal colon cell (a cell lining the inside of the large bowel) may take 300 days before it duplicates, whereas a cancerous colon cell may take 600 days.

It would probably be a number of years before a cancer had doubled, say, twenty times from the original cell. Twenty doublings would be a cancer with approximately one million cells in it (10^6). That may sound like a lot, but cells are quite small to begin with. A one-million-cell cancer would be only one millimeter in size (less than one-sixteenth of an inch). You would miss detecting a cancer that small even if it were growing on the tip of your nose. Undetected, it would keep growing.

By thirty doublings, it would be a 100 million cancer cell tumor (10^9), one centimeter in size (about a third-of-an-inch). You would notice a cancer that size if it were on your nose, but how about if it were in your breast? Maybe you'd find it, but only if you were really good at doing breast examination. If it were in a hard-to-examine organ like your stomach or liver, you wouldn't notice it—and it probably wouldn't yet be causing symptoms. It would just keep growing, as it already had been for perhaps twenty or more years.

At forty doublings you've got trouble. By now it would consist of over one trillion cells (10^{12}) and weigh over one kilogram (2.2 pounds). A cancer that size would result in death.

To accept waiting to find a cancer between the one centimeter and one kilogram size is to invite failure. At that stage, cancers become large in such a relatively short period of time. Any delay in diagnosis could be disastrous.

With colon cancer, four to six months is the average delay from when symptoms appear to when a physician is first seen. The person will explain that they thought the blood in their stool (the usual symptom of colon-rectal cancer) was from hemorrhoids. Unfortunately, it is often up to two more months before the physician finally makes the diagnosis of cancer, not hemorrhoids.

The cancer education level of the public and of physicians will determine where on the wellness-death time continuum a cancer will be detected. Cancer is detected later in those with limited education.

In the past, cancer education efforts were directed towards alerting the public to the early symptoms, or "warning signs" of cancer. However, for virtually all cancers, by the time they are symptomatic (causing problems) the chance for cure is already significantly reduced. The challenge is to find cancers as early as possible—before there are symptoms, when they are still small.

The frontier of secondary prevention can now be tackled. Cancers can be found early by screening examinations such as breast self-examination, testicular self-examination, skin self-examination, oral self-examination, and other self-exam techniques. Modern technology has given us excellent early detection tools such as mammography (breast x-rays), fiberoptic endoscopy (i.e., flexible sigmoidoscopy for examining the rectum and colon), biochemical screening methods (such as the guaiac, or stool hidden blood test), and cytological techniques (the Pap smear, sputum cytology).

Primary prevention and secondary prevention have always been the focus of the public health fields. But the field of medicine and most people's health practices are still generally at the level of "wait until it breaks before fixing it." It should be obvious that there needs to be a shift of emphasis towards early detection and primary prevention.

CANCER PREVENTION IS UPSTREAM THINKING

I heard a story as I was finishing medical school. It described just what I was feeling, and what I hoped to do. It directly pertains to cancer prevention. A friend related the story of a physician trying to explain the dilemma in the modern practice of medicine:

> "You know," he said, "sometimes it feels like this: there I am standing by the shore of a swiftly flowing river and I hear the cry of a drowning man. So I jump into the river, put my arms around him, pull him to shore, and apply artificial respiration. Just when he begins to breathe, there is another cry for help. So I jump into the river, reach him, pull him to shore, apply artificial respiration, and then just as he begins to breathe, another cry for help. So back into the river again, reaching, pulling, applying, breathing and then another yell. Again and again, without end, goes the sequence. You know, I am so busy jumping in, pulling them to shore, applying artificial respiration, that I have no time to see who the hell is upstream pushing them all in."

3

History of Cancer

Mark Renneker, M.D.

The following is a brief look at the historical findings, early guesses, research formulations, and landmark experiments concerning cancer. Although many research mistakes were made, some of the first theories have proven surprisingly accurate. Recent trends and events are also included.

125,000,000 B.C.

Cancer in dinosaurs: earliest known cancer is presumed to be the hemangioma (blood vessel tumor) of a vertebra reported in the fossil remains of a dinosaur from the Comanchean period of the Mesozoic era of geologic time.

1,000,000 B.C.

Cancer in early man: traces of cancer found in bone remains of Java man (Pithecanthropus), unearthed in 1891.

2500–1500 B.C.

Egyptians and cancer: bone cancer identifiable in mummies in the Great Pyramid of Gizeh; also, ancient Egyptian writings refer to clinical tumors and primitive means of treatment (by knife).

400 B.C.

Hippocrates: clinically recognized and described cancer of the breast, uterus, stomach, skin, and rectum; he coined the term *carcinoma* in reference to spreading tumors that destroy the patient, as opposed to benign tumors which he classed with hemorrhoids and other chronic ulcerations. The latter were called *carcinos*. For treatment he used caustic pastes and cautery (the burning away of tissues with a hot iron), but advocated no treatment for occult (deep-seated) tumors. He put forth the humoral theory of disease (four humors: *blood* from the heart, *phlegm* from the head, *yellow bile* from the liver and *black bile* from the spleen), in which he regarded disease as the result of imbalance of the four humors, with cancer resulting from too much black bile.

100 A.D.

First cancer surgery: by Celsus, a Roman physician. Roman surgeons were, in fact, doing mastectomies. (Remember, anaesthesia hadn't been invented yet.)

200 A.D.

Galen's theories: Galen (a Greek physician who practiced and taught medicine in Rome) distinguished "tumors according to nature" (such as enlargement of the breast with normal female maturation) and "tumors contrary to nature" (cancer). His distinctions, for the most part, hold true today. Galen also advocated the black bile theory of cancer, in which he thought that the more pungent the black bile, the more vile its effect. Galen taught that mel-

ancholy women, as opposed to sanguine women, have a tendency towards breast cancer. This is a view supported today by psychological research. Galen's theories dominated medical thinking through the Renaissance. In fact, Jean Astruc, a French physician in the 18th century (1600 years after Galen) went so far as to test Galen's bile and melancholy theories by comparing the tastes of the burnt ashes of a breast tumor with that of a beef steak, looking for a more pungent taste in the cancer ashes.

1700s

Cancer developments in France: the first cancer hospital was founded in Reims, France at a time when persons with cancer were regarded as being contagious like lepers. The French surgeon, Henri Ledran, demonstrated that cancer can spread through lymphatic channels to secondary sites. Also, Ledran advocated surgery as the only treatment for cancer, discarding all pastes and ointments.

1775

First identification of occupational-environmental cause of cancer: in England, Sir Percivall Pott published a paper on scrotal cancer in chimney sweeps. He reported that his patients had been forced as children to climb within the narrow chimneys to clear soot away. Unfortunately most of them wore no clothes and the prolonged irritation from contact with the soot eventually caused many of them to develop cancer of the scrotum.

During the same year, the Academie des Sciences et Beaux Arts in Lyon, France established a contest for investigations into the "causes of the cancer virus" and awarded first prize to a French physician, Bernard Peyrilhe, for his work involving the inoculation of dogs with human tumors to induce new "growths." Much later it was shown that these weren't really tumors, but merely pus-containing abscesses. At that time, microscopes hadn't been invented and so inflammatory swellings were often mistaken for malignancies.

Late 1700s

Theoretical work: Marie Françoise Bichat described cancer as being an "accidental formation" of tissue built up in the same manner as any other portion of the organism.

Early 1800s

Cancer as seen through the microscope: Johannes Müller, (from Germany) demonstrated that cancer tissue was made up of cells.

1858

Similarity of animal and human tumors: LeBlanc reported that animal tumors were composed of cells similar in every respect to those that made up tumors in man.

1863

Further studies: Rudolf Virchow (a student of Müller's) declared that "every cell is born from another cell" ("omnis cellula e cellula"), and also he maintained that cancers were caused by irritation (the Irritation Theory), concurring with Pott's work.

1873

Cancer in tar workers: in Germany, Richard von Volkmann recognized that tar workers frequently developed cancers on their hands and forearms (the parts of their bodies primarily exposed to the tar).

1876

Health in the U.S.: average life expectancy of only forty years of age; tuberculosis is the leading cause of death; twice as many women as men die of cancer. Stomach is the leading cancer site in both sexes.

1877

Embryonal rest theory of cancer: advanced by Julius Cohnheim. He held that malignant tumors arose from fragmented embryonic tissues. Also during this time, many thought that cancer was the result of parasites (the parasitic theory of cancer), such as worms.

1884

First U.S. cancer hospital: the New York Cancer Hospital, in New York City, which in 1899 became the Memorial Hospital (still one of the major cancer hospitals in the east).

1894

The radical mastectomy: William S. Halsted, of the Johns Hopkins School of Medicine, initiated the en-bloc removal of a breast with cancer, its lymphatic attachments, and muscle attachments. This becomes the principal method of breast cancer surgery.

1895

X-rays: Wilhelm Roentgen discovered a new "penetrating ray;" and in 1898, Pierre and Marie Curie isolated radium—opening the way for the development of radiology. In the early years, the "magic rays" were somewhat indiscriminately applied to cancers, usually bathing the radiologist as much as the patient. Many of the early radiologists later died of radiation-induced tumors. Clinical radiation therapy was really established in France in 1922 when C. Regaud and his associates presented evidence that cancer of the larynx could be cured by irradiation without disastrous consequences. Radiation therapy received less emphasis as a primary treatment until after World War II.

Early 1900s

Transplantable tumors: when it became possible to transplant and grow tumors in laboratory animals, cancer research blossomed. Also, during this time the science of genetics was coming into its own.

1910

Viruses and cancer: F. Peyton Rous began his now classic studies on viral-induced tumors in chickens.

1913

American Cancer Society founded: in an attempt to educate the public about cancer, this voluntary organization came into existence. Samuel Hopkins Adams, a layman, wrote: "Be careful of persistent sores or irritations, external or internal. Be watchful of yourself, without undue worry. At the first suspicious symptoms go to some good physician and demand the truth. . . . The risk is not in surgery but in delayed surgery."

1915

Chemical carcinogenesis demonstrated: in Japan, Katsusaburo Yamagiwa and Korchi Ichikawa induced the first experimental tumors by applying tar to the inside of rabbits' ears. Research then turned to investigation of what was in the tar that caused the tumors, and, in 1930, Ernest L. Kennaway and his associates (in England) isolated polycyclic hydrocarbons and proved that they were the carcinogenic agent.

1928

George Papanicolaou describes a way to detect cervical cancer early, but it isn't until the mid-1940s that his "Pap Test" becomes a part of medical practice. By the late 1940s, the incidence of cervical cancer is steadily dropping.

1935

First cancer registry: in Connecticut, it was initiated to give continuous population-based information for clinical, etiologic, and epidemiological studies. In 1935, less than 20% of cancer patients are alive five years after diagnosis.

1947

First leukemia remissions: Sidney Farber, in Boston, successfully tested a new synthetic drug (aminopterin) on children with leukemia. Prior to that time, leukemia was uniformly untreatable and fatal. Thus began the modern era of chemotherapy and since that time many more drugs have been proven to be successful in the treatment of cancer.

Early 1950s

Owing to the fact that over 90% of breast cancers are detected by women themselves, the American Cancer Society introduces the idea of a breast self-examination (BSE)—hoping that women will find smaller, earlier cancers. However, despite intensive education efforts, to this day the percentage of women who perform BSE has never exceeded 30%. Lack of knowledge, a low level of confidence, and, paradoxically, a fear of finding a cancer are reasons given by women for not performing BSE.

1962

Henry Kaplan is using Stanford's linear accelerator to successfully treat Hodgkin's Disease. Radiation therapy has entered a new era. Even so, the cure rate for cancer continues to be less than 30%.

1964

The Surgeon General's Report on Smoking and Lung Cancer: At the turn of the century, lung cancer was such a rare disease that medical students were gathered in to see a case. With the world wars came the epidemic of smoking, and by 1950 lung cancer was the leading cancer killer in men. In 1964, the Surgeon General issued a landmark report alerting the public to the hazards of smoking. While smoking in men began decreasing, in women and teenagers it increased. In 1979, it was again time for the Surgeon General to state: "Cigarette smoking is the single most preventable cause of death in the United States."

1969

From the 1940s until this year, the synthetic estrogen, diethylstilbesterol (DES), has been widely used to prevent miscarriages. Arthur Herbst, at Massachusetts General Hospital, determines that female offspring are developing a previously rare type of vaginal cancer, and DES becomes a prime example of iatrogenesis (physician-caused illness). But, well into the 1970s, physicians widely prescribe estrogens, particularly to stave off menopause, until, again, they are shown to cause cancer—this time cancer of the uterus.

1970

Reverse transcriptase, the means by which RNA type retroviruses are able to replicate, is discovered by Temin, Mizutani, and Baltimore. Tumor virus research begins accelerating.

1971

The United States Congress passes the National Cancer Act, declaring war on cancer. The National Cancer Institute is given priority status and cancer research funding is substantially increased. At this time, about 33% of cancers are being cured.

1975

A new chemotherapeutic drug, cis-platinum, has recently been discovered. It is found to be highly effective in treating usually fatal germ cell tumors (like testicular cancer), practically changing overnight how those tumors are treated. It is a model for the hope that cancer research (and chemotherapy) can produce miracles.

1975–79

In the early to mid-1970s, there is heightened fear of breast cancer as it strikes Senator Birch Bayh's wife, Ambassador Shirley Temple Black, Governor Nelson Rockefeller's wife, and First Lady Betty Ford. In 1975, the five-year Breast Cancer Detection Demonstration Project, an ACS/NCI nationwide project involving over one-quarter million women, ushers in the era of effective screening for breast cancer. Mammography proves to be effective, but controversy erupts over risks of radiation—a belief that persists well into the 1980s, long after safer, lower-dose methods are instituted.

1977

Colorectal cancer is the number one cancer in the United States, but is soon overtaken by lung cancer.

1978

Molecular biology has developed to the extent that the ethics of genetic engineering has been the subject of the now famous Asilomar Conference in the early 1970s. In 1978, by recombining DNA, the first monoclonal antibodies are produced in a laboratory in London. This facilitates and accelerates cancer research, making it possible, for instance, to produce large quantities of natural cancer-fighting substances like interferon and interleukin-II.

1980

Robert Gallo, at the National Cancer Institute, announces that, after twelve years of work, he and his group have proof of the first human cancer virus—HTLV, which causes adult T-cell leukemia.

1980/81

The American Cancer Society issues their guidelines for cancer-related checkups, challenging traditional medical practices by recommending, among other things: healthy people under the age of 40 only need to see a doctor for a checkup every three years, but every year after 40; stopping doing routine chest x-rays, annually or otherwise, because it is practically worthless as a screening method for lung cancer; that, the Pap test needn't be performed yearly, that all women after age 35 should have periodic mammograms; and that all people after age 50, men and women alike, should be screened annually for colorectal cancer, including periodic sigmoidoscopy.

1981

With the sudden appearance in otherwise healthy young men of a previously rare cancer of elderly men, Kaposi's Sarcoma, the AIDS epidemic is discovered. It would be almost three years before

its cause would be determined, a virus named HTLV-3, or, as it is now called, human immunodeficiency virus (HIV). The history of the AIDS epidemic is like a condensed history of cancer, starting with fear and helplessness, but moving to understanding and hope.

1981/82

Few cancer researchers gave credence to the role of diet in cancer until Sir Richard Doll and Richard Peto publish their report on "Causes of Cancer," in which they indicate diet to be the probable number one cause of cancer deaths in the United States. Quickly following suit, the National Academy of Sciences, the National Cancer Institute, and the American Cancer Society begin recommending diet as a means to reduce cancer risk. The cancer and medical institutions have finally caught up with what the public has believed all along.

1985

As a result of screening with the stool occult blood test and a flexible fiberoptic sigmoidoscope and colonoscope, polyps and then an early colon cancer is found in President Reagan. For the first time, the American public becomes aware of polyps and colorectal cancer, and how they can be detected early by screening tests.

1988

Largely due to smoking, the total number of cases of cancer continues to increase, but public education combined with advances in research, early diagnosis, and treatment has, for the first time in history, brought the cure rate for cancer to 50%.

References

1. Breslow, Lester and Devra: "Historical Perspectives (in Cancer Control)," in *Cancer Epidemiology and Prevention,* Schottenfeld and Fraumeni (Eds.), W.B. Saunders Co., 1982.

2. Pitot, Henry C. Lecture notes for his course, Introduction to Experimental Oncology, University of Wisconsin, 1974.

3. Richards, Victor, M.D. "The History of Cancer." *Cancer: the Wayward Cell.* (Berkeley: University of California Press, 1972), pp. 81–92.

4. Shimkin, Michael B., M.D. "Neoplasia." *Advances in American Medicine: Essays at the Bicentennial.* Vol. 1. Edited by John Z. Bowers, M.D. and Elizabeth F. Purcell. (New York: Josiah Macy, Jr., Foundation, 1976), pp. 210–250.

4

The Cancer Field

Mark Renneker, M.D.

How does "progress" against cancer come about? When we speak of "cancer research," where does that take place, who is doing it, and who is paying for it? How is the American Cancer Society different from the National Cancer Institute?

The field of cancer is composed of a large number of organizations, institutions, and specialists from many fields. It can be quite confusing. To get to first base in understanding cancer requires first learning who the "players" are in the cancer field.

THE AMERICAN CANCER SOCIETY

The American Cancer Society (ACS) was founded in 1913 by lay members of the public. It is now the largest voluntary health organization in the world. Though it works closely with the Federal Government's National Cancer Institute, the American Cancer Society is completely independent from it. The mission of the American Cancer Society is the ultimate control of cancer.

The activities of the ACS are supported by donations from the public, which amounts to about 300 million dollars per year. Less than one-fourth of that money is spent on the organization itself and for raising further funds. The rest is divided almost equally between its three major activities: supporting cancer research, public and professional education, and service and rehabilitation for cancer patients and their families.

Broad policy is determined by the Board of Directors at the National level (the National office is in New York City). These policies are translated into action through 58 ACS Divisions (usually organized by states, e.g., the California Division of the ACS), and 3,252 Units (usually representing cities and centers of population), and Branches (local neighborhoods and suburbs). There are more than 2.5 million ACS volunteers—about one out of every 100 Americans.

The ACS supports only about one-fifth of the cancer research in this country, with the National Cancer Institute supporting most of the rest. However, the ACS has often proved itself venturesome and timely in its research allocations. For instance, the ACS funded the landmark epidemiologic studies on tobacco in the 1950s (Hammond, 1954), the first national cancer prevention study in the early 1960s (called CPS-I), and now the second national cancer prevention study (CPS-II), which is focusing on life style and environmental causes of cancer. The ACS has also developed quite a good track record in identifying and sponsoring beginning researchers, whose research and careers later gain major prominence.

Lester Breslow, M.D., M.P.H., a long-standing leader in the cancer control field and himself an active volunteer with the ACS, has at times been critical of the ACS, referring to its "conservatism when more activism seemed warranted," with regard to its sluggishness in translating research findings on tobacco use and other environmental carcinogens into genuine social action. However, in recent years the American Cancer Society has become more active, even so far as to lobby legislative bodies on issues relating to cancer.

The least obvious—but perhaps biggest—contribution of the American Cancer Society has been in removing much of the fear and stigmata that historically has surrounded the word "cancer." They have been pivotal in promoting their own and others' self-help programs for breast cancer patients (Reach to Recovery), throat cancer patients (laryngectomies), children with cancer (Candlelighters), colorectal or bladder cancer patients requiring ostomies (United Ostomy Association), and for cancer patients, in general, and their families (CanSurmount and I Can Cope).

To become a volunteer with the American Cancer Society, you need only call or walk into the ACS Unit in your town and say, "I'd like to volunteer. . ."

THE NATIONAL CANCER INSTITUTE

It wasn't until the 1920s that governmental cancer control activities began—and that was only at the state level. Congress followed suit in 1937 by passing the National Cancer Institute Act—which established the National Cancer Institute (NCI) as one of the National Institutes of Health (the largest). Others are devoted to heart disease, mental health, and so forth. The NCI, then, is the Federal government's official agency for research on cancer and its treatment.

The NCI was initially only minimally funded. For instance, in 1956 the entire appropriation for the NCI was under $25 million, compared to the ACS's $26 million raised that year. However, in 1971 the "war on cancer" was declared when Congress passed the National Cancer Act, and NCI funding has since increased to where it now tops $1.2 billion per year. An additional $800 million of Federal money supports cancer research at other institutions around the country. Over 5000 studies on cancer are supported by the Federal government, with the NCI conducting the majority of them—and overseeing the rest.

All aspects of cancer research take place at the NCI, from basic research on cells and viruses, to the application of that research in developing and testing new cancer therapies. The NCI attracts young, promising physicians and researchers and has, like the ACS, launched many in highly successful careers.

As with any government agency, a charge can be made that the NCI is sometimes slow and bureacratic. In some areas, however, the NCI has been quicker to respond than, for instance, the ACS. Recent examples are in the area of diet and cancer prevention, and with AIDS—both of which the ACS was slow to become involved with—but which the NCI took an earlier and more aggressive role in.

COMPREHENSIVE CANCER CENTERS

One of the activities of the National Cancer Institute has been to stimulate the regional consolidation and development of cancer research and treatment facilities. 25 institutions have been designated and funded by the NCI as Comprehensive Cancer Centers. To qualify, an institution must already have strong research and treatment programs, including advanced diagnostic and treatment programs, and be willing to participate in nationwide clinical trials of new treatment modalities.

The distribution of the 25 Comprehensive Cancer Centers is less in accordance with geography or population density, and more in terms of institutions' abilities to unify diverse and often disharmonious programs and personnel. For instance, there are two Comprehensive Cancer Centers in Los Angeles (at UCLA and USC) but none in Northern California (despite an abundance of cancer research and treatment programs at the University of California, San Francisco, and Stanford University).

STATE CANCER CONTROL SERVICES

States vary as to the range of cancer-related services they provide. The NCI depends on states to cooperate in implementing many of their cancer control programs. State-funded cancer programs may be comprehensive, or spotty and inconsistent, reflecting the character and temperament of the state and its governing bodies. However, state cancer resources can be far more accessible and responsive than the Federal government's.

UNIVERSITY RESEARCH CENTERS AND HOSPITALS

Almost every medical school in the United States has a university-affiliated faculty, and teaching hospital(s) in which cancer research is being conducted. Funding comes from the Federal Government (NCI), the American Cancer Society, private foundations, or the university itself.

Cancer research and treatment advances are always newsworthy, and local media will often carry news items on cancer-related activities of nearby universities and hospitals. Occasionally there will truly have been a breakthrough discovery, but it often only represents a successful public relations campaign on behalf of the university (public visibility equals more funding support). On the other hand, some of the most significant advances in cancer have come from tiny, seldom heard from cancer research labs.

CANCER FOUNDATIONS AND INSTITUTES

Scattered around the country are many non-governmental, non-university cancer foundations and institutes. They may have sponsorship or funding from the government, universities, or the American Cancer Society, but usually they are dependent on philanthropic funding—and may carry the name of the principal funder. They often have a special focus, for instance on leukemia, breast cancer, or cancer prevention. Unfortunately, there are also fraudulent "cancer foundations," often with a name deliberately similar to the American Cancer Society or the National Cancer Institute, that trick the public into giving them money.

CANCER RESEARCHERS

Any physician or scientist conducting research in an area of medicine or science that relates to cancer can be considered a cancer researcher—particularly if their funding is coming from the NCI or ACS. However, much of cancer research is simply basic scientific research (called "bench research"). For instance, investigations into the fundamental biochemistry of cells, or the development of techniques to produce monoclonal antibodies, do not involve cancer cells at all—but the outcome of research in those areas could contribute significantly toward major advances in cancer research per se.

In truth, much of the basic biomedical research in this country could as appropriately be funded in the name of, for instance, heart research or AIDS research (a shift which is, in fact, taking place). It just so happens that since the early 1970s the biggest pool of research money has been for programs targeted specifically at cancer. But cancer research cannot progress without progress in fundamental scientific research.

Another area of cancer research, albeit indirectly, has been through research funded by the Department of Defense. For instance, the linear accelerator used in radiation therapy can be viewed as a product of atomic bomb-related particle physics research.

CANCER SPECIALISTS

Cancer specialists are physicians who specialize in cancer. They are called oncologists, oncology being the name for the study of cancer. A surgical oncologist operates on cancers, and can be further specialized as, for instance, a gynecological oncologist (treating gynecological cancers only) or a urological oncologist (treating genitourinary cancers). A medical oncologist is an internist who took additional training in cancer, and is skilled in the use of drugs to treat cancer (cancer chemotherapy). Pediatric oncologists are generally pediatricians with special training in how to use chemotherapy to treat childhood cancers. And, there are radiation oncologists, who treat cancer with radiation. Nurses specializing in the care of cancer patients are called oncology nurses. Social workers working with cancer patients are oncology social workers.

Those are the common uses of the word "oncologist," but it could as well be applied to all other health professionals who primarily work with cancer. For instance, a psychiatrist or psychologist who specializes in seeing cancer patients and their families is certainly a cancer specialist, and could be called a psychiatric oncologist—but isn't. A specialist in cancer prevention can be said to work in the field of preventive oncology, but isn't generally called a preventive oncologist.

PATIENTS

The cancer field is spoken of as being multi-disciplinary (involving people and ideas from many different backgrounds). In recent years, the cancer patient has been increasingly considered a member of the cancer team—for obvious reasons. How true that is will vary from case to case, largely depending upon the team's "captain"—who is ideally the patient's primary physician. Remember, too, that every cancer case, every cancer patient is unique—as different as one person can be from the next. The cancer field, then, is varied and enormous.

"ALTERNATIVE THERAPY" PROPONENTS

There are a number of organizations and individuals in the United States who advocate methods of cancer treatment which have either been proved ineffective or have never been studied and tested by traditional scientific methods. These are called "unproven methods" by the American Cancer Society, or "alternative" and "nontoxic" therapies by their proponents.

These proponents include such organizations as the Cancer Control Society, the Committee for Freedom of Choice in Cancer Therapy, and the International Association of Cancer Victims and Friends. The John Birch Society has actively supported these groups. Advocated therapies include laetrile, Gerson and Hoxsey therapy, and Immune Therapies.

While most cancer researchers or cancer specialists would not consider the proponents of alternative or unproven methods to be part of the cancer field, they nevertheless see and attempt to treat substantial numbers of patients.

INTERNATIONAL UNION AGAINST CANCER

The International Union Against Cancer is the most significant world-wide cancer organization. Formed in the 1930s, it is an international non-governmental organization composed of 185 institutes and national cancer associations of scientific, medical, and lay members in 79 countries. In varying locations, every four years it holds the major cancer conference in the world.

Suggested Reading

1. Breslow L, Breslow NE. Historical Perspectives (in Cancer Control). In Schottenfeld D, Fraumeni JF, ed. *Cancer Epidemiology and Prevention.* W.B. Saunders Co. 1982; 1039–1048.

2. Holleb AI, ed. The American Cancer Society Cancer Book. Doubleday and Co. 1986. (See Part 1, "Where we stand in the battle against cancer.")

3. American Cancer Society. Cancer Facts and Figures—1987.

* Consult the appendices in this book for a complete list of cancer information services.

5

Introduction to Cancer Pathology— Terms and Concepts

Mark Renneker, M.D.

Confusion abounds in the cancer field—particularly between physicians and patients—because of differing terminology and faulty understanding of the basic principles of cancer pathology. The purpose of this chapter is to establish a common set of terms and concepts about cancer.

Pathology is the study of disease. The pathologist is concerned with describing and classifying the various forms of cancer and studying how they arise, grow, spread, and kill. Pathologists decide which tissues are benign and which are malignant. They perform the autopsies. The view of the pathologist is vital in the field of cancer medicine. Parts of this chapter are adapted from an excellent book used by virtually all medical students, *Pathologic Basis of Disease,* by Stanley L. Robbins (Philadelphia, W.B. Saunders, regularly updated).

ONCOLOGY: THE STUDY OF TUMORS (NEOPLASMS)

All cancers can correctly be called tumors, but all tumors are not cancers. The word tumor simply refers to swelling, which could be from inflammation, hemorrhage (bleeding), edema (accumulation of fluid), or a growth (benign or malignant). In general use, though, the word tumor generally refers to a growth.

Confusion arises when physicians tell patients they have a tumor. The physician may be only thinking about a non-cancerous tumor, but patients may hear the word tumor and automatically think they have cancer. In our culture, particularly in film and on television, the word tumor is frequently used in place of the word cancer.

In the field of oncology, the word tumor is used interchangeably with the word neoplasm. Neoplasm means new growth (neo- means new or strange, -plasm means structure or growth). As with a tumor, a neoplasm can be benign or malignant. The word cancer refers only to a malignant neoplasm.

WHAT'S BENIGN AND WHAT'S MALIGNANT

The diagnosis of a "benign tumor" brings great relief. Deciding whether a tumor is benign or malignant is the most important judgment the pathologist is called upon to make. Once that decision is made, it decides the course of treatment, and the prognosis. Often it is not clearcut whether a tumor is benign or malignant. The following general criteria are used to help decide. (See Figure 5-1.)

Differentiation

Benign tumors consist of cells and tissue that are usually differentiated and typical of the part of the body in which they appear. Cancers range from being well differentiated to poorly differentiated. Well differentiated means that the cancer consists of relatively normal looking cells. These cancers tend to be less aggressive, less dangerous. Poorly differentiated cancers are more aggressive and have a worse prognosis. Poorly differentiated cancers are said to have de-differentiated, meaning that they have reverted to a more primitive embryonic state. That type of cancer is said to be anaplastic.

Mode of Growth

Benign tumors are usually encapsulated, meaning they are enclosed within a fibrous capsule. They rarely spread beyond that capsule. Malignant tumors are almost never encapsulated. They are characterized by invasive, erosive growth, and spread easily into other tissues and organs.

Rate of Growth

In general, malignant tumors grow more rapidly than benign tumors. The rate of growth generally parallels their degree of differentiation. Poorly differentiated cancers tend to have a greater number of cells actively dividing (in mitosis). The doubled-up chromosomes to begin that division process are called mitotic figures.

In the course of a cancer's growth, there may be long periods where it grows hardly at all, and it is said to be dormant. And then they can enter explosive growth phases. Some cancers may suddenly shrink in size, usually due to ischemic necrosis—when the cancer has outgrown its blood supply (decreased blood flow to a tissue is called ischemia), and part of it dies (tissue death is called necrosis).

Metastasis

The single biggest difference between benign and malignant tumors is that malignant tumors can

Figure 5-1 Comparisons between Benign and Malignant Tumors

Characteristics	Benign Tumor	Malignant Tumor
Differentiation	Structure often typical of the tissue of origin	Structure often atypical, i.e., differentiation imperfect
Mode of growth	Growth usually purely expansive, and a capsule formed	Growth infiltrative as well as expansive so that strict encapsulation is absent
Rate of growth	Usually progressive, slow growth which may come to a standstill or retrogress; mitotic figures scanty, and those present are normal	Growth may be rapid with many abnormal mitotic figures
Metastasis	Absent	Frequently present

metastasize. Cancers have the ability to be carried to other parts of the body, implant, and begin growing there. The implant is called a metastasis. That metastasis may give rise to others. Metastatic growth is discontinuous, as though it leaped from one place in the body to the other without leaving a trail. Benign tumors never metastasize.

There are four major routes by which cancers metastasize, of which blood vessel and lymphatic spread are the most common:

1. Spread by blood vessels: cancers often invade veins, and cancer cells may spill into the blood and be carried off to other parts of the body. Usually this will be to the lungs and the liver, where all blood is eventually routed. Occasionally, spread can be via arteries, but they are less often penetrated due to their thicker, more muscular walls. Blood vessel spread is typical of sarcomas (cancers arising in the soft body tissues, such as connective tissues, muscles, fat, tendons, vessels, and lymphoid tissue). It is also not uncharacteristic of carcinomas (cancers arising in epithelial tissues, such as the skin, mucosal linings of the mouth, throat, GI tract, and lungs) to spread via blood vessels.

2. Lymphatic spread: the lymphatic system is the body's drainage system, whereby fluid (lymph) passes from tissues through lymphatic vessels to lymph nodes and eventually into the body's circulatory system. The distribution of the lymphatic spread tends to follow natural channels of drainage. For instance, carcinoma of the breast spreads via the axillary (underarm) lymph nodes. Carcinomas mainly spread by lymphatics, sarcomas less so.

3. Spread by transplantation: this refers to cancers that are spread by mechanical means, for instance a surgeon's hands or instruments. Meticulous care is taken to not cause tumor spread by this route, and "no touch" techniques are employed by surgeons wherever possible. Cancer can also spread along the track of a needle inserted for the purposes of biopsy. Fortunately, this type of spread is rare. In laboratory conditions, cancers can be transplanted from one animal to another, and there are reports of laboratory workers, having acquired cancer by mishandling animal cancer cells.

4. Spread by seeding of body cavities: a cancer may penetrate a natural open field, such as the abdominal space or the lung cavity, and seed itself throughout that area. Examples would be with a stomach or ovarian cancer.

IDENTIFYING A CANCER CELL

The pathologist can spot a cancer cell because of its appearance under the microscope:

1. cell size is often increased;

2. cell shape is often distorted (called pleomorphism);

3. the cancer cell's nucleus is usually enlarged, even to the extent that the nucleus is as large as the rest of the cell (called an increased nuclear/cytoplasmic ratio);

4. deviation in the normal number of chromosomes (aneuploidy), so that there might be twice the normal diploid number (tetraploid) or less than the normal number (hypoploid);

5. hyperchromic nuclei, meaning that with certain stains the nucleus appears darker or more stained than normal cells;

6. abnormal mitoses are present (called mitotic figures).

On occasion, cells having the above characteristics can occur normally. For instance in the placenta and in healing tissues and bones.

DYSPLASIA, OR PRE-CANCER

Dysplasia is a type of growth that is the step before cancer, and it is called pre-cancer. In dysplasia, there is a disturbance in the orderly organization of cells and tissues. Particularly abnormal cells that don't quite fit the above criteria for a cancer cell are called dysplastic cells. Dysplasia is sometimes reversible.

CARCINOMA IN SITU

Carcinoma in situ is the step after dysplasia, where there is disturbed tissue growth in which cells can be found that fit the criteria of cancer, but where spread hasn't occurred from the tissue of origin. Carcinoma in situ is not reversible. It is the earliest stage of cancer. When the cancer has spread through the tissue it began growing in, it is called an invasive cancer.

THE DIAGNOSIS OF CANCER

The only definite way to diagnose a cancer is to examine tissue from it. This is done by means of a biopsy. The major types of biopsies are:

1. Incisional biopsy: cutting into a tumor and removing a portion of it. A specimen should be taken from the junction of the tumor and normal tissue so that normal and malignant tissues are included for comparison. A specimen taken from the center of a cancer may only show dead, necrotic tissue.

2. Excisional biopsy: for tumors that are small enough to be entirely removed, the entire growth is excised and sent for microscopic examination. If the growth doesn't extend beyond the specimen's borders, it is said to be an excisional biopsy and may be adequate treatment in and of itself.

3. Needle biopsy: by inserting a wide enough hollow needle into a tumor, a plug of tissue often can be obtained to diagnose cancer. However, it will not reveal the degree of spread.

4. Aspiration biopsy: using a needle with a suction device to aspirate cells and tissue can also provide the diagnosis of cancer, but, again, doesn't reveal the degree of spread.

CYTOLOGICAL DIAGNOSIS

The most reliable method of diagnosing cancer is by examining tissue, which is called a histological diagnosis (histology is the study of tissues). Next best is a cytological (cell) diagnosis. This is the method that Papanicolaou first described in 1928. In the "Pap smear," cells are obtained by scraping the opening to the cervix with a small spatula. Other methods of obtaining cells are by collecting secretions or discharges (breast secretions, sputum, stool, urine, etc.).

The categories commonly used to classify cells, for instance with Pap smears, are:

Class I: normal cells.

Class II: probably normal, but slightly atypical or abnormal cells (as might occur from inflammation or infection).

Class III: abnormal cells, possible dysplasia, suggestive of malignancy.

Class IV: probably cancer.

Class V: cancer.

A Class IV or V smear necessitates a formal biopsy.

STAGING OF CANCER

The stage of a cancer refers to the extent of its spread. Traditionally, a four stage system of assessment has been used. The exact definition of each stage varies for each type of cancer, but, in general, the staging system is as follows:

Stage I: a small, localized cancer that hasn't spread beyond its site of growth. The cancer is almost certainly without nodal (lymph nodes) or vascular spread (blood vessels). These are highly curable, usually by surgery alone. Carcinoma in situ is considered by some to be a stage I cancer, but others see it as preceding Stage I, causing confusion in cancer reporting.

Stage II: the cancer has spread locally through the organ it began in and may have reached adjacent lymph nodes. This is still considered to be a cancer with a good chance for cure.

Stage III: the cancer has spread into adjacent tissues and has definitely spread into the adjacent lymph nodes. Cure is still possible, but less likely.

Stage IV: the cancer has metastasized. The presence of metastases means that there is little chance of survival, but there are notable exceptions.

Because of inherent vagueness in the above system, oncologists developed a more specific method of describing the stage of a cancer, called the TNM system. T stands for Tumor, and refers to the primary site of the cancer. N stands for Nodes. M for Metastases. These symbols are further quantified by defining the primary site as T1, T2, T3, and T4 for advancing disease; N0, N1, N2, and N3 for advancing nodal involvement; and M0 or M1 for those without or with metastases.

NOMENCLATURE—CLASSIFICATION OF TUMORS

In order to discuss the phenomenon of neoplasia, it is important that certain aspects of currently-accepted nomenclature be understood. It should be noted, however, that there is no world-wide accepted nomenclature of neoplasms. In this country, nomenclature has revolved around the use of the suffix, "-oma," which literally means "tumor." With few exceptions, words with this suffix refer to neoplasms. An exception is the term, "granuloma," which is a non-neoplastic "tumor" of inflammatory tissue.

Tumor classification is based on:

a. histogenesis: tissue of origin and cell type.

b. biologic behavior: benign or malignant.

c. degree of differentiation: well differentiated, partly, or poorly.

d. anatomic site: organ or region.

e. descriptive adjectives relating to form or function, e.g. papillary (nipple-shaped elevation or projection), psammomatous (containing granular material).

f. eponyms: some tumors are named after the person who first characterized them, e.g., Ewing's sarcoma, Hodgkin's disease, Brenner's tumor, Wilms' tumor. Much of medical language is fraught with such non-descriptive eponyms, and there is a deliberate movement toward replacing them with more precise terms, but some of them are so firmly entrenched in common usage that they'll probably always be with us.

Cancers of the connective tissues are called *sarcomas*. A sarcoma is often referred to as a "soft-tissue" tumor, which, strange as it may seem, includes cancers of the bone. The sarcomas also include cancers of the muscles, blood and lymph vessels, cartilage, fibrous tissues, and fat. Sarcomas are of "mesenchymal" origin, referring to the embryonic tissue type from which the body's variety of connective tissues arose.

Cancers arising from the cells that line the body's internal and external surfaces are called *carcinomas*. This would include skin, the linings of the mouth, throat, bronchi, lungs, stomach, and the other body organs as well. If the organ is glandular, the tumor is referred to as an adenoma (benign) or an *adenocarcinoma* (malignant).

Because of long-standing usage, the following terms always mean malignancy, even though they don't follow all the rules of tumor classification: *lymphoma* (cancer of lymphoid tissue), *hepatoma* (cancer of the liver), and *melanoma* (cancer of the melanocytes, the cells that give the skin its color and that lead to tanning). Melanoma is more properly prefixed with the word "malignant" (i.e., malignant melanoma), and lymphoma is more properly affixed with the word "sarcoma" (i.e., lymphosarcoma).

There are upwards of 300 types of benign and malignant tumors, but only the major ones are listed in Figure 5-2. This list is for reference purposes only.

WHAT ARE THE MAJOR HISTOLOGIC TYPES OF CANCER?

Most body structures are composed of tissues made up of many different types of cells. Any one of these different cell forms may give rise to cancer. Thus, the common term "lung cancer" refers to a group of cancers, certain ones being more common than others. Figure 5-3, again, is for reference purposes only, and obviously needn't be memorized. It is included so that you can better appreciate what are the truly common forms of cancer and what are the more rare forms—a distinction which, in many cases, will dictate the degree of clinical knowledge available for diagnosis, treatment, and prognosis.

WHAT DO CANCER PATIENTS DIE OF?

There is no easy answer to this question. The effects of cancer that lead to death are poorly understood and involve direct and indirect effects both locally and systemically (throughout the body). The following factors are generally recognized:

1. *cachexia:* (from *Cancer Medicine,* "Cachexia and the Systemic Effects of Tumors," by Giovanni Costa, 1973). "The growth of cancer in a human host leads to profound alterations of organs and organ functions as consequences of destruction, attempted repair by the body's natural processes, and disrupted homeostasis. The result is the widely recognized but poorly understood syndrome known as cachexia."

". . . The patients appear chronically ill, often emaciated. Their skin is pale and atrophic. Their faces express the unspoken fear of a disease sensed at times only as the distant thunder of an all-encompassing storm, at times more fully as the progressive disintegration of one's physical wholeness continues. Edema, ulcerations, tumor masses, fractures, and abnormal drainages, when present, can completely subvert familiar shapes, habit, and frames of reference. . . .

"Besides the more obvious physical manifestations of cachexia, apathy, torpor, detachment,

Figure 5-2   A Combined Classification of Neoplasms

Tissue of Origin	Benign	Malignant
1. Epithelial Neoplasms		*Carcinomas*
Epidermis	Epidermal papilloma	Epidermal carcinoma
Stomach	Gastric polyp	Gastric carcinoma
Biliary Tree	Cholangioma	Cholangiocarcinoma
Adrenal Cortex	Adrenocortical adenoma	Adrenocortical carcinoma
Glandular (in general)	Adenoma	Adenocarcinoma
2. Connective Tissue Neoplasms		*Sarcomas*
Fibrous Tissue	Fibroma	Fibrosarcoma
Cartilage	Chondroma	Chondrosarcoma
Bone	Osteoma	Osteogenic sarcoma
Fat	Lipoma	Liposarcoma
Smooth muscle	Leiomyoma	Leiomyosarcoma
Skeletal muscle	Rhabdomyoma	Rhabdomyosarcoma
3. Neoplasms of the Hemopoietic and Immune Systems		
Lymphoid Tissue	Brill-Symmer's Disease	Lymphosarcoma (lymphoma)
		Lymphocytic leukemia
		Reticulum Cell Sarcoma
		Hodgkin's Disease
Granulocytes	—	Myelogenous leukemia
Erythrocytes	Polycythemia vera	Erythroleukemia
Plasma cells	—	Multiple Myeloma
Bone Marrow (in general)	—	Leukemias
4. Neoplasms of the Nervous System		
Glia	Astrocytoma	Glioblastoma Multiforme
	Oligodendroglioma	—
Meninges	Meningioma	Menigeal Sarcoma
Neurons	Ganglioneuroma	Neuroblastoma
Adrenal Medulla	Phaeochromocytoma	—
5. Neoplasms of Multiple Tissues		
Breast	Fibrodenoma	Cystosarcoma phylloides
Kidney	—	Wilms' Tumor
Ovary, testis, etc.	dermoid (benign teratoma)	Malignant teratoma
6. Miscellaneous Neoplasms		
Melanocytes	Pigmented nevus	Malignant Melanoma
Placental	Hydatiform mole	Choriocarcinoma
Ovary (Trophoblast	Granulosa cell tumor	Granulosa cell tumor
(Epithelium)	Cystadenoma	Cystadenocarcinoma
Testis	—	Seminoma

and anxiety are well known to physicians. They represent the participation of the mind in the gradual annihilation of metabolic processes and oncoming death."

2. *organ failure:* organ failure at the primary site of a cancer is uncommon. For instance, a lung or colon may still function despite the presence of a cancer. However, in the case of the liver or kidney, failure can occur easily. This may be as a result of a primary cancer, metastatic spread, or the accumulation of toxic byproducts. Obviously, failure of any of the other vital organs, such as the heart, could lead to immediate death.

3. *obstruction:* the sheer size and mass of a tumor could physically obstruct a vital organ such as the intestine, or an air passage or major vessel.

4. *increased intracranial pressure:* either because of a brain tumor or from intracranial bleeding because of disturbances in blood homeostasis (e.g., low platelet level in leukemia).

5. *hemorrhage, stroke, pulmonary embolus:* a major vessel could burst, there could be a slow bleed that couldn't be controlled, or a piece of tumor could detach and be carried through the blood vessels and come to lodge in the brain or lung—thus blocking blood flow and leading to fatal damage.

6. *infection:* the impaired defense mechanisms of a cancer patient, particularly those with leukemia, provides the opportunity for infection by *bacteria* (pseudomonas, salmonella, serratia, listeria, clostridia, tuberculosis), *fungi* (candida, asper-

Figure 5-3 Frequency Distribution of Histologic Types in Some Major Sites of Cancer: United States, 1969–1971 (TNCS, microscopically proven cases only).

Site	Histologic Type	Percent	Site	Histologic Type	Percent
Lung Bronchus & Trachea (20,255 cases)	Epidemoid Carcinoma	34.7		Lymphosarcoma	1.9
	Adenocarcinoma	16.5		Reticulum Cell Sarcoma	2.5
	Oat Cell Carcinoma	13.4		Other & Unspecified Lymphomas	1.0
	Broncholar Carcinoma	3.2		Other & Unspecified Cancer	0.9
	Other & Unspecified Carcinomas	29.9	Prostate (13,206 cases)	Adenocarcinomas	98.6
	Sarcomas & Lymphomas	0.4		Medullary Carcinoma	0.3
	Other & Unspecified Cancer	1.8		Transitional &/or Squamous Cell	0.3
Breast (23,630 cases)	Duct Carcinoma & Paget's Disease	51.0		Clear Cell Carcinoma	0.2
	Adenocarcinomas	38.6		Other Specific Carcinomas	0.4
	Medullary Carcinoma	3.5		Sarcomas & Lymphomas	0.1
	Lobular Carcinoma	2.8		Other & Unspecified Cancer	0.2
	Colloid Carcinoma	2.2	Uterine Cervix (5,169 cases)	Epidemoid Carcinoma	84.1
	Other Specific Carcinomas	1.3		Adenocarcinoma	6.1
	Stromal Sarcomas & Lymphomas	0.4		Other & Unspecified Carcinomas	9.1
	Other & Unspecified Cancer	0.2		Sarcomas	0.7
Colon & Rectum (24,430 cases)	Adenocarcinomas	87.0	Uterine Corpus (6,593 cases)	Adenocarcinomas	79.5
	Colloid Carcinomas	7.8		Papillary Adenocarcinoma	6.4
	Papillary Carcinoma	2.2		Adenocanthomas	7.6
	Squamous Cell Carcinomas	1.6		Other & Unspecified Carcinomas	2.9
	Other Specific Carcinomas	0.1		Mixed Mullerian Tumors	1.5
	Malignant Carcinoids	0.5		Leiomyosarcoma	0.9
	Sarcomas & Lymphomas	0.4		Stromal Sarcoma	0.7
	Other & Unspecified Cancers	0.4		Other Sarcomas	0.5
Stomach (5,085 cases)	Adenocarcinomas	70.9		Unspecified Cancer	0.2
	Mucinous Carcinomas	6.6			
	Signet Ring Carcinomas	1.3			
	Other & Unspecified Carcinomas	12.8			
	Leiomyosarcoma	1.9			

Source: Department of Health, Education and Welfare, *Cancer Rates and Risks,* second edition (Washington, D.C., U.S. Government Printing Office, 1974) p. 21.

gillus, cryptococcus, phycomycetes, nocardia), *viruses* (cytomegalovirus, herpes simplex, herpes zoster, measles), and *protozoa* (toxoplasma, pneumocystis). Often these will be drug-resistant organisms unique to the hospital environment (hospital or nosocomial infections).

This list of possible causes of death is not conclusive, but should illustrate that there can be a variety of factors involved, most of which fall within the syndrome known as cachexia.

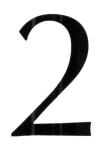

Biologic Aspects of Cancer

The Cancer Cells

Today I saw a picture of the cancer cells,
Sinister shapes with menacing attitudes.
They had outgrown their test-tube and advanced,
Sinister shapes with menacing attitudes,

Into a world beyond, a virulent laughing gang.
They looked like art itself, like the artist's mind,
Powerful shaker, and the taker of new forms.
Some are revulsed to see these spiky shapes;
It is the world of the future too come to.
Nothing could be more vivid than their language,
Lethal, sparkling and irregular stars,
The murderous design of the universe,
The hectic dance of the passionate cancer cells.
O just phenomena to the calculating eye,
Originals of imagination. I flew
With them in a piled exuberance of time,
My own malignance in their racy, beautiful gestures
Quick and lean: and in their riot too
I saw the stance of the artist's make,
The fixed form in the massive fluxion.

I think Leonardo would have in his disinterest
Enjoyed them precisely with a sharp pencil.

—Richard Eberhart

6

The Biology
of Cancer

Laurie Garrett

As an undergraduate biology major at the University of California, Santa Cruz, Laurie Garrett was a student in the first Biology of Cancer class in 1973. She went on to the University of California, Berkeley, to do graduate work in immunology. While doing her doctoral research she also served as science editor for KPFA-FM (Berkeley) radio news, and eventually fled the test tubes for the microphone—feeling a commitment to demystifying science for the public. She won a Peabody Award for science programming in 1977. Since 1980 Garrett has been a Science Reporter for National Public Radio's "All Things Considered" and "Morning Edition."

The following section on The Biology of Cancer represents a somewhat unconventional approach to presenting basic biology. It is offered as an alternative to the often unimaginative and dry "university" approach that frustrated too many of us, including Ms. Garrett.

This section assumes no biology or science background. It should be of particular value to non-science students and community members. (For those with scientific training, it should serve as a review.) Read not to memorize, but rather to enjoy, and to gain an appreciation of the beauty and simplicity of the biology of cells.

The artwork for this section is by Daniel Ziegler, a San Francisco Bay Area freelance artist.—*M.R.*

INTRODUCTION

At the basis of all diseases, no matter how terrifying or mystifying they may be, lies a set of biological facts. What may be viewed as symptoms by the physician and pains by the patient is ultimately discerned as a series of biological events. Cancer is biology gone astray, a maverick anarchistic biology which defies the rules of cellular behavior. To understand what has gone wrong, it is first necessary to comprehend the order of things; which leads us to basic biology.

"Cancer" has become a powerful word in our society—a word which evokes a wide range of emotional, scientific, economic, and political responses. The disease—or, more properly, the over one hundred different diseases which comprise cancer—has affected nearly every family in our country and dominated the very fabric of our society. And yet, surprisingly few people understand it.

When cancer is reduced to its most basic biological elements, it can be better understood and more effectively prevented and cured. The estimate that some 70–90% of all cancers are caused by exposure to environmental and dietary agents provides a crucial link between the public and science. If environmental agents can cause cancer, control of these agents may reduce the incidence of the disease. Therefore, cancer must be seen as a public health problem.

As with all public health issues, the successful control of a health problem is dependent upon an informed public. The American Cancer Society Biology of Cancer course is intended to provide the public with the essential information needed to understand and cope with the cancer problem.

BRIEF PREVIEW

In the following chapter you will learn that all living organisms are composed of cells, and that in higher organisms (such as human beings) the cells provide the building blocks for each of the body's organs (such as the heart, lungs, skin, and eyes). Cells contain tiny organelles which do most of the work for them. The organelles are discrete bodies, located throughout the inside of cells, which perform the task of digesting "foods" (proteins, sugars, water, oxygen) that come into the cell, converting them into energy and proteins to serve the cell's needs.

Protein is the key. Contrary to Madison Avenue images, protein is not just something found in a hair cream or a food supplement. It might be there, but it's more important and complex than hair cream. If something is wrong with the protein balance or function in an organism, illness or death can result.

Proteins are molecules which carry out most of the work essential to life. You will learn that proteins play critical regulatory roles in relation to other molecules. Finally, you will learn about DNA, RNA, and how proteins are made.

Then, the differences between normal cells and cancer cells will be discussed. The essence of cancer is damage to the DNA, or genetic integrity, of the cell. That damage may be caused by a wide variety of natural and synthetic agents (carcinogens) in our environment.

Cancer can, in many cases, be cured.

It can also, in many cases, be prevented.

LET'S GET SMALL

As we begin to grapple with the basic building blocks of biological systems, we start small. Let's get small. Really, really small. We'll start with the *atom*, which is literally out of sight (microscopically speaking). The tiniest atom, hydrogen, weighs 1.66×10^{-27} kg, or is 1,660,000,000,000,000,000,000,000,000 times smaller than a human being. Now that's small. (It may be small but it's mighty: 63% of the human body is hydrogen.) Every type of atom is different in size, weight, and internal composition.

Atoms combine through a special process known as bonding. Chemical bonds linking one atom to another are the basis of the entire discipline of chemistry, and are a bit much for us to discuss here. Suffice it to say that when two hydrogen atoms merge with one oxygen atom to form a water molecule (which is written in chemical shorthand as H_2O), the key is bonding. The bonding reaction is the result of portions of the involved atoms interacting in a manner that is to the energetic advantage of both parties. (It's kind of like pulling Kuwait and Saudi Arabia together to set oil prices every year. As long as it's to their energetic advantage, those countries will be tightly bonded.)

Groups of atoms bonded tightly together are called *molecules*. A molecule can be extremely small, composed of only two atoms, or enormous, ranging in size from a thousand to several million times larger than the tiny hydrogen atom. Proteins, for instance, are large molecules.

Protein molecules are themselves made out of smaller, linked-together molecules, called *amino acids*. It's like stacking hundreds of small blocks to form a giant wooden cube which is, itself, a large block. There are twenty different types of amino acid building blocks. The way they are stacked together determines the type and function of the particular protein molecule.

Proteins perform a variety of functions in biological systems. They serve as the principal material from which our cells are made. They are the building blocks for the many thousands of compounds produced by cells for the varieties of life processes. Some are structural, forming such things as hair and muscle fiber. Other types of proteins simply sit still and serve as chemical sign posts to the rest of the body, demarking skin from blood, liver tissue from kidney, and so forth. And finally, there are proteins called *enzymes*. Most of the transportation, communication, degradation, construction, and chemical control in biological systems is carried out by enzymes.

There is another major group of large molecules called *polymers*. Polymers are groups of small molecules linked together in monotonous repeating patterns to form huge sugars, fats, or lipids (i.e., fatty acids). Polymers form critical boundaries and structures in biological systems and provide adhesion to hold various body structures together.

YOU'RE JUST A TRILLION CELLS TO ME

A normal cell in a living organism contains millions upon millions of molecules of all types and sizes. All living organisms, with the exception of viruses*, are composed of cells. At one extreme are the simple, single-celled bacteria—at the other, homo sapiens (you and me), composed of millions of highly specialized cell populations organized into tissues and organs.

There are two basic cell types in the living world: *procaryotic* and *eucaryotic*. (See Figures 6-1 and 6-2.) Procaryotic cells have no nucleus, are single-celled creatures, and have tough cell walls surrounding them. Bacteria are procaryotic. Eucaryotic cells have a nucleus, are surrounded by a cell membrane instead of a wall, are part of a larger organism, and often exist in highly specialized cell populations. It is estimated that the human being is composed of from 5 billion to 1 trillion eucaryotic cells, averaging 10 microns (1/25,000th of an inch) in size.

The best understood cell in the world is the procaryotic Escherichia (E.) coli bacteria. This is because E. coli is a simple life form, multiplies rapidly and adapts well to laboratory life, and so it has been the subject of much molecular and cell biology research. A great deal of what is now known about human cell functions and biochemistry was originally derived from research on the E. coli bacteria.

E. coli has served humanity well, but there are important distinctions between the bacteria and

*As you will learn later in this book, viruses are organisms which in many ways defy the basic biochemical definitions of "life."

human cells, which demand caution when applying the results of bacterial research to humans. For example, E. coli grows well in the laboratory, generation after generation. In contrast, eucaryotic cells grown and reproduced under laboratory conditions most always become cancer cells. This implies that eucaryotic cells require the complex interactions of the whole organism in order to remain normal.

There are procaryotic cells in humans, many residing happily in our guts digesting food for us. And, of course, when we are ill, bacteria are all too ready to leap upon us. But the majority of the human body is composed of eucaryotic cells.

Viewed from the outside, a cell is a rounded, oblong or cubic object with protruding proteins and, often, microvilli and cilia (cell "antennae," "feelers" and "absorbers") projecting from the surface. Some cells are large enough to be seen without the aid of a microscope—the biggest of which is the ostrich egg. (Believe it or not, an ostrich egg is a single cell!) Remember the example of the ostrich egg to remind yourself that a cell is a well-defined three-dimensional object with three-dimensional subcomponents inside. (There is a tendency after viewing pictures of cells and microscopic photographs to think of cells as flat lifeless objects. Nothing could be further from the truth.)

Inside of cells are special subcomponents, or *organelles*, discrete well-defined bodies which perform highly specific functions. They are tiny organs, breathing, digesting, and regulating for the cell. Mitochondria, lysosomes, endoplasmic reticulum, Golgi apparatus—these are all organelles, and will be described later in this chapter.

The Membrane

The cell is surrounded by a *membrane* (see Figure 6-3), which does several things: It serves to protect the cell from the surrounding environment, maintains traffic control into and out from the cell, identifies the cell type, and ensures that the cell grows only to the boundaries of its neighboring cells.

The membrane is ingeniously constructed to serve its several purposes. Basically, it is a *lipid* bilayer. Lipids are organic fatty substances, such as oils, which do not like water. They are termed *hydrophobic* (hydro = water; phobic = afraid). Compounds which are chemically hydrophobic will do anything to avoid contact with water, and will cluster together with other hydrophobic molecules, to form grease (lipid) spots. The classic example of a hydrophobic interaction is salad dressing. Hydrophobic salad oil and water-containing vinegar, as the saying goes, don't mix; the interface between the oil and vinegar layers represents a hydrophobic interaction.

Figure 6-1 The Procaryotic Cell

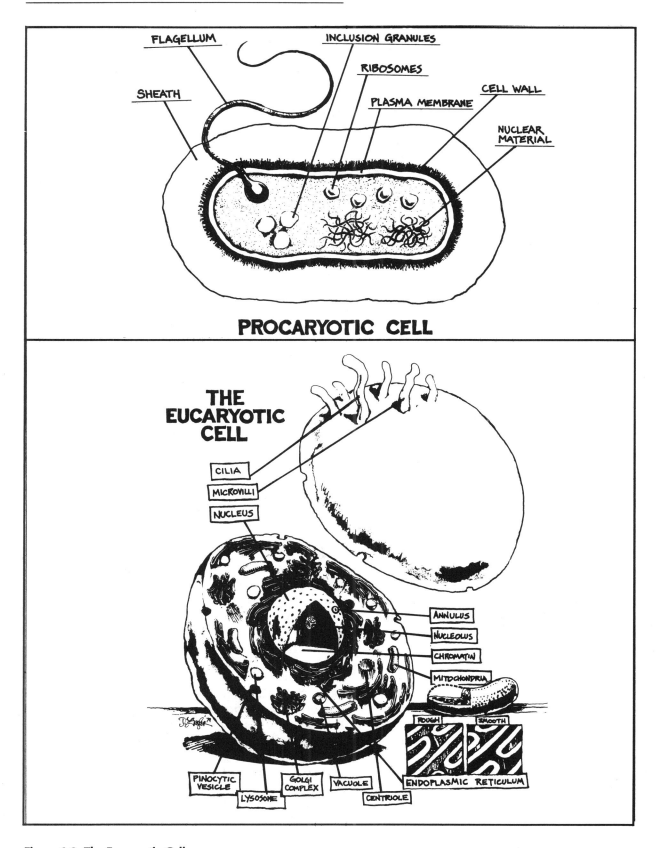

FLAGELLUM   INCLUSION GRANULES

RIBOSOMES

SHEATH

PLASMA MEMBRANE   CELL WALL

NUCLEAR MATERIAL

PROCARYOTIC CELL

THE EUCARYOTIC CELL

CILIA

MICROVILLI

NUCLEUS

ANNULUS

NUCLEOLUS

CHROMATIN

MITOCHONDRIA

ROUGH   SMOOTH

PINOCYTIC VESICLE

LYSOSOME

GOLGI COMPLEX

VACUOLE

CENTRIOLE

ENDOPLASMIC RETICULUM

Figure 6-2 The Eucaryotic Cell

Figure 6-3 The Cell Membrane

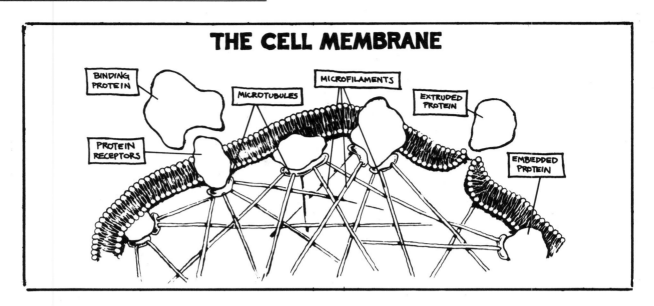

THE CELL MEMBRANE

In the case of the cell membrane the situation is more sophisticated than with salad dressing. The lipid molecules of a membrane are actually *phospholipids*, which means they have phosphate groups at one end. Phosphate likes water, which makes it hydrophilic. The membrane phospholipids are lined up in a double layer, with the phosphate "heads" sticking out into the watery seas which both surround and fill the cell, and the lipid "tails" standing in rigid hydrophobia, protected by their phosphate ends from the water. (Artificial membranes of oil or grease have been created and used industrially, following precisely the principles observed in natural cell membranes.)

Throughout the membrane are special proteins arranged in seemingly random groups, often protruding through the inner and outer cell surfaces. The arrangement of the proteins and the specific details of their relationship to the lipid bilayer has been explained theoretically by what is called the *Fluid Mosaic Model*. That model, forwarded by S. J. Singer and Garth Nicolson in 1972, postulated that the proteins are anchored in place within the lipid bilayer by a network of microtubules and microfilaments. The *microfilaments* are the "muscle" of the cell, and can move the proteins around the cell surface. The *microtubules* are the cells' "skeleton," and interact with the microfilaments to maintain the cell shape and movement. Stimulation of the microtubules or of the microfilaments will result in movement of the proteins through the cell membrane.

Proteins on the membrane surface serve as markers to alert the outside world that this is a liver cell, lung cell, red blood cell, or whatever, and more generally, that you are a human and not a lizard.

When membrane proteins of one cell make contact with membrane proteins of a neighboring cell, this is a signal for the cells not to grow into each other's territory. This signal, which is called *contact inhibition*, will prove very important in our later discussion of cancer. In this way, therefore, membrane proteins serve a communication role, receiving chemical information from outside the cell and relaying the message to the inside.

The membrane also serves an important transportation role, allowing the passage of molecules in and out of the cell. Most cells produce molecules which are intended to be secreted outside the cell. (They run an export business.) The secretion process often requires active support from membrane proteins. Many molecules which the cell requires for survival may be too large to pass freely through the lipid bilayer, and the membrane proteins can facilitate transportation.

Diffusion is the simplest form of transport. It is a non-energy-requiring process in which molecules pass through the membrane from areas of higher concentration to areas of lower concentration. It's like the flow of traffic on a highway: if a fourth lane opens up on a crowded three-lane freeway, half the motorists will risk life and limb to get into it. They're looking for a lower automobile concentration to flow into. In the case of the cell, if molecular concentration is higher outside the cell than inside, the tendency will be for molecules to flow into the cell—and vice versa, in each case tending toward a balance.

There are some molecules that can't go with

the flow. They want to, but their chemistry won't let them pass freely through the membrane. Most of these molecules are hydrophilic, so they have trouble getting through the hydrophobic midsection of the membrane. They are aided by membrane proteins, called carriers, which grab them and tug them through, either in or out. The proteins facilitate their transport across the membrane. So, no surprise, the process is called *facilitated transport*. The process requires no energy and seems to operate on the same principle as diffusion—that is, the molecules move to the area of lowest concentration.

Finally, there are situations in which the cell wishes to absorb or secrete molecules against the concentration gradient. In other words, the cell wants to move something from an area of lower concentration to an area of higher concentration. For this the cell has to pay a price. This movement process is called *active transport*, and does require exertion of energy—and again, in many cases, the involvement of membrane proteins. If diffusion is simply floating downstream effortlessly, active transport is swimming upstream, against the current, expending loads of energy, and taking whatever help can be gotten.

The Cytoplasm

The majority of cell space is filled with a gelatinous mess of water, sugars, proteins, salts, and other molecules. This is the *cytoplasm*. In the center of the cytoplasm rests the nucleus, and throughout the cytoplasmic mess float the organelles. The cytoplasm has a high water content (50–90%) which allows the water-loving hydrophilic molecules to float freely through it.

The Mitochondria

The active transport of molecules across the cell membrane and the maintenance of the cell membrane and its "skeleton" require energy. The key form of biological energy is *ATP* (adenosine triphosphate). The major ATP refineries for the cell are the *mitochondria*. (See Figure 6-2.) Most eucaryotic cells have numerous mitochondria floating throughout their cytoplasm. Present scientific thought has it that the mitochondria are procaryotic creatures which have been co-existing within eucaryotic cells for millions of years. It's one of those "you scrub my back and I'll scrub yours" deals. The mitochondria happily crank out enormous amounts of energy for the cell, breathe for the cell, fuel every critical biochemical reaction, and only ask in return for a home and some protein. They have their own membranes (similar to the cell walls of E. Coli), carry out their own reproduction (independent of the cell), and move about

freely in the cell cytoplasm. It is the mitochondria which do much of the "eating" for us, digesting molecules down to useful sizes. Their major job, however, is "breathing"—taking in oxygen and using it to produce energy.

The mitochondria maximize their possible surface area for exposure to oxygen and other molecules by having layers upon layers of a folded internal matrix. It is in the matrix that the energy-producing process known as *oxidative phosphorylation* occurs. Don't let the long name blow your mind; oxidative phosphorylation is simply a biochemical process involving oxygen and phosphorous in which a phosphate group is tacked onto the sugar, making it the energy-rich ATP. The ATP is ultimately shuttled out of the mitochondria to pockets of the cell where it is needed.

Suicide Bags

The mitochondria don't do all the work of chomping up massive proteins—there are also the *lysosomes*. (See Figure 6-2.) Sadly nicknamed "suicide bags," these organelles fill the essential role of breaking down proteins into constituent parts which can be used for various bodily processes. They are actually small packages of powerful enzymes, which can, if released into the cell's cytoplasm, destroy the cell from the inside out—thus the name "suicide bags." It is the means by which a cell can self-destruct, particularly if subjected to extremes of environmental stress (i.e., temperature, chemical imbalance, and certain digestive states.) The lysosomal enzymes are destructive in nature; they carry out hydrolysis (big-time demolition work) of proteins unfortunate enough to come within the lysosome's clutches. We are thus potentially at the mercy of our own organelles!

What's All This Destruction For?

Building New Proteins in the Endoplasmic Reticulum. Just to show you that all this digestive and respiratory work isn't for nothing, it's time to take a look at the *Endoplasmic Reticulum*, or ER. (See Figure 6-2.) If the mitochondria are the power plants, the ER are the factories for the cell, cranking out proteins and special molecules to order. The molecular parts created by the degradative processes of the mitochondria and lysosomes, and the energy provided by the mitochondria, are used in the ER to construct special molecules, such as hormones, and proteins.

The ER are located throughout the cell, but are generally concentrated around the nucleus. Their proximity to the nucleus facilitates their crucial work as producers of protein. There are two types of ER, *smooth ER* and *rough ER*, so named because of their differing appearance under the microscope. The concentrations of these two ER types vary from cell to cell. Protein production is the key function of the rough ER. Cells which have the job of non-protein production and secretion have high concentrations of smooth ER. An example of this is an estrogen-producing cell (estrogen is a non-protein hormone). The "roughness" refers to the microscopic appearance of large numbers of special protein clusters called *ribosomes*, which are lined up along the rough ER membrane like beads on a chain.

While the ER can be considered the factory for protein production, the ribosomes represent the actual assembly lines. Without ribosomes there would be no protein production.

The Golgi

The full process of protein synthesis will be described following this introduction of the principal players. When the job of protein production is completed, the ER still have to transfer the new molecular products out to the *Golgi apparatus*. (See Figure 6-2.) The ER moves its products from the ribosome on to the Golgi by clustering them together and surrounding them with portions of the ER membrane. The membrane in a sense "swallows" the new molecules, creating a neatly enclosed package of protein (or hormones, or whatever). The package detaches itself from the ER membrane and migrates to a neighboring Golgi.

The Golgi apparatus suffers unfairly from its strange name. Any organelle which does all the work it does ought to be dubbed something fancy like endoplasmic reticulum. But no such luck for the Golgi. The organelle was first spotted at the turn of the century by an Italian histologist named Camillo Golgi, and originally it was called Golgi's complex. I think people thought that sounded like an unfair Freudian slur on Nobel Laureate Golgi, but until recently nobody really knew what a Golgi did. So a safe nondescriptive word was used—*Golgi apparatus*. I'd like to think of them as Golgi's Distribution and Marketing Center.

As we said, Golgi receive the packaged proteins and other molecules from the ER and prepare them for distribution. The first step involves changes in the shape and appearance of the proteins. Although the proteins may have the right parts, their shape (or conformation) is wrong for their intended roles. And that can be critical. Remember, many proteins operate by highly specific mechanisms like a lock and key: if the shape of the lock is wrong, the key won't fit. Some proteins require the attachment of sugar or carbohydrate molecules to make them active.

So the Golgi manufacture these large complexes of sugars (polysaccharides).

Once the product is prepared for distribution, it is surrounded by a Golgi-made membrane similar to that used by the ER. In some cases the Golgi packages a number of different types of powerful enzymes, surrounds them with a membrane, pops them into the cytoplasm of the cell, and—voila!—a lysosome is born. (Remember those "suicide bags"?) In other instances the packaged molecules are budded off into the cytoplasm of the cell, where they migrate either to destinations inside the cell, or to the outer cell membrane, where they are actively secreted.

The Godfather (the Nucleus)

The intense activities within the cell have to be directed from somewhere. In the procaryote that "somewhere" is a bit amorphous; the control of procaryote activity lies among certain molecules floating in the cytoplasm along with everything else. But the eucaryote is more sophisticated; it has a central controller, a single, discrete membrane-coated organelle called the *nucleus*. (See Figure 6-2.) It controls virtually all the cellular activity—it's the Washington D.C., it's the Godfather.

Inside the nucleus is the genetic control material, *DNA* (deoxyribonucleic acid). (Try saying deoxyribonucleic acid sixteen times real fast and you'll never be blown away by big scientific names again. I personally have a lot of respect for deoxyribonucleic acid—after all, it is the basis of life. So let's say it right: dee-ox-ee-rye-bow-new-clay-ick-acid). In procaryotes the DNA is loosely associated with other molecules in the cell and floats freely through the cytoplasm. In eucaryotes, however, the DNA is packaged and protected inside the nucleus, in material called chromatin. The chromatin is simply a mass of molecules wrapped around each other, two thirds of which are protein, and one third the DNA.

When cells are preparing to reproduce, the chromatin bunches up into discrete groupings of 23 pairs, forming chromosomes.

The nucleus also contains tiny organelles called *nucleoli* (singular: *nucleolus*), whose function is still poorly understood. It is known, though, that the nucleolus is involved in rRNA synthesis and ribosome formation.

DNA CONTAINS THE GENETIC CODE

As early as the 1800s it was felt that the nucleus was the cellular control center, and that the chromosomes must play a key role. In the early 1900s, it was shown experimentally that the blueprints which result in specific individual traits are located at particular positions on the chromosomes, called genes.

A *gene* is really more of a concept than an actual "thing." As indicated, it refers to an area of the DNA molecule, which can be discrete or diffuse, that contains information which, if carried into the next generation, will result in an identifiable trait. So the code for a specific trait is also called a gene.

The location of the gene on a particular chromosome is called a site. In human chromosomes each of the 23 pairs carries different genetic information. One pair, for example, carries the genes which determine sex. Finding out where particular genes are located on chromosomes is called "mapping." When a gene is experimentally turned on and the protein it codes for is produced, the gene is said to have been "expressed." The first direct link between genetic expression and protein production was found with research on the genetic disease, sickle cell anemia.

But what proves that DNA, rather than the chromatin proteins (which also make up the chromosomes), are responsible for the genetic code? Four things:

• In 1944 researchers showed that when a particular cell extract from bacteria was transferred into other bacteria it caused them to express genes they didn't normally express. That cell extract was pure DNA (without the proteins).

• Every species has a constant amount of DNA, regardless of the cell type, unless there is something wrong (i.e., most cancer cells have abnormal amounts of DNA).

• Some viruses contain nothing but DNA (or RNA, which we'll learn about later). If Master Control is the bottom line for "life," and viruses are a form of life and have nothing but DNA in them, then DNA must be Master Control.

• The final and most conclusive piece of evidence came in 1953 when James Watson and Francis Crick discovered the structure of DNA. With the elucidation of the DNA structure, understanding of the relationship of that structure to its function quickly followed. And with that, the Biology Revolution was full steam ahead!

One of the key concepts in modern molecular biology is called the *Central Dogma*. This refers to (1) the basic relationship between DNA, RNA, and protein; (2) the concept that DNA is a template for both its own duplication and the synthesis of RNA; and (3) the concept that RNA is then used as the template in protein synthesis. In the following pages the Central Dogma will be more fully explained.

What's Longer Than a Football Field, So Thin It Can Only be Seen with a Powerful Electron Microscope, and Looks Like a Twisted Ladder?

DNA is a molecule which is made of three types of smaller molecules: nucleotides, deoxyribose, and phosphates. The DNA molecule is two strings of these molecules wound together in a helical formation. The deoxyribose and phosphate link together; the nucleotides pair in specific relationships. If the DNA molecule is viewed as a twisted ladder, the deoxyribose-phosphate linkages form the parallel sidebars, and the nucleotides are the rungs.

The key is the *nucleotides*. These are small molecules. They may not look like much, but their sequences along the deoxyribose chain constitute the basis of the Genetic Code.

In DNA there are four types of nucleotides: adenine, guanine, cytosine, and thymine, or A, G, C, & T. Adenine and guanine are larger and have molecular similarity; they are designated the *purines*. Cytosine and thymine, which are smaller, are the *pyrimidines*. The secret that Watson and Crick discovered in 1953 is found in the chemistry of the pairing of nucleotides. Chemically, cytosine will bond only to guanine, and adenine to thymine.* If guanine is on one side of the DNA ladder, cytosine is directly opposite it. In this way the two DNA chains are chemically complementary to each other. If the sequence on one side is ATGAACTT, the other side is TACTTGAA. (See Figure 6-4.)

The important point here is that nucleotides are functionally important in threes (triplets). The entire genetic code is designed to be read in threes. If the sequence of the nucleotides on a given DNA molecule is AATCGTCCGTAGCGT, it is read as a code of AAT CGT CCG TAG CGT. The triplets code for specific amino acids. The last triplet (CGT) tells the translator the code is over—the gene is completed, and the protein is completed.

RNA (ribonucleic acid) is similar to DNA in that it has a phosphate-ribose (not deoxyribose, just plain ribose) backbone with nucleotides on it. The only difference between DNA and RNA is one oxygen molecule. (See Figure 6-5) RNA is not double-stranded and helical like DNA. Generally it's a single-stranded curled up mess compared to the tidy DNA molecule. Also, RNA doesn't have any thymine; it uses uracil (U) instead (so U pairs with A). So what does RNA

---

*There are deviations and bizarre nucleotides which can insert themselves where they don't belong in the DNA. This usually results in mutations.

Figure 6-4 DNA

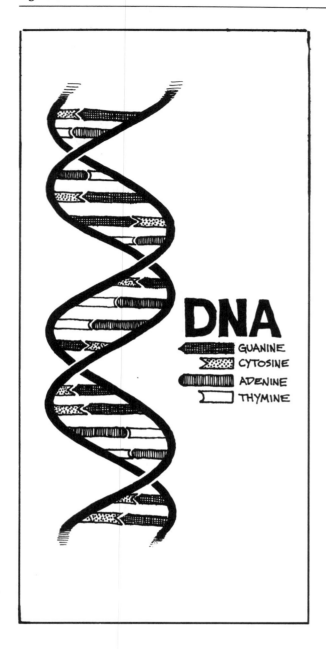

DNA

- ▶ GUANINE
- ▶ CYTOSINE
- ▶ ADENINE
- ▶ THYMINE

The nucleotides' sequences along the phosphate-ribose backbones of DNA determine the sequence of amino acids in the making of proteins. But as we said, it determines a lot more than how and when to make which proteins. The DNA genetic code includes messages telling the cell when to divide, how to take care of repairing the membrane, and how to make organelles.

Some proteins are only supposed to be made when the cell is embryonic, while others are intended to be manufactured by an adult cell. Every cell has the same DNA inside its nucleus as every other cell in the same organism. Obviously, however, if the cells of your toes begin to read out only the portions of DNA which code for production and secretion of hair proteins, you would soon have hairy toes. Therein lies the rub—Control. DNA is the control for the cell, but what determines which portions of the DNA are read and which aren't? Why is a pancreatic cell busy making insulin while a stomach cell secretes digestive enzymes? Or, more to the point, why don't things go wrong so bone cells make hair?

BACK TO THE FACTORY LINE

Protein Synthesis

To get to the bottom of the mystery of control, we need to focus on the mechanisms involved in the synthesis of proteins. The process proceeds stepwise from the copying of the triplet DNA code onto messenger RNA (transcription), the movement of messenger RNA out of the nucleus to the ribosomes, and the reading of the code (translation). Remember, the code is in triplets, each of which specifies a particular amino acid, the components of proteins.

One way to think of the role of DNA in the process of protein synthesis is as the president of a corporation, stuck in his office (DNA stays in the nucleus), and dependent upon messengers (messenger RNA) to carry his orders out to the protein synthesis factories (ribosomes).

Let's look more specifically at the steps. (They are diagrammed at the end of this section.)

Step 1 Transcription. Before mRNA synthesis can begin, a special enzyme called *RNA polymerase* must find the correct gene on the DNA and attach to it. The details of how RNA polymerase knows when and where to attach are not clear (but there is evidence that the RNA polymerase must first undergo biochemical activation before it is ready for mRNA production). Once the RNA polymerase is bound to the DNA, it orders up nucleotides in a mirror image of the DNA, links them together, and then,

do? Since it's the mirror image of the DNA, it can copy a DNA message and carry it out of the nucleus. (The DNA stays in the nucleus.)

There are three types of RNA, each of which is made in a different place in the cell and used for a distinct purpose. *Messenger RNA (mRNA)* is the largest form, and is made right on the DNA as a direct mirror copy of the DNA. *Ribosomal RNA (rRNA)* is made in the nucleoli inside the nucleus and can be found inside the ribosomes. (Remember them? They're on the endoplasmic reticulum.) *Transfer RNA (tRNA)* has the job of rounding up amino acids and bringing them to the ribosomes to be inserted in newly forming proteins.

Figure 6-5

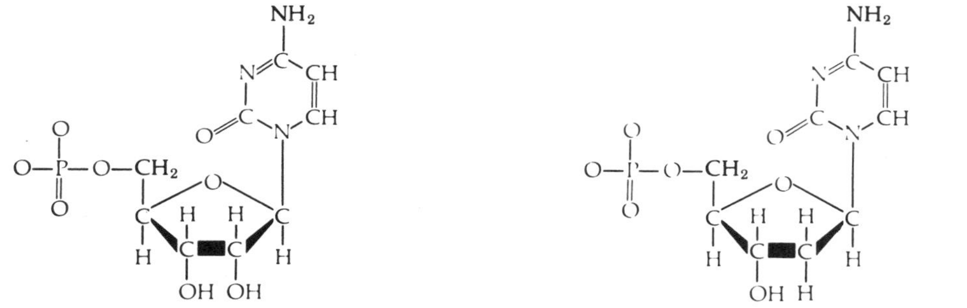

RIBONUCLEOTIDE   DEOXYRIBONUCLEOTIDE

when the DNA gene has been completely transcribed, releases them as an mRNA.

Step 2 Translation. The mRNA is now carrying a code that must be translated. It moves out of the nucleus to the ribosome, where *translation* will take place. As you will recall, the ribosomes are primarily clustered in and around ER where they work under arduous conditions cranking out proteins day and night. The mRNA provides them with their work orders.

The ribosomes are giant conglomerations of protein and rRNA (ribosomal RNA)*, which are separated into two subunits when inactive. (Every time a ribosome finishes a protein production job it falls apart into two subunits. Sort of takes a breather.) But once the mRNA starts pacing about impatiently with the work orders, the ribosomal subunits come together and prepare for action. The mRNA positions itself at one end of the ribosome awaiting the arrival of the tRNA molecules, with their appropriate amino acids.

There are twenty different amino acids, and twenty types of tRNA. Coincidence? Not on your life. Each tRNA bears the triplet genetic code for one amino acid, and it is the task of the tRNA to drag that particular amino acid into place on the ribosome according to the mRNA blueprint. Basically tRNA just transfers amino acids from outside the ribosome to their correct positions for the construction of a protein. Thus the name—transfer (t) RNA.

The tRNA with its correct amino acid enters the ribosome and attaches to the mRNA. (The tRNA is a mirror genetic code of the mRNA for three nucleotides.) When the attachment has been made,

the amino acid binds itself to the one before it with a peptide bond. The tRNA then jumps off the ribosome, another tRNA comes in, and the whole mRNA template* shifts over three nucleotides. Zip! Ready for the next one.

Here it is again:

Amino acid-tRNA in place on the mRNA template.

Amino acid attached to the previous amino acid on the new protein.

tRNA is released.

mRNA shift over three spaces.

Wow! Ready for the next one. Bring on the amino acids! Before you know it, the complete mRNA template is translated from nucleotides into amino acids, and a new protein has been made.

The New Protein. Before the production process has finished, the new protein has already begun to coil about, taking on its particular shape. Once the last amino acid is in place, special enzymes release the protein from the ribosome, sending it on its way to the Golgi apparatus for packaging and distribution.

The entire process of protein synthesis is dependent upon ready access to amino acids, plenty of biochemical energy, and a large number of specialized enzymes. If a cell is suffering from a deficiency in any of these items, it will be unable to make proteins.

WHAT CONTROLS WHAT?

Getting back to the original question of control of DNA transcription, a few points have already been answered. There are stop and start signals on the

---

*The role of the rRNA is completely unclear—obviously the cell makes it for some reason, but nobody knows what that is. (Now there's a potential research project for you!)

Template means a pattern or mold.

Figure 6-6 Protein Synthesis—Step 1

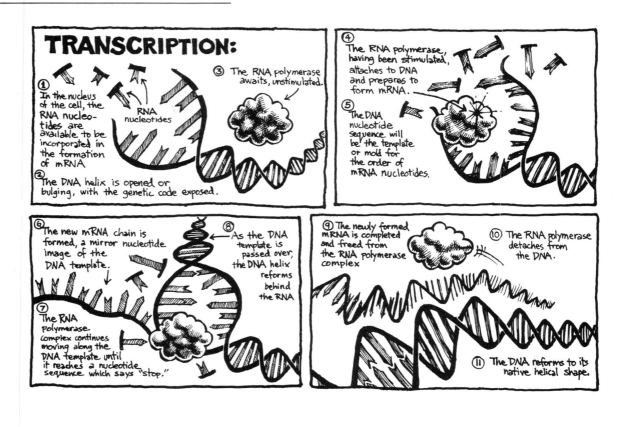

Figure 6-7 Protein Synthesis—Step 2

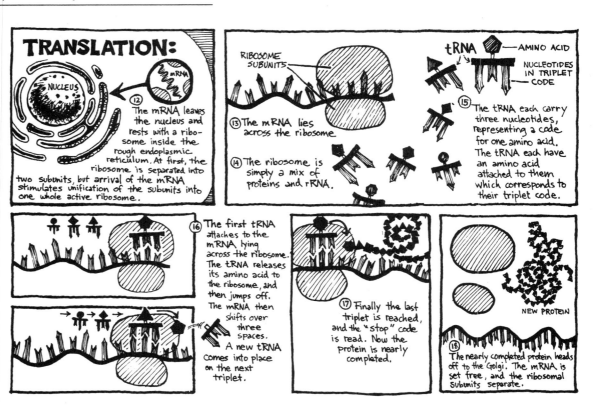

Figure 6-8 Protein Synthesis—The New Protein

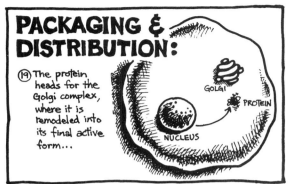

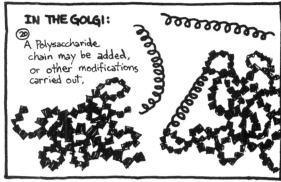

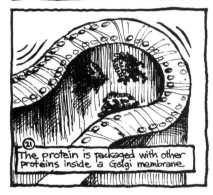

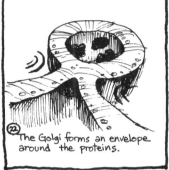

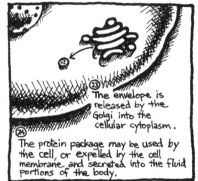

DNA. The RNA polymerase must be turned on, and the stimulus seems to involve a number of factors. But remember, the issue is a rather profound and complicated one. What makes liver cells read those portions of the DNA designed for liver, while skin cells read skin DNA? Both contain precisely the same DNA.

There are indications that for at least some genes there are actually enzymes coded for that simply hang around and either turn on or turn off any polymerase that comes within spitting distance. These special enzymes regulate transcription of a specific gene coding for a particular protein, and are sensitive to the levels of that protein in the cell. If the specific protein concentration drops, these special enzymes turn on the RNA polymerases in the neighborhood. If the concentration gets too high, they block further transcription. It's kind of like having someone running downstream all the time to find out whether it's time to lower the dam.

ZIP! DNA REPRODUCES ITSELF

At a specific point in its life, a cell receives a signal to reproduce. When the cell reproduces, it does so by stretching itself outward, duplicating its con-

tents, and dividing into two cells. The two resulting cells are called *daughter cells.*

The tenet that all living organisms (with the exception of viruses) are composed of cells, and that the cells reproduce by dividing to form daughter cells, is called the Cell Theory. Until 1839, when Schleiden and Schwann put forward the Cell Theory, scientists and physicians thought human beings were variously composed of everything from opposing metaphysical forces to tiny animals. The elucidation of the Cell Theory provided science with the first logical building block for our current Biological Revolution.

From the perspective of the biochemist the most intriguing aspect of cellular reproduction is the synthesis of DNA. This is the trigger for over-all cellular reproduction, and the source of potential errors in the transmission of genetic information from one generation to the next.

The major elements of DNA replication are DNA polymerase, unwinding protein, and a number of specialized enzymes. To some degree, the events of DNA synthesis are similar to those described for mRNA synthesis. The DNA itself is used as the template for the construction of the new DNA. Construction takes place on both strands of DNA simultaneously, and is guided by polymerase enzymes. But that is about where the similarity stops.

The DNA strands are separated by special enzymes called unwinding proteins. Once the helix is unzipped, it is available to use as a template. All synthesis on a DNA template must proceed in the direction in which the order of the nucleotides is intended to be read. Since the two strands are mirror images of one another, one strand will be in straight-ahead order and will be synthesized smoothly in the wake of the path opened by the unwinding protein—but the other strand must be synthesized in the opposite direction, and this makes for an awkward proposal. The cell conquers the problem by synthesizing the opposite strand in chunks.

The pump has to be primed, as it were, with a little RNA every step of the way. (The reason for this totally escapes everybody, although there are plenty of theories floating around.) RNA polymerase places the RNA primer pieces on the DNA template, kicking off the DNA synthesis process. Then a DNA polymerase attaches to the newly formed RNA chain and, using it as a template, starts the new DNA chain. Another DNA polymerase takes care of making DNA directly on the original DNA template, following closely behind the first DNA polymerase. Finally a ligase enzyme follows up at the rear, sealing up the holes between newly formed DNA pieces. In the end there are two DNA double-stranded helixes, each composed of one old chain and one new one. (See Figure 6-9.)

Our understanding of DNA synthesis has expanded so rapidly in the past few years that it is now possible to synthesize entire genes in a test tube, place them inside of bacterial DNA, and have the bacteria produce the protein that the newly implanted gene codes for. This process is called genetic engineering, or *recombinant DNA*. Despite concerns about the possible hazard of creating an uncontrollable, mutant infectious bacteria through genetic manipulation, the research in the area has been moving at an astonishing rate. In 1975 it was only beginning, but by 1978 researchers had succeeded in creating new mutant strains of bacteria that produce insulin, growth hormone, and numerous other proteins. Genetic engineering represents the frontier of the biological revolution—a frontier which poses both wondrous and troubling possibilities for the future.

The most obvious effect of the new step in the biological revolution is the change in perspective it has brought to the fields of biology and medicine. Where once DNA was a mystery, it is now a molecule under the control of science. It can be manipulated. It can be changed. Researchers hope that further experiments in the manipulation of DNA synthesis will reveal details about the creation of cancer cells. To understand this new era of genetic manipulation, and the possible applications it may have to cancer research, you must understand DNA synthesis.

Figure 6-9 DNA Synthesis

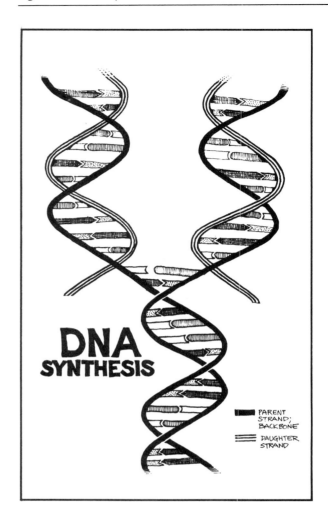

DNA Pitstops

DNA Repair. Special enzymes ensure that no errors are made in DNA synthesis. The right nucleotides must be in the correct order, or the gene will no longer code for the correct amino acids. If a mistake is made, an exonuclease or endonuclease enzyme (the repair enzymes) simply chomps off the mistake and the DNA polymerase replaces the nucleotide correctly. A similar mechanism operates throughout the life of the cell for the repair of DNA.

There are many ways in which DNA can become altered, or mutated, so that it no longer bears the correct genetic code. Agents which are capable of mutating DNA are called *mutagens*. One of the best understood mutagenic processes involves exposure of nucleotides to ultraviolet (UV) light. Sunlight contains UV light. Most human cells have little appreciation for UV light. This is primarily because UV light causes a chemical reaction in thymine nucleotides. Thymine, which usually only pairs with adenine, becomes altered so that it incorrectly pairs with another thymine. This causes two problems: The genetic code is now incorrect (there is a T where an A should be); and the pairing of two small nucleotides instead of a small and a large one causes a change in the shape of the DNA molecule.

Depending on where in the genetic code this thymine-thymine pairing occurs (the strange pair is called a thymine dimer), it can be very serious. The cell has developed elaborate enzyme mechanisms for the removal of thymine dimers and replacement with correct nucleotides. Endonucleases and exonucleases both play a role in such repair.

But there are other forms of mutations which are not as easy to repair. Some are totally irreparable and will be passed on to every subsequent generation of the cell's lineage, and may be lethal. A good example is a frameshift mutation. During DNA synthesis, DNA repair, or some other time not clearly understood, a single nucleotide is either eliminated from the DNA or added. The insertion or deletion of a nucleotide causes the entire genetic code to be off by at least one nucleotide digit. If, for example, a DNA sequence normally read

GTTACAGA
CAATGTCT,

and the nucleotide C were inserted thusly:

GCTTACAGA
C AATGTCT

. . . the change in the reading of the triplets for the amino acid codes would be from the original

GTT ACA GA...
CAA TGT CT...

to the newly mutated

GCT TAC AGA
C A ATG TCT.

The change would go all the way down the DNA chain unless the repair mechanisms spotted the error. Because the insertion or deletion of a nucleotide on one chain of the DNA helix causes a shifting of the genetic frame (ergo the name "frameshift mutation"), the other side has a gap in it. This can result in a bulge in the DNA, which may be easily spotted by the DNA repair enzymes, and be excised and repaired. Or it may be missed, and result in total breakdown of DNA transcription and eventual cell death. In between the two extremes is a scenario of possible altered cell behaviors and functioning.

There are many other mutagenic examples. Some are environmental, arising from exposure of the organism to radiation or chemicals. Others are caused by certain viruses which insert themselves into the DNA of cells they infect. And finally, the cells are themselves capable of making mistakes which can ultimately be self-damaging.

THE CELL CYCLE

Every cell type has its own biological clock, a schedule programmed in the DNA which, partially in response to biochemical changes in the cell's environment, tells the cell when to enter a new phase of development or reproduction. Some procaryotic cells go through their biological clock so fast that it is difficult to tell when they are entering one stage and leaving another. Most eucaryotic cells take a more civilized, relaxed approach to life, strolling from one stage to another. Some, like the nerve cells, are downright boring and never seem to change much.

Although the biological time clock for each cell type differs, the general phases of eucaryotic cell lifespan are consistent. The "average" cell has a life cycle similar to that pictured in Figure 6-10. Immediately following cell division and the formation of a new cell, the new cell is in its G_1 period. During this time (which lasts, on the average, 6 hours) the cell primarily produces RNA and protein. At the end of the G_1 period the signal is given to start reproduction, and the cell enters S period (S as in Synthesis). This time phase, which is the longest in the cell's lifespan (6 to 8 hours, on the average), is when DNA synthesis and the synthesis of many critical cell components takes place.

When DNA synthesis is completed, the cell enters G_2 period. Although no DNA synthesis takes place during G_2, it is an active time of protein and RNA synthesis in preparation for division of the cell.

Finally there is a hypothetical period which, for the lack of any other name, is called G_0. (The "0" as in nothing, zilch . . . the cell sits around and waits for some action . . . no reproduction.)

The demarcations of the cell cycle help our understanding of the events which take place in the cell, and have proven invaluable in cancer chemotherapy, which takes advantage of the specific susceptibilities of cancer cells at key points in their cell cycles.

Mitosis

Xeroxing Cells. The sum of G_1, S, and G_2 is referred to as *interphase*. Following the completion of interphase the cell begins its division, called *mitosis*. (See Figure 6-11.) The steps of mitosis are as follows: First, the cell enters prophase, the stage at which the chromosomes condense into tight doubled packages. Next, the cells enter *metaphase* and begin to prepare directly for division of the nucleus

Figure 6-10 Cell Life Cycle

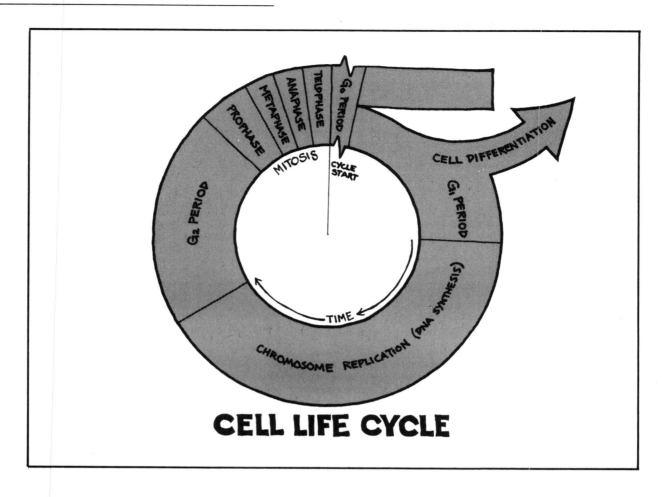

CELL LIFE CYCLE

of the cell. The chromosomes line up in parallel arrangements along a center axis representing the future splitting point for the nucleus. The movement of the chromosomes is guided by special polar areas on the chromosomes called *centromeres*. After the centromere has succeeded in lining up the chromosomes in tandem parallel arrangements, the pairs are split and pulled apart to opposite sides of the nucleus. This is *anaphase*. (It is aided by special spindle fibers which act like muscles pulling the nucleus in half.)

While the nucleus is splitting and polarizing, so is the rest of the cell. Finally, during *telophase* the spindles pinch the two polarized halves of the nucleus apart, forming two daughter nuclei. This happens simultaneously with the splitting of the rest of the cell. Once the two new daughter cells have been formed, they immediately enter the G_1 period of interphase and the cycle begins again.

Many cells are frozen somewhere in interphase, and due to their specialized functions in the organism, will not advance to prophase. Still others

may have to undergo profound developmental changes which will alter the protein content and cell appearance. These cells may spend a long time in the G_1 period.

The Sex Life of a Cell

Meiosis. The other type of cellular reproduction, meiosis, is essentially a small part of the larger process of reproduction of the entire organism. Meiosis is the prelude to sexual reproduction. In humans, meiosis converts one normal cell containing 23 pairs of chromosomes (a total of 46) to four cells, each bearing 23 individual chromosomes. These four new cells are destined to take part in sexual reproduction, and are called *gametes*. Sperm and egg cells are gametes.

The individual steps involved in getting from the single-celled 46-chromosome stage to the final four-cell stage are well understood. Figure 6-12 shows the beauty of the process graphically. (The details are not necessary for this discussion.)

Figure 6-11 Mitosis

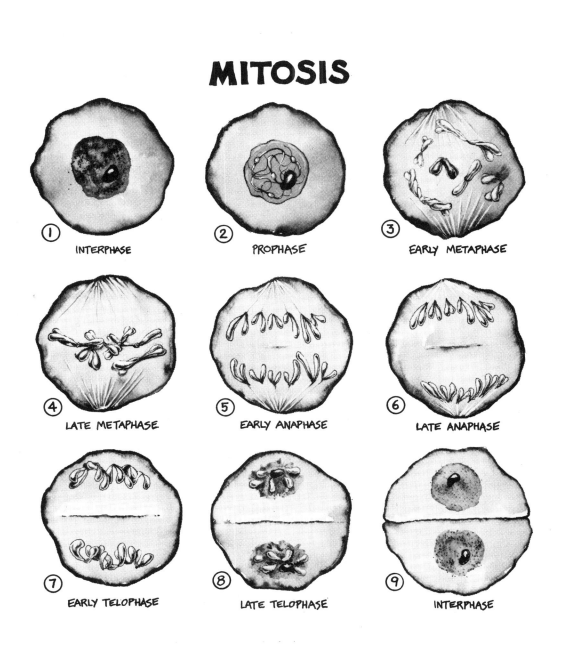

MITOSIS

① INTERPHASE

② PROPHASE

③ EARLY METAPHASE

④ LATE METAPHASE

⑤ EARLY ANAPHASE

⑥ LATE ANAPHASE

⑦ EARLY TELOPHASE

⑧ LATE TELOPHASE

⑨ INTERPHASE

Figure 6-12 Meiosis

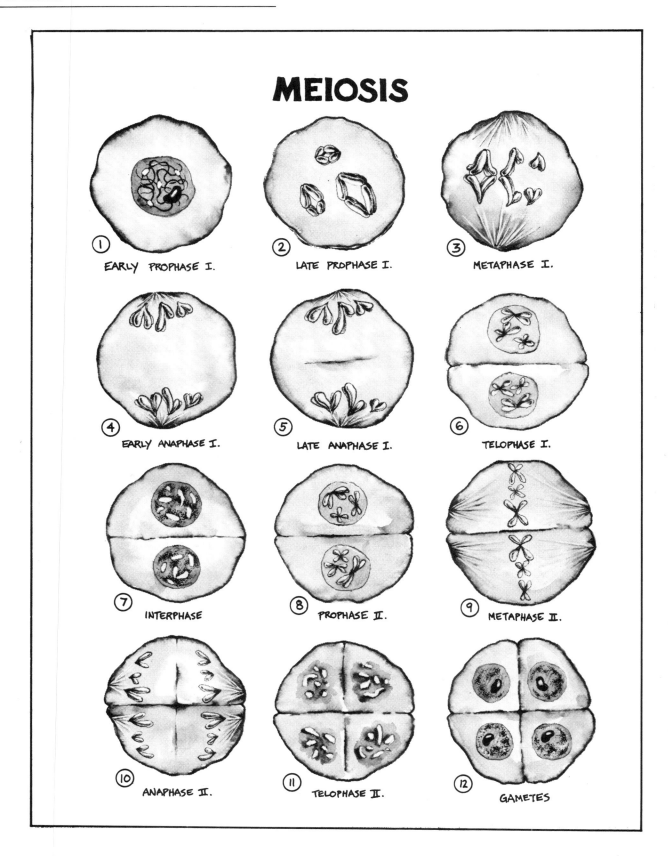

MEIOSIS

① EARLY PROPHASE I.

② LATE PROPHASE I.

③ METAPHASE I.

④ EARLY ANAPHASE I.

⑤ LATE ANAPHASE I.

⑥ TELOPHASE I.

⑦ INTERPHASE

⑧ PROPHASE II.

⑨ METAPHASE II.

⑩ ANAPHASE II.

⑪ TELOPHASE II.

⑫ GAMETES

THE ULTIMATE DEVIANT—THE CANCER CELL

Now that we have all that basic biology under our belts, it's time to take a look at the abnormal cell, the cancer cell. (See Figure 6-13.) There is no average "cancer cell," or neoplasm. Cancer cells vary tremendously. They may look something like their original cell types and still do some things normally, like secreting appropriate proteins or other molecules, but they are not the same. Each population of cancer cells has its own "personality," as it were. Each has a different biochemical composition, reproduces at a different rate, and varies greatly in the degree to which it is dangerous to the organism in which it resides. Hence, it is often said there are over 100 different kinds of cancer, each requiring a different understanding, and a different treatment.

The least dangerous growths are those considered *benign*. These growths are confined in space, tend to limit themselves to the area in which they begin to grow, and reproduce slowly. The *malignant* growth, on the other hand, tends to reproduce rapidly, grows beyond the tissue areas from which it is derived, shows abnormal mitosis, invades other organs, and has the capacity to *metastasize* (spread through the bloodstream, implanting cancer throughout the body). The spreading into neighboring tissue is called *invasive* behavior. The original cell growth is termed a *neoplasia*, or new growth, which results from the *transformation* of a normal cell. (Be sure to read Chapter 5—Introduction to Cancer Pathology—Terms and Concepts for a firmer grasp of the terminology and concepts of cancer.)

Despite their diversity, there are certain basic observations about cancer cells which can be considered rules of thumb (realizing that it is the exception which makes the rule). Most cancer cells reproduce more rapidly than the other cells in the tissue or organ from which they are derived. For example, if a particular type of normal liver cell has a complete life cycle of five days, the cancerous version of that same liver cell may complete its life cycle in just one or two days.

As we saw earlier, normal cells have very clearly defined cell membranes, and strong cell "skeletons" and "muscle" which keep the cell in a well defined space and shape. Cancer cells do not. Some cancer cells go so haywire it's hard to tell where their membranes stop, or even if they are living cells.

Normal cells observe the rules regulating which cells belong where in an organism (called *contact inhibition*). The surface proteins on the cell membranes tell their cells to grow only to the limits of their defined space and then stop. Cancer cells do not. They never know when to quit. They will grow over other cells, and expand into tissues and organs which bear no resemblance to the tissues from which they are derived.

Normal cells have only one nucleus and divide to form two daughter cells with equal sets of chromosomes and one nucleus each. Cancer cells do not. Some cancer cells have two, three, or more nuclei. Some have none. Some cancer cells have too few chromosomes, while others may have three or four complete sets.

Normal cells have protein markers on their membranes which indicate that they are part of the body ("self") and should not be attacked by the immune system. Cancer cells often have markers on their membranes which say just the opposite (and identify them as "foreign"), and the immune system may try to eliminate them in the same way it tries to eliminate invading bacteria. On the other hand, cancer cells sometimes disguise themselves from the immune system, by secreting a protective coating or polysaccharides and carbohydrates.

Cancer cells have a biochemistry that is different from normal cells. One of the most well-known differences is described as the Warburg Effect. Poor old Warburg was a German biochemist who, about fifty years ago, noticed that cancer cells use more glucose and secrete higher amounts of lactic acid than normal cells. For the life of him, he couldn't figure out why, though he spent a career looking for the answer. Console yourself, Warburg, nobody else has figured it out either.

Generalizations about cancer cells are difficult, and it would be wrong to view them categorically as a form of altered biology which is inevitably dangerous to the organism. It isn't. It's completely possible for an organism to have cancer cells for its entire lifetime and suffer no ill effects. It is not uncommon to find a cancer in a routine autopsy.

A group of neoplastic cells is called a *neoplasm*. There are many common neoplasms which are basically harmless: warts; scar tissue; hormone-induced over-growths of tissue; and so on. (The three examples are interesting because they highlight three different and important types of transforming agents: viruses, environmental exposure and hormones.)

The "how" of cancer can appear simple on one level, while on another it is profoundly perplexing. For example, a transformed cell is able to reproduce itself and pass its defects on to subsequent generations—so there must be damage to the DNA or to some aspect of the reproductive process. When the problem is viewed in terms of the several functions of the cell we have discussed, it can be seen that there are a number of vulnerable "transformation" points.

Figure 6-13 Carcinogenesis

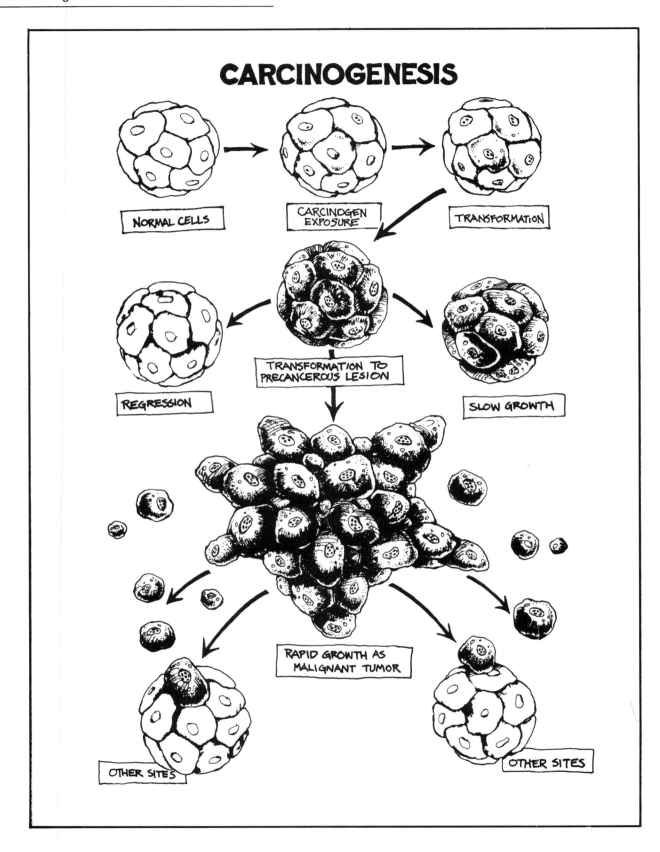

Let's look at some possibilities. Once again, the distinguishing characteristics of cancer cells are:

- rapid reproduction rate

- loss of membrane integrity

- loss of respect for growth limitations (no contact inhibition)

- ability to "deceive—the immune system, despite the presence of tumor markers on the cell membrane

- changes in cell biochemistry and character (e.g., Warburg Effect)

- loss of nuclear integrity and chromosomal stability

POSSIBLE EXPLANATIONS

The increased reproduction rate suggests that something is wrong with the control of reproduction in the G^1 period. Perhaps the key lies there. Some researchers have suggested that cancer cells simply don't have an "off" switch anymore. But other researchers point out that the "off" switch ultimately rests in the DNA—which leads to the conclusion that the damage is in the DNA itself.

Loss of membrane integrity can be induced through a number of mechanisms in normal cells cultured in the laboratory. The microtubules and microfilaments which anchor the membrane components in place are highly sensitive to changes in the levels of ions such as magnesium, calcium, sodium, and potassium. Some hormones and neural chemicals can also alter the structures of the cell's "skeletons" and "muscles." Finally, many aspects of the maintenance of the membrane and active transport through the membrane are dependent upon ATP for energy. ATP can, itself, be altered if the levels of ions change in its environment. All this would seem to indicate that cells are transformed in concert with "nutritional" changes in their environment which prompt alterations in the membrane structure. But the nutritional argument fails to explain why changes in the membrane alone can be transmitted genetically to daughter cells, and why the cells undergo rapid reproduction. In fact, any argument based solely on the membrane alterations observed in cancer cells fails to account for the genetic changes these cells undergo.

Alterations in the membrane may account for the invasive growth patterns of cancer cells and the ability of the cells to "deceive" the immune systems. Changes in protein markers on the surface of the membrane may be related to both the characteristic of random growth, and to its peculiar relationship to the immune system. When a cancer cell is attacked by the immune system, it may secrete polysaccharides and glycolipids to cover the proteins on the membrane and provide a protective barrier. The problem here is control. What tells the cell to stop making some proteins for the membrane and start making altogether new ones which stimulate the immune system? Again, as we have seen, most aspects of control go back to protein synthesis, and ultimately, to DNA.

The altered protein content and general biochemistry of cancer cells would seem to indicate that something is wrong with the mechanisms responsible for control of protein synthesis. The problem could be either at the point of transcription, translation, packaging in the Golgi, production of RNA, production of polymerases for RNA and DNA production, DNA synthesis, or the genetic code itself. The most tempting choice is the genetic code (i.e., mutagenesis).

Although most mutations in the genetic code are either repaired or are lethal to the cell, some slip by unnoticed. Nearly every agent which is known to cause cancer has also been shown to cause mutations in the genetic code.

GOING FROM BAD TO WORSE: ENVIRONMENTAL CARCINOGENESIS

Sunburns and Hair Sprays

As we discussed, ultra-violet light causes DNA changes, and therefore mutations. UV light is also thought to be responsible for most skin cancer in humans. There is concern among scientists and the public that the depletion of the ozone layer in the earth's atmosphere, through pollution and the use of fluorocarbon aerosol sprays, will increase our exposure to UV light (ozone shields us from UV light), and result in a correspondingly increased rate of skin cancer.

As you will soon learn, more and more chemicals are being suspected (or proved) of causing cancer. But there are thousands and thousands of new chemicals manufactured and introduced into the environment each year. There isn't time and money to test all of these chemicals (in test animals) for possible mutagen cancer-causing effects.

In the 1970s Bruce Ames at Berkeley developed a clever assay system for testing the mutagenic potential of chemicals in bacterial cells. Ames cultures Salmonella bacteria on special laboratory plates, exposes them to a test chemical, and then waits to see if mutant colonies of bacteria develop. To bring the test a little closer to home, Ames adds human liver enzymes to the plates, so that the bacteria have the same chance to safely break down (detoxify) the chemicals that we have in our livers. So far the Ames test method has found hundreds of chemicals to be mutagenic and there is a close relationship between the chemicals he finds mutagenic and those the National Cancer Institute finds carcinogenic in test animals.

Radiation exposure is primarily harmful by virtue of its damage to DNA. Most studies on radiation exposure have been concerned with nuclear radiation, x-rays and UV light (light is a form of radiation), although there is beginning to be concern about microwaves and other types of radiation as well. High dose radiation causes burns and severe immediate harm, while lower doses cause relatively gradual, long-term harm through damage to the DNA. Radiation exposure which has been demonstrated to be carcinogenic in test animals, and in many cases, humans, has also been shown to be mutagenic.

Gotta Virus?

In the late 1970s scientists at the National Cancer Institute discovered a virus that causes a rare type of leukemia in humans. Long before this discovery was made an outspoken minority of cancer researchers had argued that some types of human cancer had to be caused by viruses. After all, they said, Mammary Tumour Virus causes breast cancer in mice, Feline Leukemia Virus causes leukemia in cats, and dozens of other viruses have been found to directly transform various types of animal cells into cancer cells. Why should humans be spared the viral attack?

It turned out human cancer viruses had been hard to find because they are part of an entire family of viruses science didn't even discover until the 1970s: *retroviruses*. These bizarre viruses are much smaller than the more familiar of our viral enemies, such as influenza and chicken pox. And they are backwards, genetically speaking. Retroviruses don't have any DNA. Instead, they have mRNA and a special trick enzyme, called *reverse transcriptase*, that allows the viral mRNA to reverse itself into its mirror image, and then insert these viral genes into the DNA of the infected cell. In this way, the virus completely commandeers the cell, forcing its entire genetic machinery to go into high gear making viruses.

Scientists have been studying a range of possible cancer-causing viruses at a furious pace in recent years, and in test tubes it seems a large list of viruses

are capable of transforming normal human cells into cancer cells. Now it's a long way from a test tube to a human being, and there is good reason to think that most of the time our bodies' immune systems successfully fight off such viruses before they have the opportunity to transform healthy cells into cancer cells. Still, there is increasing enthusiasm among basic biologists for viral explanations of at least some types of cancer.

In the process of studying how cancer viruses affect cells, scientists found many contain special signals in their genes that help them to take over the DNA of cells they infect. These signals seem to tell the various components of the transcription system, "Come on over here and read me. Now!" It's as if somebody were intercepting all the boss' factory production orders and sending out totally different commands, leading to the fast-paced manufacture of a whole different line of products. Even more astonishing, when the "boss" catches on, there doesn't seem to be anything that can stop the pirating of the system by the virus.

Well here comes the truly amazing part of the virus story. It turns out those take-over signals found in the viral genes actually exist NORMALLY in our cells. A tremendous amount of research is underway now to identify what those genes are expected to do normally. They have been named *oncogenes* (onco = cancer, genes). Some of these oncogenes seem to code for growth factors; special proteins that are supposed to promote rapid cell growth or protein production at certain stages in the life of the cell or human being. For example, human beings grow at an extraordinary pace during the nine months of fetal development, and some of these special factors are responsible for that growth. But normally all the genes for embryonic growth are supposed to be shut off when the growth spurt is over. Many scientists believe oncogenes are simply growth signals that, for unknown reasons, got switched back on, causing rapid cell growth and eventually cancer.

So some viruses may cause cancer because they possess those same oncogene signals, and trigger the same set of rapid growth responses. And it is possible, although hard science is glaringly missing here, that environmental carcinogens are most lethal when they cause damage to DNA at the site of an oncogene. The tar or nicotine in a cigarrette, for example, may be relatively benign to lung cells until its mutational damage happens to hit an oncogene site on the DNA.

DES and You

Researchers who search for human cancer viruses continue to operate on the assumption that the key to cellular transformation is alteration of DNA. Similarly, there are efforts to understand the biochemistry of hormone-induced cancer. For a while there were theories floating around which asserted that hormone-induced cancer had absolutely nothing to do with the genetic code. The case of diethylstilbesterol, or DES, casts a shadow on such theories, however.

DES is an artificial estrogen drug which was given to pregnant women (particularly in the early 1950s) to prevent miscarriage. Some twenty to twenty-five years later, some of the female offspring of the DES recipients developed rare forms of vaginal cancers. Because the cancers developed at a common site, and because the types of neoplasms appear quite distinct from other vaginal cancers, a strong finger is pointed at the genetic code. Once again, it appears the mechanism involves damage to DNA. (The male DES offspring have also been studied, and show a higher rate of structural and developmental abnormalities.)

Let's go back, for a moment, to the last of our list of characteristics generally observed in cancer cells: chromosomal and nuclear abnormality. Abnormal chromosomes implicitly indicate damage to the genetic code. Nuclear malfunctions, particularly malfunctions in the division of the nucleus, indicate damage to either the centromere or spindle mechanisms, both of which are under genetic (DNA) control. The proof of the pudding lies in reproducibility. There are human tumor cell lines which have been maintained in laboratory cultures for generation upon generation. These cells change over time, but when they do, the change is passed on to the subsequent generation. Again, this has indicated direct changes in the DNA.

The Genetic Link

The susceptibility of a given individual in a population to a particular carcinogen may deviate strongly from the norm. Although a compound may be labelled a "strong carcinogen" (e.g. asbestos), there are individuals who have spent entire cancer-free lives working with the material. At the other extreme, there are cases of short exposure to the substance leading to lung cancer. This variation, which is seen in test animals and humans for all carcinogens, was puzzling for a long time. Obviously, there appeared to be a genetic link to cancer susceptibility; but what was it? The answer isn't clear; many theories have been tried and cast aside over the years. Today, the main point is that genetic variation does exist, and provides further proof that carcinogenesis is a genetic process.

Summary of the Environment and Cancer

Let's leave the summary on this point to Nobel laureate James Watson:

> In general, compounds which are transformed into strong carcinogens likewise become strong mutagens, and vice versa. There thus seems little doubt that much if not most carcinogenesis is the result of changes in the DNA. From, *Molecular Biology of the Gene* (3rd edition, 1976, pp. 645–646).

The assumption that changes in the DNA are the basis of carcinogenesis, and that there is a link between mutagenesis and carcinogenesis, leads to a critical question: how much carcinogenic (cancer-causing) material does it take to transform a cell and cause cancer? Or, when does a mutation lead to cancer? Those questions are prompting the most heated scientific-governmental-industrial debate our country has ever witnessed.

The ramifications of the debate are staggering. On the one hand it can be argued that only extremely high doses of exposure to mutagens will lead to cell transformation and then human cancer. From a regulatory point of view, this would mean that few, if any, potential carcinogens would require banning or tough regulation. That point of view argues from a biological perspective that the liver takes care of the job well enough to prevent cancer. One of the primary jobs of liver cells is breaking down incoming chemicals in the bloodstream. These researchers feel that the enzymes present in the liver are more than adequate to handle the job under normal conditions of exposure. The cancer problem, they believe, only arises when the levels of carcinogen exposure are so high that the liver cannot adequately handle the traffic. Then carcinogens slip through the liver without being detoxified, ending up somewhere else in the body where they transform cells.

Completely on the other side of this debate is the "no safe level of exposure" position. From a regulatory standpoint, this point of view would hold that the use of any compound demonstrated to cause cancer or mutations in test animals should be severely restricted with respect to human exposure. This argument operates on two levels. First, with respect to the liver: the liver was never designed to detoxify most of the chemicals which have been shown to be carcinogenic, because most of these chemicals are man-made. Cigarette smoke, benzene, asbestos, benzpyrene, nitrosamines—these are all part of our environment because of some form of human manipulation. The liver does not possess the enzymes for

Figure 6-14 Summary: Environmental Carcinogenesis

SUMMARY: ENVIRONMENTAL CARCINOGENESIS

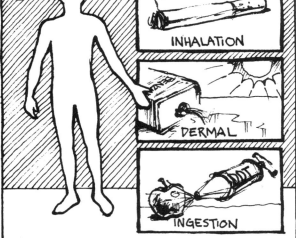

①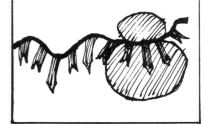

INHALATION

DERMAL

INGESTION

A HEALTHY PERSON IS EXPOSED TO CARCINOGENS

② CARCINOGENS ATTACK INDIVIDUAL CELLS BY DIRECTLY ATTACKING THE DNA MOLECULE.

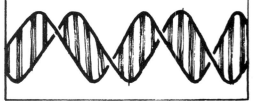

③ EITHER THE DNA IS MUTILATED, OR THE PROCESS OF DNA TRANSLATION IS ALTERED.

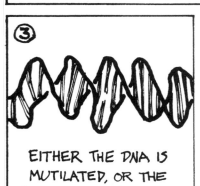

④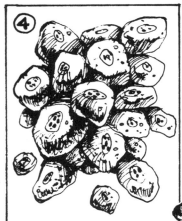

THE CELLS CONTAINING ALTERED DNA ARE TRANSFORMED AND A TUMOR DEVELOPS. THE TUMOR METASTASIZES INTO THE BLOOD STREAM.

⑤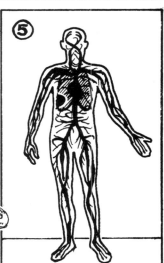

THE PERSON HAS MALIGNANT CANCER

effective detoxification of chemicals which were never intended to be part of the natural human environment.

In some cases the liver actually makes the situation worse by converting a minor problem into a big one. Aflatoxin for example, is a natural carcinogen which is relatively harmless until liver enzymes convert it to a more potent mutagenic chemical. Similar liver and digestive action is seen with nitrates used as food preservatives. (Also, there is great variation in liver function from one individual to the next.) The argument ultimately asserts that the liver does a fairly poor job of protecting us from mutagens.

The second part of the argument is cellular—that the nature of the disease indicates that even low levels of mutagenic exposure pose an unreasonable risk. It starts with the proposition that it usually takes ten to twenty years for a small group of transformed cells to result in a tumor large enough to be medically detected. Further, it has been proposed that every cancer case begins with a single cell or small group of cells being exposed to a mutagen. That single cell or small group of cells is transformed and begins to divide. Twenty years of cell division ultimately results in a visible tumor. Because, as was pointed out above, there is generally a specific genetic character to any tumor, many researchers believe that cancer may arise from a single altered cell which passes on its misfit identity to its progeny, ultimately resulting in a tumor full of genetically similar cells.

If the theory is correct, the problem of mutagen exposure becomes immense. There are over 5 billion cells in the average human body, any one of which could potentially be transformed. Some researchers feel the probability of transformation of at least one cell (given that there are billions to choose from) in the face of mutagen exposure is too great to risk. According to their argument, even very low doses of carcinogens could be sufficient to transform a single cell, which will multiply to form a tumor.

Somewhere in the middle is another viewpoint, the compromise. Because of the economic realities of chemical use in our society, it can be argued that statistical probabilities of exposure must be weighed against economic need. In essence, the biological arguments are countered by economic arguments.

From the point of view of the biologist it appears that the future for cancer research rests with further basic biological research. But there are limitations. And there have been mistakes.

Biology and cancer research have developed together. Invariably, at each stage, the characteristics of the cancer cell have been ascribed to some defect in whatever branch of biology happens at the time to be fashionable and exciting; today it is molecular genetics. Even if the various advances in biology have not thus far provided the key to understanding cancer, they have at least provided an explanation for some of the puzzling phenomena discovered by people doing cancer research.

—John Cairns (*Cancer—Science and Society*), page 63 (San Francisco, W. H. Freeman & Co., 1978)

WHERE DO WE GO FROM HERE?

The Future Biology of Cancer

It is tempting to beg for technical solutions to technical problems. If a jet airplane is creating air pollution, bring in an engineer to change the exhaust system. If the pollution index drops by 1%, you can always brag about how much better the pollution is than what it would have been.

Nobody is certain how much cancer is environmental in origin, but it is a generally accepted estimate that 70 to 90% of all cancer is environmentally derived. Some of this involves natural carcinogens (like aflatoxin), but most is man-made (particularly, cigarette smoking). A technical solution for a technical problem? Can we find a cure for the cancer we have spread all around us?

In his State of the Union Address on January 22, 1971, President Richard M. Nixon called for a "war on cancer." It was felt that since pouring lots of federal money into the space industry had put a man on the moon, the cure for cancer could be approached in the same manner. The war was to be fueled by an additional $100 million in the cancer research pot. Almost a year later, on December 23, 1971, President Nixon signed the National Cancer Act. In 1971 the National Cancer Institute was given separate agency status (it had been a subsidiary of the National Institutes for Health), and received a budget hike of 29%. Since 1971 the NCI budget has climbed steadily from $233 million to over $1 billion for 1988.

And what have we got to show for it? There are those who say the war on cancer has been fruitless; that there have been no significant changes in the overall cancer picture in the U.S. since 1971. It is true more people are getting cancer today. In the 1960s, about 25% of all Americans had cancer at some point in their lifetime. By the late 1970s, more than a third of all Americans had cancer during their lifetime. And by the Year 2000, your odds will be fifty-fifty of getting some type of cancer during your lifetime. That is a grim forecast.

The optimists look at those numbers another way. They say the War on Cancer is being won because while more people may be getting cancer, fewer are dying of it. Treatment has improved dramatically, as you will read in later chapters, and some types of cancer thought terminal twenty years ago are cured 70 to 90% of the time today. In addition, they say, the numbers are skewed because people are living longer and cancer is a disease that most often strikes in old age.

Still, it does appear that pouring massive amounts of federal dollars into a War on Cancer has not been the key to the fundamental biological breakthroughs that have helped us understand the disease. Research on genetic repair mechanisms, the signals involved in transcription and translation, oncogenes, ways viruses infect cells, fundamental cellular biochemistry, recombinant DNA: these are the areas that have had the most profound impact on our understanding of cancer.

As a society we will continue to wage war on cancer. And few would disagree that the war will be most effectively waged if it combines a strong commitment to basic biology research with regulation of environmental, occupational and dietary carcinogens.

Bibliography (Annotated by Laurie Garrett)

1. Agran, L., 1977. *The Cancer Connection,* Houghton-Mifflin Co. *Agran's more complete study of job-related cancers. He did his research well, drew fair conclusions, and had a rough time coming up with solutions. Easy reading.*

2. American Chemistry Society and National Cancer Institute, 1976. *Proceedings of Symposium on Environmental Carcinogens.* ACS. *This is full of technical reports, but is very informative and will supply the critical reader with a shopping list of potential carcinogens.*

3. Bailer J. C., Smith E. M. Progress Against Cancer? N Eng J. of Med. 1986; 314:1226–1232. *"They argue that we are losing the war against cancer."*

4. Blumer, M. et.al., 1977. "Polycyclic Aromatic Hydrocarbons in Soils of a Mountain Valley: Correlation with Highway Traffic and Cancer Incidence," Env. Sci Tech. 11:1082. *A good specific example of the environmental carcinogen problem. Advanced reading.*

5. Braun, A. C., 1974. *The Biology of Cancer,* Addison-Wesley Publishing Company. *Braun is a plant physiologist who has been carrying out cancer research. The book is general and slightly supplementary to this text.*

6. Braun, A. C., 1977. *The Story of Cancer,* Addison-Wesley Publishing Company. *Another general overview for the intermediate reader.*

7. Cairns, J., 1975. "The Cancer Problem," Sci. Amer., Nov. '75, pg. 64. *Another classic, and a pathbreaker.*

8. Cairns, J., 1978. *Cancer, Science, and Society,* W. H. Freeman & Company. *Excellent! Read it!*

9. Diet, Nutrition and Cancer, Committee on Diet, Nutrition and Cancer, Assembly of Life Sciences, National Research Council, National Academy Press, 1982. *This is the most comprehensive analysis ever written of the relationship between the food you eat and cancer.*

10. Epstein, S., 1976. "The Political and Economic Basis of Cancer," Tech. Rev. July/Aug. (1976), pg. 35. *It is what it claims to be, and worth reading. General audience.* Also by Epstein, *The Politics of Cancer,* Sierra Club Books, 1978.

11. Grobstein, C., 1977. "The Recombinant DNA Debate," Sci. Amer. 237:22. *More of the debate. Easy reading.*

12. Hiatt, H. H.; J. D. Watson & J. A. Winsten, 1977. *Origins of Human Cancer,* Books A, B, & C., Cold Spring Harbor. *For the advanced student, this is an excellent resource for nearly all cancer issues and answers (or at least hints).*

13. Holliday, R., 1977. "Should Genetic Engineers be Contained?", *New Scientist,* Feb. 17, 1977, pg. 399. *The author thinks the answer is "yes."*

14. Hopson, J. L., 1977. "Recombinant lab for DNA and my 95 days in it," *Smithsonian,* June, 1977. *This reporter walked into the most gung-ho high pressure recombinant DNA research labs in the world, and loved every minute it.*

15. Kornberg, A., 1974. *DNA Synthesis,* W. H. Freeman & Co. *This is definitely for advanced students only, and even then only molecular biology freaks. There's more detail on DNA synthesis in this book than you could possibly want to know. Great pictures.*

16. LaFord, R., 1977. "of principals, crabs, and stars," *Chemistry,* Jan/Feb, 1977. *Part of a series of special American Chemistry Society papers on cancer. This is an overview. Excellent beginning reading.*

17. Lehninger, A. L., 1975. *Biochemistry,* 2nd edition. Worth Publishers, Inc. *If you're serious about understanding biology in the 1980s, you're simply going to have to read this.*

18. Levine, A. J., 1977. "Cancer and Viruses," *Chemistry,* May, 1977. *Part of a series of a special American Chemistry Society papers on cancer. This is an overview. Excellent beginning reading.*

19. National Cancer Institute *Technical Reports Series These reports, which are constantly being released, detail the results of carcinogenicity tests for particular substances on mice and rats. Check your library for them. This is the best way to get quick information on a particular suspected carcinogen.*

20. Nature 312:6 (1984). *The skeptical British doubt life expectancy has really improved for cancer patients.*

21. Nature 315:190 (1985). *Good overview on how tumours arise from oncogenes.*

22. Nature 321:112 (1986). *This paper was written by the King of Oncogenes, Michael Bishop. In it he links oncogenes and steroids.*

23. Nature 323:488 (1986). *The British science journal asks, "Are we losing the war on cancer?".*

24. New England Journal of Medicine 316:1044 (1987). *Excellent analysis of the relationship of benzene to leukemia*

25. Rettig, R. A., 1977. *Cancer Crusade: The story of the National Cancer Act of 1971,* Princeton University Press. *If you really want to understand why the Nixon Administration's War on Cancer didn't yield victories, read this. Tough investigation by a Rand Corporation fellow.*

26. Richards, V., 1978. *Cancer: The Wayward Cell, Its Origins, Nature, and Treatment,* 2nd edition. University of California Press. *He has a way with words. General overview, written by an M.D.*

27. Sauter, D. Y., 1975. "Synthetic Fuels and Cancer," Emergency Task Force on Energy Options, Scientists Institute for Public Information, 49 E. 53rd Street, New York, NY 10022. *A good specific example of the environmental carcinogen problem. Easy reading.*

28. Science 226:1199 (1984). *Cancer cells show very specific chromosomal abnormalities that can actually be used to diagnose cancer without biopsies.*

29. Science 228:669 (1985). *Peter Deusenberg casts doubt on the oncogene model, and says other factors are involved in carcinogenesis.*

30. Science 229:37, 54, 69, 74 (1985). *Excellent series of research papers demonstrating how the HTLV family of oncogenes are involved in carcinogenesis.*

31. Science 233:1061 (1986). *Remember contact inhibition and its role in cancer? Well this research paper shows oncogenes may be affecting cancer cell membranes.*

32. Science News 127:10 (1985). *Report of an oncogene involved in retinoblastoma.*

33. Science News 127:346 (1985). *Report that the National Cancer Institute is increasingly turning to viral explanations for carcinogenesis.*

34. Shimkin, M. B., 1973. *Science and Cancer,* DHEW Pub. No. (NIH) 74-568. *Short monograph. Very basic information.*

35. Singer, S. J. & G. Nicolson, 1972. "The Fluid Mosaic Model of the Structure of Cell Membranes," *Science* 175:720. *This paper is a classic. For advanced students interested in membrane problems, this is a must.*

36. Stellman, J. & Daum, S., 1973. *Work is Dangerous to Your Health,* Vintage. *Provides a glimpse of the problems and complications surrounding potential occupational carcinogens. Easy reading.*

37. Suss, R. et al., 1973. *Cancer: Experiments and Concepts.* Springer-Verlag New York. *This is for advanced students interested in cancer research problems and approaches. It's somewhat out-of-date, and the techniques have moved past this book. Provides good background, however.*

33. Thomas, L., 1974. *The Lives of a Cell: Notes of a Biology Watcher,* Macmillan Co. *This is fun. And worth reading.*

39. Watson, J. D., et al. 1987. *Molecular Biology of the Gene,* 4th edition, The Benjamin/Cummings Publishing Company, Inc. *This is the Numero Uno in biology books. If you read and understand this one, you're ready to tackle anything. But be forewarned—real appreciation requires a previous background in basic chemistry and cell biology.*

7

Immunology

The following two pieces concern immunology and cancer. In the first one, Isaac Asimov takes you through the immune system in person. In the second, William R. Clark, Professor of Biology, University of California, Los Angeles, provides an introduction to immunology as it relates to cancer.—*M.R.*

Fantastic Voyage
(Through the Immune System)

Isaac Asimov

Owens' voice sounded from the bubble, "Dr. Michaels, look ahead. Is that the turnoff?"

They could feel the *Proteus* slowing.

Michaels muttered, "Too much talk. I should have been watching."

Immediately ahead was an open-ended tube. The thin walls facing them were ragged, almost fading away into nothingness. The opening was barely wide enough for the *Proteus*.

"Good enough," called out Michaels. "Head into it."

Cora had left the workbench to look forward in wonder, but Duval remained in his place, still working, with infinite, untiring patience.

"That must be a lymphatic," she said.

They had entered and the walls surrounded them, no thicker than those of the capillary they had left some time back.

As in the capillaries, the walls were made up, quite clearly, of cells in the shape of flat polygons, each with a rounded nucleus at the center. The fluid through which they were passing was very similar to that in the pleural cavity, sparkling yellowish in the *Proteus* headlights, and lending a yellow cast to the cells. The nuclei were deeper in color, almost orange.

Grant said, "Poached eggs! They look exactly like poached eggs!" Then, "What's a lymphatic?"

"It's an auxiliary circulatory system in a way," said Cora, explaining eagerly. "Fluid squeezes out of the very thin capillaries and collects in spaces in the body and between the cells. That's interstitial fluid. These drain off into tiny tubes, or lymphatics, that are open at their ends, as you saw just now. These tubes gradually combine into larger and larger tubes until the largest are the size of veins. All the lymph . . ."

"That's the fluid about us?" asked Grant.

"Yes. All the lymph is collected into the largest lymphatic of all, the thoracic duct, which leads into the subclavian vein in the upper chest, and thus the lymph is restored to the main circulatory system."

"And why have we entered the lymphatic?"

Michaels leaned back, the course momentarily secure. "Well," he put in, "it's a quiet backwater. There's no pumping effect of the heart. Muscular pressures and tensions move the fluid and Benes isn't having many of those right now. So we can be assured a quiet journey to the brain."

"Why didn't we enter the lymphatics to begin with, then?"

"They are small. An artery is a much better target for a hypodermic; and the arterial current was expected to carry us to target in minutes. It didn't work out and to make our way back into an artery from here would delay us badly. Then, once we reached the artery, we would receive a battering which the ship might no longer be able to take."

He spread out a new set of charts and called out, "Owens, are you following Chart 72-D?"

"Yes, Dr. Michaels."

"Make sure you follow the path I've traced. It will take us through a minimum number of nodes."

Grant said, "What's that up ahead?"

Michaels looked up and froze. "Slow the ship," he cried.

The *Proteus* decelerated vigorously. Through one portion of the wall of the widening tube a shapeless mass protruded, milky, granular, and somehow threatening. But as they watched, it shrank and vanished.

"Move on," said Michaels. He said to Grant, "I was afraid that white cell might be coming, but it was going, fortunately. Some of the white cells are formed in the lymph nodes, which are an important barrier against disease. They form not only white cells but also antibodies."

"And what are antibodies?"

"Protein molecules that have the capacity to combine specifically with various outside substances

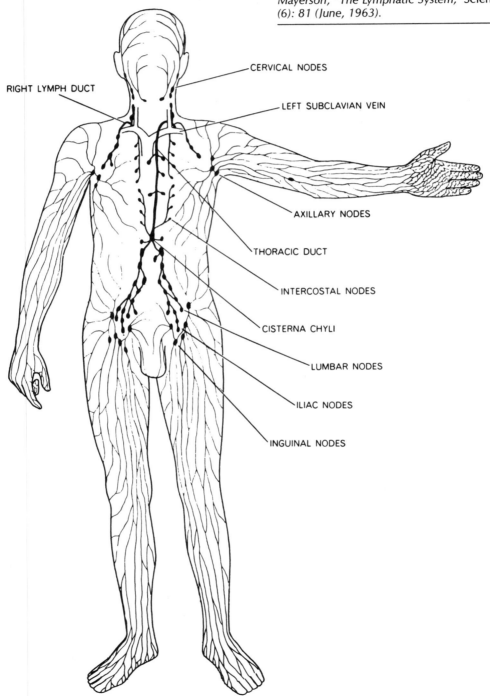

Figure 7-1 The Lymphatic Vessels. Lymphatic vessels drain the entire body, penetrating most of the tissues and carrying back to the bloodstream excess fluid from the intercellular spaces. This diagram shows only some of the larger superficial vessels (*light color*), which run near the surface of the body, and deep vessels (*dark color*), which drain the interior of the body and collect from the superficial vessels. The thoracic duct, which arises at the cisterna chyli in the abdomen, drains most of the body and empties into the left subclavian vein. The right lymph duct drains the heart, lungs, part of the diaphragm, the right upper part of the body and the right side of the head and neck, emptying into the right subclavian vein. Lymph nodes interspersed along the vessels trap foreign matter, including bacteria. *Source: H.S. Mayerson, "The Lymphatic System,"* Scientific American, *208 (6): 81 (June, 1963).*

RIGHT LYMPH DUCT

CERVICAL NODES

LEFT SUBCLAVIAN VEIN

AXILLARY NODES

THORACIC DUCT

INTERCOSTAL NODES

CISTERNA CHYLI

LUMBAR NODES

ILIAC NODES

INGUINAL NODES

invading the body; germs, toxins, foreign proteins."

"And us?"

"And us, I suppose, under proper circumstances."

Cora interposed. "Bacteria are trapped in the nodes, which serve as a battleground between them and the white cells. The nodes swell up and become painful. You know, children get what are called swollen glands in the armpits or at the angle of the jaw."

"And they're really swollen lymph nodes."

"That's right."

Grant said, "It sounds like a good idea to stay away from the lymph nodes."

Michaels said, "We are small. Benes' antibody system is not sensitized to us, and there is only one series of nodes we need pass through, after which we have clear sailing. It's a chance, of course, but everything we do now is a chance. Or," he demanded, challengingly, "are you going to set policy by ordering me out of the lymphatic system?"

Grant shook his head, "No. Not unless someone suggests a better alternative."

●

"There it is," said Michaels, nudging Grant gently. "See it?"

"The shadow up ahead?"

"Yes. This lymphatic is one of several that enters the node, which is a spongy mass of membranes and tortuous passages. The place is full of lymphocytes . . ."

"What are those?"

"One of the types of white cells. They won't bother us, I hope. Any bacteria in the circulatory system reaches a lymph node eventually. It can't negotiate the narrow twisting channels . . ."

"Can we?"

"We move deliberately, Grant, and with an end in view, whereas bacteria drift blindly. You do see the difference, I hope. Once trapped in the node, the bacterium is handled by antibodies or, if that fails, by white cells mobilized for battle."

The shadow was close now. The golden tinge of the lymph was darkening and turning cloudy. Up ahead there seemed a wall.

"Do you have the course, Owens?" Michaels called out.

"I have, but it's going to be easy to make a wrong turning."

"Even if you do, remember that at this moment we are heading generally upward. Keep the gravitometer indicator on the line as steadily as you can, and in the end you can't go wrong."

The *Proteus* made a sharp turn and suddenly all was gray. The headlights seemed to pick up nothing that was not a shadow of a deeper or lighter gray. There was an occasional small rod, shorter than the ship and much narrower; clumps of spherical objects, quite small, and with fuzzy boundaries.

"Bacteria," muttered Michaels. "I see them in too great detail to recognize the exact species. Isn't that strange? Too much detail."

The *Proteus* was moving more slowly now, following the many gentle sweeps and turns of the channel almost hesitantly.

Duval stepped to the door of the workroom. "What's going on? I can't work on this thing if the ship doesn't hold a steady course. The Brownian motion is bad enough."

"Sorry, Doctor," said Michaels, coldly. "We're passing through a lymph node and this is the best we can do."

Duval, looking angry, turned away.

Grant peered forward. "It's getting messy up there, Dr. Michaels. What is that stuff that looks like seaweed or something?"

"Reticular fibers," said Michaels.

Owens said, "Dr. Michaels."

"Yes?"

"That fibrous stuff is getting thicker. I won't be able to maneuver through them without doing some damage to them."

Michaels looked thoughtful. "Don't worry about that. Any damage we do will, in any case, be minimal."

A clump of fibers pulled loose as the *Proteus* nudged into it, slipped and slid along the window and vanished past the sides. It happened again and again with increasing frequency.

"It's all right, Owens," said Michaels, encouragingly, "the body can repair damage like this without trouble."

"I'm not worried about Benes," called out Owens. "I'm worried about the ship. If this stuff clogs the vents, the engine will overheat. And it's adhering to us. Can't you tell the difference in the engine sound?"

Grant couldn't, and his attention turned to the outside again. The ship was nosing through a forest of tendrils now. They glinted a kind of menacing maroon in the headlights.

"We'll get through it soon," said Michaels, but there was a definite note of anxiety in his voice.

The way did clear a bit and now Grant could indeed sense a difference in the sound of the engines, almost a thickening hoarseness, as though the clear echo of gases bubbling through exhaust vents was being muffled and choked off.

Owens shouted, "Dead ahead!"

There was a soggy collision of a bacterial rod with the ship. The substance of the bacterium bent about the curve of the window, sprang back into shape and bounced off, leaving a smear that washed off slowly.

There were others ahead.

"What's going on?" said Grant in wonder.

"I think," said Michaels, "I *think* we're witnessing antibody reaction to bacteria. White cells aren't involved. See! Watch the walls of the bacteria. It's hard by the reflection of miniaturized light, but can you see it?"

"No, I'm afraid I can't."

Duval's voice sounded behind them. "I can't see anything, either."

Grant turned. "Is the wire adjusted, Doctor?"

"Not yet," said Duval. "I can't work in this mess. It will have to wait. What's this about antibodies?"

Michaels said, "As long as you're not working, let's have the inner lights out. Owens!"

The lights went out and the only illumination came from without, a ghostly gray-maroon flicker that placed all their faces in angry shadow.

"What's going on outside?" asked Cora.

"That's what I'm trying to explain," said Michaels. "Watch the edges of the bacteria ahead."

Grant did his best, narrowing his eyes. The light was unsteady and flickering. "You mean those small objects that look like BB shot."

"Exactly. They're antibody molecules. Proteins, you know, and large enough to see on our scale. There's one nearby. See it!"

One of the small antibodies had swirled past the window. At close quarters it did not seem to be a BB shot at all. It seemed rather larger than a BB and to be a tiny tangle of spaghetti, vaguely spherical. Thin strands, visible only as fine glints of light, protruded here and there.

"What are they doing?" asked Grant. "Each bacterium has a distinctive cell wall made out of specific atomic groupings hooked up in a specific way. To us, the various walls look smooth and featureless; but if we were smaller still—on the molecular scale instead of the bacterial—we'd see that each wall had a mosaic pattern, and that this mosaic was different and distinctive in each bacterial species. The antibodies can fit neatly upon this mosaic and once they cover key portions of the wall, the bacterial cell is through; it would be like blocking a man's nose and mouth and choking him to death."

Cora said excitedly, "You can see them cluster. How . . . how horrible."

"Are you sorry for the bacteria, Cora?" said Michaels, smiling.

"No, but the antibodies seem so vicious, the way they pounce."

Michaels said, "Don't give them human emotions. They are only molecules, moving blindly. Interatomic forces pull them against those portions of the wall which they fit and hold them there. It's analogous to the clank of a magnet against an iron bar. Would you say the magnet attacks the iron viciously?"

Knowing what to look for, Grant could now see what was happening. A bacterium, moving blindly through a cloud of hovering antibodies seemed to attract them, to pull them in to itself. In moments, its wall had grown fuzzy with them. The antibodies lined up side by side, their spaghetti projections entangling.

Grant said, "Some of the antibodies seem indifferent. They don't touch the bacterium."

"The antibodies are specific," said Michaels. "Each one is designed to fit the mosaic of a particular kind of bacterium, or of a particular protein molecule. Right now, most of the antibodies, though not all, fit the bacteria surrounding us. The presence of these particular bacteria has stimulated the rapid formation of this particular variety of antibody. How this stimulation is brought about, we still don't know."

"Good lord," cried Duval. "Look at that."

One of the bacteria was now solidly encased in antibodies which had followed its every irregularity, so that it seemed to be exactly as before, but with a fuzzy, thickened boundary. Cora said, "It fits perfectly."

"No, not that. Don't you see that the intermolecular bindings of the antibody molecules produce a kind of pressure on the bacterium? This was never clear even in electron microscopy, which only shows us dead objects."

A silence fell upon the crew of the *Proteus,* which was now moving slowly past the bacterium. The antibody coating seemed to stiffen and tighten and the bacterium within writhed. The coating stiffened and tightened again, then again, and suddenly the bacterium seemed to crumple and give way. The antibodies drew together and what had been a rod became a featureless ovoid.

"They killed the bacterium. They literally squeezed it to death," said Cora, with revulsion.

"Remarkable," muttered Duval. "What a weapon for research we have in the *Proteus.*"

Grant said, "Are you sure we're safe from the antibodies?"

Michaels said, "It seems so. We're not the sort of thing for which antibodies are designed."

"Are you sure? I have a feeling they can be designed for any shape, if properly stimulated."

"You're right, I suppose. Still, we're obviously not stimulating them."

Introduction to Immunology

William R. Clark, Ph.D.

Adapted with permission from a lecture to the 1983 UCLA Biology Cancer Class, and updated in 1986 by William R. Clark, Ph.D. (Professor of Immunology, UCLA).

What is the immune system? What does it do?

The immune system is the body's major defense against foreign substances. *Foreign* means anything that is not a natural part of the self.

The immune system is the main line of defense against infection by bacteria and other microorganisms ("germs"). It is also the body's natural defense against cancer, which the immune system regards as foreign, even though they arise from "self" cells and tissues.

But the immune system can also work *against* you—for example, a kidney transplant, which could save your life, may be attacked and rejected just as vigorously as any other foreign substance. The immune system cannot discriminate between "good" and "bad" foreign substances. Also, there are certain conditions in which the immune system cannot discriminate between "self" and "non-self," and turns against the body itself. This is thought to be the basis for autoimmune diseases such as rheumatoid arthritis, lupus, scleroderma, and myasthenia gravis, among others.

In recent years, the study of immunology has blossomed. New concepts and terminology arise almost daily. The essentials of the immune system are presented in the following sections.

ORGANS OF THE IMMUNE SYSTEM

Bone Marrow

The marrow of primarily the long bones (femur, ulna, etc.), but also the vertebrae and sternum, is the site in the body where the cells of the immune system (see below) are replenished. Both red and white blood cells have short life times, and new cells must be generated daily to take their place. This happens in the bone marrow. Because there are so many rapidly growing cells in the bone marrow, it is very sensitive to the drugs and radiation used to treat cancer. Bone marrow toxicity is often the limiting factor in these treatments.

Thymus Gland

Located in the center of the upper part of the chest, above the heart, this very important organ is where some of the bone marrow cells go to mature into T cells. These cells are very important in fighting viral infections and in defending against tumors. The thymus gradually shrinks and disappears as we get older.

Spleen

This large organ in the upper abdomen, with many red and white blood cells, is important for good immune function, but can be removed with no major harm to the system. It functions somewhat like a lymph node, filtering foreign antigens out of the bloodstream and supporting immune reactions against them.

Lymph Nodes

These small, white, bean-shaped structures located throughout the body are sometimes referred to as "lymph glands." They are the major site of response against infection, transplants, cancer, etc. They usually swell when they react against something foreign. Bacteria and other foreign objects are trapped and destroyed here. Cancer cells that break away from a primary tumor (metastasize) often localize here.

Accessory Organs

The appendix, tonsils (Waldeyer's ring) and "Peyer's patches" on the intestine are also lymphoid in character, although their function in the immune system is not yet clear.

CELLS OF THE IMMUNE SYSTEM (WHITE BLOOD CELLS)

Granular Leukocytes

These are the eosinophils, the neutrophils and the basophils. The *neutrophils* (polymorphonuclear leukocytes, or "PMN"s) are the most numerous and important. They quickly arrive at the site of a wound or infection, and help to clear away dead cells and bacteria. The *basophils* are involved in certain allergic responses (e.g., asthma). *Eosinophils* are involved in the defense against parasites.

Lymphocytes

These are the most "sophisticated" cells of the immune system. B lymphocytes (B cells) produce antibodies (see Figure 7-2). T lymphocytes do not produce antibodies. They directly attack and destroy cancers and transplants, on a cell-to-cell, one-on-one basis.

Macrophages

Important as "scavenger" cells in the body. They help to clear away foreign substances killed or neutralized by the immune system (i.e., bacteria, cancer cells, etc.).

MOLECULES OF THE IMMUNE SYSTEM

Antibodies

Antibodies are protein molecules made by "B" lymphocytes and secreted into the bloodstream, where they circulate throughout the body. Antibodies will attack and destroy or neutralize foreign substances such as bacteria, toxins, and other harmful molecules that get into the bloodstream. In order to actually kill a bacterium or a cancer or a transplanted cell, the antibodies need the help of other proteins collectively called "complement" (see Figure 7-3).

There are two major classes of antibodies, IgG and IgM. "Ig" stands for "Immunoglobulin," which is a more formal name for antibodies. The other classes of antibodies are IgA, IgD, and IgE.

Antigen

The part of the foreign substance that the antibody or T lymphocyte recognizes and attaches to. For example, bacteria have specific proteins and carbohydrates on their surfaces that the human immune system recognizes as being foreign. These bacterial antigens trigger the immune response, mostly antibodies. Similarly, cancers have antigens on their cell surfaces. These "tumor antigens" also trigger an immune response, which in most cases, leads to suppression of the cancer. This response consists of both antibodies and T cells.

Complement

A group of proteins which help the antibody kill foreign cells. The antibody combines with the cell (bacteria, transplant, cancer) surface antigens. After this step has occurred, complement proteins attach to the antibody, leading to cell death.

ORGANIZATION OF THE IMMUNE RESPONSE

The immune system has two branches: The antibody or B cell response (spoken of as "humoral immunity"), and the T cell-mediated or "killer cell" response (spoken of as "cell-mediated immunity").

In the antibody response, B cells, with the aid of a special type of T cell called a "helper" or T_4 cell, come into contact with antigen. As a result of this contact, the B cell matures to another special type of lymphocyte called a plasma cell, which makes and secretes antibody (IgM at first, then IgG).

In the T cell-mediated response, a different type of T cell, the "pre-killer" cell, contacts antigen on its own, and matures to a "killer" cell. These cells then directly attack and destroy the original antigen, which is usually a cancer cell or a transplant cell. T cells do not make or secrete antibody.

In both types of response, memory cells are produced. When the body contacts the antigen a second time, the memory cells react much more quickly and strongly than the original cells. This is what is meant by being "immune" to a disease.

THE IMMUNE RESPONSE TO A CANCER

The immune response could start as the result of a "T" cell directly contacting the cancer, recognizing the cancer's antigens as foreign and returning to the lymph node via a lymphatic vessel. The T cell would divide and produce daughter cells that are mature killers. These killer T cells would then recirculate to the cancer and begin to destroy it.

Alternatively, one of the cancer cells could break away (metastasize), travel via the lymph fluid to the regional lymph node, and trigger T cells to respond. These T cells (killers) would then recirculate to the cancer and begin to destroy it. This latter pattern is dangerous because once a cancer cell has

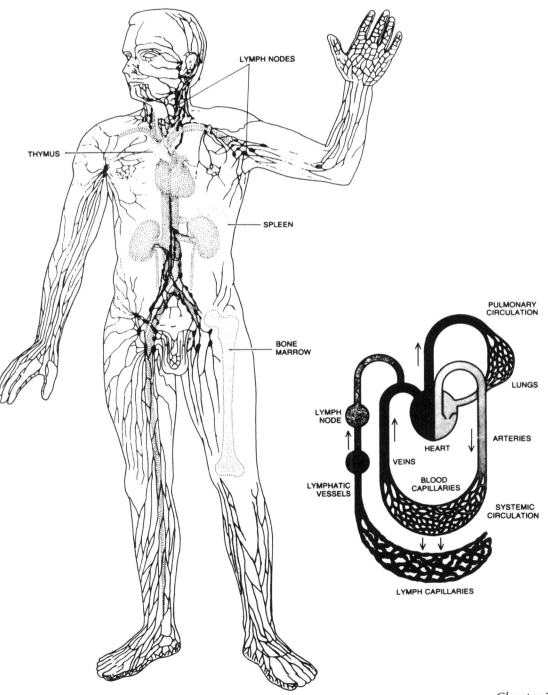

Figure 7-2 The Immune System. Immune system consists of the lymphocytes and the antibody molecules they secrete. The cells and antibodies pervade most of the tissues, to which they are delivered by the bloodstream, but are concentrated in the tissues shown in color: the tree of lymphatic vessels and the lymph nodes stationed along them, the bone marrow (which is in the long bones, only one of which is illustrated), the thymus and the spleen. The lymphatic vessels collect the cells and antibodies from the tissue and return them to the bloodstream at the subclavian veins. Lymphocytes are manufactured in the bone marrow and multiply by cell division in the thymus, the spleen and the lymph nodes. The relation of the blood vessels and the lymphatic vessels is shown highly schematically in the illustration at right. *Source: Neils Jerne, "The Immune System,"* Scientific American, *229 (4): 52−61 (July, 1973).*

LYMPH NODES

THYMUS

SPLEEN

BONE MARROW

PULMONARY CIRCULATION

LUNGS

ARTERIES

HEART

LYMPH NODE

VEINS

BLOOD CAPILLARIES

SYSTEMIC CIRCULATION

LYMPHATIC VESSELS

LYMPH CAPILLARIES

Figure 7-3
Source: Max Cooper and Alexander Lawton, "The Development of an Immunoglobulin," Scientific American, 231 (5): 58–72 (November, 1974).

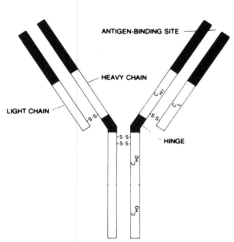

IMMUNOGLOBULIN MOLECULE consists of four polypeptide chains, each made up of many amino acid units. Two of the chains are longer and are designated heavy chains; the smaller ones are called light chains. The molecule is held together by disulfide bonds (-S-S-) but can flex in the region of the hinge. In part of each chain the amino acid sequence is the same in all molecules of the same type; this is called the constant region. There are three or four constant domains in each heavy chain (C_{H1}, C_{H2}, C_{H3}) and one in each light chain (C_L). The genes specifying the constant region may have evolved through the duplication of a primordial gene the size of a single domain. In the variable regions (*color*) the amino acid sequence differs from molecule to molecule. The immunoglobulin binds antigens at clefts formed by folds in the variable regions of the heavy and light chains.

IMMUNO-GLOBULIN	LIGHT CHAIN	HEAVY CHAIN	OTHER CHAINS	STRUCTURE
IgM	KAPPA OR LAMBDA	MU	J	
IgG	KAPPA OR LAMBDA	GAMMA 1 GAMMA 2 GAMMA 3 GAMMA 4		
IgA	KAPPA OR LAMBDA	ALPHA 1 ALPHA 2	J, SC	
IgD	KAPPA OR LAMBDA	DELTA		
IgE	KAPPA OR LAMBDA	EPSILON		

CLASS OF AN IMMUNOGLOBULIN is determined by the type of heavy chain in the molecule. There are five types—mu, gamma, alpha, delta and epsilon—and subclasses of gamma and alpha. In addition each immunoglobulin can have either of two kinds of light chain: kappa or lambda. Some of the immunoglobulins form oligomers, or associations of a few subunits in a single molecule. IgM is ordinarily a pentamer, with five subunits and with an additional "joining" chain, or J chain, shown here as a black dot. IgA occurs as a monomer, dimer and trimer, with respectively one, two and three subunits. The J chain is present in oligomeric forms, and the dimer, when found in secretions such as saliva and tears, is bonded to yet another polypeptide: the secretory component (SC), shown here as a gray disk.

entered the immune system, it can travel via the lymph circulation system to other sites in the body (metastases).

In recent years, another type of lymphocyte has been discovered that is important in resisting cancer. This type of lymphocyte is called a "natural killer," or NK cell. NK cells do not produce antibodies, and so they are quite different from B cells. They are also different from T cells, in two basic ways: T cells resist many different foreign invaders—viruses, bacteria, funguses, parasites, transplanted organs, and cancer. NK cells have only one target—cancer cells. The second major difference between T cells and NK cells is that T cells require from 1–3 days to mature into potent killer cells. NK cells are ready to attack instantly. T cells, once activated by the tumor, may produce a chemical substance called α-interferon. NK cells, although always in an activated state with regard to attacking cancer cells, go into a hyperactivated state under the influence of α-interferon.

T cells and NK cells, together with antibodies, are the principal forms of immunity to cancer. One other form of immunity involves macrophages, which produce something called tumor necrosis factor.

IMMUNE SURVEILLANCE

It is believed that immune surveillance normally works to help control cancer. Some scientists theorize that cancers arise continuously throughout life in all people, but that the immune system eliminates them before they become apparent. Older people, who have weaker immune systems, have a high incidence of cancer. If one interferes with the immune system in even a young patient, the patient is more likely to get malignant tumors. For example, kidney transplant patients receiving medications that suppress their immune system to prevent rejection of the transplant, have up to 400 times the chance of getting certain types of cancer, compared to the normal population.

Additional Reading

1. Roitt, I. Essential Immunology—6th edition. Blackwell Scientific Publications, 1988. (Technical but accessible.)

2. Benjamini, E, Leskowitz, S. Immunology—A Short Course. Alan R. Liss, Inc., 1988. (Basic, well-illustrated.)

8

Viruses and Cancer

Kevin Starr

Fourth Year Medical Student, University of California, San Francisco

Doll and Peto estimated that perhaps 10% of cancer deaths in the United States are attributable to infection by viruses, bacteria, and parasites. And of those three, viruses were felt to account for the lion's share. This chapter presents a broad overview of viruses: what they are, what they do, and how they are involved in cancer causation. Illustrations in this chapter are by Ken Miller, a San Francisco medical illustrator.—*M.R.*

WHAT IS A VIRUS?

A virus is a tiny bundle of RNA or DNA wrapped in a protective protein jacket. Viruses don't eat and they don't move. They have but one function: to enter cells and use the cells' biochemical machinery to produce copies of themselves.

In doing so they can cause a number of diseases, such as measles, colds, the flu, hepatitis, rabies, AIDS, and even cancer. This chapter will help you understand viruses and their role in cancer.

WHAT ARE VIRUSES MADE OF?

Viruses are a varied and heterogeneous group. They range from tiny bits of bare DNA—called viroids—to complex assemblies of varied macromolecules, following a progression of increasing complexity and size. (Macromolecules include proteins, nucleic acids, fats, and carbohydrates and are the basic building materials of all living things.)

At the core of all viruses is a string of nucleic acid, which is in the form of either DNA *or* RNA. This nucleic acid is the same as the nucleic acid found in cells: it is a string of chemical information that controls what the virus is and what it does. As in cells, there are areas along the nucleic acid string in viruses which control specific aspects of their structure and function. These areas are called genes, and just as we might say that a person carries the genes for red hair and freckles, we also speak of a virus as having the gene to make a certain enzyme or specific protein.

The nucleic acid in a virus may be double or single stranded and contains only a few genes; between 3 and 30, compared to about 50,000 in a human cell. These viral genes contain instructions for the manufacture and assembly of new virus copies.

All viruses infecting animal cells have a protein coat surrounding their nucleic acid. This protein coat is important for three reasons:

1. It provides protection, allowing the virus to survive outside the cell.

2. The composition of the protein coat serves as a kind of mailing label, determining what type of cells the virus can enter.

3. The proteins in the coat act as antigens to trigger the immune system of the host.

In addition to a protein coat, some viruses have an outer envelope which is a piece of cell membrane acquired when the virus passes out of the cell. The envelope allows the virus to enter and exit cells without damaging them.

Viruses will occasionally contain enzymes. These enzymes facilitate viral replication in the cell, but like all other viruses, enzyme-containing viruses use the cell they take over in order to reproduce, to make copies of themselves—a process called *replication.*

HOW IS A VIRUS DIFFERENT FROM A CELL? A BACTERIA?

A virus differs from a living cell in many ways. The most obvious difference is size: the biggest virus is about the same size as the tiniest cell. The average cell dwarfs the average virus like an ocean liner next to a rowboat. They differ in the amount of DNA and RNA: the cell has an enormous amount while the virus has comparatively little. They differ in what they have inside: the virus lacks *organelles* (i.e., mitochondria, golgi bodies, ribosomes) which are abundant and essential in the cell. This means that a virus cannot produce energy (the function of the mitochondria) or synthesize proteins (carried out by ribosomes).

Outside of a cell, a virus can't do anything—it's an inert bag of chemicals. Once inside the cell, it becomes active only in its ability to direct its own replication. Unlike cells, which usually have a whole range of different functions and activities, viruses act only to replicate.

Bacteria, in contrast, are single-celled organisms performing the entire range of cellular functions. They can move, metabolize nutrients, synthesize their own proteins—they can even serve as hosts for viruses! While some bacteria must live within another cell to survive, they are largely inde-

Figure 8-1 Schematic Diagram of Viral Structural Levels.

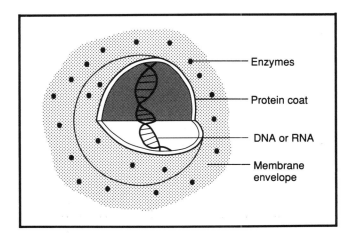

pendent, relying on the host cell for certain nutrients or energy. Like other cells, bacteria contain both DNA and RNA, while viruses have only one or the other.

IS A VIRUS LIVING?

Viruses test our definition of "what is life." Some scientists argue that a virus is not living because it cannot reproduce independently. Others argue that a virus is a living organism because it does direct its own replication—even though it needs a cell in which to do it. Whether or not we define them as living, viruses affect life—the way we live.

TYPES OF VIRUSES

Traditionally, viruses have been classified as DNA or RNA viruses. An additional class has recently emerged, commonly called the *retroviruses* (strictly speaking, retroviruses form only a part of this class, more properly referred to as retroid or retroposon viruses). These retroviruses, while containing either DNA or RNA, use the opposite nucleic acid as a template when making copies of themselves. The tra-

ditional DNA and RNA viruses make their copies directly from the same kind of nucleic acid as the original.

REPLICATION PATHWAYS

DNA viruses: DNA original → DNA copy
RNA viruses: RNA original → RNA copy

Retroid viruses:

1. DNA original → RNA template → DNA copy

2. RNA original → DNA template → RNA copy

The major subgroups of these three classes of viruses are presented in the diagram below. Keep in mind as you read: **1.** The size of a virus determines the number of genes and hence the degree of complexity of the virus; **2.** Having an envelope allows a virus to replicate and exit a cell without destroying it. Viruses without an envelope are trapped inside by the cell membrane and must eventually blow up the cell to get out; and **3.** This diagram is highly simplified and there are important exceptions in each subgroup.

Figure 8-2 The World of Viruses.

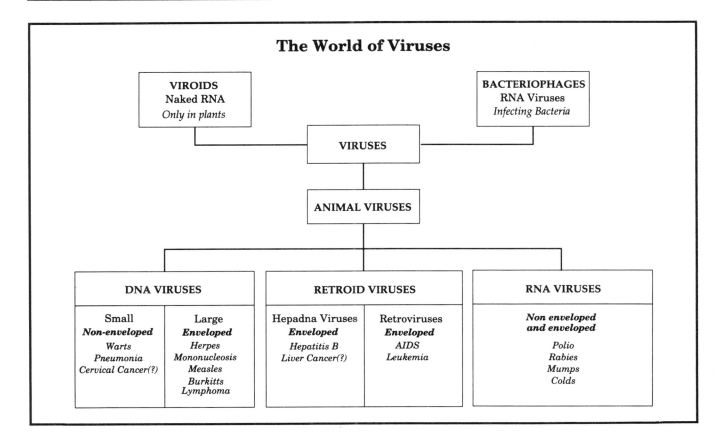

DNA viruses are able to plug directly into the cell's protein synthesizing apparatus and viral DNA is treated the same as cellular DNA. The fact that these viruses use the same kind of nucleic acid as cells has two important implications: 1) the virus, able to use cellular enzymes, need not carry or make enzymes for its own replication, and 2) viral DNA can be inserted into the cell's DNA, becoming a permanent part of the cell's genetic code. Because the cellular DNA is copied each time a cell replicates, changes in a cell caused by insertion of viral DNA will also be seen in future generations of cells.

RNA viruses replicate by making RNA copies from viral RNA. Cells have no enzymes capable of this task (cells can make either DNA or RNA copies from DNA originals, but can't make copies from RNA originals). The virus must direct the cell to make the necessary enzyme. Once this enzyme is made, the cell makes RNA copies, which then direct it to make viral proteins.

Retroviruses were thus dubbed (retro means backward) because they, unlike any other cell or virus, can make DNA copies from RNA originals. Retroviruses are RNA viruses which direct the cells in which they replicate to produce an enzyme known as *reverse transcriptase*. This enzyme makes DNA copies of the virus' RNA.

Retroviruses replicate by making a DNA template of their own RNA and then inserting this DNA template into the DNA of the cell, where it is expressed as though it were cellular DNA—except that the products are viral RNA and proteins. This integration into the cellular DNA is an essential part of the viral replication cycle and can have important consequences for the cell. The viral DNA does not leave the cell, but rather becomes a permanent part of the cell's DNA. If this insertion has deleterious effects on the cell, those effects are permanent and will also be seen in the cell's descendants. Furthermore, if a mistake is made as the reverse transcriptase makes DNA copies, bits of cellular genes or even entire cellular genes can find their way into new virions. This can have disastrous consequences when the new altered viruses infect other cells.

Another group of viruses related to the retroviruses are the *hepadnaviruses,* which include the virus responsible for hepatitis B in humans. These are DNA viruses which replicate by copying their DNA to RNA and back again to DNA—a novel mechanism only recently discovered and not yet completely understood. While integration into the cellular chromosomes is not an essential part of their cycle, these viruses can insert bits of their DNA into the cell's DNA.

HOW DO VIRUSES INFECT CELLS?

Because viruses have no means of independent movement, their world is one of random collisions. A virus floats along in the bloodstream or in a mucus droplet from a sneeze until it bumps into a cell with protein receptors which happen to fit the contour of its viral proteins. When this contact is made, the virus sticks to the cell membrane. This is how a given type of virus comes to infect a particular type of cell.

Once the virus adheres to the appropriate cell, it must still get inside. Typically, what happens is that the virus is enveloped by the cell membrane and taken intact into the cell. Inside the cell, the virus loses its outer coat and the remaining nucleic acid has the task of commandeering the cell's machinery to begin making more viruses.

OUTCOMES OF INFECTION

There are three possible results of a virus taking over a cell (infection). These are:

1. **Acute Cell Death or Damage.** This is the usual outcome. A single virus entering the cell may result in the production of hundreds, perhaps thousands, of perfect and complete copies of that one virus—called virions—within a few hours. The cell is damaged as the pirate virus diverts cellular machinery away from essential cellular functions toward the production of virions. As if this were not enough, cellular damage and the swelling numbers of virions may cause the cell to rupture, releasing the new viruses. These new viruses will invade other cells, repeating the cycle, eventually producing many thousands of additional viruses. In this way, the virus infection spreads throughout the body, generating the symptoms of disease (such as fever, aching muscles and joints, fatigue, and headache) when enough cells are affected.

2. **Chronic Infection.** Here the virus remains in the cell for a long period of time, during which it may produce virions and may not. Sometimes this chronic viral presence does no harm to the cell, but usually there is eventual cell damage. In other cases, the presence of virus in a cell for a long time can lead to the third possible outcome of infection: *transformation.*

3. **Transformation.** This is when the presence of virus in the cell causes a change in the genes of the cell, leading to a change in the structure or function of the cell. Transformation is pos-

Figure 8-3 Steps to a Virus Infecting a Cell. This illustrates how a virus infects (gets inside) a cell. In this case, the virus is a *retrovirus,* which goes on in Steps 4 and 5 to insert its DNA into the cell's DNA.

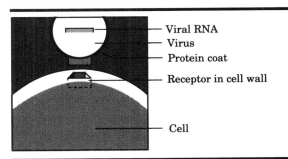

— Viral RNA
— Virus
— Protein coat
— Receptor in cell wall

— Cell

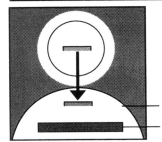

Step 3

Inside the cell, the virus is enveloped in a coating from the cell's membrane. The virus loses its protein coat.

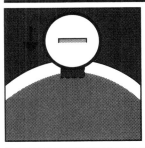

Step 1

The virus, carrying viral RNA, attaches to the cell wall with the matching protein receptor.

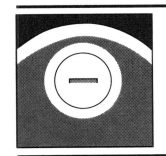

Step 4

The viral RNA enters the cell nucleus.

— Nucleus of cell
— Cellular DNA

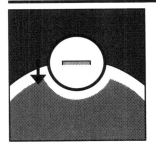

Step 2

The cell is enveloped by the cell membrane.

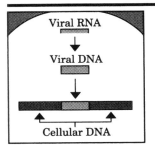

Viral RNA

Viral DNA

Cellular DNA

Step 5

Once inside the cell nucleus, the viral RNA forms viral DNA and inserts itself into the cellular DNA.

sible because viruses use the same nucleic acid—DNA—as the cell and can, in many cases, insert or remove DNA in the genes of the cell. Transformation refers to any change produced in the cell, and transformed cells exhibit a wide range of changes. In some cases, transformation causes a relatively insignificant change, but at the other end of the spectrum is malignant transformation, where the genetic alterations have led to uncontrolled growth and division of the cell.

Of the three possible outcomes of viral infection—acute, chronic, and transformation—it is important to note that a given virus can have differing outcomes depending on the sort of cell it infects. For example, Simian (monkey) Virus 40, a small DNA virus, causes immediate viral replication and cell destruction in monkey cells but results in transformation without virus production in the cells of mice.

NEOPLASTIC TRANSFORMATION

Neoplastic transformation is a specific type of transformation which causes cells to grow abnormally. Often when scientists speak of cell transformation, they are referring only to neoplastic transformation. The ability to cause neoplastic transformation in laboratory culture cells (culture simply refers to cells grown in a laboratory test tube, outside a living organism) is a feature common to all identified tumor-causing viruses.

Neoplastic transformation is not the same as malignancy—neoplastic transformation can lead to

Figure 8-4 Outcomes of Viral Infection.

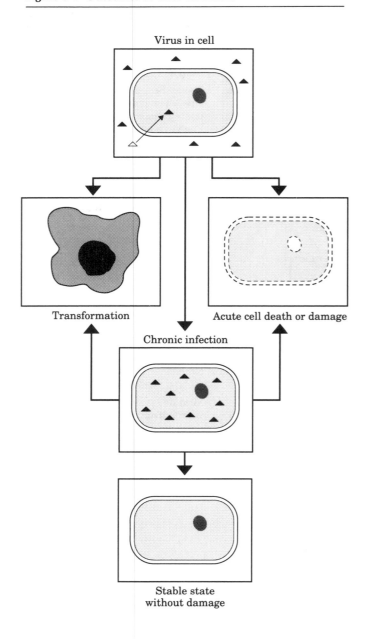

Virus in cell

Transformation

Acute cell death or damage

Chronic infection

Stable state
without damage

cells, like cancer cells, can grow and divide indefinitely.

3. *Appearance*—Transformed cells just look more like cancer cells—surface proteins and cell morphology are altered so that these cells take on the appearance of cancer cells.

FROM TRANSFORMATION TO MALIGNANCY

Unlike transformation, which can be accomplished by one or two alterations in the genes of a cell, malignancy requires multiple "hits" to the cell's DNA. Scientists estimate that four to six different changes in the cell's genes must occur for the cell to become malignant. These successive changes can occur as a result of another virus infection, exposure to certain chemicals, or anything else capable of DNA alteration. They endow a cell which has undergone neoplastic transformation with the properties essential for malignancy:

1. The ability to invade other tissues.

2. Some ability to evade the immune system.

3. The ability to grow and divide without hormonal stimulation—to "immortalize."

ONCOGENE THEORY

The most widely accepted theory on the relationship between viruses and cancer is the theory of *oncogenes*. There is a small number of genes within the cell controlling growth and division. *Oncogene theory* states that alterations within these genes, such as the changes caused by viruses, may lead to a loss of growth control in the cell and its descendents, i.e., cancer. Altered genes which lead to cancer are called oncogenes.

This rather simple theory, which only recently gained wide acceptance, has been a long time in the making. Its history begins in 1906, when Peyton Rous discovered a virus which caused tumors in chickens. Decades later, this virus was identified as an RNA retrovirus and its genes were mapped out. Since the virus only contained a few genes, it was possible to determine which gene was responsible. This gene was named "src" (for Rous sarcoma virus: pronounced sark).

A gene nearly identical to src was then found in a wide range of normal cells, where it apparently played an essential role in normal cell functioning.

benign or malignant growth. The process leading to malignancy involves a number of different steps. Neoplastic transformation is only the beginning.

Transformed cells share a number of characteristics with cancer cells. Among these are:

1. The loss of *contact inhibition*—normal cells stop growing and dividing upon contact with other cells, growing in a single layer. Transformed cells grow right over one another and form disordered layers.

2. *Immortality*—while normal cells in lab cultures die out after a few divisions, transformed

Soon, other retroviral oncogenes were identified, and by the time 40 or so of these retroviral oncogenes with cellular counterparts had been identified, a coherent picture emerged. These retroviruses were carrying cellular genes picked up at some earlier point in their evolutionary history. The presence of these genes in the retroviruses was probably only an accident—an accident noticed only because they cause tumors.

Little is known of the functions of these counterpart genes in normal cells. What is known is that they play a role in the regulation of growth. The striking thing is just how few of them there are—scientists estimate that within a human cell of perhaps 50,000 genes there are probably not more than 100 concerned with the regulation of cell growth and division. In a normal cell, they are referred to as *proto-oncogenes* because, in theory at least, they can become oncogenes if something happens to alter the way they function.

Oncogene theory has been supported by other experiments in which these same genes have caused cancer. For example, researchers who isolated bits of DNA from tumors found that this DNA could transform normal cells. The transforming DNA from the tumor was identical to DNA from a retrovirus oncogene. Other researchers looking at tumor cells have found that the genes which have been altered are the same as retroviral oncogenes.

Only rarely can a single oncogene cause malignancy; more often it is the product of multiple oncogenes working in concert.

VIRUSES AND ONCOGENES

Viruses, with an ability to insert their DNA into the cell's DNA, can bring about the emergence of oncogenes in two ways. First, if a virus contains its own oncogene it can insert it into the host DNA. This is referred to as *acute transformation* because it happens quickly. The oncogene is expressed along with the other viral genes as the virus attempts to replicate. Usually these viruses are not good at replicating because the oncogene has taken the place of some essential viral gene. Most viruses identified as carrying their own oncogene are retroviruses, but oncogenes can be found in DNA viruses as well.

The second way involves viruses which are carrying no viral oncogene—these can be either retroviruses or DNA viruses. These viruses somehow turn on cellular proto-oncogenes to bring about transformation. This is referred to as *chronic transformation,* as it is much more hit-and-miss and usually requires a lengthy period of viral infection. In effect, these viruses act as random mutating agents, inserting viral DNA in key locations to turn on cellular oncogenes.

ONCOGENIC (TUMOR CAUSING) VIRUSES

There are many viruses that transform cells in laboratory culture, cause tumors in animals, or are strongly associated with cancer in humans. These tumor-causing viruses are referred to as oncogenic viruses. These are either DNA or retroviruses; none of the RNA viruses has been associated with cancer in any species.

Oncogenic DNA viruses belong to one of three families: the *papovaviruses,* the *herpesviruses,* or the *adenoviruses.* DNA viruses, with few exceptions, only transform cells in which they are unable to replicate. The retroviruses, in contrast, can often replicate and transform the same cell. They can also transform cells in which they are unable to replicate.

Most cases of infection by oncogenic viruses do not result in neoplastic transformation: transformation is a relatively rare event and progression to malignancy even more rare. Also, viral oncogenesis usually requires a lengthy period of time—decades, in many cases—and a particular set of circumstances to come about.

However, viral induced malignancy can be rather dramatic, as in the case of leukemia in cats. Feline leukemia, like human leukemia, is a type of cancer and is one of the leading causes of death in domestic cats in the U.S. Infection with the virus can lead to leukemia in a relatively short time and the virus is contagious: veterinarians advise owners to keep their leukemic cats in isolation, away from other cats. Feline leukemia, for other cats at least, is a contagious disease. However, there are no known cases of cats passing the disease on to humans.

VIRUSES AND HUMAN CANCER

Scientists have long known that viruses cause cancers in animals, but it has been difficult to prove for humans. A set of criteria known as *Koch's postulates* has traditionally been used to ascertain whether a certain disease is caused by a given infecting agent. Koch's postulates are:

1. The agent is always found in diseased individuals.

2. The agent, once isolated, must be able to be grown in culture.

3. The agent, once cultured, must produce the same disease when introduced into healthy, susceptible individuals.

4. The agent must again be recovered from the experimentally infected individuals.

You can see why it is difficult to prove that a virus is the cause of tumors in man. Scientists can't very well inject the suspected virus into human subjects to satisfy Koch's third postulate. To overcome this obstacle, A. S. Evans later proposed a set of criteria with respect to cancer, making use of techniques only recently available to supply indirect proof of viral causation. The main features of *Evan's postulates* are as follows:

1. Exposure to the suspected virus is more common in cancer patients than in comparable healthy people.

2. Specific immune response to the virus is seen in patients (i.e., patients have antibodies to the virus in their blood).

3. The disease comes after exposure to the suspected virus.

4. Virus and/or viral DNA is found in cancer tissue.

5. The virus and/or its DNA is shown to induce neoplastic transformation in lab cell culture.

Koch's postulates are a rigid protocol for proving causation. Evan's postulates, in contrast, are simply a set of guidelines to help scientists reach consensus. A virus need not fulfill every one of Evan's postulates to be accepted as cancer-causing. By these new criteria, a number of viruses have gained acceptance as tumor viruses. The following examples illustrate the current state of evidence for a viral role in human cancer.

ADULT T-CELL LEUKEMIA

Leukemias are malignancies of white blood cells. Arising from the bone marrow, leukemias crowd out the normal blood-cell producing marrow and flood the bloodstream with enormous numbers of abnormal white blood cells. For example, in normal blood there are 5000 to 10,000 white blood cells (WBC) per cubic centimeter, but in the blood of leukemia patients there may be 80,000 to 100,000.

Adult T-cell leukemia (ATL) is an uncommon type of leukemia which often occurs in clusters of cases within a small geographical area. The cancer cells in ATL are T-lymphocytes of a certain type called T_4 or helper cells. The disease has a characteristic set of clinical features including spleen, liver, and lymph node enlargement, and is often rapidly fatal.

The fact that ATL often occurs in clusters led scientists to suspect that an infectious agent might be responsible. In 1980, Robert Gallo and his colleagues at the National Cancer Institute announced that, after twelve years, they had finally isolated a previously unknown virus from the blood of two ATL patients in the United States. This virus turned out to be a retrovirus—the first ever isolated in man. Gallo et al. named the virus *Human T-Lymphocyte Leukemia Virus (HTLV-I)*. (When the virus responsible for Acquired Immune Deficiency Syndrome—AIDS—was discovered, it was thought to be a relative of HTLV I and so was called HTLV III. It is now known that they belong to different virus subfamilies and the AIDS virus has been renamed Human Immuno-deficiency Virus HIV).

A study in southwest Japan provided further evidence of HTLV I as the cause of ATL. Close to 100% of Japanese ATL patients had antibodies showing past infection with HTLV-I. Furthermore, researchers were able to determine that the areas within southwest Japan with the highest incidence of HTLV-I infection correlated well with the distribution of ATL cases. Soon after, Japanese researchers isolated HTLV-I from the blood of ATL patients.

The evidence from Japan was subsequently corroborated by studies of ATL in the Caribbean, Latin America, and Africa. Further evidence of HTLV causation in ATL has since accumulated and includes:

1. Leukemic cells from ATL patients contain HTLV-I DNA integrated into their chromosomes.

2. Malignant blood cell tumors in monkeys are sometimes caused by a retrovirus very closely related to HTLV-I.

3. HTLV-I can transform T-lymphocytes in cell culture. This evidence fulfills Evan's Postulates completely.

The transformation of T-lymphocytes in culture is probably the single most convincing piece of evidence. Cells transformed by HTLV-I grow without the hormonal stimulation needed by normal T-lymphocytes and closely resemble leukemic cells from ATL patients—clearly a fully malignant transformation.

HTLV-I is the first proven human cancer virus. It fulfills all of Evan's Postulates. HTLV-I causes adult T-cell leukemia.

BURKITT'S LYMPHOMA

Burkitt's lymphoma is a tumor of the lymph nodes in the jaw. Rare in the United States, it is very common in children in tropical Africa and New Guinea. In Nigeria, Burkitt's lymphoma accounts for more than 60% of all cancer in children, with a higher than 50% mortality rate.

Extensive epidemiological studies in areas of high incidence of the disease have demonstrated a strong association between Burkitt's lymphoma and *Epstein-Barr virus (EBV),* a member of the herpesvirus family. Findings linking the two include:

1. 100% of Burkitt's lymphoma patients show immunological (antibody) evidence of EBV infection. Studies in Uganda showed that those with elevated amounts of antibody to EBV had a 30-fold risk of developing Burkitt's lymphoma.

2. All tumor cells examined thus far have contained EBV DNA.

3. Tumor cells in lab culture can be made to produce EBV virions, although virions do not appear in fresh samples of tissue from human tumors.

4. EBV can immortalize and stimulate growth in B-cells (the type of lymph node cell in which Burkitt's lymphoma arises) in lab cultures.

This evidence satisfies most of Evan's Postulates, but there are arguments against the role of EBV in Burkitt's lymphoma. First, EBV is a common virus (80–100% of the world's population have been exposed to EBV: EBV causes mononucleosis—"mono"), but the cancer occurs mainly in geographically limited areas. Second, although EBV can transform cells, it does not by itself make them malignant.

Clearly, if EBV does play a role, there must be other factors involved. Two factors that have been proposed are malaria and chromosome translocation.

There are only two areas in the world where malaria is hyperendemic (meaning that virtually everyone gets it): tropical Africa and New Guinea—the same areas where Burkitt's lymphoma occurs in high frequency. Researchers have suggested that malaria may depress the part of the immune system which is responsible for the body's defense against viral infection, while at the same time stimulating the growth of B-cells. Repeated bouts of malaria may then lead to a large population of EBV-infected B-lymphocytes, the type of cells which become cancerous in Burkitt's lymphoma. As proposed, the increase in numbers of infected cells eventually leads to the next stage in the generation of Burkitt's lymphoma: chromosome translocation.

Chromosomes are the individual strings of DNA in the cell. Normal human cells each contain 46 chromosomes. Genes are sections of DNA located along the DNA string of the chromosome. Each gene belongs in a specific place on the chromosomes. A gene in the wrong place or on the wrong chromosome can mean trouble for the cell.

Chromosome translocation is when pieces of chromosomes are moved to a new location in the cell's DNA. In all Burkitt's lymphoma cells there is a translocation in chromosome number 8: a piece of chromosome 8 breaks off and moves to another chromosome, usually chromosome 14. It appears that, in the process, a proto-oncogene in chromosome 8 is activated and begins to act as an oncogene.

EBV may play a direct role in the actual translocation, or it may play an indirect role by stimulating B-cell proliferation—rapidly proliferating cells are more likely to contain mistakes like chromosome translocations. Chronic malaria may aid the process of oncogenesis by suppressing the immune response which usually destroys transformed cells before they become malignant.

It seems clear that EBV does play an important role in Burkitt's lymphoma. The details must still be worked out, but one thing is clear: the presence of EBV alone is not enough to cause the disease. Burkitt's lymphoma is probably the result of a number of factors working in concert.

PRIMARY HEPATOCELLULAR CARCINOMA

Primary hepatocellular carcinoma (PHC), a cancer of the liver, is one of the world's most common and deadly cancers. While uncommon in the developed nations, it is one of the leading cancers in Asia and Africa. In Mozambique, for example, PHC makes up 70% of all cancers. It is quite lethal: average survival after diagnosis is about six months. Hepatitis B virus is suspected of causing PHC.

Hepatitis B virus (HBV) causes a disease of the liver characterized by fever, fatigue, and a yellow coloration of skin and eyes (jaundice). Of those who get acute Hepatitis B, 80% recover with no significant liver damage, while 5% experience severe disease leading to serious liver destruction or death. The remainder experience varying forms of chronic infection in which the virus remains within liver cells.

As far back as 1950, pathologists had noted that PHC usually occurred in livers affected by cirrhosis (a form of liver damage). Workers in Africa suggested that the cirrhosis was of a type associated with viral hepatitis. By the late '60s, improved blood testing techniques made it possible to detect chronic carriers of HBV. Soon after, large-scale epidemiologic studies showed that high incidences of chronic HBV infection and PHC were occurring in the same geographical areas.

More evidence has since emerged pointing to HBV as a causative agent in PHC, including:

1. Evidence of persistent HBV infection is more common in PHC patients than in comparable healthy people. A lengthy study in Taiwan has found a 250-fold risk of PHC in those who show evidence of chronic HBV infection.

2. HBV infection in PHC patients precedes the development of PHC. Patients infected with HBV at birth develop the tumors at a younger age than those infected later in life.

3. HBV DNA is found in most PHC tumors, without evidence of viral replication within the tumor cells.

The HBV DNA within tumor cells does not appear to be inserted into a consistent spot in the cellular chromosomes. In different tumors it appears in different sites. HBV carries no known oncogene and is inserted next to no known proto-oncogene. If HBV does cause transformation, it is probably of the chronic transformation type and requires a lengthy period of infection, apparently as long as 30 years. It is likely that malnutrition during this period also plays a role.

Some scientists believe that the cycle of liver damage and repair (cirrhosis) caused by chronic HBV infection may combine with viral effects in the nucleus to bring about malignant transformation. Attempts to uncover the mechanism of transformation in PHC were hampered by the fact that scientists were unable to grow HBV in laboratory culture. However, recent successes in growing HBV in the lab should soon lead to further elucidation of the role of HBV in PHC. In addition, the development of a hepatitis B vaccine holds out the possibility of being able to test the hypothesis that lowered rates of chronic HBV infection will lead to lower rates of PHC.

CERVICAL CARCINOMA

Cervical carcinoma is the number one reproductive tract cancer in premenopausal women. It develops slowly through a series of recognizable stages over a period of ten to thirty years. Because the early precancer stages are detectable using the Pap smear, cervical cancer is a largely preventable disease.

In the 1970s, a number of risk factors were identified for cervical carcinoma. Chief among these was young age at onset of sexual activity, and having multiple sexual partners. Women having sex with men whose other partner(s) developed cervical carcinoma showed an increased incidence of cervical carcinoma themselves. For example, Kessler, in 1976, found that second and third wives of men whose first wife had died of cervical carcinoma also had a higher than normal incidence of the disease. This identification of "high risk males" led to a search for a sexually transmitted infectious agent responsible for cervical carcinoma.

The first suspect was *herpes simplex II virus (HSV),* the virus which causes genital herpes. Initial research showed that HSV infection was more frequent in cervical carcinoma patients, but subsequent studies revealed that this was probably just coincidental: the same patterns of sexual activity that put a woman at risk for cervical carcinoma also make her more likely to be infected with the herpes virus.

More recently, attention has focused on *human papilloma viruses (HPV),* a large group of DNA viruses. Of the 42 different types of HPV, some cause common warts in humans (growths on the skin which are essentially small benign tumors). Others cause venereal warts—called condyloma accuminatum—which are the third leading venereal disease in the U.S., behind chlamydia and gonorrhea.

The incidence of venereal warts has risen dramatically in the past 15 years, paralleled by a striking increase in the number of women diagnosed as having precancerous cervical changes. This alerted researchers to a possible role for HPV in cervical carcinoma. Evidence of a primary role for HPV in cervical carcinoma has mounted steadily, including:

1. Women with cervical carcinoma have a higher incidence of HPV. One British study showed that 93% of cervical carcinoma patients in a given group had evidence of past HPV infection.

2. 90% of all cervical carcinomas examined for evidence of HPV infection have contained HPV DNA.

3. HPV DNA has been found in over 80% of precancerous cervical lesions examined.

4. Studies following women with HPV infection have shown a 16-fold increased risk of cervical carcinoma. Women infected under the age of 25 have a 38-fold increased risk.

Although researchers cannot yet grow HPV in lab culture, it is clear that HPV plays a major role in cervical cancer. Some researchers feel that cervical HPV infections should be regarded as precancerous lesions. While this is the subject of controversy, it is obvious that venereal warts are not a harmless annoyance as once believed.

Other factors probably work together with HPV to cause cervical carcinoma. One of these is cigarette smoking; another may be herpes simplex virus infection. Various conditions causing suppression of the immune system may also play a role.

It was estimated in 1981 that there were a million people in the U.S. infected with genital HPV; there are probably far more today. Women who are sexually active should be examined for HPV infection as part of their regular yearly pelvic exam. If you or a sexual partner suspect venereal warts, both of you should go to a physician or other health professional who is experienced in dealing with them. (Venereal warts look a lot like common warts. The most common locations for them are the shaft and head of the penis and the outside of the vagina, but they often appear inside the vagina, around the anus, or even on the inner thigh. A good rule is that any wart-like growth between hips and mid-thigh should be examined by a health professional.) Treatment is usually quite simple, although careful follow-up, including more frequent Pap smears, is important.

Genital HPV infections are very contagious and are transmitted sexually: sexual partners need to be treated together to avoid "bouncing" the infection back and forth. As with the AIDS virus, condoms help prevent the spread of genital HPV. With careful prevention and treatment of genital HPV infection, we may be able to halt and even reverse the rising incidence of precancerous cervical changes in young women.

CONCLUSION

With proof of HTLV-I as the cause of adult T-cell leukemia, the question of whether or not human cancer viruses exist was finally resolved. A great deal has been learned about how viruses can cause cancer, but it is all too clear that what is not known about viruses greatly outweighs what is known. While we know that viruses can cause certain cancers, we do not know what role, if any, they play in the majority of cancers. It may be that viruses provide a common pathway for certain steps in all malignant processes; or, it could be that in most cases non-viral mutagens are sufficient to induce cancer.

It is frightening to think that a contagious agent can cause cancer. Perhaps that is why the idea of tumor viruses has met with a great deal of resistance. However, acceptance of a viral role in human cancer may bring hope for the future. Once an agent of a disease is identified, strategies against it can be devised. New vaccines and drug therapies may reduce both the incidence and consequences of viral infection. A greater understanding of the interaction between virus and cell may allow us to prevent viral transformation and perhaps even reverse it.

References

1. Alberts, Bruce, et al. *Molecular Biology of the Cell.* NY: Garland Press 1983, especially pp. 232–240.

2. Baird, Phillip John. The causation of cervical cancer, Part II. *Clinical Obstetrics and Gynecology* 1985 March; (12) 19–32.

3. Beasley, R. Palmer, et al. Hepatocellular carcinoma and hepatitis B virus: A prospective study of 22,707 men in Taiwan. *Lancet* 1981; 1129–1132.

4. Bishop, Michael J. Viruses, genes, and cancer: Retroviruses and cancer genes. *Cancer* 1985; 55: 2329–2333.

5. Bishop, Michael J. Cellular oncogenes and retroviruses. *Ann Rev Biochem* 1983; 52: 301–54.

6. Blumberg, Baruch S.; London, W. Thomas. Hepatitis B virus and the prevention of primary hepatocellular carcinoma. *N Engl J Med* 1981; 782–84.

7. Fields, Bernard, et al. *Virology.* NY: Raven Press, 1985.

8. Gross, Ludwik. The role of viruses in the etiology of cancer and malignant lymphomas. *Resident and Staff Physician;* 31: 35–38.

9. Reid, BL. The causation of cervical cancer, Part I. *Clinical Obstetrics and Gynecology* 1985 March; (12) 1–18.

10. Robbins, Stanley L., et al. *Pathologic Basis of Disease.* Philadelphia: W. B. Saunders Co. 1984, especially chapter 8.

11. Rothschild, Henry; Cohen, J. Craig. *Virology in Medicine.* New York: Oxford University Press, 1986.

12. Singer, Albert, et al. Genital wart virus infections: nuisance or potentially lethal? *Br Med J* 1984; 288: 735–736.

13. Spriggs, Dale R. Cofactors in disease: Epstein-Barr virus, oncogenes, and Burkitt's lymphoma. *J Infectious Diseases* 1985; 151: 977–988.

14. Varmus, Harold E. Viruses, Genes, and Cancer: The discovery of cellular oncogenes and their role in neoplasia. *Cancer* 1985; 2324–2328.

15. Watson, JD et al., *Molecular Biology of the Gene,* 4th edition, CA: The Benjamin/Cummings Publishing Company, Inc. 1987.

16. Wong-Staal, Flossie; Gallo, Robert C. The family of human T-lymphotropic leukemia viruses: HTLV-I as the cause of adult T cell leukemia and HTLV-III as the cause of Acquired Immunodeficiency Syndrome. *J Amer Soc Hematology* 1985; 65: 253–263.

9

Evolution and Cancer

Clyde J. Dawe, M.D.

Excerpted with permission from Clyde J. Dawe, "Comparative Neoplasia," James F. Holland, M.D., and Emil Frei, III, M.D., editors, Cancer Medicine (Lea & Febiger Publishing Company, Philadelphia, PA 1973).

Why is there cancer? Does it have a role in life and evolution? Does it accomplish more than just "population control" (i.e., kill people)? There is a fascinating corner in the field of cancer that deals with the above questions. It's called comparative neoplasia, and is presented below. Dr. Dawe is Head of the Comparative Oncology Section at the National Cancer Institute. This section consists of excerpts from his longer chapter on "Comparative Neoplasia" in Holland and Frei's Cancer Medicine, 1973. It's elegant in using a systems theory approach—and approaches pure philosophy. Get ready!—*M.R.*

Comparative oncology is that branch of oncology seeking to improve understanding of neoplasia by identifying the differences and similarities among neoplasms in man, in other animals, and even in plants. Experimental carcinogenesis, experimental cancer therapy, and the epizootiology of animal neoplasia are primary branches from the mainstem of comparative oncology, and these in turn have secondary branches, such as experimental cancer immunology, viral oncogenesis, chemical oncogenesis, radiation oncogenesis, studies of neoplasia in vitro, studies of cell population kinetics, and many others. . . .

. . . It is the unique advantage of the comparative oncologist to be able to take a nonpragmatic view of neoplastic diseases. His is not only the prerogative, but also the responsibility, to examine "neoplasia" in its totality and to conceive questions heretical to the orthodox medical mind, which is traditionally oriented to the view of preventing, curing, or alleviating human disease. For example, the comparative oncologist can ask, with all candor: Is neoplasia, from the broad biologic point of view, necessarily "bad"? Does neoplasia serve some useful function in the overall scheme of life and evolution? Could neoplasia be a phenomenon or group of phenomena that merely reiterate the fundamental biologic laws in ways that *appear* novel or aberrant, simply because science chooses to define norms in statistical terms? Indeed, are we justified in perpetuating the concept that events leading to "true neoplasia" are distinct from those occurring in related phenomena such as hyperplasia, regeneration, asexual speciation, embryogenesis, dysontogenesis, and borderline situations still not well understood? Is it not possible that the most primitive forms of life were more akin to "neoplastic cells" than to the obedient, well-ordered and highly coordinated cells belonging to the communities we recognize as "normal" metazoan individuals? In contemporary individuals there can be no question that neoplasia stems from non-neoplasia, but is it not possible that, phylogenetically, non-neoplasia evolved from neoplasia?

These are challenging but difficult questions to answer. Certainly the answers could not be found through information on neoplasia in man alone, or in any other single species. In the following discussion an attempt will be made to take into account the main pieces of information available regarding animal neoplasms. While plant neoplasia is indeed pertinent to comparative oncology, it is beyond the scope of this chapter. A cogent consideration of the similarities and differences between plant and animal tumors is available in the concise treatise by Braun.[17]

State of the Science

The Question of the "Universality" of Neoplasia. How universal is the occurrence of neoplasia among multicellular animals? To answer this question first requires the solution of semantic problems, for the terms "universal" and "neoplasia" must be defined. The term "universal" can be defined for present purposes to mean distribution of the phenomenon within every known taxonomic category of multicellular life form, extending to the species level. . . .

The definition of neoplasia is far more difficult. At best it represents a major stumbling block in practical identifications, and at worst it represents an enigma in conceptual thinking. Some views expressed on this subject in a previous essay may warrant repetition here.[39] These merely illustrate the problem, without solving it.

First, a highly desirable and practically acceptable definition of neoplasia would be a constitutive one. That is, if a structural common denominator could be demonstrated for a particular group of cell population disorders, such a structural denominator would serve well as a definition of that group, which could then be designated neoplastic disease. Unfortunately no such common denominator currently exists for even a small segment of the conditions that are currently called neoplasms. . . .

At the cellular level, as well as at the molecular level, it is as yet impossible to identify a qualitative constitutive feature that permits definition of neoplasia. True enough, the medical pathologist can perform a feat that is both practically important and intellectually satisfying in identifying and grouping "neoplasms." But this is an empiric art-science, depending heavily on accumulated past experience. Pathologists of long experience generally agree that no two examples of "neoplasia" are exactly alike, and that the identification of "neoplasms" is essentially an exercise in matching, more or less precisely, the histologic features of a given lesion with those of similar lesions that one has previously chosen to call neoplasms on the basis of clinicopathologic correlations. Specific morphologic atypicality in individual cells of the disorder may or may not be present. Further, historically it is well demonstrated that conditions once widely thought to be "neoplastic" are no longer accepted as such on behavioral grounds, though the morphologic features at cell and tissue levels have not changed.

We shall admit the present lack of a constitutive definition of neoplasia, and proceed to the search for an operational definition, considering such concepts as autonomy, cellular proliferation uncontrolled by normal restraints, invasiveness, lethality, lack of useful function to the host, clonal derivation, and irreversibility. Such definitions are much more elusive than the desirable but nonexistent constitutive definition, for they depend heavily on something in the mind of the observer rather than on a measurable and absolute property of the lesion. For example, autonomy and uncontrolled proliferation are relative and often transient features of processes that are useful to the host, such as regeneration, wound healing, and even embryogenesis. If it can be argued that a fetus is not invariably useful to its nurturing parent, but is useful to the perpetuation of the species, it can also be argued that certain neoplasms, allegedly resulting from expression of oncogenes, "could be viewed like senescence itself as providing survival advantages to species."[99] Ecologists consider that predators are in a sense beneficial to prey species, as well as to ecologic balance, in that they exert constant selective pressure which results in the gradual evolution and selective survival of individuals with new or better defense and escape capabilities. We do not know to what extent neoplasia, like a form of predator, may have influenced certain phases of phylogeny.

The matter of "unregulated growth" is also relative. Neoplasms of endocrine target organs (mammary gland, prostate, thyroid) are sometimes dramatically responsive to endocrine therapy. Though it may be correctly argued that such responsiveness occurs only to abnormal levels of hormone, this argument only emphasizes the relativity concept. The feature of "lack of useful function to the host" holds true with few exceptions, such as the rare occurrence of a functioning thyroid carcinoma that temporarily relieves a pre-existing hypothyroid state. The weakness of the "useful purpose" feature is that, of itself, it is not unique to "neoplasia," since the same can be said for a myriad of totally dissimilar conditions. The same is true for the feature of lethality or even morbidity. . . .

. . . [It] can be advanced that neoplasia may have existed even in pre-life forms, and that neoplasia, by an operational definition, was the first form of life on earth. In a previous essay,[39] environmental conditions and events favorable to the evolution of regulatory mechanisms were outlined (Figure 9-1). It was postulated that the first pre-life replicating macromolecular systems existed in a sea of "primordial soup" that initially provided, for practical purposes, an infinite quantity of substrates. In such an environment, the primitive replicating forms would gain no selective survival advantage if they randomly acquired, through primitive mutations, the ability to replicate more slowly under one set of conditions, and more rapidly under another. Since one set of conditions prevailed universally, no selective pressure would be exerted.

However, with the appearance of land masses creating tide pools, a pre-life form, with the ability to grow at variable rates, would have an advantage over fixed-rate replicating forms competitive for the same substrates. It seems reasonable to believe that by replicating at slower rates during low tides, the forms with regulating mechanisms relating to substrate depletion or end-product accumulation would be able to survive until the ensuing high tide replenished the supply of substrate.

Then, with a high replication rate turned on by the renewed concentration of substrate, the regulated form could return to a replicative phase again.

Figure 9-1 Concept of the influence of a cyclic phenomenon (tide) on the evolution of growth-regulatory mechanisms in primitive life forms. Fine stippling represents substrates in "primeval broth." Large solid black spots represent a replicable pre-life form. A, Tide pool has just been filled and the pre-life form is in process of assimilating substrate and replicating. B, Tide has fallen and begun to rise again. This pre-life form with feedback inhibition mechanisms has multiplied but has regulated its generation time so that substrate is not exhausted and is sufficient to permit continued limited replication until the incoming tide replenishes substrate. C, Pre-life form lacking feedback inhibition mechanisms has completely exhausted the substrate and all individuals of this form have undergone degradation (open circles). Through exhaustion of the ecosystem, this form has not survived in the tide-pool niche. The pre-life form in B is analogous to "normal," regulated cells; that in C is analogous to neoplastic, unregulated cells. The tide pool with its substrates is analogous to the metazoan host. (From Dawe.[39])

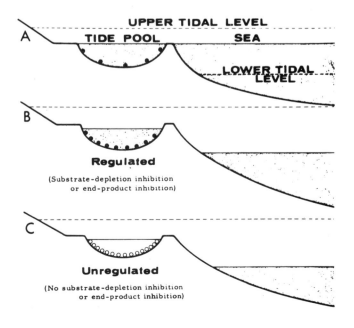

Thus it would have exercised a successful mechanism for survival under cyclic conditions. A cyclic environmental change, it is postulated, was the initial selective factor favoring the evolution of regulatory mechanisms. Today we see highly developed and complex regulatory responses to multiple cyclic environmental conditions. Circadian rhythms, rhythms related to light periodicity, and to temperature periodicity, are well known. Endocrine cycles, intimately tied into these environmental rhythms, have profound effects on proliferative activities of particular cells. One may think of the neoplastic endocrine target cell (e.g., mammary epithelium) as a cell that has reverted to a state of partial nonresponsiveness to an environmental cycle analogous to the tide pool cycle. Incompletely regulated, the neoplastic cell relentlessly proliferates until it destroys the ecosystem (the animal host, analogous to the tide pool and its contents) upon which it depends for its own existence.

Viewed in this way, neoplasia might indeed be considered a reversion of cells to a "primitive" type of behavior. The only kind of "primitivity" involved, however, is the absence of a critical regulatory device, making the cell comparable only in an operational sense to the hypothetically unregulated first life forms. There would be no analogy between the cancer cell and the normal cells of primitive or lower metazoan species, since even in these animals, smoothly functioning regulatory mechanisms were well developed and continue to operate effectively today. Further, in keeping with this concept, which embodies certain aspects of the deletion theory of cancer, one would not expect to find any single constitutive common denominator in cancer unless deeply hidden from our knowledge there exists in all cells some central molecular pathway through which all regulatory mechanisms pass. Although some regulatory mediators, such as cyclic AMP, are widely distributed in diverse cells and organisms, there is as yet no evidence that a specific disorder of this "second messenger" is universally and primarily at fault. The concept of oncogenes, which may be triggered into active transcription by a variety of stimuli, has been put forward.[98,97] Such universal capacity to induce neoplastic disease by a viral mechanism, if true, suggests there could be a final common pathway, but much variation in the triggering stimulus.

The almost limitless diversity of genetic and epigenetic patterns that serve as afferent and efferent centers and pathways for reception and response to environmental input offer only too abundant opportunities for regulatory disruption by chemical, physical, and viral reactants. The wonder is not that neoplasia occurs, but that it occurs at frequencies still permitting the continued existence of a magnificent world of orderly and highly complex plant and animal life. The forces of selection favoring development and preservation of reliable regulatory systems are strong; otherwise life would still be confined to a chaos in the primitive soup.

As noted earlier, an understanding of neoplasia in the broadest comparative sense encourages use of an operational definition of neoplasia. Such a definition can cut across the several levels at which we customarily recognize individuality, as well as across the several levels at which we recognize individual ecosystems. An ecosystem at one level is an individual when viewed from the next higher level. We recognize individuality at species levels, at organismal levels, at cellular levels, and even at subcellular levels, in which viruses, organelles, or molecular species may be considered to have individuality. In customary medical usage, definitions of neoplasia regard the individual animal as the ecosystem, and in this context it is the cellular level of individuality with which the definitions happen to be concerned. Thus one operational definition confined to this level might state that neoplasia includes those disorders in which selected cell populations, whether clonally derived or otherwise, undergo disproportionate increase to the point where the usual characteristics of the host are modified and the existence of the host is threatened or terminated. . . .

If there is a grand lesson or principle to be learned from comparative oncology, it is that the ways of neoplasia are as protean as the ways of life in all its forms. Every ecosystem is an individual within a greater ecosystem. The ways through which a relatively steady-state ecosystem can be rapidly thrown into jeopardy may well be more numerous than the interactive mechanisms responsible for the ecosystem's original organization. To hope for a simplistic cause and an equally simplistic solution to "the" problem of cancer, is to live in a fool's paradise. To harvest specific information on specific neoplastic processes in ever-increasing depth is to divide and perhaps ultimately to control. A comprehension of comparative oncology enables the individual investigator to survey the roles available in the drama of cancer research, to choose his own part wisely, and to play it spiritedly but with a due sense of humility.

References

17. Braun, A. C. (Ed.): Progress in Experimental Tumor Research. V 15. Plant Tumor Research. New York, S. Karger, 1972, 275 pp.

39. Dawe, C. J.: Phylogeny and oncogeny. Nat. Cancer Inst. Monogr., 31:1, 1969.

97. Huebner, R. J.: Identification of leukemogenic viruses: specifications for vertically transmitted, mostly "switched-off" RNA tumor viruses as determinants of the generality of cancer. In Comparative Leukemia Research, 1969. Bibl.

Haemat. No. 36. Edited by R. M. Dutcher, Basel/Munich/New York, Karger, 1970, pp. 22–44.

98. Huebner, R. J., and Todaro, G. J.: Oncogenes of RNA tumor viruses as determinants of cancer. Proc. Nat. Acad. Sci. U.S.A., *64:*1087, 1094, 1969.

99. Huebner, R. J., Sarma, P. S., Kelloff, G. J., Gilden, R. V., Meier, H., Myers, D. D., and Peters, R. L.: Immunological tolerance to RNA tumor virus genome expressions: significance of tolerance and prenatal expressions in embryogenesis and tumorigenesis. Ann. N.Y. Acad. Sci., *181:*246, 1971.

3

The Causes of Cancer

10

Overview—
Everything Does Not
Cause Cancer

Mark Renneker, M.D.

How would you answer the question: "What are the causes of cancer?" Those who feel pessimistic about cancer might answer "EVERYTHING—everything causes cancer." Those who have little understanding about cancer might answer "NO ONE KNOWS." Both would be wrong, for their answers and for their hopelessness.

It is true that newspapers and magazines seem always to be carrying scary stories about yet another cause of cancer having been discovered. The purpose of this section is to put all of the known and unknown causes of cancer into perspective.

Much of what you will read is based on the work of Sir Richard Doll and Richard Peto. Both are preeminent for their pioneering work in cancer epidemiology. In 1981, they published the landmark "The Causes of Cancer," in the Journal of the National Cancer Institute, and later that year as a monograph with Oxford Press. The impact on the cancer field is still being felt. For instance, many had previously spoken of diet as a cause of cancer, but when Doll and Peto said so, it was like the E.F. Hutton commercial—everyone listened.

Here is what they said, in the preface to their book, *The Causes of Cancer:* "The truth seems to be that there is quite good evidence that cancer is largely an avoidable (although not necessarily a modern) disease, but, with some important exceptions, [there is] frustratingly poor evidence as to exactly what are the really important ways of avoiding a reasonable percentage of today's cancers. Perhaps because of this uncertainty, the number of different ways of avoiding cancer is enormous. As a convenient framework in which to seek an overview of them all, we have divided the various hypothetical ways of increasing or decreasing cancer onset rates into a dozen groups, and for each group we have attempted to review what is known about the percentage of current U.S. deaths that might thereby be avoidable."

They then trace all lines of thinking and past cancer research done worldwide to come up with their best estimates as to the major causes of cancer.

Each of the major causes of cancer described above will be taken up in this section. However, first there are a few points to be made as to the overview Doll and Peto's estimates provide.

1. Everything doesn't cause cancer. In fact, very few things cause cancer. Most of the causes of cancer are listed above. All of the factors still not known, together with the causes you can think of that aren't on the above list, probably account for less than 1%. Far outshadowing all other factors are diet and tobacco, which together account for almost two-thirds of cancer deaths.

Factor	Percent of cancer deaths	
	Best Estimate	Range of estimates
1. Diet	35	10−70
2. Tobacco	30	25−40
3. Infection	10?	1−?
4. Reproductive/Sexual	7	1−13
5. Occupational	4	2−8
6. Alcohol	3	2−4
7. Geophysical Factors (sun/radiation)	3	2−4
8. Pollution	2	<1−5
9. Medicines/medical procedures	1	0.5−3
10. Food Additives	<1	−5−2 (may be protective)
11. Industrial products	<1	<1−2
12. Unknown	?	?

2. The "environment" is everything outside of your genes. If you're not born with the probability of getting cancer, then it comes about because of things that happen to you as you go through life—things you were exposed to. In that sense, there are only two causes of cancer: genetic and environmental. And there are very few cancers that are purely attributable to heredity. The vast majority—at least 90%—of cancers are therefore environmentally caused.

3. The role of heredity in cancer is overestimated by most people. Many feel that because someone in their family had cancer, they will, too. But if you realize that one in three people in this country get cancer, that means that in a family of four you'd expect to see one cancer. Add in blood relatives and you easily have twelve people—of which you'd expect four to get cancer. Remember, three in four families are affected by cancer—the family that has not had cancer is the exception.

4. The cancers where heredity plays the largest part are: skin cancers (inheriting a fair skin, for instance), breast cancers that occur in a family member before menopause, and colorectal cancers that occurred before age 50 (particularly if associated with polyps).

5. Stress and emotional factors aren't on the list, but stress is thought by many to be a major cause or contributor to cancer. Stress is difficult to

study, and difficult to quantify as a factor in causing cancer. But let's remember that the causes of cancer overlap with other diseases and it is well-known that stress is a major factor in heart disease—and heart disease kills twice as many people as cancer.

6.   Age and immune function could be thought of as causes of cancer, but really they are contributing factors common to all the cancer causes. It is true that more cancers occur in older people, and that cancer patients have poorer immune function—but advancing age only implies a longer potential time to have been "hit" by carcinogenic agents, which also may have weakened the immune system.

7.   Doll and Peto estimated that about 10% of cancers are due to infections, which would imply that some cancers can be "caught," i.e., that it is like an infectious or contagious disease. This is a tough issue to discuss because it has only been in the past few years that the educational efforts of groups like the American Cancer Society have resulted in the public not treating cancer patients like lepers, teaching that you can't, for instance, get cancer from touching a person with cancer. That is true. However, it is also true that you can catch from other people, cancer patients or healthy people, certain infections that, if they become chronic and persistent, may lead to cancer. Hepatitis is a good example; it can lead to liver cancer if the person remains infected over a period of years.

8.   Many people mistakenly believe that the act of performing surgery may cause cancer: that a swelling or lump doesn't become cancer until it is cut open (i.e., by some form of surgery). Also, there is no evidence that trauma or a blow to your body leads to cancer—only that it may draw attention to a part of the body where a pre-existing cancerous lump is then noticed.

9.   A chronic irritation can be thought of as a cause of cancer, but Doll and Peto saw that as a process common to many cancer-causing substances, or else within the category of geophysical factors. In this book, the geophysical factors that are presented are limited to sun and radiation. However, it is true that, for instance, a poorly fitting denture—chronically irritating the gum—can lead to the development of a cancer.

If it becomes apparent to you that not everything causes cancer, then the real work can begin of determining your own risk factors for cancer. Consider how you might reduce or control them. Devote time to risk factors of highest magnitude (i.e., for smokers to worry less about preservatives in their bread and more about how they're going to stop smoking).

Accordingly, this section of *Understanding Cancer* will focus on the major avoidable causes of cancer: diet (including alcohol), tobacco, infection, occupational, radiation, medical causes, and pollution.

11

Diet and Cancer

Lorelei K. DiSogra, Ed.D., R.D. and
Charles A. DiSogra, M.P.H., Ph.D.

Lorelei DiSogra (formally Lorelei Groll) has been one of the trailblazers in the area of diet and cancer. While it was still largely heretical in academic medicine to speak of diet as a cause of cancer, she forged ahead and developed the booklet the National Cancer Institute eventually began using to educate the public about cancer and diet. She and her husband, Charles, are presently coordinating the State of California's Nutrition and Cancer Prevention Program. They regularly lecture at Biology of Cancer courses throughout California.—*M.R.*

Diet and nutrition are increasingly being recognized as major factors influencing the development of many types of human cancer. Thirty-five percent of all cancer deaths in the United States have been attributed to the typical American diet (1). Nine of the ten leading cancers in the United States are associated with dietary practices. In 1984, both the American Cancer Society (ACS) and the National Cancer Institute (NCI) issued dietary recommendations to the public to reduce the risk of cancer (2–3). The ACS and NCI recommendations are based on the *Diet, Nutrition and Cancer* report by the National Academy of Sciences and are consistent with the well-known Dietary Guidelines for Americans and with dietary recommendations for heart disease prevention (4–6).

Research on cancer risk now justifies prudent recommendations concerning dietary factors, such as fat, fiber, vitamins A and C, nitrites, cruciferous vegetables, charred foods, and alcohol. Strategies to change the way Americans eat are central to NCI's cancer prevention awareness campaign. The potential exists to significantly reduce cancer mortality in the United States if all Americans adopt a diet that is lower in fat, higher in fiber and contains generous daily servings of fruits and vegetables (7).

CANCER RISK ATTRIBUTED TO DIET

If the risk of various cancers can be reduced by changing dietary patterns, an exciting potential exists to prevent some types of cancer. Although this concept has been around since the middle of the nineteenth century, the most convincing scientific data has been produced during the past 20 years. With this accumulation of evidence, and an increased level of research activity, epidemiologists have been involved in what Ernst Wynder and Gio Gori have called the "epidemiological exercise" of quantifying the overall contribution of diet to cancer risk. Gori's own estimate in 1977 was that 30–40% of all cancers in men and 60% of all cancers in women are related to diet (9).

In 1981, British epidemiologists, Richard Doll and Richard Peto estimated that 35% of the risk for all cancer in the United States was attributed to diet (1). Doll and Peto's quantitative estimates (Figure 11-1) illustrate the attributable risk associated with the two primary risk factors for cancer, smoking (30%) and diet (35%), compared to other known factors. This risk also varies greatly for different types of cancer (Figure 11-2); for example, diet accounts for 90% of the risk for bowel cancer, 50% for breast cancer, and 20% for lung cancer. Admittedly, these percentages for individual types of cancer are "guesstimates." However, the overall estimate that 35% of all cancer deaths are attributable to diet is now a widely accepted figure.

THE EMERGENCE OF DIETARY RECOMMENDATIONS

Prior to 1981, dietary recommendations to reduce cancer risk were chiefly those written by individuals. The occasional, and usually overcautious, article in scientific journals tended to focus on the dietary component(s) of interest to the author and was not written as guidance for the public. The mass media, by default, became the primary guiding source for public information related to diet and cancer. Unfortunately, this did not always prove reliable or accurate. Research findings are too often reduced by the press to newsworthy headlines that overstate conclusions. Press reports generally present the results of one study and usually emphasize a single dietary component. Undoubtedly, this has caused both alarm and confusion among people concerned about a relationship between food and cancer.

An unjustified belief persisted that just about everything caused cancer and that nothing could be done to avoid the disease. Such a fatalistic attitude displaced informed preventive action. Since everyone has to eat, and some would like to take steps to reduce their risk of cancer, an environment existed that was ripe for charlatanism. Many individuals promoted their own prescription for diets to prevent cancer while the government and private agencies remained silent.

In light of this, one might have asked what the scientific community could reasonably tell the American public. With billions of dollars spent on cancer research, what had been learned about preventing cancer? Such a question, aimed at NCI, was raised by the U.S. Congress in the late 1970s. In 1980, NCI responded by requesting the National Academy of Sciences to appoint a special committee to review the literature, develop interim guidelines for the public, and provide recommendations for further research in the area of diet, nutrition, and cancer.

Also in 1980, ACS funded a small research project to produce and field test a prototype public education booklet on nutrition and cancer prevention. It is important to note that in 1980 ACS did not have a position or policy on diet and cancer. In 1981, the project successfully produced a 28-page consumer booklet entitled *Nutrition and Cancer Prevention: A Guide to Food Choices* (10). This booklet made specific nutrition recommendations to reduce the risk of cancer. These recommendations were, in substance, similar to the NAS interim guidelines released the following year. Despite very limited project publicity, over 250,000 booklets were requested from 1981 to 1983. Besides demonstrating public interest, this project illustrated that scientific information on nutrition and cancer prevention could be successfully translated and packaged for the public.

In 1982 the National Academy of Sciences released its pivotal report, *Diet, Nutrition, and Cancer,*

Figure 11-1   Proportions of Cancer Deaths Attributed to Various Major Factors

| | Percent of All Cancer Deaths | |
Factor	Best Estimate	Range of Acceptable Estimates
Diet	35%	10 to 70%
Tobacco	30%	25 to 40%
Occupation	4%	2 to 8%
Alcohol	3%	2 to 4%
Pollution	2%	<1 to 5%
Food Additives	<1%	−5 to 2%

Source: Adapted from Doll, R. and R. Peto, *"The Causes of Cancer: Quantitative estimates of avoidable risks of Cancer in the United States today"* J. National Cancer Institute 66:1191–1308, 1981

Figure 11-2   Risk Attributed to Diet for Various Cancers

Type of Cancer	Risk Attributed to Diet
Stomach, large bowel	90%
Uterus, gallbladder, pancreas, breast	50%
Lung, larynx, bladder, cervix, mouth, pharynx, esophagus	20%
Other types of cancer	10%
All cancers	35%

Source: Doll, R. and R. Peto, *The Causes of Cancer: Quantitative Estimates of Avoidable Risks of Cancer in the United States Today.* JNCI 66:1191–1308, 1981

which concluded that the American public has the option of adopting a diet that could reduce its incidence of cancer by approximately one-third (4). The NAS proposed an interim set of dietary guidelines for cancer risk reduction. These guidelines suggested that diets high in fat and low in fresh fruits, vegetables, and whole grains increase the risk of certain types of cancer. The NAS concluded that there was sufficient scientific justification to issue prudent dietary guidelines for the public, and that these would be updated as significant new research became available.

In early 1984, NCI launched a major new cancer prevention awareness program for health professionals and the public. Dietary modification became a legitimate strategy within NCI's cancer control activities. NCI's free consumer booklet, *Diet, Nutrition and Cancer Prevention: A Guide to Food Choices,* recommended that Americans reduce their fat intake to no more than 30% of total calories, increase their dietary fiber to 20–30 grams per day, and increase the consumption of fresh fruits and vegetables, particularly those high in vitamin A and vitamin C (3).

Also in the wake of the NAS report, the American Cancer Society announced its dietary recommendations in early 1984 (2). The ACS guidelines were similar to those of the NAS and NCI. The ACS also provides a free professional education document on nutrition and cancer (11), and has developed a slide tape presentation, entitled "Taking Control," which emphasizes dietary risk factors and dietary protective factors.

Figure 11-3 summarizes and compares the NAS, NCI, and ACS cancer risk reduction dietary guidelines. These recommendations have become a reference point for health professionals and the public.

The combination of research findings, public interest, and support of key scientists and policy-makers were important factors in the rapid emergence of die-

tary guidelines for cancer risk reduction. Another significant factor was that these recommendations were consistent with those of the American Heart Association for the prevention of heart disease (5), and the well-known *Dietary Guidelines for Americans* (6). The similarity of these dietary recommendations should help avoid public confusion, and should reinforce a consistent nutrition message for promoting good health and preventing chronic diseases.

In Chapter 73—Diet and Cancer Prevention, each dietary recommendation is explained and suggestions are given for how to implement the guidelines.

References

1. R. R. Doll and R. Peto, The Causes of Cancer: Quantitative estimates of avoidable risks of cancer in the United States today. *J. Natl. Cancer Inst.,* 66, 1191–1308 (1981).

2. American Cancer Society, *Nutrition and Cancer: Cause and Prevention.* American Cancer Society, California Division, Inc., Oakland, Calif., 1984 (pamphlet).

3. National Cancer Institute, *Diet, Nutrition, and Cancer Prevention: A Guide to Food Choices.* National Institutes of Health, 1984.

4. Committee on Diet, Nutrition and Cancer; National Research Council, *Diet, Nutrition, and Cancer.* National Academy Press, Washington, D.C., 1982.

5. U.S. Dept. of Agriculture and U.S. Dept. of Health, Education, and Welfare, *Nutrition and Your Health, Dietary Guidelines for Americans.* U.S. Government Printing Office, Washington, D.C., February 1980.

6. American Heart Association. Rationale for the diet-heart statement of the American Heart Association. *Circulation* 65:839A, 1982.

Figure 11-3   A Summary and Comparison of Cancer Risk Reduction Dietary Recommendations Issued by the National Academy of Sciences (NAS), the National Cancer Institute (NCI), and the American Cancer Society (ACS)

Risk Factor	Agency (Year)		
	NAS (1982)	NCI (1984)	ACS (1984)
Total fat (% of calories)	Reduce to 30%	Reduce to 30% or below	Reduce to 30%
Fiber (vegetables, fruit, whole grains	Daily	Increase to 25–35 g/day (several servings per day)	Eat more
Vitamin A/β-carotene foods	Frequently	Daily	Daily
Vitamin C foods	Frequently	Daily	Daily
Cruciferous vegetables (indoles)	Frequently	Several servings per week	Include in diet
Charred or smoked foods (benzopyrene)	Minimize	Choose less often	Moderation in smoked foods only
Alcohol	Moderation	Moderation	Moderation
Nitrites (cured/pre-served foods)	Minimize	—	Moderation
Obesity	—	—	Avoid

Note: a dash (—) indicates that no recommendation has been made.

12

Tobacco as a Cause of Cancer and Death

Craig Wilson, M.D., M.P.H. and Mark Renneker, M.D.

This chapter provides an overview of the role of tobacco in causing deaths—from cancer and other diseases. Dr. Wilson is a specialist in preventive medicine and practices in San Francisco.—*M.R.*

Cigarette smoking is clearly the largest single preventable cause of illness and premature death in the United States.

> J.B. Richmond, M.D.,
> Surgeon General, 1979

Tobacco use in the United States, mainly cigarette smoking, is currently responsible for:

30% of all cancer deaths

30% of all heart disease deaths

80% of all chronic lung disease deaths

There are more than 350,000 deaths per year in the United States caused by tobacco use. It's hard to fathom the magnitude of such large numbers, so consider this—it's the equivalent of three fully-loaded jumbo jetliners crashing every day for a year. If three jets crashed in one week—much less in one day—the American public would be outraged, they would demand an explanation, and a solution.

WHAT ARE SMOKERS SMOKING?

There are thousands of chemicals in cigarette smoke. Both smokers and second-hand smokers (e.g., children of smoking parents) are exposed to all of the chemicals. Pipe and cigar smokers expose themselves to a somewhat different array of chemicals, but they include the same major ones found in cigarette smoke. The many chemicals in all forms of smoking can be divided into three groups: nicotine, tar, and carbon monoxide.

Nicotine

Smokers won't habitually smoke cigarettes unless they contain nicotine. Marketing non-nicotine low-tar lettuce cigarettes failed in 1977.

Besides causing addiction, nicotine is highly poisonous. One cigar contains enough nicotine for two lethal oral doses to an adult; one cigarette, if eaten, can be lethal to a child. However, only a small portion of the nicotine in a cigarette is absorbed from smoking it. Tobacco ingestion seldom kills people because it is a powerful emetic (induces vomiting).

Nicotine causes adrenaline release, increased heart rate and blood pressure, and other often unpredictable physiological effects. The amount of nicotine exposure from tobacco smoke is proportional to the amount of tar contained in the smoke, and both are dependent on the amount and manner of smoking.

Tar

Tar is the particulate matter derived from burning organic compounds, and the leading cancer-causing chemical in tobacco smoke. Tobacco tar is a complex mixture of thousands of chemicals, primarily polycyclic aromatic hydrocarbons, which are powerful carcinogens and mutagens.

Carbon Monoxide

Carbon monoxide is one of the many gases inhaled in tobacco smoke. It binds to the red blood cell's hemoglobin with greater affinity than oxygen, and therefore reduces the amount of oxygen carried by the red blood cells. This reduces the supply of oxygen to body organs like the brain, heart, and placenta—even in passive smokers.

Other Chemicals

Other tobacco by-products inhaled or swallowed include ammonia, formaldehyde, phenols, creosote, anthracene, pyrene hydrocyanic acid, arsenic, and lead.

Tar's disease-causing effects are chiefly associated with cancers, whereas the effects of nicotine and carbon monoxide relate to cardiovascular disease especially atherosclerosis (hardening of the arteries).

CANCERS FROM SMOKING

Lung Cancer

Cancer of the lung is the number one cancer killer, accounting for more than 135,000 deaths/year, or about 25% of all cancer deaths. Eighty-three percent of lung cancer is caused by cigarette smoking.

Lung cancer is fatal for 87% of its victims within five years, and there is no effective method for its early detection. The risk is dose related, and much higher when the smoker is also exposed to asbestos, uranium, nickel, chromium, coal, graphite and other industrial carcinogens.

There has been an epidemic of lung cancer among women. In the early 1950s it was correctly predicted that lung cancer would overtake breast cancer in the early 1980s as the leading cause of cancer death.

Exposure to cigarette smoke increases the incidence of lung cancer in nonsmokers as much as 30%, and may account for as many as 5,000 deaths per year.

Smokeless tobacco includes both chewing tobacco and snuff. Manufacturing and sales of these products now total over $1 billion, with over 12 million Americans reporting using smokeless tobacco in 1985. Three million are under 21. One million are under 15.

Smokeless tobacco may be of greater appeal to young people because it is sweet like candy (it's mixed with molasses and other sweeteners, flavorings, and scents), it can be used where they are not supposed to smoke (e.g., school), and because the tobacco industry has targeted its advertising to reach their age group.

With chewing tobacco ("chew") the tobacco may be shredded (looseleaf), pressed into cakes (plugs), or dried and twisted together (twists). The user either chews it, or wedges a wad between their lip and gum.

Snuff comes in either a dry or moist form. It is a finer, powdery cut of tobacco that is either sniffed through the nose or used in the mouth ("dipped").

Smokeless tobacco contains full-doses of nicotine, but lots more. Chemical analysis of the carcinogens in smokeless tobacco reveals polonium-210 (which is as bad as it sounds—it's radioactive!), polycyclic aromatic hydrocarbons (i.e., tars), and nitrosamines. The nitrosamines are suspected of accounting for the majority of cancers among smokeless tobacco users.

Of 19 nitrosamines identified in smokeless tobacco, the types known as NNN and NNK are in the highest concentrations. Snuff contains 1.6 to 135 mg/kg of NNN and 0.1 to 14 mg/kg of NNK; chew contains 0.2 to 8.2 of NNN and 0 to 1.0 mg/kg of NNK. By comparison, food and beverages in the U.S. may not legally contain more than 0.01 mg/kg of nitrosamines.

In addition to cancers and precancers (leukoplakia) of the lip, mouth, tongue, and throat, smokeless tobacco causes gum disease, tooth decay, and bad breath.

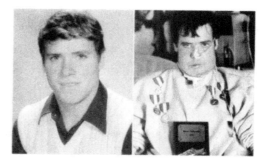

A budding track athlete and a popular student, Sean Marsee started dipping when he was 13 because he thought it was safer than smoking. After five years of dipping a can or more a day, he got mouth cancer. He had part of his tongue removed. At age 19, he died, after writing a simple message on a pad of paper: "Don't dip snuff."

Photo courtesy of the American Cancer Society

Head and Neck Cancers

There are about 18,000 deaths per year from cancers of the head and neck: cancers of the lip, tongue, oral cavity, pharynx, larynx, and esophagus. The risk of these cancers is higher if tobacco is used with alcohol (synergism). The risk of these cancers is particularly high for users of smokeless tobacco, (snuff, chew) which contains n-nitrosamines (a powerful carcinogen).

Bladder Cancer

Many of the chemicals found in tobacco smoking are eliminated via the urinary tract, so the kidneys and bladder are exposed to high concentrations of smoking by-products. Nearly one-third of all bladder cancers are attributable to smoking. Like oral cancer, there are fewer recurrences of bladder cancer if the patient-smoker quits.

Other Cancers

Pancreas, cervix, and stomach cancers, and probably some leukemias, are also associated with tobacco use.

TOBACCO AND CARDIOVASCULAR DISEASE

Heart Attacks, Strokes, High Blood Pressure, and Hardening of the Arteries

There are more than 170,000 deaths per year from heart attacks caused by cigarette smoking alone—accounting for nearly one-fourth of the yearly deaths from heart disease. Cigarette smoking is an independent risk factor for heart attacks. It increases blood pressure and raises the levels of fats in the blood (hyperlipidemia).

In particular, smoking causes increased atherosclerosis (hardening of the arteries), which leads to peripheral vascular disease (bad circulation—which can result in gangrene and amputations), aortic aneurysm, and decreased blood flow to the kidneys and brain. At least 20% of all senile dementias (multi-infarct dementia) are caused by atherosclerosis. One study reported a marked improvement in mental functioning of seemingly demented nursing home residents after getting them to quit smoking.

Smoking increases carbon monoxide in the blood, alters platelet function (causing blood clotting), increases the demand of the heart muscle for oxygen, and may upset the heart rhythm.

CHRONIC BRONCHITIS, EMPHYSEMA, ASTHMA, AND NON-CANCEROUS LUNG DISEASE (also called COPD—Chronic Obstructive Pulmonary Disease)

There are more than 50,000 deaths per year from chronic lung conditions. They are a leading cause of Social Security disability claims, with an estimated 10 million people disabled due to tobacco use. Smoking also increases the damage from other respiratory pollutants.

The chemical ingredients of tobacco smoke damage and irritate the respiratory tract and lungs in a variety of ways. Goblet cells in the respiratory tract respond to the irritating chemicals in cigarette smoke by increasing in number, and by producing mucous which clogs the lining of the delicate respiratory passages.

Nicotine kills scavenger cells of the lung (macrophages), paralyzes cilia which protect the airways, alters protease-antiprotease (lung enzyme) activity—which causes auto-digestion and destruction of the lung tissue itself—and inhibits white blood cell function (reducing immune function).

All smokers have some degree of chronic bronchitis. A morning cough is not normal—it signifies increased mucous production and decreased ciliary function. Smokers have more pneumonias and allergies.

OTHER DISEASES ASSOCIATED WITH SMOKING AND TOBACCO USE

Smoking doubles the risk of stomach ulcers from either coffee or alcohol consumption. It also aggravates allergies, reactive airway disease (asthma), vitamin B-12 deficiency, amblyopia (dimness of vision), osteoporosis (thinning of bones), increased wrinkling of the face (to the extent that one study showed people can easily identify heavy cigarette smokers by their appearance), bad breath, and periodontal disease.

SMOKING MARIJUANA

While marijuana does not contain tobacco (or nicotine), it does contain tars and other carcinogens. All available evidence indicates that smoking marijuana is harmful to the lungs and may cause cancer. Studies show that one "joint" is equal to up to twenty cigarettes.

SMOKING AND THE PILL

Smoking doubles the risk for thromboembolism (blood clots) of women who take birth control pills. Obviously, women who smoke should not be on the pill.

SMOKING AND THE FAMILY—PASSIVE SMOKING

Smoking increases the risk of cancer for exposed nonsmoking family members. It may account for as many as 5000 lung cancer deaths a year.

Cigarette smoke exposure worsens symptomatic coronary heart disease and increases the risk of cardiac death. It lowers fertility and also causes infant pneumonia, asthma, and upper respiratory tract infections. Smoking during pregnancy is associated with more still births, lower birth-weight infants, and more newborn deaths.

SMOKING AND THE COMMUNITY

Cigarette smoking is estimated to cause more premature deaths than do all the following together: acquired immunodeficiency syndrome, cocaine, heroin, alcohol, fire, automobile accidents, homicide, and suicide. That means that 350,000 individuals each year, if they did not smoke, would realize a life-expectancy gain of 15 years.

The Office of Smoking and Health released the results of their Adult Use of Tobacco Survey (August 1987) which reported the lowest prevalence of current cigarette smoking among adults ever recorded in the United States.

Ten states and more than 260 communities already have laws that restrict smoking in public places, due to increased evidence that environmental tobacco smoke (ETS) is harmful to non-smokers.

Smoking-restriction programs work. The point is not to attack the smoker, but to create a smoke-free work place for the majority of non-smok-

---

Adult Use of Tobacco

Present Smokers
29.5%—Men Smokers
23.8%—Women Smokers
26.5%—Overall (down from a high in 1966 of 42%)
Former Smokers
24.6%—Former Smokers
    30.4% Men
    19.3% Women

ers. 80% of smokers who quit do so on their own. The others do so on the advice of their physician or by participating in a formal quit-smoking program. It is speculated that environmental regulation of ETS will reduce further the number of smokers—perhaps to a greater extent than the extensive public education on the health hazards of smoking for over 30 years. However, as more smokers quit on their own, those remaining are bound to be more heavily addicted and will need special help.

In 1984, treatment of diseases caused by smoking, coupled with lost earnings from tobacco-related illness and premature death, cost the country almost $60 billion—a cost to every tax-paying American of $454 per year.

Yet, the tobacco industry, which has been heavily subsidized by the Federal Government, is still 35-billion-dollars-per-year strong. Tobacco earned between 9 and 13 billion dollars in tax revenues. However, the writing is on the wall . . . there was a 2% drop in tobacco sales in 1986, and a 3–5% per year drop is expected over the next five years. The percent of tobacco that is exported to third world countries is going up, as is prices per pack of cigarettes in the United States:

1980	$ .60	1984	$ .90
1981	$ .63	1985	$ .97
1982	$ .70	1986	$1.15
1983	$ .78	1987	$1.35

SUMMARY

Tobacco does more than just cause cancer—it is, as the Surgeon General has said, "the largest preventable cause of illness and premature death in the United States."

References/Additional Readings

Read Chapter 74—Understanding Smoking, later in this book.

13

Parasites, Bacteria, and Cancer

Mark Renneker, M.D.

Doll and Peto estimate that 10% of the cancers in the United States are due to infections by viruses, parasites, and bacteria. The majority of those infection-related cancers are due to viruses, which have already been presented in this book. This chapter focuses on parasites and bacteria.

It's easy to forget, living as comfortably as most of us do in the United States, that close to fifty percent of the people in our world are infected with parasites. And those parasites, particularly if they are affecting the liver or bladder, cause large numbers of cancers. There are parts of Africa where the incidence of parasite-related liver cancer is equal to that of breast or lung cancer in this country.

EFFECTS OF INFECTION

Our world abounds in parasites. Among the better known parasites are the protozoa, which includes malaria, leishmaniasis (kala-azar), trypanosomiasis (African sleeping sickness—from the Tsetse fly, and Chaga's Disease—from the Kissing bug), amoebiasis (amoebic dysentery), giardiasis, trichomonas (common vaginal infection), and pneumocystis carinii (the AIDS-related pneumonia). Then there are the various worms, roundworms (strongyloides, ascaris, trichuris, and loa loa—the eye worm), tapeworms, and flukes (schistosomiasis—"Bilharzia").

What all of these organisms have in common is that in the course of their life-cycle they, temporarily or permanently, live, feed, or reproduce within other living organisms. The effects of parasites on host organisms (i.e., man), as relates to cancer, include: (1) possible release of toxins, enzymes, secretions, and eggs; (2) direct physical interference with the function of an organ, for instance obstructing the outflow of the liver's bile; (3) direct and chronic damage to tissues; (4) decreasing the nourishment available to the host; and (5) causing abnormalities of the immune system.

EXAMPLES OF PARASITIC INFECTIONS LEADING TO CANCER

An easy way to think of how a parasite could lead to cancer is to consider that chronic irritation—from whatever cause—is related to cancer causation. A poorly fitting denture, for instance, is associated with the development of pre-cancerous leukoplakia lesions in the mouth. A liver parasite, like one of the liver flukes (clonorchis) can live in the liver and biliary passages for more than 40 years—that's 40 years of abnormal, chronic irritation. However, most people who are infected with this parasite would probably die of other more immediate effects of the parasite, such as malnutrition.

Schistosomiasis results from infection by the blood fluke (schistosoma), and is an enormous problem world-wide—particularly in Africa and Asia. It occurs as close to the United States as Puerto Rico. The eggs of the blood fluke are extremely toxic to human tissue, resulting in a chronic, fibrotic, foreign-body like reaction, particularly in the liver and bladder. Cancers are then more likely in those sites. Schistosomiasis also has been shown to cause some colorectal cancers (first causing widespread polyps), lymphomas, and gynecological cancers.

Malaria has been strongly implicated in Burkitt's lymphoma, but it may not be a direct cause of that cancer. It appears to involve a co-factor, the Epstein-Barr Virus (EBV). It has been suggested that EBV infection is an early initiator and malaria a later promoting factor. Again, though, the primary disease of malaria causes far more deaths than the secondary cancers that may result.

The possible cancer-causing role of bacteria has been suggested for intestinal cancers. Your entire gastro-intestinal tract is naturally inhabited by bacteria, and they play an important role in digestion. However, they also may play a role in the conversion of foodstuffs to nitrosamines (a carcinogen), and in bile acid breakdown (suspected to play a role in the cause of colon cancer). Bacteria-caused chronic bronchitis has been associated with an increased risk of lung cancer in smokers, possibly because it allows more direct and prolonged contact of the inspired carcinogens with the denuded lining of the bronchi.

IS CANCER AN INFECTIOUS DISEASE?

One consideration that must be raised is: "If 10% of cancers are due to infection, is cancer an infectious disease?" The answer to that question lies, again, in the understanding that there are over 100 different kinds of cancer—differing as to their cause, treatment, and prevention. Though 10% of those cancers are thought to be caused by infections, according to Doll and Peto's estimates, the cancer itself is not what is infectious. People who have a great deal of contact with cancer patients—nurses, doctors, and spouses of patients—have not been found to develop more cancers because of that exposure. There are no known or proven cases of the common cancers—lung, breast, and colon—having been "caught" by anyone.

It would be accurate to say, however, that there are cancer-causing infections that can be "caught." AIDS infection leading to AIDS-related cancers, and hepatitis B infection leading to liver cancer are good examples. Also, when a person has malnutrition and/or weakened immunity, infectious agents that they have been carrying in a dormant state for all of their life may take on a more aggressive nature—and then lead to a cancer. Again, hepatitis is a good example of this.

IN THE FUTURE

In the years to come there will be discoveries of new microorganisms. For most, it will be realized that they were present all along, but were either so rare or led to such minor illnesses, or were so hard to detect, that we were unaware of them. Recent examples are Legionnaire's Disease (caused by a bacteria), Toxic Shock Syndrome (also caused by a bacteria), Chlamydia (an extremely common, often sexually-transmitted disease caused by a bacteria-like organism), and HBLV (human B-cell lympho-trophic virus—implicated in what is called "chronic fatigue syndrome"). And there will be discoveries of seemingly new-on-this-planet microorganisms, such as the AIDS virus.

In fifty years, medicine today will look as primitive as medicine fifty years ago looks to us now. Whole new classes of microorganisms will be discovered that were affecting us all along. Taken in total, the presently known and the future likely-to-be-discovered parasites and other infectious agents will continue to account for a substantial number of cancers.

References and Additional Reading

1. Brown H. W. *Basic Clinical Parasitology.* Appleton-Century-Crofts. 1975.

2. Burton, G. J. Parasites, In Schottenfeld and Fraumeni, ed. *Cancer Epidemiology and Prevention.* W.B. Saunders and Co. 1982: 408–418.

3. Doll R, Peto R. *The Causes of Cancer.* Oxford University Press. 1981.

4. Mustacchi P. Parasites. In Holland J. F. and Frei E, ed. *Cancer Medicine.* Lea and Febiger. 1973: 106–112.

14

Reproductive and Sexual Behavior as a Cause of Cancer

Sir Richard Doll and Richard Peto

from The Causes of Cancer, *Oxford University Press, 1981.*

In *The Causes of Cancer,* Doll and Peto succinctly explained the range of considerations appropriate in evaluating the role of reproductive and sexual factors in cancer causation. You will also see how they arrived at their estimate of what percentage of cancers these factors account for. Bear in mind that their summary below is from 1981, and doesn't include AIDS-related cancers—which for many are a result of sexual behavior.—*M.R.*

. . . Changes in the body resulting from sexual intercourse, pregnancy, childbirth, and lactation* are in a different class from those produced by exposure to chemicals in the ambient atmosphere. They are, however, environmental in origin, insofar as they are not solely the product of the individual's own genetic material, and they were certainly regarded as "extrinsic factors" by the WHO (1964) expert committee on the prevention of cancer, which defined extrinsic factors as including "modifying factors" that favor neoplasia of apparently intrinsic origin (e.g., hormone imbalances). The impact of these factors varies greatly from community to community, and study of the way the processes of reproduction affect the incidence of cancer may well throw light on the mechanism of carcinogenesis in the relevant organs, perhaps indicating ways (short of encouraging or discouraging reproduction!) in which an important group of cancers can be prevented.

The most obvious relationship is that observed between sexual intercourse and the development of cancer of the cervix uteri. This disease occurs in virgins, but only with extreme rarity. It is more common in women who have had several children than in women who have had only one, and it was for a long time thought to be due to the trauma of childbirth. Now, however, it appears that the number of children is not directly relevant and that the risk of developing the disease is chiefly related to the number of sexual partners. Whether the risk for women who had had only one sexual partner is also increased if that partner had previously had multiple partners remains to be proved, but the present evidence strongly suggests that one of the primary causes of the disease is an agent passed between partners in intercourse, quite possibly a virus. If this is indeed so, it may eventually be possible to protect against the disease by immunization, by treatment of the infection, by closer attention to personal hygiene, or by the use of obstructive methods of contraception. Meanwhile, of course, the impact of the disease can be greatly reduced by regular vaginal examination and the treatment of women in whom a smear shows evidence of pre-malignant change.

Pregnancy and childbirth, for their part, seem to play a significant role in the prevention of cancers of the endometrium [uterus], ovary and breast, all these conditions being somewhat less common in women who have borne children early than in women who have had no children. The relationship with cancer of the breast, which has been reviewed by MacMahon et al. (1973), is particularly striking, breast cancer in parous** women becoming progres-

sively less likely to develop as the age of first pregnancy decreases. A pregnancy leading to abortion does not have the same protective effect as one that goes to term, and it is probable that the effect is produced by the first stimulus to lactation which somehow diminishes the risk of the subsequent initiation of a cancer. Lactation itself, however, seems to have no material effect, irrespective of whether it is suppressed or prolonged. Finally, the risk of cancer of the breast is diminished by a late onset of menstruation (made more likely by undernutrition) and by an early menopause.

Cancer of the cervix currently accounts for some 1.5% of all U.S. cancer deaths, but the number is decreasing due at least in part to the more widespread use of cervical screening and to the increasing proportion of women who, having had a hysterectomy some time previously, have no uterus and so no risk of uterine cancer. Comparison of the total number of deaths from cancer of the uterine cervix with the small number that would have been expected if the low rates typical of nuns had prevailed throughout the United States suggests that the large majority of cases of cancer of the uterine cervix are due to the (presumably infective) processes reviewed above, prevention or treatment of which might, therefore, reduce total cancer mortality by 1%.

It is not clear how far it will be possible to reduce the incidence rates of cancers of the breast, ovary, and endometrium (which together account for 29% of all U.S. female cancer deaths) when we understand the mechanisms whereby reproductive factors influence them. It is difficult to believe that no preventive strategies will be discovered for these cancers, since reproductive activity affects them so profoundly. Whether practicable preventive strategies will emerge within the next decade or two is, however, so uncertain that neither pessimism nor optimism can yet be refuted. These cancers collectively account for 13% of all U.S. cancer deaths, and estimates of the percentage that will be avoidable by mechanisms related to the mechanisms whereby reproduction exerts its effects might range between 0 and 12%. We have arbitrarily taken a middle figure of 6% and have added to it the definite 1% of deaths that would be avoidable by control of the causes of cervical cancer, to get an estimate of 7% thus avoidable. Note, however, that reproductive and dietary factors might well interact multiplicatively in the production of these cancers, unless diet affects them by a hormonal mechanism, and in either situation, this estimate of 7% and the percentage preventable by dietary modification will overlap. . . .

*breast feeding. *Lactation* refers to the state of a woman's breasts when they are milk-producing.

**Parous refers to a woman who has borne children.

15

Occupational Carcinogenesis

Harriet S. Page and Ardyce J. Asire,
Adapted by Greg Raymond, M.S.

Cancer Rates and Risks, *3rd edition, 1985. National Cancer Institute, Bethesda, MD*.

Doll and Peto estimate that approximately 4% of cancer deaths are due to occupational factors. In the 1970s, when data on this critical subject was in short supply, estimates ranged as high as 36%. Fortunately, in the light of recent, fairly good, comprehensive studies, the numbers are not that bad. But, if you are the worker exposed to the asbestos or uranium dust, or any of the other occupational carcinogens, that 4% could approach 100% for you.—*M.R.*

OCCUPATION

In 1775, London surgeon Percivall Pott published a report on a rare cancer of the scrotum that he found was common among chimney sweeps, a disease known at the time as "soot-wart" (Shimkin, 1977). A century later, two other scientists noted similar cancers among gas plant workers in Germany and oil shale workers in Scotland. Yet another 40 years later, certain constituents of tar, soot, and oils, known as polycyclic aromatic hydrocarbons, were found to cause cancer in laboratory animals.

This brief detective story has become a model for many later investigations of workplace carcinogens: observation of unusual cancers, or a high incidence of more common cancers, among groups of workers; a search for a responsible agent; and finally, demonstration that the agent can cause cancer in laboratory animals.

A postscript to the chimney sweep story deals with the ultimate goal of workplace cancer studies: prevention. Spurred by Pott's report, the Danish chimney sweeps guild in 1778 urged its members to take daily baths* (Clemmesen, 1951). A report in the 1892 British Medical Journal, "Why Foreign Sweeps Do Not Suffer From Scrotal Cancer," noted that the sweeps of northern Europe seemed to benefit from this hygiene measure, but English sweeps, who apparently ignored such implications, continued to develop cancer.

Industrial workers are, in a sense, flagmen for our society. In this age of chemicals, metals, plastics, and fibers, we all run the risk of exposures to industrial carcinogens in our air, water, food, and homes. But the exposures of the industrial worker may be intense and prolonged. If a substance used in the workplace is a carcinogen, the cancers it can cause will most likely be seen first in workers.

Since 1971, the International Agency for Research on Cancer (IARC), an agency of the World Health Organization headquartered in Lyons, France, has been publishing critical reviews of data on the carcinogenicity of chemicals to which humans are exposed, and IARC working groups of scientists have been evaluating these data in terms of human risk.

The IARC scientists assessed the data from epidemiologic studies of humans, from studies in experimental animals, and from short-term tests or assays. Based on these data, they assigned individual chemicals, chemical groups, industrial processes and occupational exposures to one of three categories of risk. (See Figures 15-1 and 15-2.) When

---

Carcinogens

*[Almost 200 years later,] In early 1972, a 43-year-old patient with newly diagnosed lung cancer was referred to a young pulmonary physician in Philadelphia, Dr. William Figueroa. The patient had worked at a Philadelphia chemical company, and according to the referring physician some of his co-workers had succumbed to lung cancer. Figueroa later described his first encounter with the patient: "He came in, told me he believed he had lung cancer, the same thing that had killed 13 other men he'd worked with. What excited me was that he had oat cell carcinoma, which is very rare among nonsmokers, and he'd never smoked. Oat cell is the wild, undifferentiated kind. It spreads fast. It's usually found among smokers. But [the patient] swore he'd never smoked and neither had three of the other men who'd died. Most of the others were very light smokers, he said. They were young. Cancer is an old man's disease, usually among men in their fifties and sixties who've smoked at least a pack a day for 20 to 30 years."

Figueroa recognized that an occupational carcinogen might be involved, and he determined to investigate further. Many of the workers, it turned out, were exposed to chloromethyl methyl ether (CMME), an intermediate in the manufacture of ion-exchange resins. CMME is invariably contaminated with bis (chloromethyl) ether (BCME); animal data suggesting that BCME was a carcinogen had appeared in 1967 and well-designed experiments verified this by 1971. Figueroa appealed to company management for the exposure records of a cohort of workers in order to determine if BCME was associated with human lung cancer. Unfortunately, the records were not made available to him.

Faced with a similar situation several years earlier, another Philadelphia physician had not pursued the matter. "I had a feeling that four cases in 125 was excessive. . . ." he explained. "I didn't go any further because I didn't know if it was significant. [The company] said there was no exposure data and I didn't know what to do." Figueroa, however, turned to another source of data—his patient.

"I decided to trust the memory of this guy, of one honest American worker," remembered Figueroa. "We stood next to [his] bed as he lay there, dying of cancer, in an oxygen mask. I read him all the names and he told me which had been exposed and who had died." Through this investigation Figueroa was able to document that BCME exposure was associated with a marked elevation in lung cancer mortality. His results were soon published and, together with subsequent corroborating data, produced both local and national effects. In 1974 the widows of BCME victims were informed that they could file for workers' compensation benefits based on the work-relatedness of their husbands' deaths; and in that same year OSHA promulgated a series of regulations designed to control exposure to 14 carcinogens, one of which was BCME. . . .

Occupational Health—Recognizing and Preventing Work-Related Diseases, edited by Barry S. Levy, M.D., M.P.H. and David H. Wegman, M.D., M.S. Little, Brown Company, 1982. Used with permission.

Figure 15-1

Group 1:

Industrial processes and occupational exposures causally associated with cancer in humans:

Auramine manufacture
Boot and shoe manufacture and repair (certain occupations)
Furniture manufacture
Isopropyl alcohol manufacture (strong-acid process)
Nickel refining
Rubber industry (certain occupations)

Underground hematite mining (with exposure to radon)

Chemicals and groups of chemicals causally associated with cancer in humans:

4-Aminobiphenyl
Arsenic and arsenic compounds
Asbestos
Benzene
Benzidine
N, N-Bis (2-chloroethyl)-2-naphthylamine (Chlornaphazine)
Bis (chloromethyl) ether and technical-grade chloromethyl methyl ether
Chromium and certain chromium compounds
2-Naphthylamine
Soots, tars and oils
Vinyl chloride

Figure 15-2

Group 2A:

Chemicals, groups of chemicals or industrial processes *probably* carcinogenic to humans with at least limited evidence of carcinogenicity to humans:

Acrylonitrile
Benzo(a)pyrene
Beryllium and beryllium compounds
Diethyl sulphate
Dimethyl sulphate
Manufacture of magenta
Nickel and certain nickel compounds
ortho-Toluidine

Group 2B:

Chemicals, groups of chemicals or industrial processes *probably* carcinogenic to humans with sufficient evidence in animals and inadequate data in humans:

Amitrole
Auramine (technical grade)
Benzotrichloride
Cadmium and cadmium compounds
Carbon tetrachloride
Chlorophenols
DDT
3,3'-Dichlorobenzidine
3,3'-Dimethoxybenzidine (*ortho*-Dianisidine)
Dimethylcarbamoyl chloride
1,4-Dioxane
Direct Black 38 (technical grade)
Direct Blue 6 (technical grade)
Direct Brown 95 (technical grade)
Epichlorohydrin
Ethylene dibromide
Ethylene oxide
Ethylene thiourea
Formaldehyde (gas)
Hydrazine
Phenoxyacetic acid herbicides
Polychlorinated biphenyls
Tetrachlorodibenzo-*para*-dioxin (TCDD)
2,4,6-Trichlorophenol

there was enough evidence from epidemiologic studies to support a causal association with cancer, the chemical, chemical group, process, or exposure was assigned to Group 1. The scientists placed the chemicals, chemical groups, processes, or exposures that they considered *probably* carcinogenic to humans in Group 2. Those with data to support the highest carcinogenic risk to humans appear in Group 2A; those with lower risk are in Group 2B.

To illustrate briefly how exposures occur, how risk is ascertained, and how exposures can be minimized or prevented, four types of workplace carcinogen, each from Group 1, are discussed here in some detail: a mineral fiber (asbestos), a chemical (benzene), a metal (chromium), and an industrial process (furniture manufacture).

Asbestos

Derived from the Greek word meaning "incombustible," asbestos is the generic name for a group of minerals composed of silicate fibers that are heat-stable, non-conductive and can be woven. Asbestos occurs widely in mineral formations found throughout the world and has been used since the late 1800s. In 1976, more than 5,500 tons of asbestos were produced (IARC, Vol 14, 1977), the bulk of it by Canada and the Soviet Union. About two-thirds of the asbestos produced is used in the construction industry for cement sheets and pipes, insulating materials, and floor and ceiling tiles. It is also used

for friction applications, like clutch and brake facings for cars and machinery. It is used widely in the shipbuilding industry, chiefly for insulating and fireproofing. In the past, it was often sprayed on for insulation, fire-proofing, and decorative and acoustic uses, but its use in many of these settings is now decreasing.

The presence of asbestos in various materials does not necessarily pose a health risk. The health risk arises when the asbestos fibers are set free during mining, drilling, sawing, or spraying, or when materials with asbestos in them start to decompose.

Reports linking asbestos with lung cancer and asbestosis, a lung disease, have been appearing since 1935. The earlier studies reported these diseases mostly among asbestos workers and miners, but as the uses of asbestos multiplied, particularly in shipbuilding during World War II, the numbers of workers who suffered the injurious effects of asbestos exposure continued to grow. Mesothelioma, a rare cancer that affects the lining of the chest and abdominal cavity, has been linked with asbestos exposure since the early 1960s. Inhaled asbestos fibers produce these cancers in a number of different laboratory animals.

Lung cancer and mesothelioma both have latency periods of up to 30 years or more; this means it may take that long for cancer to develop after exposure. But the duration of the exposure needed to cause cancer may be very brief. In some cases, individuals who were exposed to asbestos for only a few months have developed cancer. Men who worked in shipyards for only a few years during World War II, for instance, have been found to be at high risk of lung cancer (Blot et al, 1982). Some cases of lung cancer and mesothelioma have also been found to occur among "bystanders": the families of workers who carried asbestos fibers home on their clothing; workers who were nearby when asbestos materials were sawed, drilled, or sprayed; individuals who lived near asbestos mines or factories where asbestos was fabricated.

Cigarette smoking and asbestos exposure have a synergistic effect: smoking plus asbestos exposure creates far more risk than either one alone. Some other cancers have also been linked to asbestos exposure, including cancers of the esophagus, stomach, colon, larynx, and kidney.

Asbestos exposure is now regulated by the Occupational Safety and Health Administration (OSHA), which sets standards for the number of fibers that may be present in the workplace air. It also requires personal protective equipment for workers. The National Institute for Occupational Safety and Health (NIOSH), the research arm of OSHA, recommends that all non-essential uses of asbestos be eliminated.

Benzene

A clear, colorless liquid, benzene was first isolated by Faraday in 1825 from a liquid condensed by compressing oil gas (IARC, Vol 7, 1974). It is now produced from petroleum. Up until World War II, benzene was used chiefly in this country as a gasoline additive. Now it is also used widely as a solvent in the chemical and drug industries, and as an intermediate reactant in the synthesis of resins, adhesives, and plastics.

Case reports linking leukemia with occupational exposure to benzene have appeared in the literature since the late 1920s; such reports have come from a number of countries. The major route of absorption of benzene is through the lungs; most of the affected workers had breathed its fumes. Among those exposed who later developed leukemia were workers who made artificial leather, or made shoes using rubber cements that contained benzene. Case-control and cohort studies (IARC, Vol 7, 1974) have supported this association.

Benzene causes chromosomal abnormalities, but not mutations, in some short-term assays (IARC, 1982) and has recently been found to be carcinogenic in assays with laboratory animals (NTP, 1984).

Some two to three million workers may be exposed to benzene in petrochemical, rubber, and coke plants. Shoemakers, furniture finishers, and gas station attendants are also exposed to it. OSHA regulates workplace exposures.

Chromium and Chromium Compounds

The element chromium is the 20th most abundant element and occurs, mostly in chromite ores, throughout the world. The Republic of South Africa and the Soviet Union are now the two major producers. Chromium and its compounds are used widely in industry because of chrome's hardness, resistance to corrosion, high melting point, and wide availability. Its name is derived from the Greek word "chroma," for color, because of the reds, oranges, yellows, and blues of its salts when it is combined with other minerals.

Most chromium compounds are used in the metallurgical industry, particularly to make stainless steel and alloys. Chromium compounds are also used in the manufacture of bricks, glass, ceramics and certain iron-containing metals. The colored chromate salts of various metals, like zinc and potassium, are used in the pigment, paint, tanning and dyeing industries (IARC, Vol 23, 1980).

An increased incidence of lung cancer has been seen among workers in the chromate-producing industry. There are also indications of high risk among chromium platers and chromium alloy workers.

Furniture Manufacture

For many centuries, furniture and cabinetmaking were performed by craftsmen and artisans working at home or in small shops. With the advent of the Industrial Revolution and the development of circular saws and planers, furniture and cabinetmaking became an industry. Advances in mechanization were most rapid after World War I. With the development of bandsaws, routers, lathes, and sanders, furniture-making became an assembly-line process, a process that created more furniture and more hazards: high noise levels, accidents, and dust pollution. It was not until the 1960s that the cancer-causing effects of furniture dust began to be recognized.

An increased incidence of cancers of the nose and nasal cavities was first reported among furniture makers in England. Later reports came from Italy, Canada, the Netherlands, Denmark, France, Germany, Sweden, and other parts of England (IARC, Vol 25, 1981). A study in this country (Brinton et al, 1984) showed high nasal cancer risks among furniture workers, particularly in North Carolina. There have also been reports of high incidence of cancers of the larynx, lung, and gastrointestinal tract among furniture workers in the United States, England, and Germany, although these associations are not clear.

From the epidemiologic data available, IARC has concluded that nasal adenocarcinomas have been caused by employment in the furniture-making industry, and that the excess risk of these cancers occurs mainly among those workers exposed to dust from certain hardwoods.

Suction devices, particularly near saws and sanders, can markedly reduce the amount of airborne dust at the workplace (Hounam and Williams, 1974) and masks worn by workers can further reduce the amount of dust inhaled.

Summary

The remaining chemicals or processes listed in Figures 15-1 and 15-2 each fall into the four categories discussed above. Ways to reduce workplace exposure to them, including labeling, venting, and individual protective measures, are regulated by a number of Federal agencies. NCI studies are attempting to gain further understanding of workplace carcinogens, and are looking at ways to counter the cancer risks of workers who have already been exposed to workplace carcinogens. Also, some industries are testing substances in short-term cell-culture assays before introducing them to the workplace.

16

Radiation and Cancer

Introduction to Radiation

Mark Renneker, M.D.

Radiation is a mixed blessing. It can be used to diagnose and cure cancer, but it is also a known cause of cancer. In this chapter, we will look at the basic physics of radiation, its cancer-causing effects on cells and tissues, and its historical and prospective impact on our world.

BASIC PHYSICS

"Radiation" is an abstract term referring to energy that is transmitted through space. This radiant energy is described by physicists as occurring in two forms: (1) electromagnetic *waves*, which include ultraviolet waves (UV light), visible and infrared light, radiowaves, X-rays, and microwaves; and, (2) energetically charged atomic *particles*, including alpha particles, beta particles (electrons), protons, neutrons, pi mesons, as well as a variety of newly discovered particles with odd-sounding names such as quarks and antiquarks.

Whether as a wave or as particles, radiation can be thought of as something very small zooming through space. If you and your cells (which, in terms of radiation, are a net of atoms) stand in the way of radiation, it is possible that there will be a collision and that your body will be biochemically changed.

EFFECTS OF RADIATION ON CELLS (RADIOBIOLOGY)

Of all the components of a cell, DNA is probably the most vulnerable to radiation. To alter the DNA is to alter the genes on the chromosomes, possibly resulting in a mutational event that could lead to cancer. Radiation is thought to either directly hit the DNA (the direct hit theory) and cause linkages and bonds to be nicked or broken, or to set off a string of chemical reactions that secondarily interact with the DNA (the indirect action theory).

You will hear the distinction made between "ionizing" and "non-ionizing" radiation. The qualitative effects of either form of radiation are generally the same; suffice it to say that X-rays and gamma rays are ionizing radiation and that ultraviolet rays are non-ionizing radiation. Both can cause cancer.

The final word isn't in yet on low-level radiation, such as microwaves.

It is also important to consider the remarkable cellular processes of DNA repair, whereby there are specialized enzymes that can actually patch up damaged DNA. Cancer cells are less able to repair their DNA, making them more vulnerable to the damaging effects of radiation (as in radiation therapy). Figure 16-1 summarizes the range of radiation effects on humans and other mammals.

THE LAW OF RADIOSENSITIVITY

The Law of Radiosensitivity was first formulated in 1906 by J. Bergonie and L. Tribondeau. While investigating the effects of radiation on rat testes, they noticed that highly mitotic, rapidly dividing cells (germinal cells) were affected by radiation far more than less mitotic, less frequently dividing cells. They then considered that mature, well-differentiated cells divide less frequently than immature, poorly differentiated cells (i.e, cancer cells). Therefore, the Law of Radiosensitivity states that the radiosensitivity

Figure 16-1   Some of the Types of Mammalian Radiobiological Damage

Level of Biological Organisation	Important Radiation Effects
Molecular	Damage to macromolecules such as enzymes, RNA and DNA, and interference with metabolic pathways
Subcellular	Damage to cell membranes, nucleus, chromosomes, mitochondria and lysosomes
Cellular	Inhibition of cell division; cell death; transformation of a malignant state
Tissue; organ	Disruption of such systems as the central nervous system, the bone marrow and intestinal tract may lead to the death of animals; induction of cancer
Whole animal	Death; 'radiation of lifeshortening'
Populations of animals	Changes in genetic characteristics due to gene and chromosomal mutations in individual members of the species

Source: Coggle, J. E., *Biological Effects of Radiation* (London: Wykeham Publications, 1971), p. 17.

of tissue is directly proportional to its mitotic activity and inversely proportional to the degree of differentiation of its cells. The Law of Radiosensitivity forms one of the cornerstones of the principles of radiotherapy, and explains (together with the principle of DNA repair) why cancer cells are more likely to be eliminated by radiation therapy than normal cells.

DOSE—RAD OR ROENTGEN

The two units of radiation dose in common usage are the rad and the roentgen. The rad (radiation absorbed dose) is the most useful measurement. It refers to the amount of radiation energy absorbed by the tissues. The roentgen refers to the amount of radiation energy directed at an object, of which a fraction may be absorbed.

SUMMARY

With these basic principles under your belt, you're ready to absorb what some of the best minds in the business have to say about radiation and cancer.

Biological Effects of Radiation

J. E. Coggle, M.D.

Excerpted with permission from Biological Effects of Radiation *(London: Wykeham Publications, 1971), pp. 110–115.*

INDUCTION OF CANCER BY RADIATION

One of the first observations of cancer following radiation was the appearance of skin tumors on the hands of many of the early workers with X-rays. Since that time many systematic studies on animals have shown that radiation causes an increase in the incidence of almost all types of naturally ('spontaneously') occurring cancers. The malignant tumors do not appear until long after the exposure, and carcinogenesis is therefore one of the delayed effects of radiation. The delay may be as long as 30–40 years in the case of some human cancers. Between the exposure and the appearance of the tumor there may be no observable defect in the tissues that eventually become cancerous.

Radiation is capable of inducing tumors in almost all of the tissues of the body, although some types of tumor are more common than others. Generally speaking tissues that have a high rate of cell division are more prone to tumor induction than tissues that exhibit a low rate of cell proliferation. *The fact that radiation may induce tumors in nearly all tissues distinguishes it from the vast majority of chemical and viral agents that can cause tumors only in a few selected tissues. . . .*

Tumors most commonly appear in the tissues that have been directly exposed to radiation, but there are some cases where cancer induction is an indirect process. For example, if mice with their thymus glands removed are irradiated and a new thymus is then transplanted into them a cancer will develop in this unirradiated organ. Or again, the pituitary gland may become cancerous as a result of the irradiation of the thyroid gland with radioactive iodine (^{131}I).

Many of the experiments on radiation carcinogenesis show that at very low doses there is no detectable increase of the natural incidence of tumors. But this does *not* prove that there is a threshold dose for the induction of cancer. Two things must be emphasized on this problem. First, the delay (or latent period) between radiation exposure and the appearance of a tumor may exceed the lifespan of the short-lived experimental animals. And secondly, it must be stressed that no dose effect relationship, however large the number of mice involved, can disprove the existence of a threshold dose, as the incidence of tumors at very low doses may be too low to be demonstrable. Therefore, it is safest to assume that, however small the dose, some tumor induction may still occur.

What is the relationship between the tumor incidence and the dose of radiation? There is in fact no common pattern between radiation and tumor incidence, nor does there seem to be any instance of a tumor whose incidence increases in a simple linear fashion with increasing dose. In an American experiment called 'Operation Greenhouse' mice were exposed to a mixture of γ [gamma] rays and neutrons from a nuclear weapons test in Nevada, and the incidence of tumor at different doses was measured. The results showed that tumors of the thymus gland generally increased with increasing dose. Tumors of the liver and the pituitary gland increased to a maximum and any further increase in the dose had no effect. The incidence of tumors in breast and lung decreased with increasing dose after a certain dose level. This decrease in the incidence of cancer with increasing dose has been found by other research workers for some leukemias, bone tumors, thyroid and ovarian tumors. Figure 16-2 shows a graph of the incidence of a type of leukemia against the dose of radiation. The incidence peaks at 300 rad after which any further radiation reduces the number of leukemias induced. How can we explain this strangely shaped curve? It has been suggested that radiation is doing two things: first, it is inducing leukemia in cells and secondly it is killing cells. At low doses the induction of leukemia predominates, while at higher doses the rate at which radiation kills potentially leukemic cells overtakes this, so that a maximum is reached at 300 rad. However, there have recently been a number of theoretical and experimental objections to this hypothesis which make it an unlikely explanation.

RADIATION CARCINOGENESIS IN MAN

The induction of cancer in man by radiation has been studied since a skin cancer was first reported in 1902 on the hand of a radiation worker. This was some seven years after Roentgen's discovery of X-rays. It has been realized for a long time that large doses of radiation (several hundreds of rad) are carcinogenic; more recently, however, the United Nations Scientific Committee on the Effects of Atomic Radiation reported in 1964 that there is now evidence that quite small increases in the level of environmental radiation may add to the natural incidence of human cancers.

There can of course be no experiments on cancer induction in man, comparable with those in animals. Nevertheless, observations on people deliberately and accidentally exposed to radiation show that radiation can and does induce tumors in man.

Leukemia is perhaps the best-documented of human cancers associated with irradiation and evidence for its induction in man comes from several groups of people, and shows that all types of leukemia, except chronic lymphocytic leukemia, are associated with irradiation. The most extensive study of leukemia has been carried out on the victims exposed to the atomic bombs in Hiroshima and Nagasaki in 1945 (see Figure 16-3). The radiation from these bombs was mainly γ rays and neutrons. The survivors show an increased incidence of leukemia relative to an equivalent unexposed population. At higher doses there is a higher incidence of leukemia amongst the victims. Leukemias first appeared in the victims 1–1½ years after exposure. The different types of leukemia appeared at different times: acute lymphatic and chronic granulocytic leukemia showed a peak incidence 5–8 years after irradiation, whilst the other acute leukemias did not appear until 10–15 years after exposure. Generally, the latent period between exposure and the appearance of leukemia was shorter for higher exposure doses.

Besides bomb victims there are several groups of people who have received radiation treatment for various diseases and all these groups show an increased incidence of leukemia. In one group of 2393 children, irradiated for the enlargement of their thymuses, 9 cases of leukemia were reported where fewer

Figure 16-2 The incidence of myeloid leukaemia in RF mice as a function of whole body X or γ ray exposure at 5–10 weeks of age. The figures denote the numbers of mice used per point. *Annals of the New York Academy of Sciences*, Vol. 114, Art. 1, fig. 1, p. 573, A.C. Upton *et al.* The New York Academy of Sciences, 1964; reprinted by permission.

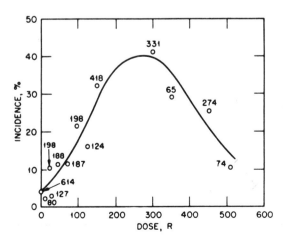

Figure 16-3 The incidence of leukaemia in three Japanese populations for the period 1946–1962. The incidence for all Japan remained relatively constant over these years. The 'exposed' group (survivors of the atomic bomb on Hiroshima) show a higher incidence of leukaemia than the 'non-exposed' group. The latter, although present in Hiroshima, were too far from the explosion (>5000 m) to have received a significant radiation dose. *The Report of the United Nations Scientific Committee on the Effects of Atomic Radiation, General Assembly document, 19th Session, Supplement No. 14 (A/5814), United Nations, N.Y., 1964.*

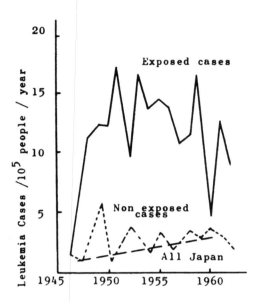

than 1 was expected. These leukemias appeared between 1½ and 14½ years after the radiation treatment.

Three-quarters of a million children in the U.S.A. whose mothers had received medical X-ray examinations whilst they were still *in utero* have been studied. The children were found to have a 40 per cent higher incidence of leukemia than a control group of children whose mothers had not been X-rayed. A similar study carried out in the U.S. on approximately 40,000 children irradiated *in utero* failed to reveal an increased incidence of leukemia— 10.5 cases of leukemia were expected and 9 cases were observed.

A final piece of evidence comes from a study of the American radiologists who use radiation daily in their work. They were found to be 2.5 times as likely to get leukemia as doctors who did not use radiation routinely. Radiologists practicing before 1950 were even more likely to get leukemia, presumably because they were less rigorous in applying safety precautions than is now the case.

This is no evidence from any of the groups that there is a threshold dose for leukemia. The data on childhood leukemia following prenatal X-ray examination, in which the average dose received by the fetus was 2.0 rad, suggests that very low levels of radiation may be leukemogenic. What then can one say of the risks involved in medical X-ray examinations? These involve doses to the skin of between 30 mrad and several rad depending on the site of irradiation and the extent of the examination. This leads to gonad doses of approximately the same order, again dependent on the site of examination. It is estimated that the mean dose to the bone marrow from medical X-ray examination is approximately 100 mrad. . . .

On the basis of the Japanese data given by the United Nations Committee on the Effects of Atomic Radiation, the International Commission on Radiological Protection (1966) has suggested that one to two extra cases of leukemia are expected each year for 13 years as a result of every million people who undergo X-ray examination. In the U.K. out of every million people some fifty to sixty cases of leukemia occur 'spontaneously' each year. The risk of one or two extra cases is held to be an acceptable risk when balanced against the enormous medical benefits of diagnostic radiation. However, the X-ray examination of pregnant women is severely restricted because of the special risk to the fetus.

Let us look briefly at some of the other radiation-induced human cancers. The data for human skin cancer following radiation are consistent with the experimental results on animals. The tumors take from 10 to 20 years to develop and a high dose rate is much more effective than a low dose rate.

There is a high incidence of tumors of the thyroid in the Japanese atomic bomb survivors and in the children of the Marshall Islands in the Pacific. These were subjected to the radio-active fall-out from an American atomic test explosion in 1954. An unprecedented change in the wind blew radio-active ash over the islands. The radio-active iodine, ^{131}I, in the fall-out induced thyroid tumors in 50 per cent of the children over 10 years of age; no previous thyroid tumors had been reported in Marshallese children of this age.

A high incidence of lung tumors is found amongst the uranium miners of Czechoslovakia and the U.S.A., due to the inhalation of radio-active dust.

Bone tumors appeared in many of the women who used to paint the luminous dials on watches. They were in the habit of licking their paint brushes and thus ingesting radio-active substances, particularly radium, which was deposited in their bones.

The above are some of the instances of human cancers following radiation, and they are consistent with the data from experimentally induced tumors in animals. Since human tumors are detectable at lower doses than was previously held to be the case, they constitute one of the real hazards of any increase in the environmental levels of radiation. . . .

Radiation Hazards in Peace and War

J. Walter, M.A., B.M., F.R.C.P., F.R.C.R., D.M.R.E.

Excerpted with permission from Cancer and Radiotherapy *(New York: Churchill Livingston Company, 1977), pp. 108–110.*

. . . In the light of our knowledge about the biological effects of ionizing radiation, we will now view the subject in a wider context. Radiotherapy is only a very minor source of radiation to mankind as a whole. We are all exposed to radiation from sources both natural and man-made. *Natural sources* of ionizing radiation are: (a) cosmic rays and (b) naturally occurring radioactive elements on the earth.

a. *Cosmic radiation* bombarding the earth from outer space includes electrons, neutrons and other particles. Most of it is filtered off by the earth's atmosphere, but the small fraction which gets by is highly penetrating and irradiates the whole body uniformily.

b. *Terrestrial radiation* comes from radioactive chemical elements which are distributed over most of the earth in minute quantities in rocks and soils, especially granite rock. From these, gamma rays arise so that building bricks and stone are liable to be sources of radiation. Radon gas diffuses from the earth into the atmosphere where it is normally present in extremely low concentration. The normal human body itself contains traces of radioactive carbon and potassium as well as radium etc., absorbed from food and water and deposited in bone.

In considering the effects of natural radiation on mankind, our first concern must be the dose to the gonads. The average dose from all the above sources has been estimated at roughly 0.1 rad per year, or about 3 rads per generation of 30 years.

Genetic effects. Gene mutations have been mentioned. . . . Biologically they are of fundamental importance, as they provide the 'raw material' on which the evolutionary processes of natural selection can work. Mutations occur naturally and continually in genes at a definite but very low rate.

All genes are subject to possible mutations, but the causes are not clear. Genes are complex molecules, and structural disturbances can arise from random chemical influences as well as ionizing radiation. Natural background is responsible for only a fraction of ordinary mutations—perhaps 10 per cent. There is no reason to think that radiation, natural or otherwise, produces any novel type of change—its effect is simply to increase the rate or *frequency of mutation.*

Since the biological effects of gene mutations are generally harmful, the consequences are serious. They may be apparent as congenital abnormalities in the next generation or may not appear for several generations. Note that there are no serious consequences for the individual originally irradiated, only for his/her descendants. They are therefore of no importance if that individual cannot or does not have children.

Man-made sources of ionizing radiation. These include the increasing uses of radiation in industry and medicine. *In medicine,* diagnostic X-rays contribute a far greater dose to the population as a whole than radiotherapy. *In industry,* radiography is widely used for e.g., examination of castings. Physicists, chemists, engineers, and others engaged in the production of X-ray tubes or radioactive isotopes are similarly exposed. Isotopes are employed in a wide variety of industrial processes for calibration, accurate control etc. The development of *atomic energy* plants has added a new sector on the industrial front and here radiation hazards involve many thousands of workers.

There are many *historic* examples of the dangers involved and some have already been described—skin cancers in pioneer X-ray and radium workers . . . anemia and leukemia . . . sterility . . . cataract . . . after some industrial accidents, bone sarcoma in luminous dial painters . . . lung cancers in miners of radioactive ores.

THE ACUTE RADIATION SYNDROME

This is exemplified by the *atom bomb.* At Hiroshima and Nagasaki, where the bombs fell in 1945, most of the casualties were due to blast and fire, but 15–20 per cent were from gamma and neutron radiation. The effective range for serious injury from radiation was about one mile, compared with three miles for flash burns and five miles for blast.

The radiation doses have been estimated and the survivors carefully followed up and observed. Other episodes have been: unintentional exposure in the Marshall Islands in the Pacific in 1954 in the course of bomb testing, affecting nearly 300 people; over a dozen accidents involving high exposure in industrial plants, laboratories and hospitals. All these plus experimental animal work, have given us a detailed picture of the effects and mechanisms of acute radiation damage.

1. Doses of about 700 rads—i.e. to the whole body at once—leave few if any survivors.

2. Doses of 450 rads make all victims very ill, and 50 per cent die in 2–3 months.

3. 150 rads cause illness in about half.

4. 100 rads cause sickness in about one-seventh, with very few deaths.

5. 50 rads rarely cause sickness.

The effects may be summarized under three headings:
(1) the _hematological syndrome_; (2) the _gastro-intestinal syndrome_, (3) the _central nervous system_ (CNS) _syndrome_.

The typical sequence of events after a dose of about 400 rads is as follows. Nausea and vomiting within the first few hours, then a latent period of several days. Then sickness again, fever and weight loss. Intestinal ulceration now dominates the picture with diarrhea, fluid loss, dehydration and prostration. Bleeding occurs from bowels, nose etc. Deaths begin in the third week, till 50 per cent succumb by the end of the third month. The rest recover very slowly and suffer premature aging later and increased risk of cataract, leukemia, amenorrhea, sterility, etc.

At this level the chief target tissue is the bone marrow, where the parent cells of the peripheral blood cells are inhibited or killed. Lymphocytes are affected most, then the other white cells, then megakaryocytes (from which platelets are derived). The red cell precursors are also sensitive, but since the life-span of the adult red cell is about four months, anemia sets in later then leukopenia. Thrombopenia leads to hemorrhages, leukopenia to bacterial infection, especially from the bowel.

There is some direct effect on gastrointestinal mucosa which is one of the fastest-growing tissues in the body and normally renews itself every two days. This is slowed down or prevented, with resultant ulceration and bacterial invasion leading to septicemia.

At higher dose levels, over 1000 rads, the gastro-intestinal effect becomes even more important, with death in a few days from fluid loss and massive bacterial damage.

At above 2000 rads the CNS syndrome sets in, with headache, coma and convulsion. It is always fatal.

In those who survived the bomb a special hazard involved pregnant women. Abortions and stillbirths (i.e. birth of dead babies) were brought about. If the child in the womb survived, its brain development was liable to be retarded and it might be born with an abnormally small head and mental deficiency.

LATE HAZARDS OF ATOM BOMBS

The newer (thermonuclear) bombs are thousands of times as powerful. In addition to the late hazards already mentioned (aging, leukemia, etc.) there are special dangers from the 'fall-out'. This is the radio-active dust containing fission products carried to great heights in the atmosphere with the vaporized material from the bomb. The fine particles are carried in air currents, settling down gradually to earth. These dust clouds can travel enormous distances, even encircling the earth many times over, so that _no part of the world is immune_. A bomb exploded e.g. in Nevada (U.S.A.) produces fall-out detectable in England after about five days. If the firing of test bombs continues at its present rate, the gonad dose involved will be quite low, only about 1 per cent of the natural background; but any marked increase in the number of bombs could soon become significant genetically to the future world population. As it is, the fall-out from a bomb can have fatal effects over an area of 7000 square miles and be dangerous for tens of thousands of square miles.

A special danger from fall-out concerns radioactive strontium, a fission product. This is soluble and is absorbed by plants, cattle, etc., and thereby reaches humans in food and drink. It behaves chemically like calcium and is deposited in bone tissue after absorption. It is therefore potentially capable of producing late effects comparable to those in the luminous-dial painters mentioned above. So far the danger is negligible but is one of the indices that have to be watched.

Taking all the man-made sources together (radiography, industry, bombs, etc.) the total gonad dose is estimated to amount to about 20 per cent of the natural background, or rather less than 1 rad in

Figure 16-4   Radiation to Whole Population

Source of Radiation	Dose as % of Natural Background
Natural background	100%
Diagnostic radiology	14.1%
Occupational exposure (medical, industrial, atomic energy)	0.5%
Fall-out from nuclear explosions	3.7%

a generation of 30 years. This is a figure that need cause no present alarm. Constant watch is now kept on the dosage to the population from industry, atomic energy plants, fall-out, etc., and our knowledge of the potential hazards is extensive enough to give us warning of any serious risk. Complacency would be foolish, especially as regards any increased firing of atomic bombs, but pessimism would be equally unreasonable.

Figure 16-4 summarizes the present situation. Radiotherapy is not listed separately; its contribution is almost insignificant. It involves large individual doses to a few, but this is of very minor importance to the population as a whole. . . .

Additional Reading on Radiation and Cancer

1. Arena, Victor, *Ionizing Radiation and Life* (St. Louis: C. V. Mosby & Company, 1971).

2. Coggle, J. E., *Biological Effects of Radiation* (New York: Wykeham Publications, 1971).

3. Laws, Priscilla W., *Medical and Dental X-rays: A Consumer's Guide to Avoiding Unnecessary Radiation Exposure* (New York: Public Citizens Health Research Group, 1974).

4. Robbins, Stanley L. and Marcia Angell, *Basic Pathology* (Philadelphia: W. B. Saunders Co., 1976).

5. Walter, J., *Cancer and Radiotherapy*, 2nd Edition (London: Churchill Livingston Co., 1977).

Additional Reading on Nuclear Risks

1. Caldicott, H. *Missile Envy*. Morrow, 1984.

2. Schell, J. *The Fate of the Earth*. Knopf, 1982.

17

Solar Radiation

Harriet S. Page and Ardyce J. Asire (NCI)

Cancer Rates and Risks, *3rd edition, 1985. National Cancer Institute, Bethesda, MD.*

Solar radiation is the chief cause of nonmelanoma skin cancer, responsible for about 90 percent of cases. It has also been linked with skin melanoma, but that relationship is more complex.

Though nonmelanoma skin cancers are now considered to be 98 percent curable, they still accounted for as many deaths in the United States during the 1950s and 1960s as did melanomas, which are far rarer but far more lethal (Mason et al, 1975). More than 400,000 new cases of nonmelanoma skin cancer are thought to occur in the United States each year, and this number is rising. Nonmelanoma skin cancer is the most common form of cancer among Caucasians.

The relationship between sun exposure and nonmelanoma skin cancer has been clarified greatly in the past decade. Observers had noted in the late 1800s that sailors exposed to the sun developed "Seamanshaut," or "sailor's skin," and in the early 1900s an excess risk of skin cancer was observed among farmers. The greater risk for Caucasians exposed to sun had also been observed (Hyde, 1906).

By 1928, scientists were able to demonstrate the cancer-causing effects of ultraviolet radiation on the skin of lab animals, using both sunlight and artificial light sources (Findlay, 1928). These carcinogenic effects were produced by ultraviolet-B (UV-B) radiation in the 290 to 320 namometer range, the same range that produces burning in human skin.

Though latitude, or distance from the equator, generally determines the amount of UV-B radiation in a given location, altitude and sky cover are also determining factors. Atlanta, Georgia, and El Paso, Texas, for example, are in the same general latitude (32 to 33° N). But El Paso, which is higher and drier, has an annual UV-B count 38 percent higher than Atlanta.

Time of day and time of year also affect the amount of UV-B radiation in any location. The greatest amount, of course, occurs during the summer months, and a third of the day's total amount occurs between the hours of 11 a.m. and 1 p.m. (or 12 noon and 2 p.m. DST).

In 1973, special meters designed to measure UV-B radiation were set up in a number of U.S. cities by Temple University in collaboration with the National Cancer Institute and other government agencies. Data from these meters permitted precise correlations, for the first time, with NCI data on skin cancer incidence in four of these cities, thus affording observations on human populations (Scotto et al, 1976).

The most striking association was the inverse relationship between latitude and nonmelanoma skin cancer incidence: the lower the latitude (the equator is at zero), the higher the incidence. The data also indicated that nonmelanoma skin cancer is related to annual, cumulative UV-B exposure, while skin melanoma may be related to brief exposure to high-intensity UV radiation.

Other findings from the UV-B stations and NCI incidence data are that in some parts of the South, the incidence of skin cancer exceeds that of all other cancers combined, and in parts of the North it accounts for about 40 percent of all cancers.

Another factor that affects UV-B exposure is the amount of ozone (O_3) in the atmosphere (Scotto et al, 1982). Ozone gases absorb most of the UV light in the upper stratosphere and let only small amounts reach the earth. There has been concern in the past decade that the exhaust gases of supersonic aircraft, some fluorocarbons (particularly those used in spray propellants), nuclear weapons, and nitrogen fertilizers could deplete this ozone layer. A Federal task force warned in 1975 that if 1972 levels of fluorocarbon release were continued, the ozone concentration would be reduced by up to 7 percent within several decades. It also observed that there would be about a 2 percent increase in UV-B radiation near the equator for each 1 percent reduction in stratospheric ozone concentration. These concerns are now being studied by a number of Federal agencies.

Solar radiation ranks high among the "lifestyle" factors associated with cancer. Most individuals have some choice in the amount of sunlight exposure they get, and too much sun is the chief cause of nonmelanoma skin cancer.

18

Iatrogenesis and Cancer

Harriet S. Page and Ardyce J. Asire (NCI)

Cancer Rates and Risks, *3rd edition, 1985. National Cancer Institute, Bethesda, MD.*

Iatrogenesis means "physician-caused illness." In recent history, there are a number of cases in which physicians have unknowingly caused cancer—for instance, the DES story. This chapter addresses that problem. It originally appeared as a chapter titled "Drugs" in Page and Asire's 1985 Cancer Rates and Risks (NCI, 3rd edition, 1985).—*M.R.*

The development of "miracle" drugs that effectively treat a variety of illnesses has been one of medicine's major achievements. Unfortunately, when chemically altering or arresting the course of one disease, these drugs can contribute to the development of other diseases, including cancer. Estrogenic hormones, immunosuppressive agents, and, ironically, anticancer drugs designed to kill tumor cells are the classes of drugs most often linked to human cancer.

Drugs are believed to account for fewer than 2 percent of all cancers. When deciding to use drugs, the informed patient and physician must carefully weigh the benefits of a medication against its possible risks.

Hormones

Estrogens are hormones, produced mainly by the ovaries, that help regulate menstruation and pregnancy. They are also responsible for the development of feminine body features. The ovaries produce several different estrogens—estradiol, estriol, and estrone—but because they have similar functions and chemical structures, they are collectively referred to as estrogens.

Many middle-aged and older women take synthetic "replacement" estrogens to relieve symptoms of menopause that may develop when their ovaries decrease production of these hormones. Such use has been linked to cancers of the endometrium, the lining of the uterus. One study reported that women who take replacement estrogens for more than 7 years increase their risk of endometrial cancer 14 times (Zeil and Finkle, 1975). It appears, though, that women who stop taking replacement estrogens decrease their risk of this cancer to the level of a nonuser after 2 years (Stolley and Hibberd, 1982).

It is not clear if replacement estrogens increase the risk of breast cancer in menopausal women. Several studies have shown a slightly increased risk (Hoover et al, 1976; Brinton, 1981; Ross, 1980; Thomas, 1982; Hoover, 1981; Jick and Walker, 1980; Hulka and Chambless, 1982) especially in long-term users. The groups these studies looked at differed, and other investigators have failed to show an association (Kelsey et al, 1981). Thus, results are not conclusive.

Synthetic estrogens are the chief ingredient of birth control pills. The most effective and most widely used birth control pills are "combination" pills that contain both estrogen and a second ovarian hormone, progestin. Pills that contain only progestin, called "minipills," are also available.

Combination pills may actually decrease a woman's risk of developing some cancers. Women who take these pills are only half as likely as nonusers to develop cancer of the ovary or endometrium; their use is estimated to prevent 1,700 cases of ovarian cancer and 2,000 cases of endometrial cancer each year (CDC, 1983).

A different form of birth control pills, known as "sequential" pills, were available at one time. They were taken off the market by the U.S. Food and Drug Administration in the late 1970s because studies linked them to an increased risk of endometrial cancer. Sequential pills provided separate estrogen and progestin in sequence: during the first weeks of her menstrual period, a woman took the estrogen pills, and in the last week took the progestin.

One study showed a sevenfold increase in risk of endometrial cancer among women who took one brand of sequential pills, but failed to find an increased risk among users of other brands (Weiss and Sayvetz, 1980). The risk was associated with the brand that contained the most potent form of estrogen and the weakest progestin.

The link between birth control pills and breast cancer is less clear. Most of the evidence suggests that women who use oral contraceptives do not have an increased risk of breast cancer despite duration of pill use and other variables. In some studies, though, specific groups of women who use these pills have been adversely affected: those with a family history of breast cancer or those with benign breast disease. A recent study suggested a fourfold increase in breast cancer incidence among women under age 36 who were long-term users of combination pills containing a "high" dose of progestin (Pike et al, 1983). Other recent studies have linked oral contraceptives with an elevated risk of cervical cancer, even after sexual activity and other risk factors for this cancer were taken into account.

DES (diethylstilbestrol), an estrogen-like compound, has been widely publicized as a cancer-causing drug. During the 1940s and 1950s, doctors prescribed DES to pregnant women because they believed the drug helped prevent miscarriages. Although studies in the 1930s had shown that DES caused cancer in laboratory animals, the problem received little attention until the 1970s, when a rare vaginal and cervical cancer was found in a number of young women living in areas where DES had been widely prescribed. Histories showed that the patients had been exposed to DES *in utero* when their mothers took the drug (Herbst et al, 1971). It is now thought that between four and six million Americans—mothers, daughters, and sons—may have had pregnancy-related exposure to DES. The DES findings also provided the first evidence that a carcinogen could travel across the placental barrier from the mother to the fetus.

There have been few studies of the effects of DES on women who took it, and those studies produced conflicting results. One study showed some increased risk of cancer of the breast and reproductive organs in these women (Bibbo et al, 1978); another showed no such link (Brian et al, 1980).

DES has not been associated with cancers of the reproductive tract in sons of women who took it, but anatomic abnormalities of the sperm and reproductive tract have been reported in these men. Studies to see if these abnormalities affect their fertility have been delayed because, as a group, these DES sons seem to have postponed starting families (DES Task Force, 1978).

Androgens, a class of male hormones, are structurally related to estrogens. Synthetic androgens are used to treat various cancers, some genetic diseases, and some blood and endocrine disorders. Some athletes use androgens to increase body mass and athletic performance.

Studies have shown an increased incidence of liver cancer among children who received androgens for the treatment of some types of anemias (Johnson et al, 1972). It is not known, though, if the liver cancer these children developed resulted from the androgens or the disease.

Anticancer Drugs

In the last decade, anticancer drugs have prolonged the lives of many thousands of cancer patients. A number of these patients have developed second cancers.

Alkylating agents are a class of drugs used to treat a variety of cancers. They work by inserting foreign molecules into the genetic material of dividing cancer cells. These foreign molecules act like wrenches thrown into the machinery of the cell, preventing growth and division.

Alkylating agents may also cause mutations in the cell's genetic material, similar to the mutations caused by ionizing radiation, and lead to cancer. Several studies have shown that Hodgkin's disease patients treated with alkylating agents have an increased incidence of acute myelocytic leukemia (AML).

Not a single case of AML was found in more than 3,000 Hodgkin's disease patients studied before 1962 (Moertel and Hagedorn, 1957 and Berg, 1967). But a study done between 1961 and 1973 showed that Hodgkin's disease patients were developing AML at a rate of 156 cases per 100,000 population (Weiden et al, 1973). The greatest incidence of AML in this 12-year study occurred from 1970 to 1973, a few years after the MOPP regimen (nitrogen mustard, vincristine [Oncovin], prednisone, and procarbazine) was introduced in 1967. Both nitrogen mustard and procarbazine are alkylating agents. The risk of leukemias after treatment of Hodgkin's disease has

continued to increase, especially among patients who receive both MOPP and radiation therapy.

Alkylating drugs used to treat other cancers have also been linked to cancer. Epidemiologic studies showed a hundredfold increase in AML among multiple myeloma patients after the drug melphalan was introduced (Adamson and Sieber, 1977). A recent survey of women treated for ovarian cancer showed that melphalan and chlorambucil increase the leukemia risk in steps that correlate with dose (Greene et al, 1982).

The risk of acute leukemia has also been shown to rise after use of alkylating agents to treat lung cancer (Stott et al, 1977), the blood disorder known as polycythemia vera (Berk et al, 1981), and non-Hodgkin's lymphoma (Greene et al, 1983).

The alkylating agent methyl-CCNU (semustine), used to treat cancers of the stomach, colon, and rectum, was recently shown to increase a patient's risk of developing leukemia by sixteenfold (Boice et al, 1983). Most surveys of chemotherapy-related cancers have focused on leukemia because it develops within 4 to 5 years after exposure. The risk of other cancers has not been evaluated in a systematic way because most exposed patients have not lived long enough to develop other cancers.

Immunosuppressive Drugs

Drugs that suppress the immune system are given to organ transplant patients to help them accept a foreign organ. Azathioprine and adrenal corticosteroid hormones were widely used in the past for kidney transplant patients, and cyclosporin A has been used recently. Non-Hodgkin's lymphoma, the most common type of cancer in these patients, occurs 32 times more often among them than in the general population (Hoover and Fraumeni, 1973). The lymphoma often arises rapidly—within a year or two—after the transplant operation, and often develops in the brain, an unusual site for this type of cancer (Hoover, 1977). Some other cancers—skin cancers, Kaposi's sarcoma, and lung cancer—also occur at a high rate in transplant recipients.

Other Drugs

Radioactive drugs contain a molecule "tagged" with a radioactive isotope so the isotope can be counted or imaged in diagnostic tests. Radioactive drugs can concentrate in body tissues and, depending on their strength and half-life, may injure those tissues. Radioactive drugs are also used to treat bone tuberculosis, thyroid cancer, and the blood disorder polycythemia vera. Some of these radioactive drugs have been shown to cause various cancers, including osteogenic sarcoma, a type of bone cancer; leukemias; and a rare form of liver cancer (Hoover and Fraumeni, 1981).

In 1964, chlornaphazine, a drug used to treat polycythemia vera and Hodgkin's lymphoma, was withdrawn from the market because it was found to cause bladder cancer. Chlornaphazine is chemically related to beta-naphthylamine, a chemical earlier associated with bladder cancer among workers in the dye industry.

Other drugs have also been found to increase the rate of human cancers. Pain-killing drugs that contain phenacetin have been linked to kidney cancers, and methoxypsoralens, used with ultraviolet-A radiation in the PUVA regimen for psoriasis, have been linked with skin cancer.

19

Air and Water Pollution

Harriet S. Page and Ardyce J. Asire (NCI)

Cancer Rates and Risks, *3rd edition, 1985. National Cancer Institute, Bethesda, MD.*

As a nation we have learned that the air around us may become contaminated with industrial and automotive emissions, and that this may happen to our seas, lakes, rivers, and groundwater supplies as well. Americans are becoming increasingly concerned with this issue, but there is still very little conclusive information about the effects of such pollution on the incidence of cancer.

Each of us, at various times, may be exposed to potential carcinogens in the air we breathe and the water we drink. Though the number of such substances is large, the levels are generally small—much smaller, for example, than the levels found in some workplaces. On the other hand, carcinogens in air and water may be harder to avoid than those found in specific workplace locations. It has been estimated that pollution accounts for at most 1 to 5 percent of all cancer deaths (Doll and Peto, 1981).

Air Pollution

There is little evidence to date that ambient air—the circulating air around us—poses serious cancer risks. The ambient air in specific areas may contain industrial plant emissions, automobile exhaust, and other pollutants linked to cancer, but in most places, the air we breathe does not contain high levels of carcinogens. In fact, the strongest link between air pollution and cancer is found among smokers, who inhale particulates in their tobacco smoke.

Much of what we know about the health effects of large amounts of pollutants in the air comes from workplace studies of coal gas, tar, pitch, and coke oven emissions. Certain workers may be at some risk but workplace exposures are often 10 to 1000 times the levels found in ambient air.

Asbestos is a known carcinogen found in the air around some workplaces. Levels vary, but are highest near asbestos mines, mills, waste dumps, and manufacturing plants. Asbestos is the only cause of mesothelioma, a form of cancer that affects the membrane lining of the chest and abdominal cavities. It is rare in the general population, but found frequently among workers exposed to high levels of airborne asbestos. Asbestos can also cause lung cancer. Studies of shipbuilders in coastal areas of Georgia, Florida, and Virginia, many of whom were exposed to asbestos insulation, showed an increased risk of lung cancer in all areas, and of mesothelioma in Virginia, particularly among employees who worked during World War II (Blot and Fraumeni, 1981). There may also be risks of exposure during demolition of buildings that contain asbestos used for fireproofing in walls and ceilings. There has been concern, for example, about children's exposure to asbestos in older school buildings. It is sometimes safer to cover interior asbestos than to try to remove it.

Benzo(a)pyrene, or B(a)P, is a combustion product. B(a)P levels in ambient air in this country have decreased since the 1930s and 1940s when oil and natural gas—which burn more cleanly—replaced coal for home heating (Shy and Struba, 1982). A study of roofers exposed to high levels of B(a)P in hot pitch showed a higher incidence of lung cancer among them than in the general population (Hammond et al, 1976).

Lung cancer incidence is higher in cities than in the country, but this is not necessarily due to urban air pollution. Workplace exposures and other lifestyle factors of city dwellers, like cigarette smoking, may be more important (Buell, 1967; Cederlof, 1975). The "urban factor" is much weaker than cigarette smoking on lung cancer incidence.

Increased death rates from chronic, non-malignant lung diseases like bronchitis, particularly among the elderly, have been linked with "brown-outs," smogs, and other episodes of serious air pollution. Sulfur dioxide from older power plants and smelters is the main component of acid rain. It can also aggravate chronic lung disease. Few cancer studies have looked at any link with acid rain, but it produces other effects like damage to trees and to aquatic life in lakes and rivers.

Exposure to radioactive emissions from radon in uranium mines has been shown to be responsible for the increased risk of lung cancer in miners. Recent concern has focused on radon exposures in homes, particularly those that have been made airtight by efficient insulation. The radon can enter the home from soil, water, or building materials. Some researchers estimate that as many as 10,000 cancers a year may result in this country from indoor radon pollution. Cigarette smoke is another form of indoor pollution that has been linked to increased lung cancer, but the extent of the hazards from both radon and passive smoking is not now clear.

Water Pollution

Drinking water contains complex mixtures of known and suspected carcinogens including asbestos, metals, radioactive substances, and industrial chemicals. Even the process of treating water may create small quantities of chemicals linked to cancer, but the levels are so small that there is probably a low risk, if any, associated with most drinking water supplies.

Trihalomethanes, or THMs, can be formed when chlorine used to purify drinking water reacts with organic compounds in water. At levels normally found in chlorinated city water supplies, there is some suspicion that THMs may increase the risk of gastrointestinal and urinary tract cancers (Crump and Guess, 1982). THMs are also used as indicators of more hazardous compounds that are difficult to measure directly. To reduce the levels of THMs, water is often filtered so that less chlorine is needed to purify it.

A few other chemicals that have been found in drinking water from a small number of supplies are known to cause cancer in humans (Harris et al, 1977). Vinyl chloride, for example, may be introduced into drinking water from industrial plants, or, in very small amounts, by seepage from polyvinyl chloride piping used in some water distribution systems. Benzene and bis(2-chloroethyl)ether are other carcinogens that are occasionally found in drinking water (Kraybill et al, 1980).

Nitrates are seldom removed during the water treatment process. Nitrates themselves do not cause cancer, but they can be transformed in the body into nitrosamines, which are powerful carcinogens. Although some studies have found a link between high levels of nitrates in drinking water and gastric cancer (Cuello et al, 1976; Geleprin et al, 1976), there is no indication that the low levels sometimes found in drinking water pose a risk of cancer.

Asbestos fibers are widely distributed in water supplies in this country, with higher levels often found near cities and industrial centers. But studies have not shown consistently that asbestos in drinking water affects cancer risk (Shy and Struba, 1982).

The trace metals arsenic, chromium, and nickel are found in drinking water in varying amounts. They may come from industrial plants, mines, seepage from soil or piping, by mineralization from rocks, or from water treatment processes. High levels of arsenic in drinking water in some other countries have been linked with skin cancer (Tseng et al, 1968; Tseng, 1976) but the much lower concentrations in U.S. drinking water have not been linked with cancer in humans.

Radioactive substances may be found in water depending on local rock type and on the use and disposal of radioactive compounds by nearby industries, hospitals, and nuclear power plants. Radioactive strontium and radium, sometimes found in some water supplies, can accumulate in bone tissue but even the cumulative dose from radium would result in so few fatal bone cancers that they would probably not be detected in epidemiologic studies. Naturally occurring radon gas is found dissolved in water in some parts of the United States. Ingestion of radon in water does not pose much of a hazard, because of its low concentration. Radon can be released, though, from water into household air via showers and washing machines. Studies are trying now to evaluate the risk of such exposures.

Water that percolates down below the earth's surface, known as groundwater, is often the source of spring and well water. Aquifers—rock formations that hold water in underground "lakes"—may also be sources for springs and wells. Contamination of these water sources with pesticides, industrial solvents, and other industrial chemicals such as polychlorinated biphenyls, or PCBs, can become a serious problem. Disposing of such wastes in lagoons or landfills can contribute to groundwater contamination.

Burying hazardous wastes on land is the most common method of disposal in this country because it is inexpensive. Disposal sites can leak, however, contaminating groundwater with toxic substances. Contamination of groundwater could become more widespread as older disposal sites begin to leak, but cleanups and better disposal methods can prevent contamination. Environmental Protection Agency regulations now require that hazardous waste disposal be completed in safer ways than in the past.

The major United States water supplies are continually monitored for carcinogens under Environmental Protection Agency guidelines. National Cancer Institute scientists have been studying the possible link between cancer and drinking water quality (Cantor et al, 1978). Except for some drinking water supplies that contain unusually high levels of carcinogens, the evidence to date suggests that our drinking water now poses little cancer risk to us.

4

Major Sites of Cancer

20

Cancer Review

Mark Renneker, M.D.

Based on the information collected for each cancer-site chapter, the following "Cancer Review" is presented as a way of summarizing and comparing the major cancers. The Cancer Review is based on my review of the cancer literature, as of early 1988. (Some people in the cancer field may quibble over, for instance, whether a given category should have received two stars instead of three. Remember, though, that the Cancer Review is just that—a review—like a review of a restaurant or movie, and using the same "stars" system.)

The principal sources for the Cancer Review (and each cancer-site chapter) are as follows:

1. American Cancer Society—*Facts and Figures, 1988.*

2. DeVita VT, Hellman S, Rosenberg SA. *Cancer—Principles and Practice of Oncology.* 2nd edition. J.B. Lippincott Co., Philadelphia. 1985.

3. Doll R, Peto R. *The Causes of Cancer.* Oxford University Press, Inc., New York. 1981.

4. Page HS, Asire AJ. *Cancer Rates and Risks.* National Institutes of Health (pub. No. 85-691), April, 1985.

5. Rubin P. *Clinical Oncology—a Multidisciplinary Approach.* The American Cancer Society. 6th edition. 1983.

6. Schottenfeld D, Fraumeni JF. *Cancer Epidemiology and Prevention.* W. B. Saunders Co., Phil. 1982.

To account for the lag-time from publication of the above books, reference was made to a wide variety of articles and professional sources, particularly *The New England Journal of Medicine, Cancer, The Journal of the National Cancer Institute,* and *Ca—A Cancer Journal.*

CANCER SITES

	Bladder/Kidney Cancer Chapter 30 page 166	Brain/CNS Cancer Chapter 37 page 182	Breast Cancer Chapter 24 page 139	Childhood Cancers Chapter 44 page 202	Colon/Rectal Cancer Chapter 23 page 135	Esophagus Cancer Chapter 33 page 174	Larynx Cancer Chapter 32 page 172	Leukemias Chapter 42 page 196
Epidemiology								
Sex (M: male, F: female)	M more than F	M more than F	F much more than M	M more or equal to F	M equal to F	M more than F	M more than F	M more or equal to F
Age (range of peak incidence)	over 60	3–12; 50–70	55–70	0–5 greater than 5–18	70–80	over 60	60–75	all ages
Cases Annually (approximately)	70,000	15,000	**143,000**	7000	**151,000**	10,000	12,000	27,000
Incidence	increasing	constant	increasing	constant	increasing	increasing	increasing	constant
Causes/Risk Factors Strength of evidence for the listed factor as a cause of that type of cancer, and the approximate number of cases attributable to that factor.								
Diet (causative, rather than preventive)	clearly implicated; significant number of cases	slightly implicated; very few cases	**strongly implicated; large number of cases**	not shown to be a factor	**strongly implicated; large number of cases**	clearly implicated; significant number of cases	somewhat implicated; some cases	not shown to be a factor
Tobacco (smoked and smokeless)	**strongly implicated; large number of cases**	not shown to be a factor	not shown to be a factor	not shown to be a factor	not shown to be a factor	**strongly implicated; large number of cases**	**strongly implicated; large number of cases**	slightly implicated; very few cases
Infection (primarily viruses, but also parasites)	somewhat implicated; some cases	somewhat implicated; some cases	slightly implicated; very few cases	somewhat implicated; some cases	slightly implicated; very few cases	slightly implicated; very few cases	slightly implicated; very few cases	somewhat implicated; some cases
Occupation (exposure at work, primarily chemical)	clearly implicated; significant number of cases	somewhat implicated; some cases	slightly implicated; very few cases	not shown to be a factor	slightly implicated; very few cases	slightly implicated; very few cases	somewhat implicated; some cases	slightly implicated; very few cases
Alcohol (alcohol alone or with smoking)	slightly implicated; very few cases	not shown to be a factor	somewhat implicated; some cases	not shown to be a factor	not shown to be a factor	**strongly implicated; large number of cases**	clearly implicated; significant number of cases	not shown to be a factor
Radiation (ionizing/medical, or non-ionizing/ sun)	somewhat implicated; some cases	somewhat implicated; some cases	somewhat implicated; some cases	slightly implicated; very few cases	not shown to be a factor	slightly implicated; very few cases	slightly implicated; very few cases	somewhat implicated; some cases
Genetics/ Heredity (inherited risk, family history)	slightly implicated; very few cases	somewhat implicated; some cases	**strongly implicated; large number of cases**	somewhat implicated; some cases	clearly implicated; significant number of cases	slightly implicated; very few cases	slightly implicated; very few cases	somewhat implicated; some cases
Unique causative factors	chemicals	whites	no children	congenital	polyps	blacks	blacks	drugs
Prevention/Early Detection								
Primary prevention (prevent from beginning)	**excellent chance of prevention**	hard to prevent	limited chance of prevention	limited chance of prevention	very good chance of prevention	**excellent chance of prevention**	**excellent chance of prevention**	limited chance of prevention
Secondary prevention (early detection)	limited chance of early detection	hard to detect early	**excellent chance of early detection**	limited chance of detecting early	**excellent chance of early detection**	hard to detect early	very good chance of early detection	hard to detect early
Treatment/Prognosis								
Treatments used (? indicates that treatment is experimental, but may be effective)	surgery radiation therapy chemotherapy ? immunotherapy ?	surgery radiation therapy chemotherapy ? immunotherapy ?	surgery radiation therapy chemotherapy immunotherapy ?	surgery radiation therapy chemotherapy	surgery radiation therapy chemotherapy immunotherapy ?	surgery radiation therapy chemotherapy	surgery radiation therapy chemotherapy ?	chemotherapy radiation therapy immunotherapy
Overall cure rate (percent free of cancer five years after treatment)	possibly curable 75%/40%	possibly curable 25%	**fairly curable 75%**	possibly curable 50–90%	possibly curable 55%	rarely curable 6%	**fairly curable 70%**	possibly curable 30%

CANCER SITES

	Liver/Biliary Cancer Chapter 36 page 180	Lung Cancer Chapter 22 page 132	Lymphoma (Hodgkin's) Chapter 41 page 192	Lymphoma (non-Hodgkin's) Chapter 41 page 192	Mouth and Throat Cancer Chapter 31 page 169	Multiple Myeloma Chapter 43 page 200	Ovarian Cancer Chapter 27 page 157	Pancreas Cancer Chapter 35 page 178
Epidemiology								
Sex (M: male, F: female)	M equal to F	M more than F	M more than F	M more than F	M more than F	M more than F	F	M more than F
Age (range of peak incidence)	over 65	55–65	20s, 70s	50–70	over 45	over 50	65–84	70–79
Cases Annually (approximately)	15,000	**155,000**	7,500	33,000	31,000	12,000	20,000	27,000
Incidence	decreasing	increasing	constant	increasing	increasing	constant	constant	increasing
Causes/Risk Factors Strength of evidence for the listed factor as a cause of that type of cancer, and the approximate number of cases attributable to that factor.								
Diet (causative, rather than preventive)	clearly implicated; significant number of cases	somewhat implicated; some cases	not shown to be a factor	not shown to be a factor	slightly implicated; very few cases	not shown to be a factor	somewhat implicated; some cases	clearly implicated; significant number of cases
Tobacco (smoked and smokeless)	not shown to be a factor	**strongly implicated; large number of cases**	not shown to be a factor	not shown to be a factor	**strongly implicated; large number of cases**	not shown to be a factor	not shown to be a factor	somewhat implicated; some cases
Infection (primarily viruses, but also parasites)	**strongly implicated; large number of cases**	slightly implicated; very few cases	clearly implicated; significant number of cases	clearly implicated; significant number of cases	not shown to be a factor	slightly implicated; very few cases	not shown to be a factor	not shown to be a factor
Occupation (exposure at work, primarily chemical)	somewhat implicated; some cases	clearly implicated; significant number of cases	slightly implicated; very few cases	slightly implicated; very few cases	slightly implicated; very few cases	somewhat implicated; some cases	slightly implicated; very few cases	somewhat implicated; some cases
Alcohol (alcohol alone or with smoking)	**strongly implicated; large number of cases**	not shown to be a factor	not shown to be a factor	not shown to be a factor	**strongly implicated; large number of cases**	not shown to be a factor	not shown to be a factor	somewhat implicated; some cases
Radiation (ionizing/medical, or non-ionizing/sun)	slightly implicated; very few cases	somewhat implicated; some cases	slightly implicated; very few cases	slightly implicated; very few cases	slightly implicated; very few cases	somewhat implicated; some cases	slightly implicated; very few cases	slightly implicated; very few cases
Genetics/ Heredity (inherited risk, family history)	slightly implicated; very few cases	slightly implicated; very few cases	slightly implicated; very few cases	slightly implicated; very few cases	not shown to be a factor	slightly implicated; very few cases	slightly implicated; very few cases	slightly implicated; very few cases
Unique causative factors	gallstones	second-hand smoke	rich	immunity	poor	blacks	no children	poor
Prevention/Early Detection								
Primary prevention (prevent from beginning)	very good chance of prevention	**excellent chance of prevention**	hard to prevent	hard to prevent	**excellent chance of prevention**	hard to prevent	hard to prevent	very good chance of prevention
Secondary prevention (early detection)	hard to detect early	hard to detect early	hard to detect early	hard to detect early	**excellent chance of early detection**	hard to detect early	hard to detect early	hard to detect early
Treatment/Prognosis								
Treatments used (? indicates that treatment is experimental, but may be effective)	surgery radiation therapy ? chemotherapy ?	surgery radiation therapy chemotherapy immunotherapy ?	radiation therapy chemotherapy	radiation therapy chemotherapy immunotherapy	surgery radiation therapy chemotherapy	chemotherapy radiation therapy immunotherapy ?	surgery chemotherapy radiation therapy	surgery radiation therapy ? chemotherapy ?
Overall cure rate (percent free of cancer five years after treatment)	rarely curable 5%	rarely curable 13%	**fairly curable 70%**	possibly curable 50%	possibly curable 50%	possibly curable 25%	rarely curable 35%	rarely curable 3%

Prostate Cancer Chapter 25 page 147	Sarcomas: Bone, Cartilage and Soft-Tissue Chapter 39 page 187	Skin Cancer (Melanoma) Chapter 21 page 123	Skin Cancer (non-Melanoma) Chapter 21 page 123	Stomach Cancer Chapter 34 page 176	Testicular Cancer Chapter 29 page 163	Thyroid Cancer Chapter 38 page 184	Uterine-Cervical Cancer Chapter 26 page 150	Uterine-Endometrial Cancer Chapter 26 page 150	Vaginal Cancer Chapter 28 page 160
M	M equal to F	M more or equal to F	M more than F	M more than F	M	F more than M	F	F	F
over 50	under 18	over 20	45 to 75	50–59	15–35	25–65	25–55	55–65	over 40
103,000	8,000	27,000	**500,000 +**	20,000	6,000	11,500	13,000	34,000	21,000
increasing	constant	increasing	increasing	increasing	increasing	increasing	increasing	increasing	increasing
clearly implicated; significant number of cases	not shown to be a factor	not shown to be a factor	not shown to be a factor	**strongly implicated; large number of cases**	not shown to be a factor	slightly implicated; very few cases	slightly implicated; very few cases	**strongly implicated; large number of cases**	somewhat implicated; some cases
not shown to be a factor	not shown to be a factor	not shown to be a factor	not shown to be a factor	somewhat implicated; some cases	not shown to be a factor	not shown to be a factor	somewhat implicated; some cases	different studies have shown both positive and negative effects	not shown to be a factor
slightly implicated; very few cases	slightly implicated; very few cases	not shown to be a factor	not shown to be a factor	not shown to be a factor	somewhat implicated; some cases	not shown to be a factor	clearly implicated; significant number of cases	slightly implicated; very few cases	slightly implicated; very few cases
slightly implicated; very few cases	somewhat implicated; some cases	slightly implicated; very few cases	slightly implicated; very few cases	slightly implicated; very few cases	slightly implicated; very few cases	slightly implicated; very few cases	not shown to be a factor	not shown to be a factor	not shown to be a factor
not shown to be a factor	not shown to be a factor	not shown to be a factor	not shown to be a factor	slightly implicated; very few cases	not shown to be a factor	not shown to be a factor	not shown to be a factor	not shown to be a factor	not shown to be a factor
not shown to be a factor	clearly implicated; significant number of cases	**strongly implicated; large number of cases**	**strongly implicated; large number of cases**	slightly implicated; very few cases	somewhat implicated; some cases	clearly implicated; significant number of cases	not shown to be a factor	not shown to be a factor	somewhat implicated; some cases
slightly implicated; very few cases	somewhat implicated; some cases	somewhat implicated; some cases	clearly implicated; significant number of cases	somewhat implicated; some cases	slightly implicated; very few cases	somewhat implicated; some cases	not shown to be a factor	somewhat implicated; some cases	not shown to be a factor
blacks	congenital	whites	whites	Japanese	undescended testes	Hawaiians	sex	estrogens	DES
limited chance of prevention	hard to prevent	**excellent chance of prevention**	**excellent chance of prevention**	very good chance of prevention	very good chance of prevention	limited chance of prevention	**excellent chance of prevention**	very good chance of prevention	limited chance of prevention
limited chance of early detection	hard to detect early	very good chance of early detection	**excellent chance of early detection**	limited chance of early detection	very good chance of early detection	limited chance of early detection	**excellent chance of early detection**	very good chance of early detection	very good chance of early detection
surgery chemotherapy radiation therapy	surgery radiation therapy chemotherapy	surgery chemotherapy radiation therapy immunotherapy	surgery chemotherapy radiation therapy	surgery radiation therapy ? chemotherapy ?	surgery chemotherapy radiation therapy	surgery radiation therapy chemotherapy	surgery radiation therapy chemotherapy immunotherapy ?	surgery radiation therapy chemotherapy	surgery radiation therapy
fairly curable 70%	**fairly curable 50%**	**fairly curable 80%**	**highly curable 95%**	rarely curable 10%	**highly curable 90%**	**fairly curable 95%**	**fairly curable 65%**	**fairly curable 80%**	**fairly curable 30%**

The major sites of cancer are presented in the following chapters. Each chapter consists of:

Description: an overview of the cancer's significance, essential anatomy of the affected site, the natural history of the cancer, and the pathological cell types involved;

Epidemiology and Risk Factors: number of cases per year in United States, male–female and racial distribution, worldwide epidemiology, and then a discussion of the role of diet, tobacco, infection, occupational, radiation, heredity, and other risk factors;

Primary Prevention and Early Detection: what steps can be taken to reduce the chance of developing the cancer, or to find it early;

Symptoms and Diagnosis: the common symptoms of the cancer, and what tests are done to diagnose it;

Treatment and Prognosis: the role of surgery, radiation therapy, chemotherapy, and immunotherapy in treating the cancer, aspects of rehabilitation, and what are the chances for survival.

21

Skin Cancer

Mark Renneker, M.D.

About one-in-seven Americans will get skin cancer. Skin cancer is classified as either melanoma or non-melanoma. The non-melanoma skin cancers are the most common of all cancers, and primarily include the highly curable basal and squamous cell cancers. The melanoma, or "black mole," kind of skin cancer is less common and more often fatal. Its full name, malignant melanoma, bespeaks its dangerous nature, but most physicians refer to it simply as melanoma.

The basal cell type of skin cancer arises from the cells underlying the skin, called basal cells, which form a kind of basement for the skin to build on. Basal cell skin cancers are also called basal cell epitheliomas, meaning that they are tumors of the epithelial layer of the body. Epithelial simply refers to skin.

The squamous cell type of skin cancer arises from layers of cells above and alongside the basal cells, called the stratified squamous epithelium, which is the "skin" that you can see and touch. Though squamous cell skin cancers are also from the epithelium, they are considered carcinomas rather than epitheliomas, reflecting their more carcinoma-like nature of spread.

Melanomas develop from melanocytes, which are highly specialized cells that produce the pigment melanin. Melanin gives your skin color and allows you to tan. Melanocytes are found in places other than the skin, for instance the eyes, mouth, and GI tract, so there can be non-cutaneous (non-skin) melanomas, but they are rare.

The basal cell type is by far the most common skin cancer, accounting for between 75 and 90% of all skin cancers. The major cause of all skin cancers is ultraviolet exposure from the sun, but heredity—your type of skin—plays a large role, too.

EPIDEMIOLOGY AND RISK FACTORS

There are over 500,000 non-melanoma skin cancers diagnosed each year in the United States, making it the most common cancer. Less than 1% of non-melanoma skin cancers are fatal, but it is a significant cause of cosmetic disfigurement and cost—over $200 million a year.

However, because non-melanoma skin cancers are curable 95 to 100% of the time, and because they so rarely act like other cancers (i.e., they seldom metastasize) they are not included in the usual cancer statistics. For instance, in 1987 approximately 965,000 cancers were reported in the United States (including 26,000 cases of melanoma, but no non-melanoma skin cancers). There were over 500,000 non-melanoma skin cancers that same year, bringing the actual number of cancers for 1987 to almost one-and-a-half-million (even though the 965,000 figure would be cited for 1987s cancer incidence).

Non-Melanoma

The incidence of non-melanoma skin cancers is in direct proportion to the degree of ultraviolet (UV) light exposure and the fairness of skin. Fair-skinned whites living in sunny places are the most susceptible, but dark-skinned people can get skin cancer, too, though blacks about 100 times less frequently. The highest incidence in the world is in white South Africans and Australians. Those people of Celtic ancestry (i.e., Irish or Scottish descent), are particularly susceptible, especially if they are exposed to a lot of sunlight.

White males get about twice as many skin cancers as white women. The cancers occur most often on uncovered sun-exposed areas: the face, head, and neck in both sexes, but consistent with patterns of dress and work in relation to sun exposure, women get more skin cancers on their legs (dress) and men more on their lips (outdoor work). Being older is not a risk factor, except for the likelihood of accumulating more years of sun-exposure. These cancers are rare in the very young.

The chief risk factor for non-melanoma skin cancer is exposure to non-ionizing radiation, like sunlight [see Figure 21-1]. Sunlight consists of electromagnetic radiation ranging from 290 to 4000 nanometers in wavelength. Infrared (760–4000 nanometers) and visible light (400–760 nanometers) are not associated with sunburn or skin cancers, but ultraviolet radiation is (200 to 400 nanometers). The shortest wavelength of ultraviolet, called UVC (200–290 nanometers) is completely screened out by the ozone layer, but we are exposed to the UVB por-

tion (290–320 nanometers) and the longer wavelength UVA portion (320–400 nanometers). The UVB portion is our primary concern in terms of skin cancer.

Tanning parlors have become popular in the past few years. At first, lamps were used that emitted chiefly UVB radiation, but when the risks became known there was a shift to UVA lamps. However, UVA radiation is not harmless. It can aggravate prior UVB skin damage, suppress immune response, harm the eyes, and increase susceptibility to the same diseases and photosensitivities as natural sunlight. A tanning parlor UVA produced tan provides only limited protection against subsequent UVB exposure. In other words, a tanning parlor-acquired-tan won't protect you on a Hawaiian vacation.

The ozone layer is our natural protection from developing skin cancers. Scarcely three millimeters thick, the ozone layer around the earth filters out most of the sun's ultraviolet light. Evidence indicates that the ozone layer is being depleted by aircraft exhaust gases, above-ground nuclear weapon use, and chlorine from the decomposition of halocarbons, which can last in the atmosphere for well over 100 years. Halocarbons include the chlorofluorocarbons used as a propellant gas in aerosolized cans, and the fluids (freon) in air conditioners and refrigerators. One molecule of chlorine gas can destroy 100 molecules of ozone. It is predicted that if the ozone layer depletion continues at the present rate, there will have been an additional 88 million cancers and 800,000 deaths by the year 2075.

Ionizing radiation is also a risk, with reports of increased skin cancer in radiation workers, uranium miners, radiologists, and people receiving radiation treatments (e.g., for acne, eczema, thyroid disease, and cancer). Various chemicals cause skin cancer, particularly squamous cell cancer, including the polycyclic aromatic hydrocarbons found in coal tars, pitch, asphalt, soot, creosotes, and lubricating and cutting oils. For instance, coal miners get more skin cancers and so do psoriasis patients, whose treatment often includes coal tar ointments. Arsenic-containing compounds, including many agricultural sprays, also cause skin cancers.

There is an increased risk of squamous cell cancer at skin sites where severe or long-term damage has occurred, for example in major scars, burn areas, chronic ulcerations, or areas of irradiation (for instance from medical treatments).

There are also increased skin cancer rates among people with skin defects, for instance the condition called xeroderma pigmentosa, in which the skin lacks the DNA repair mechanism necessary for recovery from sun-damage. Albinos or people with areas of vitiligo (white patches of skin with little or no pigment) also have a greater risk of skin cancer.

Figure 21-1 Solar Radiation: Intensity at Sea Level and Effects on the Skin in Terms of Tanning, Sunburn, Aging, and Carcinogenesis. *Source:* Reprinted by permission of *The Physical and Sportsmedicine.* McGraw-Hill Publications.

	UVC (200−290 nm)	UVB (290−320 nm)	UVA (320−400 nm)	Visible (400−760 nm)	Infrared (760−3,000 nm)
Radiation at sea level (mW/cm²)					
Sun at zenith	0	.5	6.3	48.9	56.3
Sun 20° from zenith	0	.3	5.0	41.0	49.0
Sunburn†	—	4 +	1 +	—	—
Erythema	Very high	Very high	Low	—	—
MErD (J/cm²)	—	.02−.07	20−100	—	—
Tanning†	—	2 +	4 +	—	—
Melanogenesis	Lowest	High	Moderately high	—	—
Immediate	None	Least	High	—	—
Aging†	—	4 +	2 +	—	—
Cancer†	—	4 +	2 +	—	—
Dyskeratosis	Highest	High	Least	—	—
Targets	DNA	DNA	DNA	—	—
	—	RNA	—	—	—
	—	Protein	—	—	—
	—	Cell membranes	—	—	—

†Units are on a scale of 1 to 4; 1 indicates minimal effect and 4 indicates greatest effect.

Melanoma

Whites have the highest incidence of melanoma; it is uncommon in Africans, Polynesians, and Asians. In the United States, the annual incidence is ten times higher among whites compared to blacks. Australians have an extremely high incidence. The incidence is sharply rising worldwide, and has doubled every ten years for the past thirty years. The reason for Australia's enormous increase is thought to be the combination of their largely English-stock skin types, combined with their high-sun exposure and largely coastal life style.

Melanoma can strike people of all ages, but is less common among the very young. However, highly sun-exposed babies and children are considered to be at high-risk for later developing melanoma, particularly if they have had recurrent blistering sunburns.

A melanoma can appear almost anywhere on the body. In fair-skinned people they occur most often on the trunk in men and on the legs in women, but are frequent on the head, neck, and arms in both sexes. The palms and soles of the feet are most common sites for dark-skinned people.

The highest risk area is the site of a prior severe, blistering sunburn. Overall, though, melanoma is not as strongly related to ultraviolet exposure as are the other skin cancers. Other factors are significant in melanoma, including genetics and inherited traits.

Melanomas can "run in the family," but this accounts for only about 10% of all cases. Families at greatest risk are those with both a history of melanoma and the inherited condition known as dysplastic nevi syndrome (described below).

Hormonal factors have been associated with melanoma, with some studies showing an increased risk of melanoma from birth control pills. There have been reports associating occupational exposures with melanoma, including polychlorinated biphenyls (PCBs) and petrochemical exposure.

Ionizing radiation has not been so strongly linked to melanoma as with the non-melanoma skin cancers. However, it has been suspected as a contributing factor in the more than 40 cases of melanoma that have occurred since 1972 among workers at the Lawrence Livermore National Laboratory in Livermore, California. There are similar reports with respect to other such laboratories.

PREVENTION AND EARLY DETECTION

One obvious means of primary prevention of both non-melanomas and melanomas is to avoid the damaging effects of the sun. Skin types can be characterized by their degree of sensitivity to UV light, ranging from always burns easily and never tans, to tans completely and never burns. Knowing your skin type is helpful in planning an approach to skin cancer prevention. [See Figure 21-2.]

Maximal protection is achieved by avoiding peak sun periods (between 10 and 3 pm), avoiding highly-reflective surfaces like snow, sand, and water, wearing protective clothing and covering up (especially with wide-brimmed hats, long-sleeves, and pants), and the use of sunscreens.

Sunscreens are rated as to how well they protect the skin from burning by a sun protection factor (SPF). SPF numbers range from 1 to over 30, but most sunscreen preparations are from 2 to 15. An SPF number of, for instance, 15, means that it will take 15 times longer to produce a sunburn than if no sunscreen was being used. SPF ratings have not been standardized, are usually determined by indoor testing means, and are frequently less effective than their stated sun protection factor. All are most effective if applied 30 to 60 minutes before going into the sun, to allow full skin absorption. Apart from minor skin reactions, sunscreens have not been shown to have serious side-effects. The wide range of preparations available allows you to choose the best sunscreen for your skin. If, for instance, a PABA (para-aminobenzoic acid) sunscreen causes skin irritation, you could try a non-PABA sunscreen or a sunscreen in a different vehicle (cream, lotion, or gel). (See Figures 21-3 and 21-4.)

The key to the early detection of skin cancers is skin self-examination. This is presented later in the book under Self-Examination for Cancer. Do not assume that a regular medical checkup or visit to a dermatologist will constitute a complete skin examination. Most skin cancers are found by patients themselves.

Non-melanoma

In general, the earliest signs of a non-melanoma skin cancer are loss of the normal skin markings, change in the color of the skin, and a toughening of the skin. Later signs include a roughened area of skin that scabs over, rescabs, and fails to heal (longer than a month); a persistent skin ulcer (a pit or crater, often surrounded by or covered with crust) not explained by any other cause; and any suspicious skin changes in high-risk areas such as heavily sun-exposed regions, burn sites, or scars.

With time, a skin cancer takes on a more characteristic appearance. A basal cell cancer is usually a hard, raised, red or red-gray, pearly or shiny skin growth that may have faint red veins on or around it. It may have a central depression or ulceration, and a rolled, hard border. Squamous cell cancers are usually scalier, less elevated, have an irregular border, and in their late stages will ulcerate and have persistent crusts.

Actinic keratoses (AK) are pre-skin cancers. They occur in sun-exposed areas and develop as a scaly, pale pink or reddish patch of skin. An actinic keratosis is often first felt or picked at before becoming obviously visible. They grow slowly, months or years vs. days or weeks, and have an incidence of malignant change of from between 1 to 25%. Even a 1% risk is substantial if there are multiple actinic keratoses, which is frequently the case—actinic keratoses are extremely common. If they turn into skin cancer, it will be one of the non-melanoma types.

Melanomas

Melanomas often start as small, painless, mole-like growths that increase in size, change color, ulcerate, and bleed easily. A simple way to tell a melanoma from a common mole or other skin change is the ABCD rule: "A" is for asymmetry—one half of the mole does not match the other half; "B" is for border irregularity; "C" is for color—the pigmentation is not uniform and there is usually more than one color (usually black—but not always—and red, pink, orange, blue, brown, tan, and white); and "D" is for diameter—most melanomas aren't obvious until they are larger than 6 mm (the head of a pencil eraser). But remember, all cancers start small, including melanoma. If a mole, however small, suddenly appears on your body, particularly in an area of prior severe sunburn, assume that it could be a melanoma.

Figure 21-2   Skin Types and How They Sunburn. *Source: Primary Care and Cancer,* June 1985. Dominus Publishing Company, Inc. Williston Park, NY 11596. Used with permission.

Skin Type	Sunburn Prognosis (Examples)
I	Always burns: never tans (Irish, Scots, freckled redheads)
II	Always burns, then slightly tans (Blue-eyed, fair-skinned Caucasians)
III	Sometimes burns; always tans (Average Caucasian)
IV	Burns minimally; always tans (Caucasians with Mediterranean ancestry; dark hair and eyes)
V	Rarely burns; tans well (Spanish, Orientals, Indians)
VI	Never burns; deeply pigmented (Black-skinned Negroes)

Figure 21-3 A Guide to Sunscreens: Their SPF (Sun Protection Factor) Ratings and Who Should Use Them. *Source: Primary Care and Cancer,* June 1985. Dominus Publishing Company, Inc., Williston Park, NY 11596. Used with permission.

Chemical Ingredients	Commercial Name	SPF	For Skin Type
Absorbers			
Para-aminobenzoic acid (PABA) in alcohol formulations	PreSun 15	15	I, II
	Pabanol	15	I, II
	Sunbrella	15	I, II
Broad-spectrum sunscreens containing PABA and other agents	PreSun 15	15	I, II
	Total Eclipse 15	15	I, II
	M M M What-A-Tan	15	I, II
	Clinique 19	15	I, II
	Sundown 15	15	I, II
	Elizabeth Arden 15	15	I, II
	Super Shade 15	15	I, II
	Bain de Soleil 15	15	I, II
	Blockout 15	15	I, II
Esters and derivatives of PABA	Original Eclipse	10	II, III
	Pabafilm	6	III, IV
	Sundown	6	III, IV
	Aztec	6	III, IV
	Sea and Ski	6	III, IV
	Sun Guard	6	III, IV
Non-PABA chemical sunscreens: benzophenomes, cinnamates	Piz Buin	15	I, II
	Ti Screen	15	I, II
	Uval	4–12	III, IV
	Coppertone	2–4	IV
Reflectors			
Physical sunscreens: titanium dioxide, zinc oxide, etc.	A-Fil Cream	4–8	I to IV
	Reflecta	4–8	I to IV
	RVPaque	3–8	I to IV
	Clinique	4–8	I to IV
	Covermark	4–8	I to IV
	Shadow	2–6	I to IV
Lip Screens			
PABA formulations	Chap Stick		
	PreSun		
	RV Paba		
	Bain de Soleil		

The dysplastic nevi syndrome (or what was previously called B-K syndrome, named after the first initials of the first two families it was described in) is considered to be a pre-malignant condition. Nevi is the medical term for moles (nevus = mole). A mole is a clustering of melanocytes. Most everyone is born with, or acquires by early adulthood, between 10 and 40 moles on their body (the average is 20). The dysplastic nevi syndrome is characterized by larger than normal moles that begin growing later in life. There are many characteristics that distinguish them from common harmless moles [See Figures 21-5, 21-6 and 21-7].

Large (greater than 20 cm) congenital moles have a 5 to 20% risk of developing melanoma. A fre-quently worried about pigmented lesion that doesn't have a malignant potential is the seborrheic keratosis. Common on the upper body as one gets older, they have a "stuck-on" warty appearance, can some-times be peeled off (but usually regrow) and feel rough or greasy depending upon how oily they are. A seborrheic keratosis is an overgrowth of the oil-producing part of the skin. The oil oxidizes and sometimes causes them to be dark. They may grow to be quite large and unsightly, but are usually 1 cm in size or smaller.

Moles in areas of the body that are subjected to repeated irritation, for instance at the collar-line, bra-line, and waist, have been thought to be at increased chance for becoming malignant, but the evidence for this is not compelling.

Figure 21-4 Commercial Sunscreens: Active Ingredients, Consistency, Protection Factors, and Resistance to Water.* *Source:* Reprinted with permission of *The Physician and Sportsmedicine.* McGraw-Hill Publications.

Trade Name	Ingredients	Type	Sun Protection Factor Indoor Solar Simulator	Outdoor Sunlight	Resistance to Sweating	Water Immersion
PABA sunscreens						
PreSun 15	5% PABA in 50–70% ethyl alcohol	Clear lotion	15	10	Excellent	Poor
Pabanol		Clear lotion	15	6–8	Fair	Poor
Sunbrella		Clear lotion	15	6	Fair	Poor
PABA-ester combination sunscreens						
Supershade 15	7% octyl dimethyl PABA + 3% oxybenzone	Milky lotion	15–18	6–9	Excellent	Good
Total Eclipse 15	2.5% glyceryl PABA + 2.5% octyl dimethyl PABA 2.5% oxybenzone	Milky lotion	15–18	9–12	Excellent	Good
MMM What-A-Tan!	3% octyl dimethyl PABA + 2.5% benzophenone-3	Milky lotion	15–20	10	Excellent	Good
PreSun 15	5% PABA + padimate 0 + 3% oxygenzone	Milky lotion	15–20	8–10	Excellent	Good
Clinique 19	Phenylbenzimidazole-5-sulfonic acid + 7% padi-	Milky lotion	15–19	7–8	Good	Fair
Sundown 15	mate 0 + 5% octylsalicylate + 4% oxybenzone	Milky lotion	15–20	10–11	Excellent	Good
PABA-ester sunscreens						
Block Out	3.3% isoamyl-*p*-N,N-dimethyl-aminobenzoate (padimate A)	Lotion/gel	6–8	6	Good	Fair
Pabafilm	Same as Block Out	Lotion/gel	6–8	4–6	Good	Fair
Sundown	Same as Block Out	Lotion	8–10	4–6	Good	Fair
Original Eclipse	3.5% padimate A + 3% octyl dimethyl PABA	Lotion	8–10	4–6	Good	Fair
Aztec	5% homomenthyl salicylate + 2.5% amyl-*p*-dimethylaminobenzoate	Lotion	6–8	4	Fair	Poor
Sea & Ski	3.3% octyl dimethyl PABA	Cream	7–8	4	Fair	Poor
Non-PABA sunscreens						
Piz Buin-8†	5% ethyl-hexyl-*p*-methoxycinnamate +	Cream	15–20	10–12	Excellent	Good
TiScreen	3% 2-hydroxy-4-methoxybenzophenone + 4% 2-phenyl-benzimidazole sulfonic acid	Cream	16–22	10–12	Excellent	Good
Piz Buin-8†	5% ethylhexyl-*p*-methoxycinnamate + 3% 2-hydroxy-4-methoxybenzophenone	Milky lotion	20–22	10–12	Excellent	Good
TiScreen		Milky lotion	16–20	10–12	Excellent	Good
Piz Buin-4†	4.5% ethylhexyl-*p*-methoxycinnamate	Milky lotion	10–12	4–6	Fair	Poor
Uval	10% 2-hydroxy-4-methoxybenzophenone-5-sulfonic acid	Milky lotion	10–12	4	Poor	Poor
Coppertone-4	8% homomenthylsalicylate	Lotion	3.5–4	2	Poor	Poor
Physical sunscreens						
A-Fil	Titanium dioxide + zinc oxide + talc, kaolin, iron oxide, or red veterinary petroleum	Cream	6–8	4–6	Good	Fair
RV Paque		Cream	6–8	3–4	Good	Fair
Shadow		Cream	4–6	2–4	Good	Fair
Reflecta		Cream	6–8	4–6	Good	Fair
Covermark		Cream	6–8	4–6	Good	Fair
Clinique		Cream	6–8	4–6	Good	Fair

*Reprinted from Pathak MA, Sunscreens: Topical and systemic approaches for protection of human skin against harmful effects of solar radiation. *Journal of the American Academy of Dermatology* 1982;7(September):285–312. Information was updated in 1985, but current ingredients of some products may differ.
†Not available in the United States.

Given that a percentage of melanomas are genetic, it is likely that a genetic probe will be developed that detects such a predisposition, and that a preventive treatment may be found. In the meantime, though, prevention and early detection are our chief tools against melanoma.

SYMPTOMS AND DIAGNOSIS

Skin cancers don't usually make you feel sick. You would just notice a change in your skin. Any unusual skin condition, especially a change in a mole or other

Figure 21-5 Features of Normal Moles.

Feature	Normal Mole
Color	Uniformly tan or brown; all moles on one person tend to look alike.
Shape	Round or oval with a clearly defined border which separates the mole from surrounding skin.
Surface	Begins as flat, smooth spot on skin (1a); becomes raised (1b); forms a smooth bump (1c).
Size	Usually less than 5 millimeters (size of a pencil eraser).
Number	Typical adult has between 10 and 40 moles scattered over the body.
Location	Usually above the waist on sun-exposed surfaces of the body. Scalp, breast, and buttocks rarely have normal moles.

Source: About Dysplastic Nevi, National Cancer Institute, Bethesda, MD. Used with permission. A color pamphlet is available upon request.

Figure 21-6 Features of Dysplastic Moles.

Feature	Dysplastic Mole
Color	Mixture of tan, brown, black, and red/pink. Moles on one person often look quite different from one another.
Shape	Irregular borders which may include notches. May fade into surrounding skin and include a flat portion level with skin.
Surface	May be smooth, slightly scaly, or have a rough, irregular "pebbly" appearance.
Size	Often larger than 5 millimeters and sometimes larger than 10 millimeters.
Number	Many persons do not have increased number; however, persons severely affected may have more than 100 moles.
Location	May occur anywhere on the body but most commonly on back. May also appear below the waist and on scalp, breasts and buttocks.

Source: About Dysplastic Nevi, National Cancer Institue, Bethesda, MD. Used with permission. A color pamphlet is available upon request.

pigmented growth or spot is cause for concern. Scaliness, oozing, bleeding, a growing bump or nodule, itchiness, tenderness, or pain are all symptoms of skin cancer.

By the time a melanoma is detected, it may have already spread to nearby lymph nodes, causing enlargement, or to other skin areas (called satellite lesions). Metastases from melanoma can appear in such unusual places as the back of the eye or under your fingernails or toenails.

Diagnosis of non-melanoma skin cancers is frequently a treatment (and cure) in and of itself. A standard excisional biopsy is often the only surgery required to clearly remove the cancer, which can then be verified by the pathologist's review of the specimen. For pre-cancerous conditions, like actinic keratoses, or obvious early basal cell cancers, the lesion is sometimes removed without sending it for pathological analysis.

Diagnosing melanoma is far more tricky. To accurately assess a melanoma, a wider, deeper biopsy needs to be taken. The prognosis in melanoma is determined by the depth of invasion and is described in five levels. Level 1 is those lesions less than 0.76 mm in depth; level 5 is when it has penetrated deeper than 4 mm. Level 1 melanomas have almost never metastasized, but metastases should be aggressively searched for in the deeper level melanomas.

Melanocytes are derived from the neural crest, the embryonic origin of nerve tissue. During embryonic growth, there is a brief hours-long period when the melanocytes suddenly move from the neural crest to the parts of the body that will be pigmented. Melanomas, as with most cancers, largely consist of cells that have reverted to their primitive, embryonic state; they regain that neural crest-like ability to spread rapidly throughout the body.

TREATMENT AND PROGNOSIS

Non-melanoma

There are six general methods of treatment for non-melanoma skin cancers (or pre-skin cancers): surgery (used in 90% of cases); radiation therapy; electrodissecation (tissue destruction with an electrical needle); cryosurgery (tissue destruction by freezing, usually with liquid nitrogen); topical chemotherapy (5-FU); and immunotherapy (painting a lesion with a chemical like DNCB, which causes an intense local hypersensitivity reaction*).

*Tretinoin (retinoic acid, the vitamin A-like acne-treating substance marketed in the U.S. as Retin-A®), when applied to early or pre-skin cancers (non-melanoma), appears to reverse the neoplastic (and aging) process. It is generally safe to use and readily available from physicians, however, recommendations for its use are still not final.

Figure 21-7 Melanoma Warning Signs: Learn to Recognize Early Melanoma. *Source: About Dysplastic Nevi*, National Cancer Institute, Bethesda, MD. Used with permission. A color pamphlet is available upon request.

It should be stressed that dysplastic moles are generally not cancerous and most will *never* become cancer. But, because dysplastic nevi are more likely than ordinary moles to become malignant, and since persons who have dysplastic nevi (especially those in melanoma-prone families) may be at increased melanoma risk, it is important that these individuals watch for certain characteristics that may signal developing melanoma at its earliest stages.

Moles with this appearance require prompt medical evaluation. See your doctor for a mole check.

Large Size	Most melanomas are at least 5 millimeters in diameter when they are identified; many, considerably larger. An unusually large mole may be melanoma.
Multiple Colors	The presence of a mixture of tan, brown, white, pink, and *especially black* in a mole suggests that melanoma may be present.
Irregular Border	If a mole has a border that is irregular, notched or angular, it may be melanoma.
Abnormal Surface	If a mole is scaly, flakey, oozing, bleeding or has an open sore that does not heal, it may be melanoma.
Unusual Sensation	If a mole itches or is painful and is tender, or if it has a hard lump in it, melanoma may be present.
Abnormal Skin Surrounding Mole	If pigment from the mole has spread into surrounding skin, or if adjacent skin becomes red and inflamed or has lost its pigmentation (becomes white or gray), melanoma may be present.

Figure 21-8 MOHS technique of treating a skin cancer. Diagram shows the MOHS technique of treating a skin cancer by excising, microscopically examining, and mapping successive layers of tissue until all cancer has been removed. Excised layers are cut into several pieces of convenient size, and the pieces are marked with dyes (indicated by the solid and dotted lines on the maps) to maintain the correct orientation. The shaded areas on the maps show the location of cancer present at the deep margin of each layer. *Source:* Reprinted by permission of *The Physician and Sportsmedicine*, McGraw-Hill Publications.

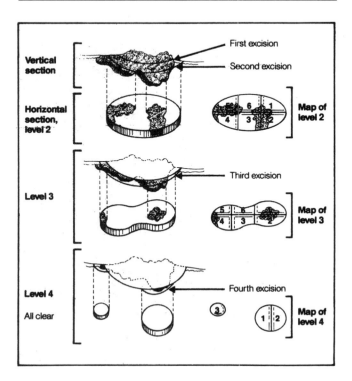

For recurrent skin cancers, large squamous cell cancers, or cancers in the "T zone" (the forehead, eyelids, cheeks, ears, and lips), a technique known as Mohs' surgery should be considered. The Mohs' technique involves the use of zinc chloride and other tissue fixing agents that stain cancer cells. Progressively deeper skin shavings and biopsies are guided by the moment to moment results of the tissue staining, so that a cancer can be followed to its roots with the least removal of normal tissue. See Figure 21-8.

Squamous cell cancer is more dangerous than basal cell. Occasionally, a squamous cell cancer will spread to lymph nodes, and rarer still, they can metastasize. Basal cell cancers almost never spread in that fashion, and instead burrow into surrounding tissues. Treatment must be planned according to the cell type. Assessment for spread of squamous cell cancers must be considered, and lymph node biopsies done accordingly.

The prognosis for non-melanoma skin cancers is excellent, with 95 to 100% cure rates for basal cell and 75 to 80% for squamous cell. And those that recur stand an excellent chance for control or cure on re-treatment. That is why there are so few deaths, less than 1% of all cases, with the non-melanoma skin cancers.

Melanoma

The treatment for melanoma is complicated. For the earliest, level 1, primary melanoma, surgical excision may be enough. But most surgeons will also recommend sampling nearby lymph nodes, and removing them if the primary melanoma is a deep one. Radiotherapy, systemic or regional perfusion chemotherapy, and immunotherapy have all been tried, with varying degrees of success, and are variously recommended on the basis of the type of melanoma and its potential for recurrence.

For melanoma that has already disseminated, surgical excision is usually inadequate, but occasional cures or palliation are possible with radiation, chemotherapy, and immunotherapy. Of these methods of treatment, immunotherapy is the most promising. Melanoma is one of the few cancers that has the potential for spontaneous regression, that is, of suddenly disappearing, even with disseminated melanoma. This is thought to be due to immunological causes, hence the potential for using immunotherapy for melanoma.

Another exciting treatment development has been the experimental use of monoclonal antibodies to carry radioactive isotopes directly to melanoma cells and kill them.

The prognosis for melanoma depends heavily on the type of melanoma, depth (level) of invasion, and the way in which it was treated. In general, level 1 melanomas have a 5-year survival rate of 95%, and the deeper level melanomas, where lymph nodes are involved, only have a five-year survival rate of 30–40%. The highest overall cure rate in the world is in Queensland, Australia, topping 90%, due to their excellent public education programs and screening campaigns.

22

Lung Cancer

Mark Renneker, M.D.

This is a horrible cancer—horrible because it's so prevalent and so few survive it, horrible because it's so preventable. In hospitals at the turn of the century, cases of lung cancer were so uncommon that, if a patient with it came in, all of the medical students and residents would gather around to see such a rare disease. Now their reaction is more like, "Oh well, another case of lung cancer." The incidence has increased fifty-fold over the past fifty years.

Lung cancer has become the number one cancer killer in the U.S. It accounts for 15% of all cancers in the U.S., but so few survive that it accounts for 25% of cancer deaths.

There are four major types of lung cancer: squamous cell (also called epidermoid) carcinoma, adenocarcinoma, small cell anaplastic (also called oat cell) carcinoma, and large cell anaplastic carcinoma.

Squamous cell carcinoma accounts for about 40% of lung cancers, is most linked to smoking and usually occurs close to the center of the lungs, where the bronchi meet the lung. Adenocarcinoma accounts for about 25% of lung cancers, are twice as common in women, and tend to occur in the periphery of the lungs. Small cell accounts for about 20% of lung cancers; large cell about 15%. Lung cancer is sometimes referred to as bronchogenic carcinoma. The lung is a frequent site of metastases from other cancers.

EPIDEMIOLOGY AND RISK FACTORS

The number of cases each year in the U.S. exceeds 150,000, about 100,000 men and 50,000 women. Blacks have a higher incidence than whites. In fact, U.S. blacks top the international charts, along with the English and the Finns.

There has been an actual drop in lung cancer incidence among white males in the U.S. since the early 1980s. This reflects the trend since the 1960s of less and less white males who are still smoking. In 1985 it was 33%, in 1987 it was 29%. The smoking rates of females and blacks is also finally dropping, so their lung cancer rates should begin dropping within the next decade or two. But, unfortunately, the overall incidence is increasing worldwide and lung cancer appears to have topped stomach cancer as the number one cancer among males in the world. Low-incidence countries include China, India, and a number of African and Latin countries. The majority of cases occur in the 35 to 75 age range, with the peak between 55 and 65.

As early as the 1920s and 1930s evidence began accumulating that cigarette smoking caused lung cancer. By the 1950s the cause and effect relationship was beyond question. There is a dose-response relationship—meaning that, for instance, a person smoking one to nine cigarettes per day has about a five times increased risk compared to a non-smoker, while someone smoking over 40 cigarettes per day (two packs) has a twenty times increased risk.

About 85% of all lung cancers are attributable to cigarette smoking. Those who smoke filtered, low-tar cigarettes are at somewhat lower risk, but their risk is still appreciably higher than non-smokers. Involuntary smokers, those exposed to second-hand smoke, for instance family members, have a higher risk of developing lung cancer than people who have no smoking exposure.

The risk of developing lung cancer quickly begins dropping after eliminating exposure (i.e., when you and/or the person around you quits smoking). After about ten years the risk has dropped to where it is about equal to non-smokers.

Exposure to airborne asbestos is a risk factor for lung cancer, and acts synergistically with cigarette smoking. (See Chapter 15—Occupational Carcinogenesis.) Lung cancer accounts for the deaths of about 20% of men exposed to asbestos for long periods during their work life. Mesothelioma, a rare, practically incurable cancer of the lining of the lung, is also more common with asbestos exposure.

Other predominantly work-related carcinogens include radon, mustard gas, polycyclic aromatic hydrocarbons, chloromethyl ethers, chromium, nickel, inorganic arsenic, beryllium, lead, cadmium, vinyl chloride, and acrylonitrile. Ionizing radiation also increases risk.

The role of air pollution in lung cancer is difficult to quantify, but one fact is clear: even when differences in smoking habits are taken into account, people living in cities have higher lung cancer rates than people living in the country.

Diet appears to play a role in lung cancer, with increased incidence when intake of beta-carotene (i.e., vitamin A) is low. Alcohol by itself doesn't appear to be a factor, except that most heavy users of alcohol also smoke.

In some cases, genetic predisposition is a factor, particularly for adenocarcinoma of the lung. Poor immunity and scarring of the lung have also been associated. Infectious etiologies have not been associated, except where they result in a scarred lung.

PREVENTION AND EARLY DETECTION

Lung cancer would again become a rare disease if cigarette smoking ceased. Start with yourself. If you smoke, stop; if you've never smoked, don't ever take it up. For maximum protection, eliminate any possible occupational or air-exposure carcinogens, minimize radiation exposure, and eat a healthy diet.

The immediate challenge in trying to deal with lung cancer is to find an effective screening procedure. It used to be recommended that every person, especially smokers, get an annual chest x-ray. But studies showed that by the time a lung cancer turns up on a chest x-ray, it's too late—it will have already spread and the chance for cure will be slight. The American Cancer Society withdrew their recommendation for an annual chest x-ray in 1980, recognizing that it was a poor screening test and that it was perhaps contributing to the smoking problem by giving smokers a false sense of security (that they could wait to quit until something showed up on a chest x-ray).

Sputum cytology as a screening test for lung cancer remains controversial. In theory at least, it makes perfect sense to do a lung "Pap test." (See Chapter 75—Sputum Cytology and Lung Health.)

There are no blood tests yet for screening, but various methods of testing for increased DNA content, tumor peptides, and lung tumor antigens using monoclonal immunoassays are under investigation. Pulmonary function testing (breathing studies) don't indicate the presence of cancer. Listening to the lungs with a stethoscope is useless; lung cancer can't be heard.

SYMPTOMS AND DIAGNOSIS

The most common symptom is hemoptysis (coughing up blood, which may be red or rust-colored). Lung cancer may be the cause of any persistent cough, whether or not there is blood. Other symptoms include shortness of breath, pneumonia, pain, wheezing, trouble swallowing, hoarseness, and weight loss. If an older smoker has any of these symptoms, lung cancer should be considered.

In 70% of cases, at the time of diagnosis the disease has spread to regional lymph nodes or distant sites. Diagnostic (and staging) tests include standard chest x-rays, tomograms (x-rays of vertical sections of the lung), CT, MRI, nuclear medicine scans of the lungs and bones, sputum cytology, bronchoscopy (using a narrow, usually flexible, fiberoptic scope to examine the airways), mediastinoscopy (using a fiberoptic scope to examine the central region of the chest, the mediastinum, which contains the lungs' lymph nodes), immunological skin testing (immunity is depressed by lung cancer), and selective blood tests. Biopsies may be taken during bronchoscopy, mediastinoscopy, and by using CT to guide a needle into the tumor. Sometimes a biopsy is taken of the scalene lymph node (located at the lower left-side of the neck) or of the bone marrow. Definitive diagnosis may depend on thoracotomy (surgically opening the lung).

TREATMENT AND PROGNOSIS

Surgery offers the best chance for cure for all types of lung cancer except small-cell (oat cell), which is better treated by radiation therapy and combination chemotherapy. Surgery for cure is only attempted in about one-third of patients—for the rest, the disease is too widespread. Palliative surgery is sometimes done, to relieve or prevent blockage of vital vessels or a major airway, but palliative radiation therapy may work just as well.

There are a multitude of considerations in deciding if and how radiation therapy and chemotherapy should be used. All lung cancer patients can benefit from their case being presented at a tumor board (see Chapter 50—Tumor Boards). There is hopeful work in the field of immunotherapy on lung cancer. One method uses a vaccine of specific active tumor-associated antigen (TAA), in which membrane portions of the same tumor type are applied to a patient to specifically boost immunity.

However, the overall prognosis for lung cancer is bleak. Less than 10% survive 10 years. For those rare cases of stage I (well-localized) squamous cell or adenocarcinoma, the cure rate can be as high as 50%.

It is unlikely that advances in the diagnosis and treatment of lung cancer will significantly improve its prognosis. The prevention of lung cancer is our real hope.

23

Cancer of the Colon and Rectum (and Anus)

Mark Renneker, M.D.

Colon and rectal cancer—cancer of the large bowel—is the second most common cancer in the United States, much to the surprise of most people, who would guess it to be far less frequent. Colorectal cancer just isn't talked about much. In the late 1970s, it was the number one cancer in the U.S., but then lung cancer passed it by. Another fact that the public is unaware of is that it's about as common among women as men—most people think women don't get it very often. Cancer of the small intestine, (duodenum, jejunum, and ileum) are quite rare, with lymphomas accounting for the majority of cases.

The hopeful things about colorectal cancer are the potential for prevention or risk-lowering through diet, and the effectiveness of sigmoidoscopy as an early detection test.

It helps to have a basic understanding of the anatomy of the large bowel (see Figure 23-1). The small bowel ends at the lower right-hand of the abdomen, where it enters the first part of the colon, called the cecum. (The appendix opens into the cecum and apparently has an immunological function.) The colon then ascends towards the liver (called the ascending colon), transverses the abdomen towards the spleen (called the transverse colon), descends to the lower left-hand side of the abdomen (the descending colon), bends into a curve (called the sigmoid—meaning "curve"—colon), flexes (called the rectosigmoid flexure), opens into the rectum, and exits the body at the anus. The entire length of the colon is about six feet; the rectum is only five or six inches long.

Fortunately, about 75% of colorectal neoplasms (polyps and cancer) occur in the rectum and sigmoid colon—which is more accessible for examination. However, it is thought that colorectal neoplasms are becoming more frequent higher in the colon, for reasons that aren't known.

The natural history of colorectal cancer is reasonably well understood. It is now recognized that at least 90% of colorectal cancers arise from polyps, and that this takes ten, twenty, or more years to occur. Polyps (and colorectal cancers) grow slowly. The doubling time (lifespan) of a typical large bowel cell is about one year, the doubling time of a cancer cell in the large bowel is about two years.

The size of a polyp predicts whether it will contain cancer. Only 1% of 1 cm polyps contain cancer, but it's 10 to 20% for 2 cm polyps, 50% for 3 cm polyps, and close to 100% for 5 cm polyps. (President Reagan's largest polyp in 1985—the one that turned out to be cancerous—was 5 cm.) Not all polyps are premalignant, most are harmless and rarely grow larger than 0.5 cm. Adenomatous or villous adenoma is the name of the pre-cancerous kind of polyp. Most all colorectal cancers are adenocarincomas.

EPIDEMIOLOGY AND RISK FACTORS

Over 145,000 cases of colon and rectal cancer occur in the United States each year, with about one-third in the rectum and two-thirds in the colon. The incidence is slightly higher among black males. It is rare before the age of 50, with a peak incidence between 70 and 80 years of age.

The incidence of colorectal cancer varies worldwide. In general, it is uncommon in underdeveloped countries, and quite common in Western countries. There are also wide variations in the United States—it's common in the Northeastern states, and significantly less common in the Southern and

Figure 23-1 Anatomy of the Large Bowel. *Source: Examinations for Preventing Colon Cancer,* Cancer Prevention Program, Wisconsin Clinical Cancer Center, Madison, Wisconsin. Used with permission.

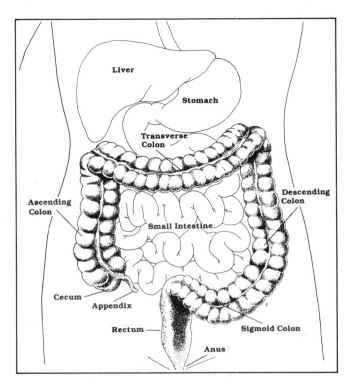

Southwestern states. Dietary habits appear to account for the different rates.

High-fiber, low-fat (low residue) diets are thought to lower risk, and low-fiber, high-fat (high-residue) diets are thought to increase risk. Denis Burkitt, the English physician who, while exploring Africa earlier in this century, first described (and had named after him) a type of lymphoma, also first described the fiber and colorectal cancer connection. There were parts of rural Africa where he simply couldn't find any cases of colorectal cancer.

It still isn't known how the fiber-fat colorectal cancer connection works. At first it was thought that the slower transit time (time for the stool to pass through the bowels) of a low-fiber, high-fat, high-residue stool lengthened the time the bowel wall was exposed to carcinogens in food. Present scientific thinking is far more difficult to understand, involving alterations of the normal bacteria in the bowel affecting bile metabolism. In addition to the helpfulness from their high fiber content, high-fruit and vegetable diets appear to provide a protective effect against colorectal cancer.

Heredity accounts for a percentage of colorectal cancers, particularly when the family member developed it before the age of 50. There are inherited polyp conditions that increase risk for colorectal cancer. Familial polyposis, in which hundreds of polyps begin growing in the bowel by age 30, invariably leads to colon cancer and prophylactic removal of the bowel is required before that occurs. Less common polyp-associated conditions include Gardner's Syndrome and Peutz-Jeughers Syndrome. There is also a non-polyposis inherited colon cancer, which favors the right-side of the colon. Again, it is notable in that it affects younger people. Research has begun to unfold the genetic map of inherited colorectal cancers.

Chronic inflammatory disease of the colon and rectum is associated with increased risk for cancer—mainly ulcerative colitis. The risk is increased according to the number of years a person has had the disease and the amount of bowel involved. Common conditions like hemorrhoids and diverticulosis are not associated with colorectal cancer, but can mimic its symptoms and appear more often in association with low-fiber, high-residue diets.

Radiation and tobacco have not been associated with colorectal cancers, but occupational exposure to asbestos has been. Beer manufacturing sometimes utilizes asbestos filters, resulting in measurable amounts of asbestos in many brands of beer.

PREVENTION AND EARLY DETECTION

It behooves everyone—particularly if there is a family history of colorectal cancer—to follow a colorectal cancer risk-lowering diet. At a minimum, be sure to have about 25 to 30 grams of fiber per day. (See Chapter 74—Diet and Cancer Prevention.)

Early detection tests include the digital rectal examination, which is usually done by a health professional but you can also examine yourself (See Chapter 70—Self-Examination for Cancer). It should be done yearly for men and women over 40.

Testing of the stool for blood, which often isn't visible because of mixing with the stool, should be done every year after the age of 50. Kits to perform these tests are available from physicians, and can be purchased in pharmacies. Remember, though, that these tests only indicate a lesion large enough to bleed.

The best colorectal cancer and polyp early detection test is called flexible sigmoidoscopy. It involves the use of a flexible tube with a light on the end of it that can safely and comfortably examine the rectum and the lower portion of the colon. If a polyp is found, it can be biopsied and removed, eliminating the possibility of it later becoming cancer.

Flexible sigmoidoscopy is recommended for people over 50, men and women alike, every 3 to 5 years.

The older type of sigmoidoscopy, called rigid sigmoidoscopy, is far less comfortable and finds far fewer neoplasms. Most physicians haven't been trained yet in the newer method of flexible sigmoidoscopy, so often only rigid sigmoidoscopy is available—but it's better than not having sigmoidoscopy at all.

X-ray studies, like a barium enema, are useful, but aren't good at finding small polyps (less than 1 cm) and miss many lesions in the anal-rectal and rectal-colon junctures. Colonoscopy is a complete fiberoptic examination of the colon that is somewhat more involved than flexible sigmoidoscopy. It is recommended when there is a likelihood of lesions on the right-side of the colon (for instance, for familial colon cancer), or when polyps are found by flexible sigmoidoscopy. (25–50% of people with a polyp in the lower colon will be found by colonoscopy to have at least one other polyp higher in the colon.)

SYMPTOMS AND DIAGNOSIS

The usual first symptom is bleeding with bowel movements. The blood may be bright red or dark, mixed throughout the stool or only appear as streaks along the outside of the stool, or it may follow the bowel movement, turning the toilet water bloody. Most people assume such bleeding to be from their hemorrhoids. Any person over the age of 50 is wrong in making that assumption. It should be checked out. Other symptoms include pain with bowel movements, change in frequency of bowel habits (increased frequency, constipation, or blockage), change in the character of the stool (narrower, fragmented, different color or odor), abdominal pain or swelling, fatigue, anemia, and weight loss.

The diagnosis is probable on the basis of appearance at the time of sigmoidoscopy and/or barium enema, but is only made definite by biopsy during sigmoidoscopy, colonoscopy, or surgery.

Bowel cancers first spread to lymph nodes on the outside of the bowel, and to the liver. Liver scans and blood tests are routinely done when bowel cancer has been diagnosed.

TREATMENT AND PROGNOSIS

Surgery is the major method of treatment, usually approached from the abdomen. Newer bowel-stapling devices have eliminated the need for a colostomy* in a large percentage of cases. Only cancers that are too low in the rectum, near the anus, require a colostomy these days.

Radiation therapy is used when the cancer has apparently spread through the bowel wall. Chemotherapy is used for advanced colon cancer, but hasn't proven very successful. Immunotherapy is still experimental.

The overall five-year prognosis for colon and rectal cancer is about 50%, ranging from almost 90% for well-localized stage I and in situ cancers, to less than 6% for advanced, metastatic cancer.

The tragedy for most cases of colorectal cancer is that, almost certainly, that cancer could have been easily seen by sigmoidoscopy some years earlier—when it would have been highly curable.

---

*Colostomy—surgical opening of the colon, usually involving loss of part of the colon and in most cases, the rectum. The end of the remaining colon is brought through the abdominal wall, and forms a stoma—through which fecal matter is eliminated (often necessitating an affixed plastic bag—pouch).

CANCER OF THE ANUS

The anus consists of the approximately one inch long muscular region where the rectum opens onto the body surface, and the skin surrounding that opening. Cancer of the anus is uncommon. Most anal cancers are of the squamous cell type. They appear to be caused by chronic irritation, such as by frequent venereal warts, abscesses (boils), fistulas (burrows), fissures (cuts), and perhaps hemorrhoids. Anal sex has been associated. Bleeding is the usual symptom. Treatment is by surgery and radiation, occasionally combined with chemotherapy. Five-year survival rates range from 50 to 85%.

24

Breast Cancer

Mark Renneker, M.D.

Breast cancer is the most common cancer among American women. Lung cancer isn't as common, but is more often lethal and accounts for almost as many cancer deaths in women. About 1 out of 10 women will develop breast cancer during her life.

Until recently, breast cancer eluded the entire cancer field. Little was known about what caused it, early detection methods didn't seem to make a difference, and treatment survival results hadn't improved in over eighty years. Now, with the advent of an effective early detection test—mammography—it appears that breast cancer may finally be brought under control.

Breast cancer is a physically and psychologically complex disease. Its physical aspects are perhaps easier to understand, beginning with learning about the basic anatomy of the breast (see Figure 24-1). Each breast is composed of 15 to 20 pie-shaped sections, called lobes, and each lobe is a separate system of milk-carrying ducts and milk-producing glandular tissue called lobules. The ducts run from the lobules to the nipple. Surrounding and supporting the ducts and lobules is dense connective tissue called stroma. The stroma consists of fibrous bands (fascia) and fat. The breast, then, is made up chiefly of glandular lobules, ducts, and stroma.

The breast is hormone-sensitive and has cyclic changes like the uterus. The lining of the lobules and ducts grow under the influence of hormones like estrogen and progesterone, which explains the pre-menstrual (high hormone) breast fullness many women experience. During pregnancy, the glandular (milk-producing) part of the breast proliferates. After menopause, the breast becomes less dense as the glandular and stromal tissue atrophies, leaving predominantly ductal tissue.

Males have minimal ductal development and usually do not develop glandular tissue. For every 100 cases of breast cancer, one will be in a male.

Almost all breast cancer is adenocarcinoma, the pathological cell type for cancer of glandular origin. Breast adenocarcinoma is classified as being ductal or lobular. Over 90% of breast cancers are ductal; less than 10% are lobular. Cancer of the stromal breast tissue is rare.

Ductal and lobular carcinomas are further classified as either non-infiltrating or infiltrating. Non-infiltrating cancer is as it sounds, an in situ, well-localized cancer. Non-infiltrating ductal cancer hasn't spread through the duct wall and is called intraductal cancer; non-filtrating lobular cancer is called lobular cancer in situ. Both are nearly 100% curable, but only account for about 5% of breast cancers—a percentage that should climb as more breast cancers are diagnosed before they have infiltrated. Infiltrating breast cancers are classified as infiltrating duct (scirrhous), medullary, mucinous, tubular, papillary, Paget's, and inflammatory breast carcinoma.

Breast cancer is more common in the left than the right breast, at a ratio of 110 to 100. This is probably because the left breast is usually larger than the right. Similarly, the upper outer quadrant of each breast (the part closest to the armpit) is where the most breast tissue lies and where the most breast cancers occur (about 50%).

The natural history of breast cancer—its pattern of growth and spread—is only barely understood. Growth from one cancer cell to where it can

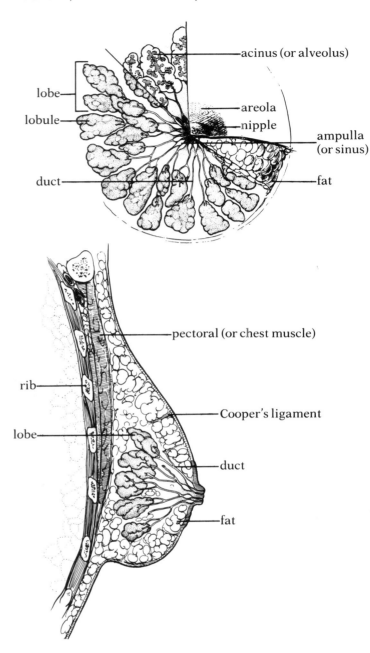

Figure 24-1 Basic Anatomy of the Breast. *Source: The Breast Cancer Digest,* second edition, National Cancer Institute, Bethesda, MD. 1984. Used with permission.

first be detected is estimated to take seven to ten years, but may be shorter or longer.

Apparently, many women harbor breast cancer without realizing it. Autopsies of elderly women who died of other causes reveals intraductal cancer (i.e., in situ, not infiltrative, not invasive cancer) to be present about twenty times more often than the reported incidence of breast cancer. This suggests that breast cancers don't grow in a continuous fashion, and that some stop at the in situ stage, remain latent or even regress. This also suggests that what initiates breast cancer growth is probably different from what promotes its later growth, i.e., breast cancer is a multi-step, multi-factorial disease.

EPIDEMIOLOGY AND RISK FACTORS

Over 130,000 cases of breast cancer are diagnosed each year in the U.S., and the incidence is gradually increasing. Whites are affected slightly more than blacks. Higher socioeconomic class is associated with a higher risk.

Increasing age is a breast cancer risk factor. Breast cancer is rare before the age of 30. The age of peak incidence is geographically related: low-breast cancer countries like Asia, Latin America, and Africa have a peak incidence at menopausal ages, at about 45 to 55. High-breast cancer countries like the U.S., Canada, Western Europe, and Australia have a peak incidence after age 65.

Breast cancer is widely regarded as a cancer that runs in families, but only about 25% of women who get breast cancer have had breast cancer in their family. Risk of developing breast cancer is increased for all first-degree relatives (female and male) of a breast cancer patient—parents, siblings, children. Having a maternal grandmother or aunt with breast cancer also increases risk.

If the family member had post-menopausal breast cancer, the risk to first-degree relatives is only slightly increased, i.e., from the American women's average of 8 to 10% to 10 to 12%. The biggest inherited risk is when a first-degree relative had pre-menopausal breast cancer, particularly if it was in both breasts—in which case the family members' lifetime risk is 50%.

Many times it isn't known whether a relative had pre- or post-menopausal breast cancer, particularly since menopause can extend over a period of years (the average age of onset is 52, and it has been increasing since the turn of the century). When a woman has had her last period, her menopause is complete and she is considered to be post-menopausal.

A woman's age when her breast cancer was diagnosed suggests what factors may have caused it: breast cancer in younger women (pre-menopausal) is less common, and appears to be due more to intrinsic factors like genetics and hormones, compared to post-menopausal breast cancer, which appears to be due more to environmental factors like diet.

A high-fat diet is associated with an increased risk of breast cancer. A diet with less than 20% of calories from fat is thought to lower risk, while over

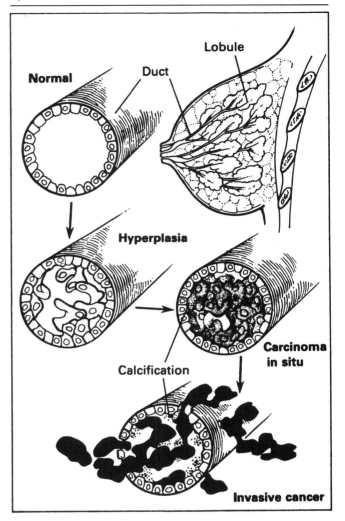

40% increases risk. Whether it's saturated or unsaturated fat doesn't seem to be a significant factor. A high-protein diet is also associated with an increased risk, though evaluation can be difficult because high-protein diets tend to be high-fat diets. Total caloric intake has been associated; obese women have more breast cancer. Exercise is being studied as a protective factor. Ingested trace chemicals can be found in breast milk, suggesting that carcinogens could concentrate in the breast—but the evidence for this is generally lacking. Selenium has been described as possibly protective. Increased fiber intake may also be protective.

Tobacco use has no effect or may perhaps lower risk, by altering estrogen metabolism. Radiation has clearly been shown to increase risk, particularly if it occurs early in life (i.e., during adolescence). Cumulative doses as low as 10 rads are thought to increase risk.

An infectious cause of breast cancer hasn't been established in humans, but has been shown in mice, with the demonstration of "Bittner" viral particles in mouse breast milk. Human breast milk is thought to be safe; having been breast-fed—even if the mother later developed breast cancer—has not been shown to increase risk.

On the other hand, a women who breast-feeds appears to lower her risk of breast cancer. Recent analysis, however, indicates that breast feeding isn't as important a factor as the fact that pregnancy took place—and the earlier the pregnancy, the lower the risk. Women who have a full pregnancy before the age of 18 have one-third the breast cancer risk of a woman whose first child is delayed until after age 30, or never has a child. One interesting angle on the breast feeding issue, is the fact that Tanka women in Hong Kong, who traditionally only nurse with their right breast, have more cancer in their left breast.

Women with increased number of reproductive years (beginning menstruation at an early age, having menopause at a later age) are at increased risk for breast cancer.

Extended and heightened estrogen exposure is the one hypothesis that may account for the various dietary and reproductive risk factors. With dietary factors, higher fat intake and obesity raise estrogen levels in the body. And with reproductive factors, an early onset of menstruation and a late menopause (risk-increasing) means there is a greater number of menstrual cycles (i.e., monthly peaks of estrogen); more pregnancies (risk-lowering) means a lower total number of menstrual cycles. The one hitch with the estrogen theory of breast cancer causation is that studies on breast cancer of women taking estrogen medications (DES, birth control pills, estrogen for menopause) haven't consistently shown a significant association.

A history of benign breast conditions, for instance a cyst or what is called fibrocystic breast disease, is somewhat associated with an increased risk of breast cancer, but the studies in this area are inconsistent. A history of multiple breast biopsies, even if they all turn out to be benign, is associated with a higher probability of developing breast cancer—particularly if the biopsies showed atypical hyperplasia or cellular atypia. Prior breast cancer clearly increases risk for the other breast.

Studies reported in 1987 on alcohol and breast cancer are alarming. Risk was shown to be significantly increased by minimal alcohol intake (as little as two drinks per week). Previous studies showed a similar association, while others including one reported in 1988, showed no association. However, the balance of results of all of the studies done on alcohol and breast cancer shows that there is a relationship.

The response of the public and the medical profession to these studies has been curiously lackadaisical, more than likely because alcohol use is so pervasive and accepted in our society. We may now be with alcohol and breast cancer where we were thirty or more years ago with lung cancer and cigarettes—it may take that long for medical opinion to sway, and for the public to act on it.

PREVENTION AND EARLY DETECTION

The first step is to take stock of your risk factors—your age, weight status, diet, family history, radiation-exposure history, and breast health. A substantial family history of breast cancer would indicate the need for the most aggressive preventive measures.

The best available evidence indicates that breast cancer risk can be lowered by dietary means: a low-fat diet, avoiding obesity, and avoiding alcohol. The National Cancer Institute believed the evidence on fat intake alone was strong enough in 1984 to justify a multi-year, multi-million dollar study (called the Women's Health Trial) to see if lowering fat intake would lower breast cancer incidence in women at high-risk, but in 1988 pulled back on their funding.

Reproductive factors can't readily be modified. However, some women, usually for non-cancer reasons, have their uterus (hysterectomy) and ovaries removed before the time of menopause—one benefit of which is a lower breast cancer risk.

The following early detection guidelines are recommended by the American Cancer Society.

Breast Self-Examination: to be done monthly by all women, beginning by age 20. Over 90% of breast cancers are found by women themselves—not by the doctor. Because only 30% of women do regular breast self-examination, most breast cancers are found when they are fairly good-sized. Only thirty years ago, the average sized breast cancer at the time of diagnosis was 4 to 5 centimeters. Now it is less, about 2.5 cm (see Figure 24-3). Breast cancer needs to be found when it is still smaller to really make a difference in survival rates. That is possible if you are really good at breast self-examination.

Physician (or health provider) examination: every three years until age 40, yearly thereafter. A physician's examination can't be relied upon to find small lesions. Most physicians don't do a thorough and extensive enough examination (five minutes is the minimum). You must learn to examine your own breasts, and do it monthly.

Figure 24-3 Tumor Sizes. *Source: The Breast Cancer Digest,* second edition, National Cancer Institute, Bethesda, MD, 1984. Used with permission.

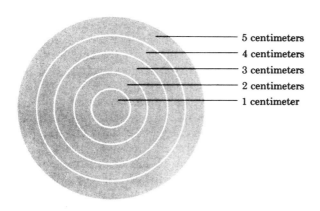

- 5 centimeters
- 4 centimeters
- 3 centimeters
- 2 centimeters
- 1 centimeter

Mammography (breast x-ray): to be done once between 35 and 40, every one to two years between 40 and 50, and every year thereafter (see Figure 24-4). Mammography was shown in 1960 by the Health Insurance Plan (HIP) of Greater New York study to successfully find breast cancer in women over the age of 50, and lower their rate of death from breast cancer. The ongoing analysis of data from 280,000 women screened by mammography (and other methods) in the National Cancer Institute/American Cancer Society five-year Breast Cancer Detection Demonstration Project (BCDDP), completed in 1979, is proving the value of mammography for women between the ages of 40 and 50, as well as those over 50. In 1987, very high survival rates were reported for as long as ten years after diagnosis. This trend is expected to continue.

For the first time in history, the number of diagnoses of in situ and well-localized breast cancer is increasing—purely due to mammography. About 40% of breast cancers in the BCDDP study were found by mammography alone—they couldn't be felt by the physician or the patient. The early fears about radiation from mammography haven't been realized, particularly since newer machines deliver 20 to 100 times less radiation than machines used in the 1970s.

Mammography has come of age. In 1983, only about 30% of women over 40 reported having had a mammogram within two years, but that percentage is increasing. In 1987, a routine mammogram found a 7 millimeter in situ breast cancer in Nancy Reagan. Appropriately so, the media proclaimed mammography to be a hero.

Other methods being studied for possible use for breast cancer early detection include thermo-

Figure 24-4 Mammography. Mammography is the most reliable method to detect breast cancer before it can even be felt. *Source: The Breast Cancer Digest,* second edition, National Cancer Institute, Bethesda, MD, 1984. Used with permission.

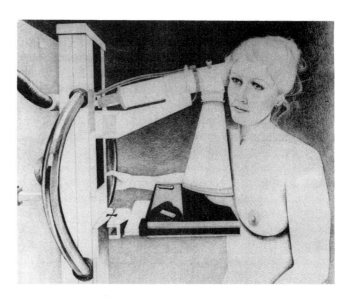

graphy (a temperature measuring process), nipple aspiration cytology (a "Pap test" of cells drawn out of the nipple), ultrasound, diaphanography (transillumination using infrared light), digital subtraction angiography (a computer study of blood vessels), computer tomography (CT), and magnetic resonance imaging (MRI). Ultrasound has shown the most promise among these methods.

SYMPTOMS AND DIAGNOSIS

Most people only think of breast cancer as being a lump, but the symptoms of breast cancer can be far more subtle: a thickening within the breast or of the overlying skin (like a thin piece of cardboard under the skin), redness of the skin, breast tenderness (though most lumps are painless), a change in the contour or shape of a portion of the breast, a slight bloody or clear-fluid discharge from the nipple, or a deviation or inward retraction of the nipple.

About 80% of all breast masses are benign, but for women over 50, only about 50% are benign. In some cases, the distinction between benign and malignant is obvious. Physicians' examinations are only accurate about 75% of the time in making the subtler distinction of whether or not the lymph nodes are involved.

A mammogram is not a diagnostic test. If a lump or breast change is found, a mammogram can't eliminate the possibility that it is cancerous: it must be biopsied. Biopsy can be done by fine needle aspiration, needle localization using radiography (particularly useful for non-palpable, mammographically discovered lesions) or surgically.

In the past, biopsies were often done when a woman was under general anesthesia, and if it was positive (determined by frozen section diagnosis, a quick pathological reading technique), surgery to remove the breast was performed immediately. Today, the usual procedure is to perform the biopsy under local anesthesia, get the results in about a week's time, and discuss treatment options. Some states have laws requiring that a woman have all possible treatment options presented to her before surgery.

Biopsy is also important for determining whether the cancer has estrogen and progesterone receptors. This is routinely tested by the pathologist, and has prognostic and treatment implications: cancers that have estrogen and progesterone receptors respond to hormone therapy. Pre-menopausal breast cancer is estrogen receptor positive only 30% of the time, compared to 60% in post-menopausal breast cancer.

Metastases are looked for in sites where they are most likely to occur, using bone, brain, and liver scans.

TREATMENT

The treatment of breast cancer depends on whether or not it has spread beyond the breast. Conventional medical wisdom has it that breast cancer spreads to the lymph nodes before spreading to the rest of the body (see Figure 24-5). For that reason, treatment has always favored surgically removing or irradiating the lymph nodes. An alternative way of thinking, though, is that the lymph nodes are protective and are needed to help eliminate the cancer. Supporting that line of reasoning is one study (Baum and Coyle, 1977) that left cancerous lymph nodes alone, only removing the breast (simple mastectomy), and the finding that 50% of the time the involved lymph nodes spontaneously regressed within three months.

Further confusing the issue is that the results of two recent large studies—the Cancer Research Campaign studies in England and the National Surgical Adjuvant Breast Project in the U.S.—failed to confirm that removing lymph nodes affected survival rates. This suggests that breast cancer may spread to the lymph nodes and to distant sites at about the same time.

Largely for that reason, breast cancer is spoken of as being a systemic disease: it affects, and is affected by, the whole body. It's this way of thinking that makes it easier to understand how breast can-

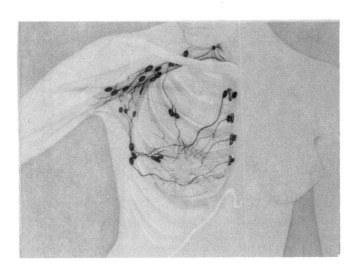

Figure 24-5 Lymph Nodes Surrounding the Breast. *Source: The Breast Cancer Digest,* second edition, National Cancer Institute, Bethesda, MD, 1984. Used with permission.

cer can appear in both breasts (10% of cases, less commonly simultaneously, more commonly sequentially), and why it can reappear after ten, twenty, or even more years.

Breast cancer treatment is controversial. Surgery is still the chief method of treatment, but the extent of surgery is subject to question. The Halsted radical mastectomy (removing the entire breast, pectoralis muscles, and axillary lymph nodes) was the standard breast cancer operation for over 75 years, but has fallen out of favor because it is unacceptable cosmetically and results in functional disability. Even the modified radical mastectomy (see Figure 24-6) (removing the breast and axillary lymph nodes, but leaving the muscles) appears to be overtreatment in most cases.

The trend in breast cancer surgery is towards performing a simple mastectomy (removing the whole breast) or partial mastectomy (also called tylectomy or lumpectomy (see Figures 24-7 and 24-8), removing just the lump and the surrounding tissue) with selective sampling of lymph nodes, often followed by radiation. The survival results appear to be equal for either of these surgical methods, even when compared to the more radical surgical procedures.

Radiation therapy is used increasingly after surgery, usually for five to six weeks. It is also highly effective for advanced breast cancer as a palliative treatment.

The effectiveness of systemic therapy—chemotherapy—depends upon the stage and type of breast cancer. For pre-menopausal women, particularly if they have positive lymph nodes, chemotherapy definitely can improve prognosis. The use of hor-

Figure 24-6 Modified Radical Mastectomy. *Source: The Breast Cancer Digest,* second edition, National Cancer Institute, 1984. Used with permission.

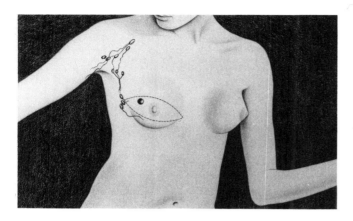

mones as chemotherapy is most often used in post-menopausal breast cancers that are estrogen and progesterone receptor positive. An anti-estrogen drug called tamoxifen is used, and/or the ovaries are surgically removed to halt the natural production of estrogen (usually only used for advanced cases). Surgical removal of the pituitary and adrenal glands may also be recommended, to eliminate signals for estrogen production.

Immunotherapy for breast cancer is still experimental. Monoclonal antibody research has yielded various tumor specific antigens, such as CA 15-3, which are being used clinically. Breast cancer is the only one of the major cancers (lung, colorectal, breast) which appears to be systemic, with microscopic spread even in its early stages, so it will be the most likely to yield to advances in monoclonal antibody treatment.

A major shift in breast cancer treatment in recent years has been towards greater recognition of the emotional consequences for the patient. Optimal breast cancer treatment should include a team approach from the start (before surgery). That team should include a social worker or psychologist who will help the woman begin dealing with her fears—fears of surgery, fears of losing her breast, fears of losing her sexuality, fears of dying. Reach to Recovery is an American Cancer Society-sponsored program in which former breast cancer patients come to the hospital to visit and talk with patients. It can make a world of difference.

Also, reconstructive surgery is increasingly being used and can be remarkably effective in restoring a breast. Discussion about reconstruction should take place before the initial breast cancer surgery, because it is often a factor in determining what type of surgical approach is best. Breast prostheses that fit into a bra are an alternative to reconstructive surgery for some women.

PROGNOSIS

Pre-menopausal breast cancer tends to be more dangerous, and has a poorer prognosis than post-menopausal breast cancer. Breast cancer in elderly women is often extremely slow-growing, and may not require much treatment.

The overall five-year survival rate for breast cancer is 60 to 75%, based on various large-scale studies. Five-year survival rates range from nearly 100% for in situ cancer, to 85% for stage I (tumor less than 2 cm, nodes free of disease), to 65% for stage II (tumor less than 5 cm, nodes positive, no distant metastases), to 40% for stage III (tumor larger than 5 cm, with extensive positive nodes, no distant metastases), to 10% for stage IV (distant metastases).

Ten-year survival, unfortunately, is about 15 to 25% lower for all stages (except in situ and very

Figure 24-7 Lumpectomy. *Source: The Breast Cancer Digest, second edition, National Cancer Institute, 1984. Used with permission.*

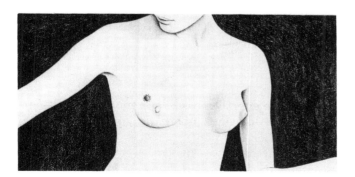

Figure 24-8 Partial or Segmental Mastectomy. *Source: The Breast Cancer Digest, second edition, National Cancer Institute, 1984. Used with permission.*

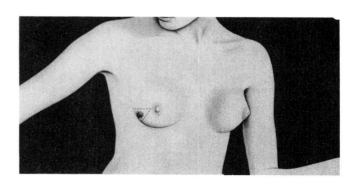

localized tumors). Twenty-year survival is still lower. Breast cancer is one of the few cancers where it is difficult to ever say that a person is absolutely cured.

It seems that the control of breast cancer in the near future will not be through improved methods of treatment, but only by prevention and early detection. Despite the fact that present research on the causes of breast cancer is inconclusive, every effort to prevent breast cancer should be undertaken—and available methods of early detection, particularly mammography, should be thoroughly utilized.

25

Prostate Cancer

Mark Renneker, M.D.

Prostate cancer is an extremely common cancer in males, ranking first among the male-only cancers (the others being testicular, penis, scrotal). It ranks third in overall cancer incidence for men, behind skin and lung cancer. The prostate is sometimes mistakenly called the "prostrate."

The prostate is a walnut-sized male organ located between the bladder and the penis, surrounding the urethra (the tube carrying urine from the bladder out through the penis). Its function is to produce and store seminal fluid. Combined with sperm from the testes, seminal fluid forms ejaculate. The prostate can be easily felt by inserting a finger into the rectum and feeling upwards towards the penis. Prostate gland growth and function depend on the male hormone testosterone, which is produced in the testes.

The prostate gland is a part of their body that most men know little about—until it causes problems. An infection of the prostate can occur in young as well as old men, but the gradual, age-related, urination-interfering enlargement of the prostate known as BPH (benign prostatic hyperplasia) is the vexing condition complained about by older men. Older men are also at high risk for cancer of the prostate.

Autopsy studies of men who have died of non-cancer causes, such as in automobile accidents, show nests of cancer cells in prostate glands of 30% of men in their 50s, 35% in their 60s, and 70% in their 70s. In other words, the incidence increases with age, and by age 100 practically all men have evidence of it. However, even if present, in most men it remains localized, a silent, asymptomatic disease.

As with cancer of other gland-organs of the body, the major type of cancer in the prostate is adenocarcinoma.

EPIDEMIOLOGY AND RISK FACTORS

There are about 100,000 cases of prostate cancer each year in the U.S. It will someday affect 1 in 11 men. It is common in American and European males, of lower incidence in the Near East, parts of Africa, and South America, and of extremely low incidence in Japan. Black men in America have the highest incidence in the world, about 14 times higher than males in Japan.

There is some evidence for its inheritability, but social and environmental factors seem to play a greater role. Japanese who migrate to the U.S. take on a higher incidence, and increased fat in their diet is the suspected cause. Also, the high incidence in blacks has only been in the past few decades, again suggesting an external factor, such as diet.

Prostate cancer is one of the few cancers for which no association with smoking have been found. Also, no association has been found for radiation exposure, but exposure to cadmium in the workplace has been shown to be a risk factor. Increased numbers of sexual partners and venereal disease have also been implicated. Men with conditions that inhibit testosterone production, such as cirrhosis of the liver (alcoholics develop atrophy of their testes), are reported to have fewer prostate cancers. Those with no testosterone production (eunuchs) have no prostate cancer.

BPH has been studied as a risk factor, and one large study showed an association with prostate cancer, but a second study showed no relationship. The issue is unsettled.

Trace elements such as aluminum and selenium have been implicated in prostate cancer: aluminum may contribute to it; selenium may protect against it. The evidence isn't strong either way.

PREVENTION AND EARLY DETECTION

Primary prevention of prostate cancer may be possible through diet, particularly a low-fat diet. (Castration, as in a sex-change operation, which virtually eliminates testosterone production, would be a means of preventing prostate cancer).

Early detection is difficult. The best and most widely available early detection method is the digital rectal examination. But by the time a prostate cancer can be felt, it is seldom in an early stage. BPH, with its multiple nodular growths, called spheroids, can confuse the exam. Early prostate cancer can feel similar to a BPH spheroid. Late prostate cancer has an obvious feel—it's hard like a knuckle.

The American Cancer Society recommends that all men over 40 have an annual digital rectal examination. It is possible to do prostate self-examination (see Chapter 70—Self-Examination for Cancer).

A recent technological breakthrough is the development of an ultrasound device that can be inserted into the rectum, aimed up to the prostate, and used to detect hard nodules that may be cancer. It is called transrectal ultrasonography (TRUS). The device is small enough to fit on the end of a flexible sigmoidoscope, permitting the prostate to be examined along with the rectum and colon.

Various blood tests have been developed that can help in detecting prostate cancer, including serum prostate antigen, and serum acid phosphatase. But both tests aren't sensitive or specific enough to be used as a general screening test. They are only generally useful to help confirm a tentative diagnosis of prostate cancer, or to check for recurrence.

SYMPTOMS AND DIAGNOSIS

Unfortunately, early prostate cancer is asymptomatic, and the symptoms of late prostate cancer are similar to other prostate conditions. These symptoms primarily relate to a disturbance in urination:

increased frequency of urination, a weakened or narrowed stream, incomplete emptying, and occasionally a feeling of irritation on urination. Bloody urine is less common. Advanced prostate cancer may present as back pain, stiffness, or pain down the legs—indicating the cancer has already spread into the bones of the back.

Diagnosis is usually by a needle biopsy through the rectum or through the perineum (the area between the anus and the scrotum). Ultrasound can be used to guide the needle more precisely. Aspiration biopsy through the rectum is gaining favor, and is in common use in Europe. Diagnosis by a transurethral approach (through the penis) is not favored, but is a common treatment for BPH.

MRI (magnetic resonance imaging) is being used to evaluate prostate cancer, and is particularly good for demonstrating extent of spread. CT is also used. A bone scan may be done, looking for bone involvement. A sampling of nearby lymph nodes is also done, sometimes by needle biopsy. If the lymph nodes are positive, surgical removal of the prostate will not be curative.

TREATMENT AND PROGNOSIS

Treatment is directed by the pathological grade of the tumor (well- versus poorly-differentiated), and the extent of spread at the time of diagnosis. Total removal of the prostate is the treatment of choice for potentially curable prostate cancer. The development of prostate operations that spare the nerves that control erections has prevented surgically caused impotency in 70% of patients. (This was a major drawback of prostate surgery in the past. Effective penile prostheses are available for those who develop impotency. They are inserted along the length of the penis, and can be pumped up like a balloon. Under investigation are various drugs that can be injected into the penis to cause an erection.)

Prostate cancer is, in general, a slow-growing cancer. Having no therapy—just observing the tumor—is sometimes an option. A stage I prostate cancer may never progress if it is well-differentiated, but a poorly-differentiated one may spread aggressively.

Radiation therapy is frequently used to treat prostate cancer, and can be given externally or by implants. Radiation may be combined with surgery or used alone, which can be curative.

Chemotherapy, single-agent or combined, is generally used for prostate cancer that has metastasized, and with limited success. But, another form of chemotherapy, using hormones, can be quite effective. It aims to suppress or eliminate the male hormones (androgens, which form testosterone). This can be done by giving female hormones (usually DES, an estrogen), anti-androgen drugs like leuprolide acetate, or a drug like ketoconazole, which blocks the male hormone cycle from cholesterol. Surgical removal of the testes doesn't totally eliminate male hormones; other parts of the body (i.e., the adrenal glands) produce some androgen.

Hormonal therapy can palliate or prevent advancing disease, with survival beyond 10 years in about 10% of patients with bony metastasis.

The prognosis for prostate cancer has significantly improved in the last 25 years. Five-year survival rates for all stages combined are up from 48% in the 1940s to 70% in the 1980s. Eighty-three percent of patients whose prostate cancer was found early (no spread beyond the gland) are alive 5 years after treatment.

26

Uterine Cancer—
Cervical and
Endometrial

Mark Renneker, M.D.

The uterus is the womb. A non-pregnant uterus is about the size and shape of an upside-down pear. The narrow end opens into the vagina and is called the uterine cervix ("cervix" means neck). The wide, upper end of the uterus is called the uterine corpus ("corpus" means body). (See Figures 26-1 and 26-2.) The lining of the inside of the uterine corpus, the womb, is called the endometrium. The cervix and the endometrium are the parts of the uterus that are most frequently affected by cancer.

The endometrium contains many glands sensitive to the female hormones estrogen and progesterone. The endometrial lining is what sloughs off with each menses—or nourishes pregnancy. Most endometrial cancers are adenocarcinomas. There are also cancers of the muscular wall of the uterus, called the myometrium, but they are uncommon.

Cervical cancer almost always occurs only at the cervical os ("os" means hole), which is where the cervix opens into the vagina. The cells on the vaginal side of the os are squamous epithelium, similar to the cells lining the mouth. The cells lining the inside of the os are columnar glandular epithelium. Where they meet is called the squamocolumnar junction (or transitional cell junction). Ninety-five percent of cervical cancers are classified as squamous carcinomas.

The Pap test involves using a thin wooden or plastic spatula to gently scrape cells from the squamocolumnar junction, and to then examine those cells under the microscope for changes suggestive of cervical cancer. It does not reliably test for cancers higher in the uterus, i.e., endometrial cancer, missing about 50% of them.

The Pap test has provided so much information about the stages of growth in cervical cancer that its natural history is better understood than any other cancer. It is known that about 95% of cervical cancers have gone through a predictable, stepwise transformation that took 15 to 35 years. To go from the pre-cancerous state known as dysplasia to carcinoma in situ is estimated to take 5 to 10 years, and to go from carcinoma in situ to invasive cancer takes 8 to 30 years. Proof of this slow growth pattern is that carcinoma in situ most commonly affects women in their 30s, and invasive cancer isn't common until women are closer to 50. Many cases of cervical dysplasia and some cases of carcinoma in situ can be expected to return to normal without treatment.

CERVICAL CANCER: EPIDEMIOLOGY AND RISK FACTORS

Each year in the U.S. there are about 13,000 cases of cervical cancer, and 45,000 cases of cervical carcinoma in situ. The incidence of cervical cancer has dramatically decreased worldwide since the advent of the Pap test. From 1945 to 1975, the incidence of cervical cancer was cut in half in the U.S. (although the rate of carcinoma in situ of the cervix went up, reflecting the effectiveness of the Pap test). The Pap test is one of the most important medical discoveries of the 20th century.

The highest incidence of cervical cancer in the world is in Columbia, where it is the most common female cancer. Religious beliefs that discourage the Pap test is a factor.

In the U.S., black women get cervical cancer far more often than white women. A black woman's lifetime risk of developing cervical cancer is 2½% compared to 1% for white women. American Indian women have an extremely high incidence of cervical cancer. Lower socioeconomic status is seen as a more significant factor than racial or genetic differences.

It was long ago noticed that nuns and virgins rarely got cervical cancer, compared to an extremely high rate for prostitutes. Sexual practices were obviously the difference. Early age of first intercourse and increased numbers of sexual partners are strongly correlated with an increased risk of developing cervical cancer. This doesn't imply rampant promiscuity: remarried women who only have had 2 partners have 2 to 3 times the one-partner risk. Early age of intercourse is a risk factor, even if monogamy is practiced from then on. This has been attributed to the cellular differences of the adolescent cervix, which has more exposed columnar epithelium than the adult cervix.

Uncircumcised partners appear to impart a slightly greater risk (Jewish women have low rates of cervical cancer; Jewish men are circumcised). Methods of contraception play a role, with barrier methods (diaphragms and condoms) reducing cervical exposure and risk of developing cervical cancer. Oral contraceptives have been associated with increased risk, but this may be due to increased numbers of partners and not having the protective effect of barrier methods. Of particular significance is the finding that pre-existing dysplasia in birth control pill users is less likely to regress and more likely to progress to carcinoma in situ. The intrauterine device (I.U.D.) has not been shown to be a significant risk factor for cervical or uterine cancer.

Sexually-transmitted disease, i.e., venereal disease, (V.D.) is associated with an increased risk of cervical cancer. Gonorrhea, syphilis, and chlamydia haven't been associated, but herpes, venereal warts, and possibly trichomonas have. Herpes genitalis (herpes simplex virus 2, called HSV 2) has been the most studied. Whereas the reports in the early 1970s strongly implicated herpes as a cause of cervical cancer, later studies did not. It probably is a co-factor.

Figure 26-1 Female Pelvic Organs (side view).

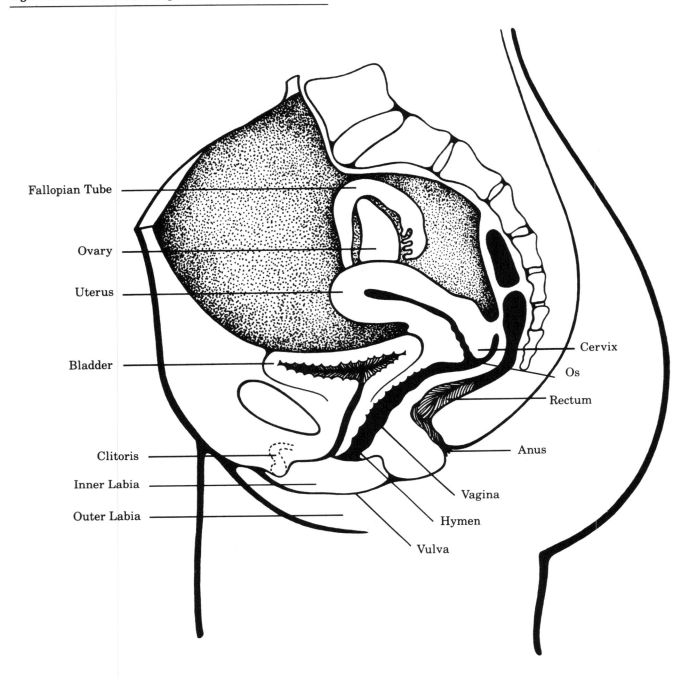

The 1980s have focused on venereal warts, the human papilloma virus (HPV), as the probable cause of many cervical cancers. Trichomonas, a protozoa that can cause vaginal infections, hasn't been studied to the extent that herpes or HPV have, but has been associated with cervical dysplasia.

Increased frequency of intercourse has not been shown to be a risk factor, but mechanical irritation and exposure to semen has been suspected. Some evidence exists to show that semen is carcinogenic, specifically seminal fluid DNA and sperm proteins. Further support of that possibility is the finding that women will produce antibodies to men's sperm.

Hygiene and douching practices have also been suspected. Earlier in this century, the use of coal tar douches was associated with cervical cancers. More recently, one study associated increased frequency of douching with an increased rate of cervical cancer. Chemical components of douches have not been well-studied.

Figure 26-2 Female Pelvic Organs (front view).

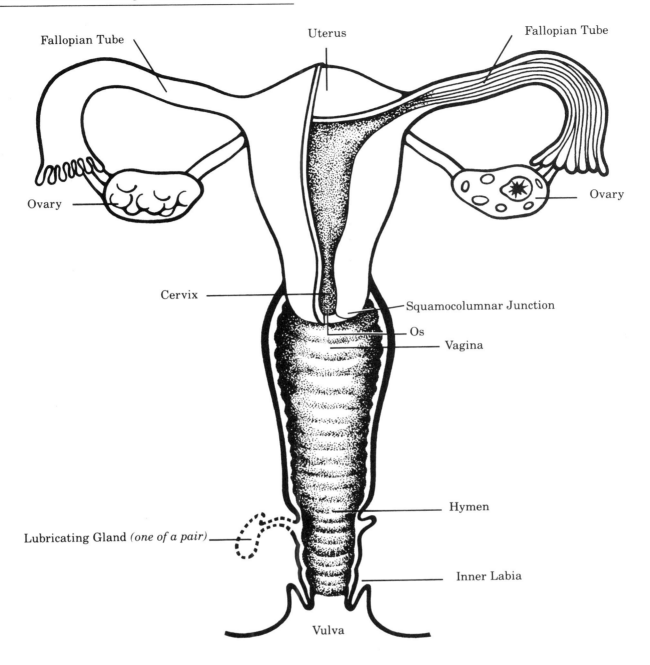

Dietary factors have been suspected, but aren't clear. Carotene may be protective. Smoking has been shown to be a risk factor for cervical cancer, and is thought to indirectly affect the squamous cells of the cervix in the way it affects the squamous cells of the mouth, throat, and lungs. Carcinogens in tobacco, perhaps benzopyrene, are thought to be transported via the blood to the cervix.

Genetic factors haven't been well studied, but aren't thought to play a major role. Radiation exposure hasn't been implicated, nor alcohol. Age when menses began or stopped, and whether menses have been regular, light or heavy, apparently isn't a significant factor.

Pregnancy, once or multiple, originally was thought to be a strong risk factor, but studies controlling for factors like early age of intercourse, numbers of partners, or venereal diseases, have shown it probably is not a highly significant factor.

Taken in total, it would appear that cervical cancer is the result of multiple, interacting factors (see Figure 26-3).

Figure 26-3 Summary Table of Risk Factors for Cervical Cancer

****strongly associated, *weakly associated, 0 not associated	
Multiple partners	****
Early age intercourse	***
Venereal diseases	***
Low socio-economic status	***
Tobacco use	**
Pregnancy	**
Uncircumcised partners	**
Oral contraceptives	*
Diet	*
Heredity	0
Age of menses	0
Character of menses	0
Age of menopause	0
Barrier methods of contraception	lowers risk

ENDOMETRIAL CANCER: EPIDEMIOLOGY AND RISK FACTORS

There are about 35,000 endometrial cancers per year in the U.S. White women have about twice the incidence of black women. Higher socio-economic status is correlated with that difference rather than racial or genetic factors.

The incidence is increasing in several countries, especially the U.S. The average age of diagnosis is about 60. In the 1960s, short-term and ill-conceived studies convinced physicians to begin prescribing estrogens to women in their 40s and 50s to prevent menopause. By the mid-1970s it became evident that their prescribing practices were causing endometrial cancers. (It is an example of iatrogenesis, a physician-caused illness.) Women at highest risk for developing endometrial cancer took estrogens for longer than 3 years. About 1% of estrogen users can be expected to develop malignant endometrial changes. Physicians' prescribing practices have shifted to what is currently reported as safe: combining the opposing hormone, progesterone, with estrogen. It remains to be seen whether there are any long-term negative consequences of combined estrogen-progesterone therapy; it just hasn't been used long enough to evaluate.

Obesity, defined as an excess 20 to 25% over ideal body weight, has been correlated with endometrial cancer. This may be due to sheer body weight, amount of calories and fat ingested, or to the fact that obese women have increased levels of natural estrogens. Hypertension and diabetes mellitus have been correlated with endometrial cancer, but it is probably more a factor of obesity and diet.

Genetic factors appear to play a role in some cases, with a familial tendency observed (apart from risk factors such as obesity).

Endometrial cancer is one of the few cancers for which a study has shown a decreased risk from smoking. However, other studies show that smoking increases risk. The issue is not yet resolved.

Menopausal age women who have never been pregnant (nulliparous), have a history of infertility, failed ovulations, irregular menses and irregular bleeding, and who have used estrogen are considered high-risk for uterine cancer. If a woman doesn't begin her menopause until after age 52 she is at higher risk.

A history of benign fibroid tumors of the uterus is not a risk factor, but adenomatous hyperplasia of the endometrium is considered in some cases to be a pre-malignant condition.

CERVICAL CANCER: PRIMARY PREVENTION AND EARLY DETECTION

Primary prevention of cervical cancer is effectively practiced by limiting the number of sexual partners, use of barrier contraceptive methods, avoidance of venereal diseases, not smoking, and getting regular Pap smears. Women at risk for venereal warts should routinely examine their external genitalia and have their cervix visualized on a regular basis by speculum examination [also see Chapter 70—Self-Examination for Cancer].

Detecting dysplasia or pre-cancerous states on a Pap smear can be thought of as a method of primary prevention of cervical cancer, but some epidemiologists consider it secondary prevention—detecting a disease already underway. The distinction is unimportant—what counts is that a Pap smear can prevent cases of invasive cancer of the cervix.

Until recently it was recommended that women have Pap smears every year. An annual frequency had been arbitrarily chosen when the Pap test was introduced in the 1940s, but now that the natural history of cervical cancer is better understood, it has become apparent that Pap smears needn't be done every year to be effective. For instance, studies show that if a Pap smear is done every three years, it will detect 92% of cervical cancers; done every year it will detect 94%. That's because, as discussed earlier, cervical cancers grow so slowly and predictably—even for high-risk women. A Pap smear done every six months wouldn't be likely to pick up the 5% of cervical cancers that are of a different cell type (adenocarcinoma and clear cell carcinoma), often aren't at the os, and grow extremely rapidly.

The 1980s were a period of flux for the Pap test. In 1980, on the basis of the evidence described above, the American Cancer Society departed from the annual Pap recommendation—instead specifying that it should be done every three years (after two normal tests done a year apart). This recommendation was heavily criticized by the American College of Obstetrics and Gynecology who feel that all women need medical care at least annually (including the Pap).

In 1988, the ACS back-pedalled their guidelines to what is essentially a recommendation for an annual Pap test. The 1988 recommendation states that women should begin having Pap smears by 18 (or younger if they are sexually active), and that it be performed annually for at least three consecutive years with normal results before a less-than-annual frequency be considered—at the physician's discretion.

In other words, the 1988 ACS Pap recommendations call for women to return to greater dependency on physicians—which some people feel is a step backwards. It certainly runs counter to the overall ACS recommendations that young people (under 40) need to have a cancer checkup only every three years. In Canada, where there is socialized medicine, the recommended interval for the Pap test is every five years, and to stop at age 60.

Medical politics aside, the important thing to realize is that cervical cancer is largely a disease of younger women, and that obtaining regular Pap smears is essential for young, sexually active women.

Only about 15% of women in the U.S. get a Pap smear every year, but about 75% have one at least every three years. Many women with cervical cancer give a history of never having had a Pap smear, or of not having had one since their last child was born. Women of lower socio-economic status are far less likely to get routine Pap smears. Until 100% of women are getting Pap smears, public education must continue to teach women about the importance of getting this important test.

ENDOMETRIAL CANCER: PRIMARY PREVENTION AND EARLY DETECTION

Primary prevention of endometrial cancer is to maintain ideal body weight, avoid unnecessary estrogens, and if at high risk to be screened for early changes of the endometrium that may lead to cancer.

The standard bimanual pelvic examination (as described for ovarian cancer) is not a good screening method for endometrial cancer. The Pap smear isn't good either, because it doesn't thoroughly sample cells from above the cervix. However, endometrial cancers do shed cells that can be picked up by a Pap test, but by then it is beyond the early invasive stage.

It is recommended that women at high-risk have an endometrial biopsy close to the time of menopause. An endometrial biopsy is a selective sampling of cells lining the uterus; it is like a mini-D&C (dilation and curettage). It can be done as an outpatient procedure with little discomfort or risk, by a gynecologist and some other primary care physicians. High-risk women are those who have a history of obesity, infertility, irregular or failed ovulation, abnormal menses, abnormal bleeding, or being on estrogens. It is recommended that women on combined estrogen-progesterone therapy have an annual or biannual endometrial biopsy.

SYMPTOMS AND DIAGNOSIS

The symptoms of both cervical and endometrial cancer only come with invasive disease, and include: painless vaginal bleeding (especially after intercourse), watery or foul-smelling discharge, and sometimes painful intercourse (dyspareunia). Bleeding between menses and especially after menopause is never normal, and should be investigated.

Preliminary diagnosis of cervical cancer is sometimes made from a routine Pap smear, but assessment of the extent of disease requires colposcopy—usually done when a Pap smear suggests pre- or early cancer. It involves the use of a colposcope, which is a visual magnification tool that is placed up against the suspected area to permit direct inspection and accurate biopsy. Biopsy is the only sure method of diagnosis, and is either done by the punch or cone biopsy method. A cone biopsy removes a wide "cone" of the cervix os and is often curative in and of itself. Biopsy is also possible with the use of a laser.

A diagnosis of endometrial cancer is likely when an endometrial cancer cell turns up on a Pap smear, but it can't be confirmed without doing an endometrial biopsy or D&C. Additional methods include hysteroscopy (direct visualization of the uterus) and other new imaging methods.

Staging of both cervical and endometrial cancer involves assessing degree of spread within the uterus and into the other organs in the pelvis (particularly the bladder) and lymph nodes. If present, metastases would be in the liver or rest of the abdomen.

TREATMENT AND PROGNOSIS

Cervical Cancer

Pre-invasive cervical cancer, including dysplasia, carcinoma in situ, and stage 1 cervical cancer can be eradicated by a properly taken biopsy (all margins clear), electrocautery, conization (removing the cone, or entire ring of squamocolumnar cells), cryotherapy, laser therapy, radiation therapy, or complete hysterectomy (removal of the entire uterus). Hysterectomy does not, however, yield a significantly higher cure rate than conization for carcinoma in situ. The overall cure rate for all of the above methods is 90 to 100%, depending on the degree of invasiveness.

Invasive cancer of the cervix is treated with varying degrees of hysterectomy, similar to the different degrees of mastectomy for breast cancer. The operation can be done from either the vaginal or abdominal approach, and ranges from a simple, modified radical, or radical hysterectomy (with stepwise degrees of tissue and surrounding organs and lymph nodes removed). For more advanced cases, surgery may be combined with radiation therapy given externally or by implants. Radiation therapy alone can be curative. For advanced metastatic disease, chemotherapy is used, but with limited success.

Immunotherapy may find a place in the treatment of cervical cancer. Streptococcal preparation (OK-432) appears to be effective in boosting immunity and lengthening survival of cervical cancer patients.

The overall prognosis for cervical cancer patients is a five-year survival rate of 66%, ranging from about 10% in advanced disease to 90% in early stages. If more women got Pap tests, the percentage of cases diagnosed in advanced stages would further dwindle, and the overall cure-rate would pass 90%.

Endometrial Cancer

Surgery is the chief method of treatment. The extent of surgery depends on the stage of the cancer. Fortunately, inoperable endometrial cancer is uncommon. Pre- or post-operative radiation therapy is an option, and is a subject of ongoing discussion and research. Radiation therapy can be given externally or by implant.

Hormonal therapy is sometimes used, depending on the presence or absence of estrogen and progesterone receptors on the cancer cells (if receptor positive, they usually respond to hormone therapy). Otherwise, chemotherapy has not been shown to be of much use in treating endometrial cancer, even for advanced stages. Immunotherapy is still experimental in treating endometrial cancer.

The prognosis is good for all endometrial cancers, with over 80% surviving 5 years—ranging from less than 25% for advanced disease to over 90% for localized disease.

27

Cancer of the Ovary

Mark Renneker, M.D.

Of the female reproductive cancers (vulvar, vaginal, cervical, uterine, fallopian tube, and ovarian), cancer of the ovary causes the most deaths—about 12,000 each year. It is difficult to diagnose early and difficult to treat.

A woman has two ovaries, one on each side of the uterus. They are quite small, about the size of an almond. The ovaries consist of an outer, epithelial shell that contains egg cells and other hormone-secreting cells important to menstruation and pregnancy. In about one-third of cases, cancer occurs in both ovaries at once.

Learning about ovarian tumors is a medical students' nightmare; there are about 50 different kinds, and many are of borderline malignancy (it's hard to tell if they're malignant or benign). There are so many types of ovarian cancer because cancer can occur in any of the ovary's many specialized cells. However, over 80% of cases occur in the outer, epithelial lining of the ovary.

EPIDEMIOLOGY AND RISK FACTORS

A white woman in an industrialized country has the highest risk of developing ovarian cancer. Each year in the United States there are about 20,000 cases diagnosed. A women in the U.S. has about a 1% chance of developing ovarian cancer during her lifetime. Risk for ovarian cancer increases with age, with the highest rates in women between 65 and 84.

As would be guessed of a reproductive cancer, child-bearing status is highly significant. Specifically, a woman who has a child is half as likely to develop ovarian cancer, and the more children, the lower the risk. Breast feeding also appears to reduce risk.

Correspondingly, rates are higher in nuns and women who have never married. Prior breast or uterine cancer increases risk two-fold. Prior colorectal cancer somewhat increases risk. Risk may be lowered by use of oral contraceptives. Genetics is, in general, not a risk factor for ovarian cancer, except for rare types. Exposure to asbestos and talc (i.e., from condoms and diaphragms) has been implicated. Radiation exposure has, too.

PREVENTION AND EARLY DETECTION

A woman's choice between having or not having children could be seen as a prevention strategy, but not many women would have children simply to lower their ovarian cancer risk. More recently, risk-lowering has been touted as a benefit of oral contraceptives, apparently to offset previous reports that they cause cancer. (Again, there are more fundamental issues in a woman's choice of contraception than lowering risk of ovarian cancer.) Avoiding asbestos and intravaginal talc is one prevention strategy that just makes good sense, even though they have not been clearly proven to cause ovarian cancer.

Just as there are no definite ways to prevent ovarian cancer, there are no good methods of detecting it early. The *American Cancer Society recommends that all women have regular (i.e. annual) pelvic examinations as a general method of early detection of gynecological cancer.*

But no study has ever demonstrated the effectiveness of a pelvic exam for detecting early ovarian cancer. By the time it can be felt, it has usually spread. The common story is that an ovarian tumor "the size of a grapefruit" was found—so much for early detection through the pelvic exam.

Ovaries are felt for during the bimanual part of the pelvic examination, in which one hand presses down on the lower abdomen while the fingers of the other hand press up from inside the vagina. Except with thin women, it's difficult with a bimanual examination to locate the ovaries, much less to assess subtleties of their surface or size. The Pap test does not detect ovarian cancer (the ovaries are anatomically distant from the uterus and cervix).

The hope for early detection of ovarian cancer lies in developing imaging methods, such as ultrasound, that can detect ovarian enlargement caused by cancer. Unfortunately, ovaries frequently have size changes in relation to menses (including what are called functional ovarian cysts), and there are many benign ovarian tumors.

Attempts to develop a blood test for ovarian cancer have had some success. Alpha feto-protein (AFP) and carcinoembryonic antigen (CEA) are tumor markers for ovarian cancer, but also for other cancers and non-malignant conditions, so they're not specific enough to use as a screening test. Monoclonal antibody research recently has led to a radioactive immunoassay called CA-125. It is now in common use in cases where ovarian cancer is suspected or to check for recurrence after treatment. A similar, simpler test using monoclonal antibodies for screening may be available in the near future.

SYMPTOMS AND DIAGNOSIS

Ovarian cancer is a "silent cancer," as are many of the cancers that originate deep within the body. When ovarian cancer has grown beyond the ovary itself, it easily and quickly spreads throughout the abdomen. Pain and abdominal swelling are the most common symptoms, with vaginal bleeding less common. All are symptoms of advanced disease.

Diagnostic tests beyond the usual physical exam include: ultrasound, needle or aspiration biopsy, laparoscopy (inserting a lighted tube into the abdomen that can be seen through), lymphangiography (taking x-rays of the pelvic and lower abdominal lymphatic system after injecting dye), laparotomy (surgically opening the abdomen) and cytological washings (washing the inside of the abdomen and examining recovered cells).

TREATMENT AND PROGNOSIS

Ovarian cancer is seldom completely removable by surgery, and when it is, the cancer is usually so aggressive that undetected spread is likely. Surgery for cure usually includes removal of both ovaries, fallopian tubes, and uterus. 5-year survival for stage I cancers is only about 60%. Surgery that reduces the amount of cancer, called cytoreductive surgery, is often undertaken and has been shown to lengthen and improve survival. Surgery is highly curative for the borderline malignant types of ovarian cancer.

Radiation therapy is often employed to treat ovarian cancer, by external beam and implants. Dysgerminoma, accounting for less than 5% of ovarian cancers, is highly radiosensitive and highly curable with radiation therapy.

Chemotherapy can be either quite effective with ovarian cancer, or quite ineffective. It is often difficult to predict which, without trying it. Patients with advanced disease have been cured with even single-agent chemotherapy, but this is the exception. Single-agent (usually alkaloid agents), combined agents, systemic or intraperitoneal (directly injecting the drug(s) into the abdomen), pre- or post-surgical, and chemotherapy as the sole treatment have all been studied, and each can be effective. Immunotherapy has been tried with limited success.

The 5-year survival rates for chemotherapy alone are less than 20%. The 5-year survival rate for all therapies is only about 22%. Finding methods of prevention and early detection of ovarian cancer is obviously needed.

28

Vaginal, Vulvar, and Less Common Gynecological Cancers

Mark Renneker, M.D.

The major gynecological cancers are of the ovaries, uterine endometrium, and cervix. Vaginal and vulvar cancers are less frequent, and still rarer are cancers of the fallopian tubes and placenta.

One of the first concerns about cancers of the sexual organs is how it will affect one's sexuality. Despite what is sometimes extensive surgery, radiation therapy, and chemotherapy, over 90% of women return to their prior level of sexual functioning. Plastic surgery and sex counseling are often important as part of the recovery process.

VAGINAL CANCER

There are less than 2000 cases of vaginal cancer a year in the U.S., and the incidence appears to be decreasing. It is largely a disease of older women, with the peak age of incidence between 50 and 70. No clear single etiology has been proven, but radiation has been implicated in about 20% of cases. A history of uterine and vaginal prolapse (where normal support is lost and the organ protrudes outside the body) and prolonged use of a pessary (a device to hold up a prolapsed organ) has been implicated in some vaginal cancers.

The major type of vaginal cancer is squamous cell carcinoma, accounting for over 90% of the cases. Malignant melanoma occasionally develops in the vagina. In young girls there is a rare tumor called sarcoma botyroides. The best-known but least frequent type of vaginal cancer is clear cell adenocarcinoma, which is almost entirely due to in-utero estrogen exposure.

Between 1940 and 1970, millions of pregnant women in the U.S. were given a synthetic estrogen called DES (diethylstilbesterol) in an attempt to prevent miscarriages—for which it was often effective. However, in 1971 it was first reported by Herbst that some of the female offspring from DES pregnancies were developing the rare clear cell adenocarcinoma of the vagina. A wide constellation of unusual growths and changes were soon discovered in the genitalia and reproductive systems of both sons and daughters of mothers who had been given DES.

The doses of DES that were given ranged from about 100 to 20,000 milligrams, and it was apparently worse if given before the fifth month (20th week) of pregnancy. Many women were unaware that they were being given DES. It was heavily prescribed in the Mid-west. The peak age when DES daughters have developed the cancer is 19 years old, and, fortunately there have only been about 400 cases in the U.S.—and the incidence is decreasing.

DES daughters should have regular exams of the vagina and cervix, utilizing special stains that highlight characteristic tissue abnormalities (called vaginal adenosis). DES sons also should be examined for abnormalities, particularly undescended testes. [See Chapter 29—Testicular and Male Genitalia Cancers.] Mothers who were given DES have not been shown to develop more cancer, nor have women who have used DES as the "morning after pill" (abortion), which involves taking a total DES dose of 250 milligrams over 5 days. In comparison, daily estrogen doses for preventing menopausal symptoms and osteoporosis is usually less than 1 mg. The duration of estrogen use appears to be the chief risk factor for those who take it.

The symptoms of vaginal cancer are bleeding or other discharges, and painful intercourse. Women who are no longer sexually active may not discover the cancer until it is quite large. Routine vaginal examinations and Pap tests often detect it. After biopsy and staging, vaginal cancer is usually treated with radiation therapy. Surgery is less often used. Overall survival is only about 30%.

VULVAR CANCER

The vulva is the soft padded skin surrounding the opening to the vagina. There are about 3000 cases of vulvar cancer a year in the U.S. 90% are of the squamous cell type. The vulva is skin covered and vulvar cancers are similar to squamous cell skin cancers. The various glands in the vulva, e.g., Bartholin's glands, rarely develop cancer. A swelling or lump in the vulva of a young woman is most often benign, and is simply a plugged gland.

The average age for vulvar cancer is 48 years, with in situ cancer at younger ages and invasive cancers in older women. No clear etiologies stand out, but for some reason vulvar cancer patients are frequently diabetics, obese, and hypertensive. Venereal diseases have been implicated.

Itching is the most common symptom, with pain, bleeding, painful urination, and a palpable mass also common. Pap smears may detect vulvar cancer, but diagnosis is by biopsy. Fortunately, many are diagnosed while still in the carcinoma in situ stage.

Surgery is the main treatment, with radiation therapy sometimes used. Early vulvar cancers can be treated by laser surgery. Chemotherapy results have been disappointing. Overall 5-year survival is about 75%. Vulvar cancers should all be diagnosed early, since examination is so easy. [See Chapter 70—Self-Examination for Cancer.]

FALLOPIAN TUBE CANCERS

These are extremely rare, with a total of only about 1000 cases reported. They are similar to ovarian cancers.

PLACENTAL NEOPLASIA

In about 1 out of 2000 pregnancies a tumor develops in the placenta. These are sometimes called molar pregnancies, but technically they are termed gestational trophoblastic neoplasia. They range from the more benign hydatiform mole to the highly malignant choriocarcinoma. Etiological studies reveal a 7 to 10 times range of incidence worldwide, with the highest rates in Asia. Socioeconomic status and diet have been associated, with one study noting that wealthy Filipinos eating more meat and protein have a far lower incidence then poor Filipinos whose diet consists mainly of rice and fish.

Gestational neoplasia is associated with high blood levels of HCG (human chorionic gonadotropin) which helps in making the diagnosis. The pregnancy is frequently interrupted by the disease. Overall, treatment is by surgery, chemotherapy, and occasionally radiation therapy. The success of methotrexate in treating gestational tumors is one of the milestones in the history of cancer treatment. Overall, the prognosis is excellent for most gestational trophoblastic tumors, approaching 90% long-term survival.

29

Testicular and Male Genitalia Cancers

Mark Renneker, M.D.

Cancer of the testis is the most common cancer for men between the ages of 15 and 35, while cancer of the penis and scrotum is rare in men of all ages. Testicular cancer will be the primary focus of this chapter.

The average testis measures 4 × 3 × 2.5 centimeters, with the left testis usually slightly larger and lower than the right—ask any good tailor. It isn't until about the 7th month of gestation that the testes move from their embryonic position in the abdomen down through the groin and into the scrotum. The testes are the male equivalent of the female ovaries. Over 90% of testicular cancers are in the testes' germ cells, the cells involved with reproduction.

There are too many types of testicular tumors and classification systems to remember—just know that every testicular tumor can be classified as a seminoma or non-seminoma. A seminoma cell is distinct under a microscope and more closely resembles the germ cell it was derived from; non-seminomas tend to be primitive bizarre growths, and include embryonal carcinomas, teratomas, and choriocarcinomas.

TESTICULAR CANCER: EPIDEMIOLOGY AND RISK FACTORS

Each year in the U.S. there are about 6000 cases of testicular cancer, and the incidence is rapidly increasing, for reasons that aren't clear. White males are at the highest risk, getting testicular cancer four to five times more often than blacks, who are at low risk. There are parts of Africa where a case of testicular cancer has never been reported. Also, when blacks do get testicular cancer, they're usually past 65. Hispanics, American Indians, and Orientals are at intermediate risk.

Genetics are apparently a significant factor in testicular cancer, but socioeconomic differences also play a role. The highest incidence for whites is among professionals. Geography is important, too: the highest incidence in the U.S. is in the San Francisco Bay area.

Undescended testes is the major risk factor for testicular cancer. Undescended testes (called cryptorchidism) is when the testes haven't fully made it into the scrotum during fetal development, and a man will apparently have only one testis or one of his testes will be tucked high up in the scrotum (and may be smaller). The degree of risk is related to the degree of maldescent: a testis that is still in the abdomen has a one-in-twenty chance of becoming malignant; if it is in the inguinal-groin area (to each side of the base of the penis, where hernias commonly appear) there is a one-in-eighty chance. About 2% of men have some degree of maldescent of the testes. The risk of malignancy is significantly reduced if cryptorchidism is surgically corrected by age 8 (the younger the better), by bringing the testicle fully down into the scrotum. Surgical correction for an adult apparently doesn't alter the risk, unless the testicle is removed.

One causation theory is that testes further from the heat of the body have less chance of malignancy. Support of that theory is: (1) the heightened risk for undescended testes in the abdomen (hotter) compared to the groin (cooler) and scrotum (coolest); (2) the statistical fact that the left testes hangs lower than the right and only has 47.7% of cancers compared to 52.3% in the right; and (3) a report that men who wear jockey shorts-underwear (which hold the testes tighter up against the body) have more testicular cancer than men who wear boxer shorts-underwear.

It is thought that DES sons are at greater risk for testicular cancer because they more often have undescended testes, as well as unusual cysts of the testes and problems with fertility. However, studies have not proven this hypothesis.

Tobacco and diet haven't been associated with testicular cancer. Nor have venereal or infectious diseases except for mumps. Mumps is a commmon childhood illness that often affects the testicles, sometimes resulting in atrophic (shrunken) testes. Mumps can be prevented by routine vaccination.

X-rays during pregnancy and at the time of delivery have been associated. Certain rare genetic and congenital conditions that affect the genitalia have been reported to have a higher incidence of testicular cancer. Cancer of the testes sometimes runs in families. Having had a cancer in one testis increases the risk for the other testis. About 50% of men with testicular cancer have a history of trauma to their testes, but the meaning of this is not clear—perhaps the trauma only brought attention to a pre-existing mass.

TESTICULAR CANCER: PRIMARY PREVENTION AND EARLY DETECTION

Primary prevention depends on identifying and correcting undescended testes in children, and avoiding radiation and estrogens during pregnancy. Common sense requires vaccination of a child against mumps.

Secondary prevention—early detection—is accomplished by testicular self-exam, a simple and easy-to-do procedure that should be performed monthly, especially by men at risk. Men at high-risk are young white males, particularly with a history of undescended testes.

TESTICULAR CANCER: SYMPTOMS AND DIAGNOSIS

Testicular cancer is symptomless in the early stages. What is usually first noticed is a painless bump on the surface of the testicle. Other conditions in the testes may confuse and scare a man, like epididymitis (soreness and inflammation of the epididymis, the attachment of the spermatic cord to the testis) or a varicocele (feels like a small bag of worms, usually above the testis). Pain is a late symptom of testicular cancer, and by then the cancer may have spread to the abdomen or lungs, causing symptoms. 96% of testicular tumors are malignant.

Diagnosis is by complete removal of the one affected testis (orchiectomy). A biopsy of the testis is not done because it is one of the few cancers where biopsy can cause a spill of cancer cells. Staging of the cancer involves looking for spread to the lymph nodes in the abdomen and the lung, the most frequent sites of metastates. Many testicular cancers produce elevations of the hormones HCG (human chorionic gonadotropin) and AFP (alpha-feto protein), which can be used to evaluate the success of treatment and to check for recurrence. They're not yet good screening tests, though.

TESTICULAR CANCER: TREATMENT AND PROGNOSIS

Testicular cancer has only recently gone from being highly fatal to highly curable, thanks to advances in chemotherapy and radiation therapy. Virtually all testicular cancers are first treated surgically by complete removal of the affected testis. The other testis is examined at that time to be sure it is free of cancer, which it usually is. Radiation therapy is usually then applied, particularly for seminomas, which are highly radiosensitive tumors. Chemotherapy is most often used for nonseminomas and disseminated seminomas. It is highly effective even in cases where the cancer has metastasized. Metastatic testicular cancer is one of the few cancers where surgery can successfully be used to remove metastases (called cytoreductive surgery), often in combination with chemotherapy.

The remaining testicle can be shielded from damage during radiation therapy, protecting its reproductive capacity. The removed testicle can be replaced with a prosthetic testicle that looks and feels real. After treatment for testicular cancer, men should expect a full return to normal sexual functioning.

Five year survival rates for all types and stages of testicular cancers is 90%, ranging from 50% for advanced cases to 96% for early cases.

CANCER OF THE PENIS

This is a rare cancer in the U.S., with less than a 1000 cases per year. However, it is an interesting cancer because of its wide geographic variation. In 1920, it was reported to account for over 20% of the cancers in China, but in more recent studies Recife, Brazil, and Bulawayo, Africa, were shown to have the highest rates—about ten times the rate among U.S. white males. Black men in the U.S. get cancer of the penis twice as often as white men. In general, lower socioeconomic classes have more penile cancer. It affects older men, being rare before the age of 25.

Most penile cancers are of the squamous cell type. There are pre-cancerous leukoplakia states. It develops into a crusting sore, most frequently on the head of the penis (glans penis). Circumcised men rarely get it. Poor hygiene has been associated with penile cancer, and smegma (the substance that collects under the foreskin of uncircumcised males) has been reported to be carcinogenic. Venereal diseases, including human papilloma virus (venereal warts) have been implicated.

Over 50% of men delay seeking medical attention for over one year after first noticing symptoms. Treatment is by surgery (partial or complete penectomy, removal of the penis) and sometimes radiation therapy. Treatment success rates are generally over 50%. Plastic surgery can help restore the penis.

CANCER OF THE SCROTUM

These are extremely rare, and are mainly of historical interest because this was the first cancer shown to be associated with occupational exposure: soot, among London chimney sweeps, as reported by Sir Percivall Pott in 1775. It has since been found with increased frequency among men who work with any kind of coal or hydrocarbon compound, such as cutting oils, shale, and so forth.

30

Urinary Tract Cancers— Kidney and Bladder

Mark Renneker, M.D.

Cancer of the kidney and bladder is common, accounting for about 10% of cancers in men and 5% of cancers in women.

The urinary tract starts with the kidneys (most people have two), located up against the inside of each side of the spine in the mid-lower back. The kidneys filter the blood to remove unneeded fluid, chemicals, and waste products from the body, and in doing so makes what is called urine. The many channels in the kidney come together in what is called the renal pelvis, which flows into the ureters (one per kidney). The ureters carry the urine down to the bladder, where it is stored until enough collects to cause the urge to urinate. The urine is then carried out of the body by the urethra. In men, the urethra passes through the middle of the prostate and seminal vessels (where a channel connects into the urethra to carry semen, when that urge comes) and exits at the tip of the penis. In women, the urethra exits just above the vagina and below the clitoris.

Cancer can occur anywhere along the urinary tract, but is most common in the kidney and bladder, presumably because that is where the most time is spent in contact with urine (which may contain carcinogens that the body is trying to get rid of, for instance the tars and other chemicals from cigarettes).

The major type of kidney cancer is adenocarcinoma, which is also called hypernephroma or clear cell carcinoma. Squamous cells line the urine pathway from the renal pelvis on through the urethra. Cancer of those cells is called transitional cell cancer.

EPIDEMIOLOGY AND RISK FACTORS

The annual number of urinary tract cancers in the U.S. is increasing, and already exceeds 65,000 (22,000 in the kidney, 45,000 in the bladder). Men get about twice as many urinary tract cancers as women. Overall, whites get urinary tract cancers more often than blacks, particularly bladder cancer. These cancers occur most often over age 60. They are common in the U.S. and Europe and rare in Asia.

Cigarette smoking accounts for a high percentage of urinary tract cancers, about 30 to 40%. The risk is highest for bladder cancer and cancer in the renal pelvis. Cigarette smokers have at least a two to three times increased risk of developing a urinary tract cancer.

Carcinogenic chemicals in the workplace, including aromatic amines (aniline dyes, benzidine, and 2,naphthylamine), have been shown to readily cause bladder cancer. Workers at higher risk for developing urinary tract cancers include: painters, chemical workers, printers, metal workers, hairdressers, textile workers, machinists, asbestos workers, truck drivers, and petroleum workers.

Fortunately, the fear from the late 1960s and early 1970s that artificial sweeteners like saccharine and cyclamates would cause increased numbers of bladder cancers hasn't been realized, but more time is necessary to be sure.

Obesity has been related to kidney cancer in women, and, as with endometrial cancer, this has been correlated with higher estrogen levels (due to increased conversion of other hormones into estrogen in their fatty tissues).

Coffee is suspected of causing urinary tract cancers, but studies of coffee intake and cancer have been inconsistent, varying with sex, age, race, cancer site, and dose. Our cultural bias in favor of coffee may influence how we choose to interpret the results of studies involving it. The balance of research on coffee and urinary tract cancers points towards a positive association.

Low intake of vitamin A foods has been associated with bladder cancer.

Radiation exposure has been associated with bladder cancers, particularly among women who have received radiation to treat uterine bleeding.

Those people using high quantities of analgesic (anti-pain) medications that contain phenacetin are considered to be at somewhat greater risk for urinary tract cancers.

Parasites like Schistosoma haematobium are thought to cause a high percentage of bladder cancers in many parts of the world.

Urinary blockage, for instance from an enlarged prostate or stones has been suspected of increasing the risk for urinary tract cancer, but studies have shown no association.

Genetic or hereditary urinary tract cancers are rare.

PREVENTION AND EARLY DETECTION

Prevention of urinary tract cancers is best accomplished by not smoking. Also, avoid dangerous chemicals, radiation, parasites, overuse of phenacetin, and, possibly coffee (or wait and see).

Early detection of urinary tract cancers is difficult. One of the first signs is often microscopic amounts of blood in the urine, and this can be picked up on a routine urine test. However, there are so many other causes of blood in the urine (menstrual contamination or bladder infections in women, kidney stones in men, etc.) that it is not a very specific screening test. However, it's worth knowing if you have blood in your urine, and you can regularly test your urine at home with easy-to-read dip sticks that change colors if there are urine abnormalities. Especially check your urine if you are at high-risk, e.g., a smoker over the age of 50.

No good low-radiation, inexpensive imaging techniques yet exist for screening for urinary tract cancers. Ultrasound holds promise. CT and MRI scans of the abdomen done for other reasons periodically detect an unsuspected urinary tract cancer. There are no good blood tests for urinary tract cancer, though it is conceivable that one could be developed. With some kidney cancers there is an elevation of an enzyme called lactate dehydrogenase (LDH); the problem is that other organs also make that enzyme.

SYMPTOMS AND DIAGNOSIS

The classic symptom of urinary tract cancer is painless bleeding into the urine. Pain is a late symptom, and might be in the back or belly. Rarely, a mass can be felt. Blood, pain, or a mass are all late symptoms of kidney cancer, with fifty percent having already metastasized by the time those symptoms are present. Fortunately, a higher percentage of bladder cancers are still localized when these symptoms begin. A subtle, mild irritation when urinating may be the symptom of an in situ bladder or urethra cancer. Cancer cells are rarely detected on routine examination of the urine.

Evaluation of symptoms usually involves an IVP (intravenous pyelogram), in which a dye (inert—rarely causes problems) is injected into the blood and x-rays are taken of the urinary tract as it is excreted. The bladder can be directly inspected by inserting a cystoscope through the urethra (done with complete anesthesia by a urologist—a specialist in the urinary tract). Ultrasound, CT, and MRI may be used; CT may be used to guide a biopsy needle. Evaluation is done for potential spread into the lymphatics and other organs.

TREATMENT AND PROGNOSIS

Surgery is the chief method of treatment, often involving complete removal of the affected organ. For the kidney that isn't a big problem (there is another kidney to take up the load of making urine), but for the bladder it may be necessary to route the ureters into the small intestines to create what is called a urostomy (bringing the ureters (usually) to the abdominal wall so that urine can be collected in an affixed bag).

Radiation may be given pre- or post-operatively, and improves survival overall. Radiation sensitizer drugs (misonidazole, oral or injected into the bladder) are being tried experimentally with these cancers. Chemotherapy hasn't proven useful. Kidney cancer occasionally responds to the hormone progesterone, but although there was early enthusiasm for its use, recent studies indicate it has limited usefulness. Metastatic bladder cancer does sometimes respond to combined chemotherapy. Immunotherapy and hyperthermia treatments are still experimental, though some kidney cancer patients appear to benefit from interferon.

The overall five-year survival rate is about 40% for kidney cancer and 75% for bladder cancer. Not enough cancers of the urinary tract are diagnosed early.

31

Cancer of the Mouth and Throat

Mark Renneker, M.D.

Cancer can develop in any part of the mouth and throat, including (from the outside in): the lips, gums, floor and roof (palate) of the mouth, tongue, tonsils, salivary glands, and back of the throat (pharynx and nasopharynx). Cancer can occur in the jaw and bony parts of the mouth, but these sites should be considered as bone cancers, different than the delicate, mucus membrane-lined oral cavity. Cancer of the larynx (voicebox) should also be seen as different, as part of the respiratory system. These oral cancers comprise the majority of what are called head and neck cancers.

Mucus membranes are composed of squamous cells, and practically all oral cancers are of the squamous cell type. Salivary gland cancers are usually adenocarcinomas.

EPIDEMIOLOGY AND RISK FACTORS

Each year in the U.S., there are about 30,000 mouth and throat cancers. The incidence is increasing: tobacco use—smoking, chewing, and dipping—is the number one risk factor. In the U.S., men have more oral cancers than women, and blacks have more than whites. 90% occur after age 45.

The site of oral cancer often directly corresponds to the site of tobacco exposure—for instance where the tip of a pipe enters the mouth, or alongside where a tobacco pinch or wad is pouched inside the cheek. The major cancer-causing chemical in smokeless tobacco is nitrosamine.

In parts of India, men and women chew "pan," a mixture of betel nuts and leaves, tobacco, and lime. The betel nut contains chemicals that cause cancer, and when combined with tobacco results in the highest rate of mouth and throat cancers in the world. (Some Indians also practice "reverse smoking," in which the lighted end of the cigarette is held inside the mouth.)

Alcohol is strongly associated with oral cancer, particularly when combined with tobacco. A person who drinks as little as one-and-a-half ounces of alcohol a day and smokes 40 or more cigarettes per day has a fifteen-fold increased risk of developing oral cancer. The inner-city alcoholic-smoker, often malnourished, has a fifty-fold or higher risk of developing oral cancer.

Poorly fitting dentures and broken teeth, causing chronic irritation, are also associated with an increased risk of mouth cancers.

Sun-exposure is associated with cancer of the outer lip, which is more accurately classed as a skin cancer.

PREVENTION AND EARLY DETECTION

Prevention of oral cancers is easy: avoid tobacco use of any kind, limit alcohol use, and maintain good dental care. All people, but particularly a person at risk for oral cancer—a smoker or drinker—should have a complete examination of their oral cavity at least once a year.

Dentists and oral hygienists are responsible for detecting a high percentage of oral cancers. Physicians, in their routine examination of the mouth and throat, are not nearly as thorough as dental health professionals. Both physicians and dental health professionals would find far more early head and neck cancers if they combined a thorough examination of the inside of the mouth and throat with a thorough examination outside for masses or changes suggestive of cancer in the glands and lymph nodes of the jaw and neck. Patients can also be taught to

examine their own mouths and necks [See Chapter 70—Self-Examination for Cancer].

Physicians and dental professionals are in a pivotal position to help smokers or drinkers to quit. During the oral examination, it should be mentioned to the patient if chronic inflammation and irritation of the oral cavity are present (which is invariably the case with smokers and heavy drinkers). They should be strongly advised to quit smoking and drinking.

Early changes in the mouth suggestive of oral cancer are white patches called leukoplakia, or red patches called erythroplasia. Leukoplakia is more common, and is a good example of a dysplastic or pre-cancerous state, similar to actinic keratosis with skin cancer or cervical dysplasia with cancer of the cervix.

Leukoplakia can result from any form of irritation, including—as mentioned above—smoking and drinking, and also tongue and cheek biting. All white lesions in the mouth are not leukoplakia, and all leukoplakia is not pre-cancerous—only about 10% is. Transformation of leukoplakia to carcinoma has been found to take from 1 to 20 years. All oral leukoplakia should be biopsied. Special staining solutions (i.e., toluidine blue) and exfoliative cytology (i.e., like taking a Pap smear of the mouth) can help in identifying pre-malignant or malignant areas in the mouth.

Treatment of leukoplakia can prevent oral cancer. Treatments include surgical excision, electrodissication, cryosurgery, and more recently a chemoprevention method in which a vitamin A analogue, 13-cis retinoic acid, is ingested or directly applied to the lesions. Chemoprevention with beta carotene and vitamin E also may be effective.

SYMPTOMS AND DIAGNOSIS

Cancer of the lip begins as a non-healing, enlarging sore that may bleed or ulcerate. There is often a history of repeated scab formation without complete healing. These sores often begin as leukoplakia.

Cancers inside the mouth are usually painless, red, slightly elevated, and have poorly defined borders. It may just be a lump you feel with your tongue.

Cancer of the tongue often begins with a mild irritation, feeling as though the tongue has been bitten. Pain will begin as the cancer grows and ulcerates. The pain may be felt in the ear, an example of "referred pain," due to shared nerve origins between the tongue and the ear. Foul breath is common.

Cancers in the throat begin as a persistent sore throat, but sometimes there is no pain until a lump is felt. Trouble swallowing is a late symptom. Again, foul breath is common.

Salivary gland cancer can occur in the parotid gland (the major salivary gland, located in front of the lower part of the ear), sub-maxillary gland (under the edge of the jaw), or other minor salivary glands or ducts. The usual symptom of salivary gland tumors, benign or malignant, is a gradual enlargement of the gland that is easily seen and felt. Approximately one-fourth of the parotid tumors and one-half of sub-maxillary tumors are malignant.

Cancers of the nasopharynx (the area where the throat and the nose meet) are rare in the U.S., but common in China. The symptoms are nasal obstruction, bleeding from the nose or down the throat, ear infections, sore throat, and a lump that may first be felt on the side of the neck and be quite tender.

Cancers of the nose and sinuses are uncommon in the U.S., and have symptoms similar to cancer in the nasopharynx.

Diagnosis of cancers of the mouth and throat is by biopsy under direct visualization. Evaluation of mouth and throat cancers that are difficult to directly visualize may require the use of special mirrored tools or fiberoptic instruments, and imaging modalities like magnetic resonance. Tumors in salivary glands are often not biopsied to avoid spread if malignant; the entire gland is removed instead. Care must be taken to preserve adjacent tissues and nerves, like the facial nerve that wraps over the parotid gland.

TREATMENT AND PROGNOSIS

The major treatments of oral cancers are surgery and radiotherapy. Early cancers in the mouth can be successfully treated with radiation alone—reserving combined radiation and surgical methods for widespread disease. Chemotherapy remains controversial for oral and other head and neck cancers. It is most often used in advanced disease. Simultaneous use of chemotherapy and radiation therapy, and regional or intra-arterial chemotherapy are other methods to consider.

The goal of treatment in oral cancers must always be to eradicate the cancer but to preserve function and appearance. Extensive surgery for an oral cancer may rid patients of their disease, but leave them with such a shocking appearance that they will never again feel comfortable in public. However, major advances have been made in maxillo-facial reconstructive surgery. Using grafts of bone and other tissues with well-crafted prostheses, a person's appearance can be significantly improved.

Radiation therapy will often leave a person temporarily or permanently with xerostomia (dry mouth), painful gums (mucositis), loss of taste, and severely increased tooth decay. Special attention must be given to preventing or minimizing these complications. Radiation therapy with accompanying hyperbaric oxygen may decrease complications; so, too, may radiation implants placed directly in the tumor, limiting irradiation of the rest of the mouth.

The prognosis for cancers of the mouth and throat varies from site to site, but in general is excellent (greater than 80% cure rate) for early, well-localized cancer and dismal (less than 10% cure rate) for advanced disease (i.e., spread to the neck's lymph nodes). Overall, 5-year survival for oral cancer patients is about 50%, ranging from 91% from lip cancer to 32% for cancer of the pharynx. Prognosis is improved by giving up smoking and drinking, and improved nutrition.

32

Cancer of the Larynx

Mark Renneker, M.D.

The larynx is the "voicebox," where the air going in or out of the trachea, bronchi, and lungs funnels through the vocal cords (the glottis) and allows us to make vocal sounds. Cancer specialists refer to laryngeal cancer as supraglottic (on the mouth side of the vocal cords), glottic (if actually on the cords), or subglottic (below the cords). The majority of laryngeal cancers are of the squamous cell type.

EPIDEMIOLOGY AND RISK FACTORS

About 12,000 laryngeal cancers are diagnosed in the U.S. each year. Males are affected more than females, blacks more than whites. Peak age incidence is at ages 60–75. The incidence appears to be increasing.

Tobacco smoking is the major cause of laryngeal cancer, and in most countries the incidence of lung cancer parallels the incidence of laryngeal cancer—but there are exceptions. For instance, female Maoris (New Zealand) have extremely high rates of lung cancer, but low rates of laryngeal cancer. Bombay Indians have the reverse pattern.

Alcohol use increases risk. Alcohol and tobacco are synergestic; smoker-alcoholics have extremely high rates. Occupational factors include asbestos, nickel, and mustard gas.

Genetics may play a role. Inheritance patterns of the enzyme aryl hydrocarbon hydroxylase (AHH) may be a factor. Herpes virus has been associated, but not proved. Dietary factors haven't been well defined, but are likely to be similar to those of lung cancer.

PREVENTION AND EARLY DETECTION

Non-use of tobacco and alcohol appear to be the best means of prevention, along with avoiding known occupational carcinogens and following a healthy diet.

Early detection can be accomplished through inspection of the vocal cord region by a physician, using a small mirror or a direct viewing optical tool. Unfortunately, most physicians do not inspect the vocal cords as part of a routine physical examination—unless there are already symptoms. High-risk individuals should ask the physician to check their vocal cords as part of a checkup. Potential premalignant changes (leukoplakia) or polyps may be found.

One innovative screening method uses a computer to find a "vocal shimmer" in voice recordings, indicating an abnormality or growth on the vocal cords.

SYMPTOMS AND DIAGNOSIS

The first symptom is almost always a change in the voice—usually hoarseness (raspier, huskier). There also may be sore throat, pain (sometimes referred to the ear), trouble swallowing, or a mass that can be felt in the side of the neck.

Diagnosis is by biopsy. Imaging modalities like CT and MRI may help in defining the extent of spread.

TREATMENT AND PROGNOSIS

Treatment depends on the extent of disease. In general, surgery is used with radiation (given before or after surgery). There has been only limited success using chemotherapy. Laser therapy is proving useful for biopsing, treatment, and palliation.

The treatment of laryngeal cancer may leave patients voiceless, but they can learn to speak by other means, including: (1) use of an electronic device held against the windpipe, (2) esophageal speech, a means of swallowing air and burping it back (only a minority develop satisfactory speech with this method), or (3) a new "duckbill" valve prosthesis that fits into the neck-exit point of the trachea (tracheostomy tube).

The prognosis for laryngeal cancer is pretty good, with an overall five-year rate of between 60–80%, depending upon the location of the cancer. The probability of survival is significantly improved for those who give up smoking.

33

Cancer of the Esophagus

Mark Renneker, M.D.

The esophagus is a muscular foot-long tube-like organ that carries food and fluids from the throat into the stomach. Esophageal cancer is a deadly squamous cell type of cancer that is too often diagnosed late, but is highly preventable.

EPIDEMIOLOGY AND RISK FACTORS

There are about 10,000 cases diagnosed each year in the U.S., with males, blacks, and people over age 60 affected most frequently. Environmental, lifestyle, and socioeconomic factors are the major etiologies.

The worldwide epidemiology has fascinated scientists. There is an Asian esophageal cancer belt, stretching from European Russia to Eastern China, where some regions have thirty times the incidence of the U.S. The overwhelming probability is that alcohol use in combination with tobacco accounts for higher rates of esophageal cancer. The type of tobacco or alcohol may make some difference, but all types increase risk.

Nutritional factors may play a major role. Risk appears to be increased by high-intake of preserved foods and low-intake of riboflavin, nicotinic acid, magnesium, zinc, and vitamins A and C. Heavily seasoned or spicy foods have been suspected, but little evidence supports that hypothesis.

A genetic susceptibility has been shown in a few cases. Chemical exposure has been associated, particularly a lye burn of the esophagus. Studies in China implicate a viral cause in some cases, probably EB virus.

PRIMARY PREVENTION AND EARLY DETECTION

Esophageal cancer can be prevented by not using tobacco or alcohol in any form. Worst of all is smoking and drinking at the same time.

There are no good early detection tests, but for some high-risk people it would be reasonable to screen the esophagus with a flexible fiberoptic scope. Barium swallow studies and cytology studies also may aid in the earlier detection of esophageal cancer.

SYMPTOMS AND DIAGNOSIS

The usual symptoms are trouble swallowing, gradual weight loss, loss of appetite, and fatigue. There may be swollen lymph nodes or a palpable mass. A presumptive diagnosis can be obtained with a barium swallow x-ray or directly visualizing the esophagus with a fiberoptic instrument. Definitive diagnosis is by surgery.

TREATMENT AND PROGNOSIS

Surgery involves extensive "radical" removal of a large portion or all of the esophagus, and much of the surrounding tissues and lymph nodes in the neck. Reconstructing the feeding passageway can be difficult. Radiation therapy may be given pre- or postoperatively or as the sole treatment. Chemotherapy regimens have been tried in many combinations, both pre- and post-operative and combined with radiation therapy. Despite aggressive multidisciplinary treatment, there are very few cures. For the majority of people with esophageal cancer, treatment is palliative. Of 100 people with esophageal cancer, no more than 10 will be alive five years later.

34

Cancer of the Stomach

Mark Renneker, M.D.

In the 1930s stomach cancer was the number one cause of cancer deaths in the U.S., but its incidence began steadily dropping to where it is now one-sixth as frequent.

EPIDEMIOLOGY AND RISK FACTORS

There are about 25,000 cases of stomach cancer each year in the U.S. It is twice as common among males as females, and twice as common among blacks as whites. The peak age incidence is 50 to 59.

Despite the declining incidence in the U.S., stomach cancer continues to be a major cancer worldwide. It is the number one cancer in Japan, with rates five to ten times that of the U.S. When Japanese migrate to the U.S., their rates begin dropping.

Suspected causes are predominantly food-related. The decline of stomach cancer in the U.S. is thought to be due to the widespread use of refrigeration in the 1920s and 1930s, with increased access to fresh vegetables and fruits (with higher intake of vitamin C) and less reliance on pickled, salted, and smoked foods. Given that sodium nitrite and nitrate (the preservatives found in most hot dogs and other prepared meats) are converted by stomach acids to nitrosamines, a powerful carcinogen, it is somewhat surprising that there aren't more, rather than less, stomach cancers in the U.S.—because of our infatuation with hot dogs. Apparently, vitamin C protects against the chemical reaction involving nitrosamines.

Lower socio-economic status is associated with increased risk, which also mirrors differences in diet. An association with cigarette smoking has been shown, and also alcohol. Radiation exposure apparently increases risk. There are some occupations at greater risk.

Stomach cancer appears to run in some families, but this may only reflect common environmental factors. People with blood type A, pernicious anemia, and gastric polyps have been shown to be at greater risk. Having an ulcer does not increase risk, but stomach cancers are sometimes misdiagnosed as an ulcer.

PREVENTION AND EARLY DETECTION

A cancer-risk-reducing diet is the most obvious precaution against stomach cancer, along with not smoking or drinking. If someone in your family has had stomach cancer, your risk is increased—so special attention should be paid to primary prevention methods.

Japan has led the way in research on methods of early detection. Their best results have been with a special mass screening x-ray technique called photofluorography; for the first time, substantial numbers of early stomach cancers were found, with corresponding improved overall survival. Another method is to directly inspect the stomachs of high-risk people with a flexible fiberoptic scope. Premalignant polyps, too small to turn up on an x-ray, are sometimes found. Various blood tests have been tried with little success, but the future holds promise in this area because of the advances in monoclonal antibody technology.

SYMPTOMS AND DIAGNOSIS

The symptoms are vague, usually beginning with minimal discomfort in the region of the stomach and some weight loss. Later symptoms are accelerated weight loss, an earlier feeling of being full upon eating, trouble keeping food down, blood in the stool, anemia, a palpable mass and a swollen abdomen. Severe ulcer-like pain is not common. If an ulcer in the stomach doesn't improve after 4 to 6 weeks of treatment, however, it may be cancer.

A presumptive diagnosis can be obtained with an upper gastrointestinal barium study (called an "upper GI") and/or gastric fiberoptic endoscopy with biopsy. Definitive diagnosis may not come until surgery.

TREATMENT AND PROGNOSIS

Stomach cancer, like esophageal cancer, is hard to treat. In half of the cases, the surgeon opens the abdomen and finds that the cancer is too widespread to attempt removal. If surgery is attempted, part or all of the stomach is removed. The post-operative course can be rough. Results with radiation therapy and chemotherapy have been disappointing, but many new combinations and approaches are being tried.

The overall five-year survival rate is only about 10%.

35

Cancer of the Pancreas

Mark Renneker, M.D.

Cancer of the pancreas is among the most deadly and frightening of all cancers; few survive and the incidence is increasing. The pancreas is obscure in most peoples' minds, but all of us should be aware of this organ, given the severity of what can go wrong with it: diabetes (the cells that produce insulin are in the pancreas), pancreatitis (a painful, often recurrent condition), and cancer.

The pancreas is a thin, narrow, six-inch long gland that horizontally straddles the stomach and intestines. The "head" of the pancreas is where it empties into the small intestine, on the right side of the abdomen, near the liver; the "body" and "tail" is what extends over towards the stomach, on the left side of the abdomen.

The pancreas has two major functions: as an exocrine gland, to produce enzymes that aid in digestion; and as an endocrine gland, to produce insulin, which regulates metabolism of glucose. Over 95% of pancreatic cancers are of the exocrine type, and are mainly adenocarcinomas; the less than 5% that are of the endocrine type are covered under Chapter 38—Thyroid and Other Endocrine Gland Cancers.

EPIDEMIOLOGY AND RISK FACTORS

Some 26,000 cases of pancreatic cancer are diagnosed each year in the U.S. The incidence has increased over 25% since the 1950s. A person born today has a 1% lifetime chance of developing pancreatic cancer. Men are affected more than women, blacks more than whites. Hawaiians and American Indians are also at higher risk. It is more common in lower socio-economic groups. Pancreatic cancer is rare before age 30, and has a peak incidence between 70 and 79.

The incidence varies worldwide, with high rates in Northern Europe, Australia, the United States, and Polynesia, and low rates in Asia, Africa, and South America. The incidence is increasing worldwide.

No one etiologic factor accounts for pancreatic cancer and its increasing incidence. Tobacco use, particularly cigarette smoking, has been associated with an increased risk (two-pack a day smokers have double the risk). Dietary factors have been implicated, including a high-fat diet, preserved meats (nitrosamines), low-intake of vitamin A, and coffee. The coffee-pancreatic association remains controversial, but on balance the studies indicate that coffee drinking does increase risk for pancreatic cancer. 80% of Americans drink coffee.

Alcohol has a weak association, but chronic pancreatitis, a condition common among alcoholics, is more strongly associated. Radiation has been weakly associated. Workers exposed to organic solvents and petroleum compounds are at higher risk. Heredity is thought to play a minimal role.

PREVENTION AND EARLY DETECTION

Given that Seventh Day Adventists and Mormons have extremely low rates of pancreatic cancer, which is consistent with the risk factors described above, steps to prevent pancreatic cancer become obvious: don't use tobacco, alcohol, and coffee.

Finding a method for the early detection of pancreatic cancer has thwarted the cancer field— the pancreas is too deep in the abdomen to find on physical examination and difficult to x-ray. Ultrasound has raised some hope but, as with lung cancer, once a pancreatic cancer is large enough to be picked up by an imaging technique, it's too late.

One new test that holds promise is a serum tumor antigen immunoassay called CA 19-9, which appears to be highly specific for pancreatic cancer. At present, it is mainly used as a diagnostic tool, but it may find application for screening.

SYMPTOMS AND DIAGNOSIS

Pancreatic cancer is insidous. Symptoms come on gradually, usually starting with loss of appetite and weight, weakness, and occasional nausea, vomiting, and abdominal pain. Later symptoms are jaundice (turning yellow, from blocked outflow of bile) and worsening pain.

Diagnosis is presumptively made by ultrasound, CT, or MRI. CT-guided needle biopsy may confirm the diagnosis, but it often comes to surgery to get a definitive tissue biopsy.

TREATMENT AND PROGNOSIS

A surgical cure is possible, but rare. Most have metastasized by the time they are diagnosed, and by that time surgery offers no chance for improved survival. Only palliation is possible. Unfortunately, these cancers aren't curable by radiation therapy, chemotherapy, or immunotherapy—though new methods will continue to be developed and tried.

Cancer of the pancreas has the dubious distinction of being the most lethal of the major cancers: of 100 people with it, 90 will be dead within one year, and the remaining ten will almost certainly die within five years—survivors are rare.

36

Cancer of the Liver and Gall Bladder

Mark Renneker, M.D.

In some parts of the world, liver and biliary tract cancer are the most common cancers, but in the U.S. they are infrequent. The most common case is a metastasis from a primary cancer elsewhere in the body. Cancers that spread by way of the blood usually seed the liver.

The liver filters and cleans the blood, then channels what it filters out into the biliary tract (the gall bladder and biliary ducts) to be passed into the intestines and transported out of the body as part of the stool. The liver and biliary tract are also called the hepatobiliary tree. Most all hepatobiliary cancers are adenocarcinomas.

EPIDEMIOLOGY AND RISK FACTORS

Each year there are about 15,000 of these cancers in the U.S. Men are affected slightly more often by liver cancer, but gall bladder cancer is far more common in women. In general, blacks have a higher incidence of hepatobiliary cancers than whites. American Indians have the highest rate of gall bladder cancer in the U.S. These are generally cancers of people over 65.

Hepatobiliary cancer occurs most often where there is pre-existing disease: for the liver, cirrhosis and hepatitis B; for the gall bladder, gallstones and parasites (liver flukes). Other associated diseases include typhoid and ulcerative colitis.

Alcohol abuse is closely linked to liver cancer (i.e., as a principal cause of cirrhosis). Aflatoxin, from moldy peanuts, is associated with liver cancer; obesity and high-fat intake is associated with gall bladder cancer. Estrogen use is associated with liver tumors, which are usually benign, and gall stones, which increases the risk for gall bladder cancer. Genetic factors are probably minor. There are a number of occupational associations with liver cancer, notably angiosarcoma from vinyl chloride. Radiation plays a minor role.

PREVENTION AND EARLY DETECTION

The best prevention of liver cancer is by avoiding alcohol abuse and hepatitis B. There is a safe and effective hepatitis B vaccine, and people in high-risk occupations (like health care) should be vaccinated. Gall bladder cancer is potentially preventable through diet, avoiding (or being treated for) parasites, and considering having gall stones removed.

Early detection is possible through awareness of potentially pre-malignant conditions like hepatitis, cirrhosis, and gall stones. However, detection of these conditions is not an objective of most health screenings, and usually depends on a person complaining of symptoms. Better early detection methods, including the broader application of ultrasound, lie in the future.

SYMPTOMS AND DIAGNOSIS

As with most gastrointestinal cancers, the symptoms of hepatobiliary cancer are subtle: loss of weight and appetite, vague discomfort in the right-upper part of the abdomen, and eventually jaundice, abdominal swelling, and sometimes a palpable mass. Symptoms may go on for weeks or months before help is sought. It is said that if you can palpate the gall bladder, it's cancer.

Imaging by ultrasound, CT, MRI, and nuclear medicine scans will usually show the cancer. Liver cancer often causes elevations of the alpha-feto protein (AFP). Needle biopsy may be attempted, but it usually comes down to surgical assessment.

TREATMENT AND PROGNOSIS

Surgery is the only real chance for cure with hepatobiliary cancers. Unfortunately, by the time most of these cancers become symptomatic, they are no longer curable. Radiation therapy and chemotherapy are mainly palliative. Direct infusion of chemotherapy by the hepatic artery may increase survival. Liver transplantation is not generally considered for liver cancer: if it is a well-localized tumor, just that part of the liver can be removed; if it has spread throughout the liver, it has almost certainly spread outside the liver, and a transplanted liver wouldn't help.

The prognosis for hepatobiliary cancers is dismal, almost as bad as for pancreatic cancer, with less than 5% surviving five years. Only the early, well-localized, surgically removable hepatobiliary cancers can be cured.

37

Brain and Central Nervous System Tumors

Also see CNS Tumors under Childhood Cancers

Mark Renneker, M.D.

The central nervous system (CNS) consists of the brain and spinal cord. The inside of the skull and spinal column is a finite space and any enlarging tumor, whether benign or malignant, can be fatal or cause permanent neurological damage. Brain tumors are one of the most feared diseases; they affect and sometimes destroy our minds.

CNS tumors occur at two age peaks, between 3 and 12, and 50 and 70. CNS cancers account for 20% of childhood cancers. See Chapter 44—Childhood Cancers for more information on childhood CNS cancers.

The many types of CNS tumors are classified on the basis of the tumor cell type and location. About one-third of brain tumors are metastases from elsewhere in the body. Of the primary brain tumors, the most common type in children is a medulloblastoma (a cerebellar tumor) and the most common type in adults is a glioma (a tumor of the neuron-support cells).

The other major type of brain or spinal cord tumors are meningioma (tumor of the CNS outer lining), medulloblastoma (a cerebellum tumor), pituitary adenoma (a tumor in the pituitary gland), neurilemoma (tumor of a nerve sheath), craniopharyngioma (tumor at the base of the skull), hemangioblastoma (brain blood vessel tumor), and pineal tumors (the pineal gland is in the mid-lower part of the brain).

EPIDEMIOLOGY AND RISK FACTORS

Each year in the U.S. there are about 15,000 new cases of CNS cancer, about two-thirds in the brain. Overall, men are affected more than women, whites more than blacks. There is a similar distribution worldwide. The cause of CNS tumors is poorly understood despite numerous investigations.

Some childhood cancers are related to congenital and inherited conditions, but it is rare for CNS tumors to "run" in the family.

Chemicals can be shown to cause CNS tumors in animals, but there is little evidence for humans. There have been reports of lead, sodium nitrite, pesticides and insecticides, and vinyl chloride in association with CNS tumors in humans.

Prenatal, childhood, and medical and dental radiation has been associated with CNS tumors in some studies.

Exposure to sick pets, Epstein-Barr virus, and the HIV virus have been associated with lymphomas in the brain; so, too, have conditions of immunosuppression (e.g., organ transplant patients).

Smoking and dietary factors generally have not been associated with CNS tumors.

PREVENTION AND EARLY DETECTION

There is no known way of preventing CNS cancer, except by genetic counseling for the rare associated inherited syndromes. Avoidance of unnecessary radiation, chemicals, and viral illnesses makes good sense.

There are also no good early detection tests for CNS cancers. Brain scanning methods are just too costly at the present time.

SYMPTOMS AND DIAGNOSIS

Brain tumors cause symptoms when their growth crowds and increases pressure inside the skull (cranium). The symptoms of increased intracranial pressure include headache, nausea, vomiting, lethargy and altered consciousness. There may also be poor coordination and balance, seizures, or weakness and changed sensation in just one part of the body.

Diagnosis of a CNS tumor usually involves CT or MRI, but other scanning and diagnostic methods can provide valuable information, too. One of the most exciting new imaging methods is called positron emission tomography (PET), which measures glucose metabolism. PET allows differentiation of the degree of malignancy, particularly with gliomas. As with all other cancers, confirmation and definition of cell type is by surgery. Only rarely can a CNS tumor be biopsied without first creating access by surgery.

TREATMENT AND PROGNOSIS

The initial treatment is virtually always surgery. There are major new developments in neurosurgery, including the use of microsurgical techniques (using a microscope to view the tissue being operated on), CT-guided surgery, and the use of lasers. However, some CNS tumors are inaccessible or too large and enmeshed in vital structures to be removed by surgery. Only rarely can CNS metastases be surgically removed, but they do usually respond to radiation therapy. Most CNS cancers respond to radiation therapy, which is used after surgery in most cases.

Used alone, chemotherapy has not been successful with CNS cancers, but when used after surgery and with radiation therapy it can make a difference. There are various steroid drugs that will reduce brain swelling and improve symptoms.

Remarkable research is underway using monoclonal antibodies to bathe the CNS tissues during surgery (intra-operative immunotherapy). Immunological methods are also being developed to better characterize the grade or degree of malignancy of tumors. This is done by culturing surgically-removed tumor cells with various immunologic assays. The results can help in making decisions about the extent of additional therapy.

The successes in treating childhood CNS cancers, which are curable more often than they are fatal, are not matched by adult CNS cancers, which are fatal more often than they are cured. Over 95% of patients with high-grade astrocytomas die within two years. Those with low-grade or "benign" astrocytomas have 5-year survival rates of about 50%. Medulloblastoma (in adults), ependymoma, and oligodendroglioma have about a 50% five-year survival rate. Craniopharyngiomas and pituitary adenomas have five-year survivals of up to 90%.

Unfortunately, too many CNS tumors recur after five years. Most CNS tumors have ten-year survival rates that are about one-half the five-year rates. It suggests a peculiar not-as-yet understood natural history of CNS tumors. Also, "successful" treatment that eradicates a tumor may be unsuccessful in terms of quality of mental and physical functioning. The treatment of brain tumors has come a long way, but has a long way to go.

38

Thyroid and Other Endocrine Gland Cancers

An endocrine gland is any gland that secretes internally, as opposed to glands which secrete externally (called apocrine glands, e.g., the breast). The major endocrine glands include the thyroid, parathyroid, pituitary, adrenal, and part of the pancreas. In general, endocrine glands are stimulated by the brain to secrete hormones and substances that regulate bodily functions. An endocrinologist is a specialist in endocrine glands.

About 12,000 endocrine gland cancers are diagnosed each year in the United States. 90% are in the thyroid, so this chapter will focus on thyroid cancers. The thyroid gland is located just below the Adam's apple (thyroid cartilage) in the neck and above the notch formed by the top of the breast bone (sternum). The thyroid gland is the size and shape of a butterfly, measures 2 to 3 inches across, and feels like tender, pounded-thin veal.

The major types of thyroid cancer are papillary adenocarcinoma, follicular carcinoma, and medullary carcinoma. Papillary and follicular are far more common and are relatively slow-growing; medullary are uncommon, often inherited, fast-growing, and metastasize early. Most thyroid cancers don't grow to be large enough to be noticed or cause symptoms. Autopsy studies of people dying of other causes show that about 6% have unsuspected cancer of the thyroid.

THYROID

Epidemiology and Risk Factors

Thyroid cancer incidence is almost equal worldwide, except in Hawaii, Iceland, Israel, and Columbia, where the rates are far higher. Women get it twice as often as men. It is one of the few cancers that occurs with any frequency in young adults (ages 20 to 35). The majority of cases are diagnosed between 25 and 65. The incidence is increasing.

The major risk factor for thyroid cancer is radiation exposure to the head and neck. Radiation was commonly used prior to the mid-1950s as a treatment for ringworm (fungus) of the scalp, acne, enlarged tonsils and adenoids, and thymus gland enlargement in children. These treatments usually involved 200 to 1000 rads. Significant risk for thyroid cancer begins at about 100 rads. The thyroid gland is sterilized by exposures over 2000 rads, and is then unlikely to develop cancer. About 25% of people who receive head and neck irradiation later develop growths in their thyroid, of which less than 25% will be cancer.

Goiter is a common benign thyroid growth that results from a low-iodine diet. It has been studied in terms of thyroid cancer, and is not felt to be a significant risk factor.

Prevention and Early Detection

Primary prevention of thyroid cancer principally involves minimizing radiation exposure. Early detection of most thyroid cancers is possible because they grow so slowly. Feeling for a lump in the thyroid gland is easy once you know how [See Chapter 70—Self-Examination for Cancer]. With a family history of medullary carcinoma, family members can have blood screening for thyrocalcitonin (a hormone produced by the tumor).

Symptoms and Diagnosis

Thyroid cancers are usually first noticed as a painless lump (nodule) in the neck, in or around the thyroid gland. Most thyroid masses are not thyroid cancer. A thyroid scan using radioisotopes (that aren't known to cause cancer) may show a "hot" nodule (benign, a functioning part of the thyroid that has overgrown, e.g., goiter) or "cold" nodule (possibly cancer). Definitive diagnosis is by biopsy, often by fine needle aspiration.

Treatment and Prognosis

Surgery is the treatment of choice, sometimes followed by radiation therapy. Chemotherapy is used for metastatic thyroid cancer. Additional treatment may include searching for and destroying remaining thyroid tissue or metastases with high-dose radioactive iodine and thyroid suppression treatment with thyroid hormones. A person can easily live without a thyroid gland if thyroid hormone pills are taken.

Prognosis for most thyroid cancers is excellent, even if it recurs. Recurrence is not uncommon, even after 10 to 20 years. Overall, 10-year survival rates are 60 to 90%.

PITUITARY GLAND CANCER

The pituitary gland is located at the base of the brain. If you put your finger in your nose you are pointing at it. Most pituitary tumors are benign but can have "malignant" consequences by causing damage to nerves and brain tissue. They apparently develop spontaneously, with only limited evidence for external causes. Birth control pills have been suspected in some cases.

Early symptoms of a pituitary tumor are varied and depend upon which of the pituitary's many hormones are affected. The disease is often not suspected for months, but can be discovered by a CT or MRI brain scan. Definitive diagnosis and treatment is by surgery. Radiation therapy can be a primary method of treatment. Chemotherapy is used in some cases. Cure rates are high, upwards of 90%. But in 50–75% of cases there is permanent damage to important nerves, such as those that go to the eyes.

ADRENAL GLAND CANCER

The adrenal glands are perched atop each kidney and are quite small. Adrenal gland cancers are rare. They can occur at any age and are most common in males. Pheochromocytoma is the major type of adrenal gland cancer. No etiologic factors have been solidly identified. They are usually diagnosed after a long search to explain a mass or pain in the abdomen, or if there are characteristic abnormalities or symptoms such as blood pressure and hormone elevations. Definitive diagnosis is by surgical biopsy, or occasionally by radiographically guided needle biopsy. Treatment is by surgery, radiotherapy, and chemotherapy. They often recur and have a poor prognosis—few survive.

ENDOCRINE TUMORS OF THE PANCREAS

The pancreas is a six-inch long, narrow, thin gland that horizontally straddles the stomach and intestines and is mainly involved with digestion. The part of the pancreas that produces insulin is called the endocrine pancreas, and it can develop tumors. However, they are rare. [See Chapter 35—Cancer of the Pancreas.]

CARCINOID TUMORS (Argentaffinomas)

These are strange, rare tumors that mainly occur in the glands lining the intestines and occasionally in the lungs. The word carcinoid means "cancer-like." They behave like cancer in all respects except for their relative inability to metastasize. They are considered to be a malignant tumor. Carcinoid tumors secrete various chemicals and hormones, like the neurotransmitters catecholamine and serotonin. Symptoms include sudden attacks of skin flushing,

blood pressure changes, diarrhea, and trouble breathing. Carcinoids are hard to diagnose (average delay from first symptoms to final diagnosis is 4 years). Fortunately, they can be treated (usually by surgery) and have a long-term survival rate of about 50%.

MULTIPLE ENDOCRINE NEOPLASMS (M.E.N.)

People with the rare familial multiple endocrine abnormality syndrome have more cancers in their endocrine glands. There are various types described. If there is a known family history, family members can be tested for chemicals and hormones associated with these cancers. Treatment can be difficult, given the multiple sites, and the prognosis is usually poor.

39

Sarcomas: Bone, Cartilage, and Soft-Tissue Cancers

Mark Renneker, M.D.

Sarcomas are cancers of the body's tissues that connect, support, and surround the parts of the body. The "hard" tissues are the bones and cartilage; the "soft" tissues include muscles, tendons, fibrous tissue (sometimes called fascia), fat, and the linings of the lung, abdomen, heart, central nervous system, and blood vessels.

Any one type of soft-tissue cancer is quite rare, but added all together the fifty or so types account for about 5000 cancers a year in the U.S.

Bone and cartilage cancers also are uncommon, accounting for less than 0.5% of all cancers in the U.S. However, bone cancers seem common because other cancers frequently metastasize to the bone. When a cancer is found in a bone it probably originated somewhere else in the body and is called a secondary bone cancer. Primary bone cancers are far less common.

Benign tumors of the bone, cartilage, and soft-tissues are quite common. Most people have found at least one strange "bump" somewhere on their body, worried it might be cancer, and showed it to a physician who probably said "it's nothing, don't worry about it" (and probably didn't feel the need to biopsy or remove it). Most often these bumps are fibrous or fatty tumors (fibromas, lipomas). They commonly appear on the fatty, fleshy, or muscled parts of the arms, scalp, belly, back, or legs. They are not known to progress to cancer, and may be inherited. Harder (more fibrous) benign tumors of the sheaths of nerves sometimes appear in the hand or wrist. These are called ganglion cysts. Again, they have no malignant potential. Sometimes they require removal if they become sore or interfere with bone and tendon movement.

The benign bone tumors have a confusing overlap with malignant bone tumors. The natural history of bone tumors is a continuum from benign to malignant. There are: (1) benign-latent tumors, which grow slowly and rarely require treatment, often disappearing spontaneously; (2) benign-active tumors, which tend to grow progressively and often recur after surgical treatment unless wide-excision is used; (3) benign-aggressive tumors, which may extend into normal bone but don't metastasize, and are hard to remove; (4) malignant-low grade tumors, which have a low potential for metastasis and can usually be cured by surgery alone; and (5) malignant-high grade tumors which grow rapidly, metastasize early, and require more treatment than surgery (i.e., radiation therapy or chemotherapy).

The major types of bone, cartilage, and soft-tissue cancers are: osteogenic sarcoma (bone), chondrosarcoma (cartilage), and fibrosarcoma (soft-tissue). As an AIDS-associated cancer, Kaposi's sarcoma is increasingly more common. Kaposi's sarcoma is a cancer of the endothelial cells (the lining of blood vessels). Whether or not Kaposi's sarcoma is a true malignancy or an aggressive benign tumor is a subject of debate—but the fact remains that it is a tumor that can kill. Kaposi's sarcoma is discussed further in the AIDS section.

Malignant myeloma is a malignancy that primarily originates in the bone, but isn't really a bone cancer or sarcoma, and is covered in a separate section.

EPIDEMIOLOGY AND RISK FACTORS

Sarcomas occur worldwide with about equal incidence. They are most common in children and adolescents [see Chapter 44—Childhood Cancers]. Males and females, whites and blacks are affected about equally.

There can be a familial tendency to develop sarcomas. They are sometimes associated with genetic or congenital abnormalities. Prior radiation clearly has been shown to be a risk factor, particularly for osteogenic sarcomas. The amount of radiation can be small, as evidenced by studies of workers exposed to radium, or children who received as little as 7 rads for treatment of scalp fungal infections. When bone cancers occur as a result of irradiation, it usually is 10 or more years after radiation exposure. Recent studies of children treated for non-sarcoma cancers with both radiation therapy and chemotherapy, who later developed bone cancer, showed significant risk began at about 1000 rads and was increased if chemotherapy with alkylating drugs had been used.

Various chemicals and infective agents have been suspected. Trauma has not been linked. Pre-existing bone defects or conditions such as Paget's disease have been associated.

PREVENTION AND EARLY DETECTION

Avoidance of radiation and chemicals whenever possible would be the logical means of preventing at least some sarcomas. Knowing of a personal or family history of possibly genetically-linked conditions may heighten prevention and screening awareness.

The main form of effective screening is through careful examination of the soft-tissues and bones of children during regular checkups. Mothers' routine examinations of their young children can also be a significant means of early detection.

SYMPTOMS AND DIAGNOSIS

The usual symptom of a sarcoma is a swelling in the soft-tissues or over a bone. The swelling will at first be only minimally sore, but usually becomes progressively tender. Benign masses or bone tumors are usually painless, but can also become sore. Evaluation is by x-ray and/biopsy.

TREATMENT AND PROGNOSIS

The presently successful treatments of sarcomas, particularly bone cancers in children, are made possible by the team approach to treating cancer. Surgery, radiation therapy, and chemotherapy all play a vital role. Each cancer requires an individualized approach, depending on the type, grade, stage, and location. Immunotherapy with interferons, transfer factor, and other agents has been shown to have some effect in a limited number of cases.

In general, the prognosis for sarcomas is good, with upwards of 50% achieving long-term survival.

40

Introduction to Blood and Lymphoid Tissue Cancers

Mark Renneker, M.D.

The lymphomas and leukemias are the hardest cancers to understand. You'll quickly bring most medical students and physicians to their knees if you ask them to explain lymphoma and leukemia—what they are, how they differ, who gets them, and how they're treated. For instance, in one short chapter on just a subgroup of lymphomas in a leading textbook for cancer specialists there were over 700 references.

Hematology is the study of the blood; oncology is the study of cancer. Hematologists are well-trained in oncology, and departments of hematology and oncology are often combined as "Hem-Onc." The true overlap of these two disciplines can be seen in studying the lymphomas and leukemias.

In a general sense, leukemia is a cancer of the blood and lymphoma is a cancer of the lymph nodes. But it's quite a lot more complicated than those simple definitions, and the distinction between lymphomas and leukemias isn't always obvious. What they have in common is that both arise from cells that originate in the bone marrow.

THE BONE MARROW

The bone marrow is the soft pulp inside the longest, thickest, and biggest bones in the body, like the femur, humerus, vertebrae, or pelvis. As the pulp within a tree produces sap, the bone marrow produces our blood. In addition to red blood cells, the bone marrow churns out white blood cells and platelets. The white blood cells, also called leukocytes, are a large group of specialized cells that are divided into two groups, based on how granular they look under the microscope. This includes the granulocytes (neutrophils, eosinophils, and basophils) and the agranulocytes (lymphocytes and monocytes).

Making these many cells is a multi-step process for the bone marrow that begins in embryonic life with the formation of multi-potential stem cells. The stem cells further differentiate to become an erythroblast (which forms red blood cells), myeloblast (which makes the granulocytes), megakaryoblast (which makes platelets), or lymphoblast (which makes lymphocytes). Each of these cell lines can become abnormal, resulting in a variety of diseases—cancer among them (see Figure 40-1).

LEUKEMIA

The onset of a cancer at any step in the differentiation from a blast cell to a mature bone marrow cell is classed as a leukemia. With leukemia, there is unregulated growth of one of the marrow cell types, eventually crowding out the other normal cells. Soon there is no room, and the leukemia and other marrow cells begin spilling into the blood. The leukemia cells may then metastasize throughout the body, often appearing first in the lymphoid tissues. The first sign of leukemia may be a swollen lymph node, though by that time the leukemic cells would almost certainly be in the blood, too.

Leukemias are classified as acute or chronic. It is a vague classification, based on a technical rather than a clinical meaning. For instance, some acute leukemias run a protracted, non-acute course, and some chronic leukemias run a rapid, acute course. In general, what characterizes acute leukemia is how poorly differentiated or immature the proliferating cells are, in contrast to the almost completely differentiated, mature cells involved in chronic leukemia.

LYMPHOMA

Early in fetal life, the lymphocytes made in the bone marrow enter the body and become part of a complex network of lymphatic channels, lymph nodes, and patches of lymphoid tissue in the spleen, liver, intestines, appendix, and thymus gland. The fetal lymphocytes are further differentiated in the thymus gland to become T-lymphocytes (the thymus gland can also make its own T-lymphocytes) and in the fetal liver (probably) to become B-lymphocytes (the "B" standing for bursa, the name of the pouch where birds' lymphocytes are made).

Figure 40-1 Illustration by Ken Miller.

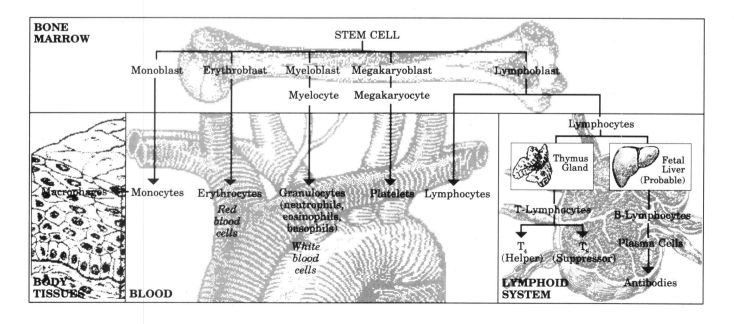

Figure 40-2   Cellular Origin of Malignant Lymphomas and Leukemias

Neoplasms of B-Cell Origin	Neoplasms of T-Cell Origin	Neoplasms of Histiocytic/Reticulum Cell Origin
Chronic lymphocytic leukemia (98%)	Chronic lymphocytic leukemia (2%)	Malignant histiocytosis (histiocytic medullary reticulosis)
Small lymphocytic (well-differentiated) lymphoma	Mycosis fungoides/Sézary syndrome	Monocytic leukemia

Lymphocytic lymphoma, intermediate and/or small-cleaved cell types	Diffuse aggressive lymphomas of adults (25%)
	  Mixed-cell type
	  Large cell, immunoblastic
		Large cell lymphomas (<5%)
		
		Hodgkin's disease

Follicular lymphomas	Adult T-cell leukemia/lymphoma	

Diffuse aggressive lymphomas of adults (65%)
  Mixed-cell type
  Large-cell type*
  Large-cell, immunoblastic
  Small noncleaved cell*
	Angiocentric lymphomas
	  (lymphomatoid granulomatosis)
	  (polymorphic reticulosis)	

Burkitt's (small noncleaved cell) lymphoma		
Acute lymphocytic leukemias (70%)	Acute lymphocytic leukemias (25%)†	
Lymphoblastic lymphomas (10%)	Lymphoblastic lymphomas (85%)	

*Majority of cases, 95%.
†These malignancies are of stem cell origin; they have an immature phenotype but are committed to B- or T-cell differentiation, respectively.
Source: Cancer—Principles and Practice of Oncology, p. 1629, DeVita T, Jaffe E, Hellman S. J.B. Lippincott, Philadelphia, PA. 1985. Used with permission.

Some B-lymphocytes then further differentiate into plasma cells—which are what make antibodies. The T-lymphocytes also further differentiate, for instance into the T4 (helper) and T8 (suppressor) lymphocytes, the T-cells affected in AIDS. The lymphocytes and antibodies are distributed through all the tissues of the body (except the central nervous system), and into what's called the "interstitial space" (the open space between vessels, tissues and organs).

If cancer occurs at a step in the out-of-the-bone-marrow differentiation of the lymphocytes, it is called a lymphoma. Lymphoma is classified as either Hodgkin's disease or non-Hodgkin's lymphoma. Hodgkin's disease is a lymphoma in which there are characteristic malignant cells, called Sternberg-Reed cells. The non-Hodgkin's lymphomas are further classified as B- or T-cell lymphomas, and then described on the basis of their size and shape as small or large, cleaved or non-cleaved (see Figure 40-2).

There is another cell line that originates in the bone marrow called the monocytes. The monocytes further differentiate in the body's tissues to become macrophages (called histiocytes), which are the body's scavenger cells. When cancer develops in these cells they are also classified as lymphoma (monocytic or histiocytic lymphoma).

MULTIPLE MYELOMA

Cancer of the final step of B-lymphocyte differentiation, the making of plasma cells, is called multiple myeloma. Multiple myeloma is a cancer of plasma cells, and is named "multiple" because it usually appears in multiple bone marrow sites at once. It also illustrates that there is obviously an entire loop in the system between the bone marrow and the lymphoid tissues, that cells and information-containing proteins must flow back and forth between the different sites.

SUMMARY

Figure 40-1 and Figure 40-2 illustrate the origin of the blood and lymphoid cells, and how they are named as lymphomas, leukemias, or multiple myeloma.

Cancers of each of these cell lines will be discussed in greater detail in the following chapters.

41

Lymphomas (Including Hodgkin's Disease)

Also see chapter on Introduction to Blood and Lymphoid Cancers

Mark Renneker, M.D.

Hodgkin's disease is a form of lymphoma, a cancer of the lymphoid system. Named after Thomas Hodgkin, who first described the disease in 1832, it is distinguished from other forms of lymphoma by the presence of Sternberg-Reed cells (also called Reed-Sternberg cells), which are large, multi-nucleated cells. Hodgkin's disease is classified as: lymphocyte predominant, nodular sclerosis, mixed cellularity, or lymphocyte-depleted.

Hodgkin's disease is less common than other lymphomas, but has received more attention—probably because it is now so curable, when only twenty or so years ago it was completely incurable. The discovery of a cure for Hodgkin's disease represents one of the most significant advances in the battle against cancer.

The non-Hodgkin's lymphomas are a varied group. What they have in common is that they aren't Hodgkin's disease. They range from B-cell lymphomas like Burkitt's lymphoma—rare in this country but common among children in central Africa—which mainly affects the lymph nodes under the jaw, to T-cell lymphomas like mycosis fungoides, a rare lymphoma affecting the skin. Together, the non-Hodgkin's lymphomas account for more cases of lymphoma than Hodgkin's alone, but in the U.S. no one type of non-Hodgkin's lymphoma outnumbers Hodgkin's.

Non-Hodgkin's lymphomas are divided into lymphocyte or histiocyte lymphomas. The lymphocytic lymphomas are further classified as well- or poorly-differentiated, and nodular or diffuse.

Hodgkin's and non-Hodgkin's lymphoma have more in common than they have differences, and for the most part can be discussed together.

EPIDEMIOLOGY AND RISK FACTORS

Hodgkin's Disease

There are fewer than 8000 cases of Hodgkin's disease per year in the U.S. It is more common in less developed countries. Males are affected slightly more often than females, whites more than blacks.

An interesting characteristic of Hodgkin's disease is its bimodal age distribution: it affects people in their early 20s and late 70s, with not many cases in between. This peculiar pattern is seen worldwide, except in Japan where only the later age group is affected. The bimodal distribution of Hodgkin's disease has led to a variety of theories of causation, none of which has been proven.

An infectious process underpins most theories, but evidence is conflicting. Hodgkin's disease sometimes occurs in clusters, for instance in one small town or school. But epidemiologists explain these occurrences as statistically possible and not necessarily proof of a contagion. One study showed health care workers who cared for Hodgkin's patients had more Hodgkin's disease than would be expected statistically, but repeat studies showed no relationship. Although, demonstrated to play a role in non-Hodgkin's Burkitt's lymphoma, the mononucleosis virus hasn't been locatable in Hodgkin's disease cases—but another study showed a two-fold incidence among people who have had mononucleosis.

A prior tonsillectomy has been shown to increase risk, but also shown to make no difference—the issue isn't settled. Hodgkin's has also been suggested in association with polio, multiple sclerosis, and Alzheimer's disease.

There have been some occupational associations, mainly with woodworkers, chemists, rubber workers, and those working with benzene.

Genetics may play a role in a small number of Hodgkin's cases, and a predisposition for it has been shown for certain rare inherited immunological disorders (such as ataxia telangiectasia). For unknown reasons, Hodgkin's disease in our country is more common in the well-educated and upper classes.

It is not inconceivable, given the tremendous push in recent years in viral research, that more evidence will accumulate for an infectious cause of Hodgkin's disease.

Non-Hodgkin's Lymphomas

There are about 30,000 non-Hodgkin's lymphomas per year in the U.S. Again, it affects males slightly more than females, and whites more than blacks. There is not a bimodal age distribution as with Hodgkin's. They become common beginning at about age 50, and maximal between 60 and 69.

Infectious agents apparently play a role in some lymphomas, but probably not in the majority. Burkitt's lymphoma, for instance, has been linked to Epstein-Barr virus. Other B-cell lymphomas have been associated with the human immunodeficiency virus (HIV). As with Hodgkin's disease, there are reports of clusters of non-Hodgkin's lymphomas, most of which haven't been related to an infectious agent and are statistically explainable.

However, consider this strange "cluster" case, which would seem explainable only by an infectious agent hypothesis. (It was reported in the December 12, 1985, *New England Journal of Medicine* by Grufferman et al., and titled "Burkitt's and Other Non-Hodgkin's Lymphomas in Adults Exposed to a Visitor from Africa"). A white South African woman visited families in the U.S. in 1982 for about 6 weeks, staying in four different households in three different parts of the country (California, Georgia, and Washington). Six to 11 months after the visit, one member of each household was diagnosed as having non-Hodgkin's lymphoma.

The South African woman's medical history was free of lymphoma and she never developed lymphoma, but a prior husband had died of a non-Hodgkin's lymphoma and she had worked in a high Burkitt's lymphoma area of Africa. However, for three days before coming to the U.S. she had had flu-like symptoms, which worsened during her visit, with a prominent sore throat and swollen lymph nodes.

In studies of all household members she had had contact with, a common infectious agent could not be identified; however, evidence of Epstein-Barr viral infection was present in some of them. The authors concluded that an unknown causative agent for non-Hodgkin's lymphoma had been transmitted from a carrier to other people.

Non-Hodgkin's lymphomas can run in families, but this can be due to genetic, infectious, or environmental factors. There are inherited immunodeficiency disorders that are clearly associated with lymphoma. The AIDS and Epstein-Barr virus led to increased lymphoma incidence. And medical conditions that require immuno-suppressive drugs have far higher lymphoma rates, for instance in kidney transplant cases.

Occupational associations have been noted for chemists and workers exposed to the herbicides phenoxyacetic acid or chlorophenol. The herbicide Agent Orange has been associated with a higher rate of non-Hodgkin's lymphomas for Marines with Vietnam service records.

PREVENTION AND EARLY DETECTION

The above discussion on risk factors would seem to suggest that one method of primary prevention of lymphomas would be avoidance of people with certain viral illnesses. That's good sense for general health reasons. As to whether or not people with lymphomas are contagious, the overwhelming balance of evidence indicates that they are not. As with AIDS patients, general physical contact with lymphoma patients is safe.

There are no good early detection tests for lymphomas—no blood tests or x-ray screening exams—only physical examination. If one is lucky, perhaps through conscious and regular self-examination of the lymph nodes, lymphomas may be caught early (see Chapter 70—Self-Examination for Cancer).

SYMPTOMS AND DIAGNOSIS

The symptoms for most lymphomas are similar: painless lymph node enlargement and constitutional symptoms (unexplained weight loss, fever, sweating—especially at night, malaise, and itching). More frequent bacterial, viral, and fungal infections are common for all lymphomas, reflecting a disturbed and depressed immune system.

Most Hodgkin's patients first notice enlarged lymph nodes in their neck. Skin, gut, and bone involvement is more common in non-Hodgkin's lymphomas. Symptoms of lymphoma may wax and wane, extending for months to years before diagnosis, with an average of five months.

Diagnosis is made by surgical biopsy of an enlarged node. Needle aspiration biopsy doesn't provide an adequate specimen. Nodes deep within the body may need to be biopsied, requiring more sophisticated means to locate and access them for biopsy. Bone marrow biopsy is sometimes done, particularly in non-Hodgkin's lymphoma.

TREATMENT

Exact staging of the extent of disease is critical to effectively treat Hodgkin's or any other lymphoma. The first determination is whether there have been constitutional symptoms. If so, it is labelled "B"; if not, it is "A." This already renders prognostic information. Standard blood studies and radiographic evaluations are done, including chest x-ray (and complete chest tomograms if the chest x-ray is abnormal), select bone films, lymphograms, and an intravenous pyelogram.

A critical determination is whether the lymphoma is on one side or both sides of the diaphragm. Until recently, virtually all cases of Hodgkin's and other lymphomas involved a staging laparotomy—a surgical exploration of the abdomen for involvement of lymph nodes, spleen, or liver. Now, however, lymphograms, combined with modern imaging methods, like ultrasound, CT, and MRI are replacing the need for a staging laparotomy. (Treatment centers vary; those that specialize in radiotherapy depend more on information from a staging laparotomy.)

One characteristic of Hodgkin's disease that separates it from the other lymphomas is that it tends to spread contiguously, moving from node to node in an organized manner. Non-Hodgkin's lymphomas are not nearly so orderly.

Radiotherapy is the treatment of choice for Hodgkin's disease and most other lymphomas that haven't spread to both sides of the diaphragm (stage I, II), or if it has, where there are no constitutional symptoms (stage IIIA). The goal of therapy is to specifically irradiate all involved lymphoid tissues, and those that may be involved. It takes about 4500 to 5000 rads to eradicate Hodgkin's disease from a lymph node. For more widespread disease, chemotherapy is combined with radiotherapy—or administered alone. When radiotherapy is used with chemotherapy for more advanced disease, it is often at lower doses (1500 to 2000 rads) and is called consolidation radiotherapy.

Treatment with combinations of chemotherapeutic drugs is more effective than single-agent therapy, but single drug therapy has its place for the treatment of patients who don't need or can't tolerate extensive chemotherapy. The drug combinations presently in use for Hodgkin's and some other lymphomas include MOPP (nitrogen mustard, vincristine (Oncovin), procarbazine, and prednisone), BCVPP (BCNU, cyclophosphamide, vinblastine, procarbazine, and prednisone), and ABVD (doxorubicin (Adriamycin), bleomycin, vinblastine, and DTIC). There are various other regimens, mostly involving the above drugs in varying combinations.

The course and outcome of treatment are well-defined for Hodgkin's disease, but less clear for the non-Hodgkin's lymphomas, which are evaluated at the time of biopsy and staging as "favorable" or "unfavorable."

Early favorable lymphomas may grow so slowly that only minimal chemotherapy is required, or no therapy. For some lymphomas, complete remission can be expected from one course of chemotherapy—but the disease may return and be less responsive, or not responsive to further chemotherapy.

Patients with advanced non-Hodgkin's lymphoma may be significantly helped by autologous bone marrow transplantation (removing one's own bone marrow to protect it while irradiating the whole body, and then replacing it).

Immunotherapy in the form of biological response modifiers have met with some success for select types of non-Hodgkin's lymphomas.

The rare (600 cases/year in the U.S.) cutaneous T-cell lymphoma, called mycosis fungoides or Sézary's syndrome, begins as a generalized, itchy rash that is easily mistaken for eczema or psoriasis. It can be treated by applying nitrogen mustard to the lesions, by photochemotherapy with oral methoxalen, radiation, and rarely, in advanced disease, with systemic chemotherapy.

PROGNOSIS

A recent article by Saul Rosenberg, M.D., of Stanford University, one of the leading radiation oncologists in the country, was titled "Hodgkin's Disease: No Stage Beyond Cure." This is another way of saying that cure is now possible even in far-advanced cases of Hodgkin's disease. The 5-year survival rate for stage I Hodgkin's is over 90%; for all stages combined it is over 70%.

The treatments for Hodgkin's disease and certain of the other lymphomas are so elaborate, and there are so few cases, that only in specialized cancer centers is there enough experience to be assured of the best prognosis.

The prognosis for the non-Hodgkin's lymphomas isn't quite as good, with the overall 5-year survival rate at about 50%. Favorable lymphomas (well-differentiated, lymphocytic, nodular) have a better prognosis.

An additional concern in treating lymphoma patients is whether the radiotherapy and chemotherapy may lead to later secondary cancers, particularly lung cancer, leukemia, and other lymphomas. The risk of developing leukemia is mainly in the first eleven years after treatment; the risk of later developing lung cancer can be reduced by not smoking.

42

Leukemias

Also see preceding chapter on Introduction to Blood and Lymphoid Cancers.

Mark Renneker, M.D.

Until recently, the word leukemia was feared as much or more than the word cancer. Leukemia, the most common childhood cancer, used to kill every child it affected. Families were devastated. It's not surprising that a widespread community movement developed to try to stop leukemia, resulting in the Leukemia Society of America, an organization similar to the American Cancer Society.

With the advent of modern chemotherapy, the grim picture of leukemia began to change. Children are now cured of it in a high percentage of cases. However, progress has not been as dramatic in treating leukemia in adults.

Leukemia is a cancer of the white blood cells. There are many kinds of leukemia and what they all have in common is they are derived from the cells in the bone marrow. The leukemias are divided into adult and childhood leukemias, but there is overlap. They are also classified as either acute or chronic, which, as described in the chapter introducing this section, refers to how well differentiated the proliferating cells are. Acute leukemias consist of primitive, poorly differentiated cells and tend to run a rapid course. Chronic leukemias are generally well-differentiated, and tend not to kill so quickly. But there are cases of acute leukemias that drag on for years, and cases of chronic leukemia that kill within days.

The four major types of leukemia are: acute lymphocytic leukemia (ALL—the childhood leukemia); acute myelogenous leukemia (AML—occurs at all ages); chronic lymphocytic leukemia (CLL—common past 50); and chronic myelogenous leukemia (CML—occurs mainly in middle life).*

Of the four major types of leukemia, CLL accounts for about 30% of cases, AML for about 15%, with ALL and CML in between.

EPIDEMIOLOGY AND RISK FACTORS

Each year in the U.S. there are about 27,000 cases of leukemia. About half are acute leukemias and half are chronic leukemias. There are only about 2000 cases per year among children, but it is the number one cancer of childhood. Men get leukemia slightly more often than women, whites more than blacks.

Worldwide variations suggest varying causes. The extremely rare acute myelomonocytic leukemia (AMML) accounts for 40% of childhood leukemias in Turkey, but only 4% here. CLL, the most common leukemia in the U.S., is rare in Japan and China.

Family "clusters" of leukemia occur, but the absence of proof for an infectious agent (except for the rare adult T-cell leukemia) argues more for a genetic cause. It has been clearly shown that some leukemias are associated with abnormal chromosomal patterns, such as the presence of a "Philadelphia chromosome." Leukemia is twenty times more common for children with Down's syndrome (mongolism), and more common for children with various other inherited conditions.

*There are two quirks in the leukemia nomenclature. Firstly, lymphocytic leukemias (ALL, CLL) are sometimes called lymphoblastic leukemias, which more accurately describes their bone marrow derivation from the blast stage of the lymphocyte. Secondly, the word granulocytic is sometimes substituted for the word myelogenous, so AML and CML become AGL and CGL. Myelogenous means "produced in the bone marrow," so granulocytic is more accurate, referring to the specific cells in the marrow that become leukemic (versus the lymphocyte cell lines in ALL and CLL).

The most impressive support for a genetic basis is the forty-fold increased incidence of leukemia for an identical twin of an infant with leukemia. The risk falls as the twins become adults, suggesting that leukemia may be caused (or prevented) by an interaction of various factors.

Other implicated factors include maternal irradiation (i.e., that change a mother's chromosomes), in utero irradiation (radiation of the fetus), or early childhood viral infections. If more than one factor is present, the incidence of subsequent childhood leukemia is greater.

There is no question that leukemia can result from ionizing radiation. All forms of leukemia except CLL increased in Hiroshima and Nagasaki after the atomic bombing, with a peak lag time of about 5 to 7 years, and increased incidence for up to 20 years. The question is really, how low a level of radiation will cause leukemia? Radiation treatments of 2000 rads or more for conditions like ankylosing spondylitis of the spine have been shown to increase the risk of leukemia. But there is persuasive evidence that even lower-dose exposure can do it.

In 1956, the major medical councils of the U.S. and England issued warnings to stop using fluoroscopy (an x-ray technique) for fitting childrens' shoes and other nonessential uses. By 1960, apparently at least in part as a result of the warnings, leukemia incidence began declining in both countries.

Workplace exposure to many chemicals, prominently benzene, is associated with leukemia. Drugs like phenylbutazone, arsenic, and chloramphenicol are reported to increase risk for leukemia. Many of the drugs used in cancer chemotherapy (particularly melphalan and chlorambucil) also increase the risk. The chemicals in cigarette smoking may be linked to acute myelogenous leukemia.

PREVENTION AND EARLY DETECTION

There is no simple primary prevention method for leukemia. Overall health vigilance is required, including avoiding viral illnesses, radiation exposure, and potentially harmful chemicals and drugs. The place to start is with precautions to insure a safe pre-natal life.

It appears at present that only rare forms of leukemia have an infectious source and that in those cases it is not the leukemia that is contagious, but the virus that caused it. How are you to know which leukemias are "safe" to be exposed to, for instance when a friend or a student at your child's school develops leukemia? Research on leukemia transmission—similar to the issue with AIDS—has shown that casual contact almost certainly does not put one at risk, even for the rare infection-caused forms of leukemia. For the other leukemias, particularly the chronic leukemias, even intimate contact is probably safe.

There are no good early detection tests for leukemia—other than being watchful for early symptoms, and aware of risk factors, such as chromosomal abnormalities.

SYMPTOMS AND DIAGNOSIS

The symptoms of leukemia can be understood more easily in terms of the bone marrow cells that are affected. Interference with production of red blood cells results in anemia, which has symptoms of weakness, fatigue, shortness of breath on exertion, heart palpitations, and pallor. Disturbed production of white blood cells results in more frequent skin and systemic infections, including pneumonia and meningitis, and fevers. Leukemia frequently causes decreased numbers of platelets (called thrombocytopenia), with a tendency to bleed under the skin and in the mouth, nose, gut, and bladder. An enlarged spleen (and liver), choked full of leukemic cells, may cause a sensation of abdominal fullness or discomfort. Leukemic infiltrations into bones and joints may cause pain.

A number of diseases of the bone marrow are called "pre-leukemic," meaning they may eventually become leukemia. There are also "pseudoleukemias" which are bone marrow conditions resembling leukemia. These are often caused by reactions to drugs.

Diagnosis of leukemia is sometimes possible by a routine blood test called a CBC (complete blood count), in which the white blood cells are counted and examined under a microscope. White blood cell counts in excess of 12,000 (the upper limits of normal) may only be due to an infection. A white blood cell count of 50-100,000 is highly suggestive of leukemia, particularly when most of the cells are lymphocytes. With the acute leukemias the white blood cell count may be normal or subnormal.

A bone marrow biopsy confirms the diagnosis of leukemia and defines its type. Chromosome studies may also be part of the diagnostic procedure.

TREATMENT

Each form of leukemia has a different treatment. The general approach with acute leukemias is to give intensive treatment to obliterate the leukemic clone that is producing the young, immature, ineffective acute leukemia cells. With chronic leukemias, treatment is directed toward suppressing the excessive production and accumulation of the mature, normal-appearing (but largely incompetent) chronic leukemia cells.

Depending on the type of leukemia, before starting treatment it is important to evaluate key body sites. For instance, central nervous system and testicular involvement is common in ALL. Lumbar puncture and, sometimes, testicular biopsy may be essential in planning treatment.

The major method of treating leukemias is chemotherapy, but radiotherapy also plays a large part. Surgical procedures have little place in treating leukemias.

Multi-drug chemotherapy is the rule—and timing is everything. For instance, for ALL there is initial "induction" therapy, with three or four different drugs, followed by "intensification" therapy in which other drugs may be used, and finally "maintenance" therapy in which, again, other drugs may be used. If there is CNS involvement, chemotherapy may be given directly into the cerebrospinal fluid (called "intrathecal" therapy).

Radiation may be given to the brain and spinal column (especially for ALL), to the spleen and other lymphoid organs (particularly for CLL), or as whole-body radiation as part of bone marrow transplantation.

Bone marrow transplantation is increasingly being used to treat leukemia, largely because of advances in the bone marrow transplantation field. It is generally reserved for high-risk or recurring leukemias. It can be successful using sibling or matched donor marrow or the person's own marrow, collected when they were in remission and presumably free of leukemia cells. Radiation is applied to the entire body at a dose sufficient to kill leukemic cells (which unfortunately also kills off most of the bone marrow; hence the need to then replace the marrow).

Immunotherapy, through the use of biological response modifiers, is used to treat some leukemias, for instance hairy cell leukemia (an uncommon, chronic-type of leukemia in which the leukemic cells have a hairy appearance).

One of the major advances in leukemia treatment has been through providing supportive therapy with transfusions of red blood cells, platelets, and white blood cells. Leukopheresis is used to help filter leukemia cells out of the blood. Also, the use of prophylactic antibiotics to prevent infections has made a significant difference.

Finally, supportive emotional therapy is vital. Leukemia patients and their families often get to feeling that there will be no end to the treatments, and need help in seeing the light at the end of the tunnel.

PROGNOSIS

The overall 5-year survival rate for all of the leukemias is about 30%. Despite the glowing press and general enthusiasm for treatment advances in leukemia, those reports mainly apply to childhood ALL. Treatment gains have related more to longer survival for the other leukemias, particularly adult leukemias. For instance, AML patients are now surviving up to two years, where before they almost all died within two to three months.

The 5-year survival rate for ALL has gone from about 5% in the 1960s, to about 25% in the 1970s, to about 50% in the 1980s. Some medical centers, able to provide optimal treatment, have achieved 5-year survival rates for ALL of up to 75 to 90%.

As with the lymphomas (particularly Hodgkin's disease), there are so few cases of ALL, and the treatments are so complicated that one should really only be treated in regional or specialized medical centers where there is the most experience.

Leukemia is one of those cancers that will sometimes spontaneously regress (i.e., suddenly vanish). Spontaneous regression is extremely rare, but has been reported for babies born with widespread leukemia, and for an uncommon adult leukemia called ANLL (acute nonlymphocytic leukemia).

43

Multiple Myeloma

Also see preceding chapter on Introduction to Blood and Lymphoid
Tissue Cancers.

Mark Renneker, M.D.

Multiple myeloma is a peculiar cancer, one most people haven't heard
of. Yet it accounts for more cases each year than the better known
Hodgkin's disease. Multiple myeloma is a cancer of the plasma cell, a
specialized type of B-lymphocyte that produces antibodies. Any of the
various classes of antibodies can be affected, and so there are many
types of plasma cell tumors. Generally, the term multiple myeloma
applies to all of the plasma cell tumors.

Plasma cells are produced in the bone marrow, lymph nodes,
spleen, upper airway passages, and the gut. Plasma cell tumors usually occur in many of these sites at once, particularly the bone marrow.
That is why it is called multiple myeloma (myeloma refers to the bone
marrow).

The most common type of plasma cell tumor produces immunoglobulins, most of which contain an unusually high amount of one type
of protein, called "M" or Bence-Jones protein. When the tumor begins
flooding the body with immunoglobulins, the M-protein can easily be
detected in the blood and urine.

EPIDEMIOLOGY AND RISK FACTORS

There are over 11,000 cases of multiple myeloma each year in the U.S. It is slightly more common in males than females, and almost twice as common in blacks as whites. It rarely occurs before age 40, with a mean age of diagnosis at 64, and the highest rates in men over 80.

Worldwide epidemiology suggests both genetic and environmental factors are involved. Blacks in the San Francisco Bay area have the highest incidence in the world, whereas blacks in Africa have a lower incidence. Whites in places like Poland and Romania have the lowest incidence.

There is an increased incidence among first-degree relatives, and cases of familial myeloma have been reported. Why blacks are more susceptible is not clear, but they do have higher average levels of immunoglobulins, suggesting a genetic difference. Also, the fact that the disease mainly affects older people implies that the aging of the immune system is a factor.

The evidence for a viral cause is not strong, although various viral particles have been recovered from some plasma cell tumors. Also, there are reports of increased rates of multiple myeloma among mink ranchers infected by a unique mink virus.

Ionizing radiation can cause multiple myeloma, as evidenced by the increased rates among survivors of Hiroshima and Nagasaki. An association with low-dose radiation has not been established, but radiologists and workers in nuclear processing plants have been reported to have higher than normal rates.

Chemical and occupational exposure is highly likely as a significant cause; increased rates have been reported among some farmers, workers exposed to heavy metals (lead, arsenic, copper), asbestos workers, petrochemical and plastics workers, furniture and wood-related workers, leather workers, and some workers in the food preparation industry.

Diseases of the immune system have been associated with multiple myeloma (systemic lupus erythematosis, scleroderma, and rheumatoid arthritis). Certain chronic diseases like recurrent rheumatic fever, chronic gall bladder disease, and chronic osteomyelitis (infection of the bone) cause a chronic antigenic stimulation (irritation) and also have been associated with multiple myeloma.

PREVENTION AND EARLY DETECTION

The above risk factors suggest primary prevention should include keeping your immune system strong and choosing a safe form of work.

Testing for Bence-Jones protein in the blood or urine can be an effective screening method for multiple myeloma, but there has been no study as to whether it makes a difference in survival. Also, finding elevated M proteins is not conclusive, because they can be elevated in other diseases, as well. However, for those at risk (e.g., an older black man with a family history of multiple myeloma who worked around radiation) it would seem logical to recommend periodic screening.

SYMPTOMS AND DIAGNOSIS

The most common presenting symptom is back pain, caused by tumor infiltration of vertebral bone marrow. Multiple myeloma will not be on the top of most people's list (or their doctors') when they have back pain, so the diagnosis is often delayed for weeks or months. Late symptoms include: infections (pneumonia, meningitis), anemia, abnormal bleeding, and poor kidney function (caused by the M proteins and other immune substances blocking the flow of the kidney).

A routine blood test for proteins may show an elevation of immunoglobulins. X-rays of the back may show pathological fractures (a pathological fracture refers to a fracture that results from a cancer in the bone) or holes in the bones.

Definitive diagnosis is by bone marrow biopsy (showing increased numbers of plasma cells) or direct biopsy of one of the tumors.

TREATMENT AND PROGNOSIS

Chemotherapy and radiotherapy are the main treatments for multiple myeloma. An alkylating drug (often melphalan), alone or with prednisone, can often bring about a complete remission. But often the disease returns. Without treatment, many patients' disease will remain dormant for some months before really setting in. It appears best to delay the start of chemotherapy until the dormant, or "chronic" phase has ended.

Radiation therapy is seldom curative with multiple myeloma, the disease is usually too widespread. Whole body radiation has been tried, with few successes. However, radiotherapy is extremely useful in helping to reduce the severe bone pain that afflicts most multiple myeloma patients. It can bring about tremendous relief if there is a tumor compressing nerves or the spinal cord.

Immunotherapy with biological response modifiers may be of some help, but is still largely experimental.

Without treatment, most multiple myeloma patients don't survive much longer than a year. With treatment, survival can be extended to three or more years. Cures are rare.

44

Childhood Cancers

Mark Renneker, M.D.

Cancer is far more common among adults than children, but it is the chief cause of death by disease for children between the ages of 3 and 14. Only accidents kill more children.

The incidence of childhood cancers varies throughout the world, but leukemias and lymphomas account for the majority of cases. The peak age among white children in the U.S. is 2 to 4; among black children there is no age peak and cancer is less common. In general, boys get cancer slightly more than girls.

The total annual incidence of childhood cancers in the U.S. is scarcely 7000. A large state like California may have only 600 or so cases in a year. Because there are so few cases, child cancer patients should be treated in specialized medical centers that have the most experience.

Most encouraging is the trend towards increasing survival rates for many of the childhood cancers. Acute lymphocytic leukemia (ALL), the number one cancer for children, has increased from a 5-year survival rate of barely 1% in the 1940s to better than 50% in the 1980s.

Some of the factors that account for the recent successes in treating childhood cancers include: new drugs; better ways of combining and giving drugs; new methods of giving radiotherapy; the development of multidisciplinary teams; combinations of surgery, chemotherapy, and radiotherapy; better identification of prognostic variables; better infection control; a philosophy of less aggressive therapy for patients with good prognosis and more aggressive therapy for patients with poor prognosis; better physical supportive therapy with blood components; and emotional supportive therapy with counseling.

Cancers that predominantly occur before the age of 18 are considered childhood cancers. They can be divided into tumors affecting (1) infants and young children, and (2) older children and adolescents. Cancers that occur during infancy and early childhood account for over half of all childhood cancers, and include leukemia, CNS tumors, Wilms' tumor, neuroblastoma, retinoblastoma, germ cell tumors, and rhadbomyosarcoma. Cancers of later childhood and adolescence include lymphomas, osteosarcoma and Ewing's sarcoma (both bone cancers), and various sarcomas and carcinomas.

Each of the major childhood cancers will be discussed in order.

LEUKEMIA

This is the most common childhood cancer, accounting for about a third, with approximately 2000 cases a year. Virtually all cases of leukemia among children are of the "acute" (vs. chronic) type. Acute lymphocytic leukemia (ALL) accounts for about three-quarters of all cases of childhood leukemia. The peak age incidence is between 2 and 6 years of age. Boys are affected slightly more than girls.

About 40% of childhood leukemia cases have been linked with chromosome defects and disorders. Genetics appears to play a role, as does radiation, chemicals, and possibly viral infections. Most childhood leukemias are highly curable. [See Chapter 42— Leukemias, which discusses both adult and childhood leukemia, including risk factors, symptoms, diagnosis, treatment, and prognosis.]

CENTRAL NERVOUS SYSTEM

Cancers of the central nervous system (CNS)—the brain and spinal cord—account for about one-fifth of childhood cancers. They tend to occur in the first ten years of life. The cause of CNS cancers is poorly understood, but for children a number of genetic disorders have been linked to increased risk, including neurofibromatosis and tuberous sclerosis.

The symptoms of brain tumors include headache, dizziness, difficulty in walking and handling objects, blurred or double vision, weakness and altered sensation in just one part of the body, nausea, vomiting, and seizure. Since many childhood brain tumors occur in the cerebellum, which is the very back part of the brain and responsible for coordination and balance, sometimes the only symptoms will be poor balance and coordination.

There are no good methods of primary prevention of CNS cancers, nor are there good screening tests to detect them early. CT and MRI scans of the brain will show early tumors, but aren't yet a feasible method of screening. CT utilizes too much radiation to be used as a screening tool for children, and MRI is too costly (about $1000).

The most common CNS tumor among children is medulloblastoma, which usually begins in the cerebellum. Medulloblastomas are treated by surgery, followed by radiation therapy and sometimes chemotherapy. They are highly curable, with 5-year survival rates of better than 50%.

Astrocytomas are also common among children. It is a cancer of an astrocyte, a neuron-support cell that can be located anywhere in the brain. For children they are frequently less malignant than for adults (called a low-grade malignancy), are most often in the posterior fossa (cerebellar area), and can be successfully treated with surgery (and sometimes radiotherapy) with a resulting 5-year survival rate of up to 90%.

Ependyomas are the third most common CNS tumor for children. An ependyoma is a cancer of the cells lining the open areas in the brain and spinal cord. Surgery and radiation (and occasionally chemotherapy) result in 5-year survival rates of about 50% overall, but up to 75% for lower-grade ependyomas.

Older children sometimes get tumors near their pituitary glands that are called craniopharyngiomas. They are usually benign, but can have severe consequences, including damage to the eyes' nerve pathways. They can be successfully treated

DOUGLAS MAURER, 15, of Creve Coeur, Mo., had been feeling bad for several days. His temperature was ranging between 103 and 105 degrees, and he was suffering from severe flu-like symptoms. Finally his mother, Donna Maurer, took him to the emergency room of Children's Hospital at Washington University Medical Center in St. Louis.

The blood tests revealed Douglas Maurer had leukemia.

During the next 48 hours, Douglas endured blood transfusions, spinal and bone marrow tests and chemotherapy. He developed pneumonia.

The doctors told him in frank terms about his disease. They said that for the next three years, he would have to undergo chemotherapy. They did not sugarcoat the side effects. They told Douglas he would go bald and his body would most likely bloat. Upon learning this, he went into a deep depression; although he was told there was a good chance for the disease to go into remission, he was smart enough to know that leukemia is often a fatal disease.

On the day he had been admitted, he had opened his eyes, looked around his room, and said to his mother, "I thought you get flowers when you're in the hospital."

One of Douglas' aunts, hearing this, called a floral shop to send Douglas an arrangement of flowers. The flower shop was Brix Florist, in St. Louis.

As the aunt placed her telephone order, she was unsure that the salesclerk would do a conscientious job. So the aunt said, "I want the planter especially attractive. It's for my teenage nephew who has leukemia."

When the floral arrangement arrived at the hospital, it was beautiful. Douglas was feeling strong enough to sit up; he opened the envelope and read the card from his aunt.

Then he saw that, in the envelope, was another card. It said:

"Douglas—I took your order. I work at Brix Florist. I had leukemia when I was 7 years old. I'm 22 years old now. Good luck. My heart goes out to you. Sincerely, Laura Bradley."

According to his mother, Douglas' face lit up.

His mother said "For the first time since he had been in the hospital, he had gotten some inspiration. He had talked to so many doctors and nurses. But this one card, from the woman at the florist's who had survived leukemia, was the thing that made him believe he might beat the disease."

I called Brix Florist and asked to speak with Laura Bradley.

"I realized what the boy must be going through," Laura Bradley said. "I wanted him to know that you really can get better. So I wrote the card and slipped it into the envelope."

I told her what her card had done for Douglas Maurer and his family. She said thank you, and then we said good-by.

It's funny; Douglas Maurer was in a hospital filled with millions of dollars of the most sophisticated medical equipment. He was being treated by expert doctors and nurses.

But it was a salesclerk in a flower shop, a woman making $170 a week, who—by taking the time to care, and by being willing to go with what her heart told her to do—gave Douglas hope and the will to carry on. The human spirit can be an amazing thing, and sometimes you encounter it at its very best when you aren't even looking.

Source: Reprinted by permission: Tribune Media Services.

---

with surgery and radiation, with 5-year survival rates of up to 90%.

WILMS' TUMOR (Nephroblastoma)

Wilms' tumor is a cancer of the kidney in which cells revert back to a more embryonic type, hence the true name for Wilms' tumor, nephroblastoma (nephro = kidney, blastoma = tumor of embryonic tissue). 90% of cases occur among children under 7, with a peak age of 1 to 3 years old. Boys get it as often as girls, and whites almost as much as blacks. Heredity is thought to account for as much as 40%. There is often an associated congenital absence of the iris of the eye. Sometimes it occurs in both kidneys.

The usual first symptom is an abdominal swelling which may appear rapidly, and be associated with pain. There may also be fever and blood in the urine. The only chance for early detection of Wilms' tumor is by routine well-child checkups with the pediatrician or family physician, with the hope that they will detect early masses in the abdomen.

Treatment is by surgery, combined with chemotherapy and radiation therapy. All stages of Wilms' tumor are highly curable, with 2-year survival rates of 97% for stage I and about 80% for later stages.

NEUROBLASTOMA

This is a strange cancer of cells derived from the embryonic neural crest, mainly in the chain of nerves that run from the neck down the inside of the back to the pelvis. It occurs almost exclusively in very young children, with a peak age of 2. It has a genetic association, being more common among siblings and certain inherited conditions. For most cases, though, it seems to represent an incomplete development of nerve tissue.

There would appear to be no way to prevent it, and early detection is difficult. Signs and symptoms include: a mass in the neck, chest, or abdomen which is rarely painful; elevated blood pressure; urine catecholamines (nerve and adrenal gland chemicals); and occasionally weight loss, fever, pallor, and weakness.

Surgery and/or radiation therapy have been very successful in curing localized disease, but less successful with advanced, metastatic disease. Chemotherapy is used, but not with the degree of success experienced with other childhood cancers. The younger the child, the better the prognosis. Overall, about 50% are eventually cured. Immunotherapy with monoclonal antibodies, and bone marrow transplantation may increase future cure rates.

Neuroblastoma has the interesting distinction of being the cancer with the highest rate of spontaneous regression—occurring in about 2% of neuroblastoma cases under 2 years of age. It's as though the body finally figures out what it was supposed to do in making those nerve tissues, and corrects it. Also interesting is the fact that autopsies of children dying of other causes show in situ neuroblastoma nodules in as many as 1 in 39 cases, and in autopsies of fetuses the rate is even higher.

RETINOBLASTOMA

Retinoblastoma is a cancer of the back of the eye, the retina. Most children who develop retinoblastoma are under 2 years old, and it is rare in children over 5. About 40% are inherited, and these are usually in both eyes at once. Specific chromosomal abnormalities have been identified for this disease, and genetic testing and counseling is important. There is also a higher risk of developing other childhood soft-tissue cancers.

Prevention of inherited or chromosome abnormal retinoblastomas is possible through genetic counseling. Early detection is through examination of an infant's eyes, looking for a white reflection or "cat's eye" reflex. (When a light is shined into a normal infant's eye there is normally a red reflection, called a red reflex). Symptoms include poor vision, or obvious malfunction or deformity of the eye.

Newer imaging modalities like MRI are excellent at determining the location and degree of spread of tumor. Treatment is aimed at preserving vision and includes surgery, radiation therapy, and chemotherapy. Long-term survival for all cases is now close to 90%, where in years past it was only

25%. Retinoblastoma, like neuroblastoma, has a significant rate of spontaneous regression.

GERM CELL TUMORS

These are infrequent, accounting for about 3% of childhood cancers. It's a group of tumors—some benign, some malignant—that have in common an abnormality in the development and migration of germ cells. The germ cells are what the gonads (testes and ovaries) use for reproduction.

These tumors occur at varying ages during childhood, and can be present in places other than the gonads, as far away as the head and neck. Any unusual mass in a child may be a germ cell tumor. Treatment includes surgery, and sometimes radiation therapy and chemotherapy. Depending on the type of germ cell tumor, the prognosis can be excellent or poor.

RHABDOMYOSARCOMA

These are cancers of the embryonic cells that form the soft tissues of the body, i.e., muscles and other flesh. It occurs in early childhood and late adolescence. In the younger age group it occurs mainly in the head and neck and GI tract; in the older age group it occurs mainly in the arms and legs, and testes. The cause of rhabdomyosarcomas is not known. As with other childhood cancers, rhabdomyosarcoma seems to represent an incomplete or incorrect process of development.

It can present as a mass anywhere in the body, causing symptoms at that site by blocking normal function or passage. When it has been verified by biopsy, there should be an extensive examination to search for other involved sites. Treatment is with surgery, radiation therapy, and chemotherapy—depending on the sites affected. Overall survival rates have increased from 20% in the 1960s to as high as 70% in the 1980s.

LYMPHOMAS

Childhood lymphomas are about equally divided between Hodgkin's disease and non-Hodgkin's lymphomas. They tend to affect older children. Genetics, viral infections, and immunological disorders are associated risk factors. They can be highly curable, especially Hodgkin's disease, which for children has an eventual cure rate of almost 90%. [See Chapter 41—Lymphomas, which discusses both types of lymphomas, risk factors, symptoms, diagnosis, treatment, and prognosis.]

OSTEOGENIC SARCOMA

This is the most common bone cancer, accounting for about 2500 cases per year in the United States. It is most common between the ages of 10 and 25. It affects males slightly more than females. The cause is not clearly understood. Irradiation is a cause in some cases. Overall, it appears to be a defect in skeletal growth.

50% occur in the femur (the thigh bone), usually at the end near the knee. The next most common sites are the humerus, tibia, pelvis, jaw, and hands. The most common first symptom is an ache in the affected part of the bone, followed by worsening pain and a palpable swelling. X-ray followed by bone biopsy confirms the diagnosis.

Surgery is the primary method of treatment, with a goal of preserving the limb whenever possible.

These tumors tend to be radioresistant, so radiation therapy isn't helpful; however, adjuvant chemotherapy has in recent years been proven quite effective. Chemotherapy can make the difference between amputation or not. Nobody wants to lose their leg or arm, especially during adolescence, the time of life when appearance is so important.

Immunotherapy protocols have been tried, but so far without significant success.

The overall prognosis for osteogenic sarcoma used to be dismal (less than 10%), but in recent years has climbed to over 50% long-term survival.

EWING'S SARCOMA

This is predominantly a bone cancer like osteogenic sarcoma, but it can also occur in non-bone soft tissues. It more frequently affects the mid-shaft of bones, whereas osteogenic sarcoma tends to be at the ends of bones. It occurs less often than osteogenic sarcoma. The affected age group is 5 to 30. It is uncommon in blacks.

Symptoms are similar to osteogenic sarcoma: pain and swelling over a bone. Treatment is by surgery, but since these tumors are quite sensitive to radiation (whereas osteogenic sarcomas are not), radiation therapy is a major part of the treatment plan. Chemotherapy is highly effective, and when combined with surgery and radiation the long-term survival rates have gone from the previously dismal 10% to upwards of 70%.

OTHER CHILDHOOD CANCERS

The other childhood cancers are generally soft-tissue tumors (sarcomas). They include fibrosarcoma (cancer of fibrous connective tissue), neurofibrosarcoma (cancer of the sheath around nerves), leimyosarcoma (cancer of the smooth muscles), liposarcoma (cancer of the fatty tissues), synovial sarcoma (cancer of the lining of joints), hemangiopericytoma (cancer of cells that surround vessels), alveolar soft part sarcoma (cancer of the skeletal muscles), and other less common tumors.

Children sometimes get one of a diverse group of cancers of the histiocyte cell-line (the phagocyte or "garbage-man" cells, like the macrophages). These are called histiocytosis X syndromes.

There are also gynecological cancers in the young, generally of the ovaries. They are most common at the time of menarche.

There will rarely be carcinomas in children, and when they occur they are usually in endocrine glands like the adrenal and thyroid.

The common cancers of adults—lung, breast, and colorectal—are exceedingly rare in children.

5

The Treatment of Cancer

45

Treatment Overview

Mark Renneker, M.D.

This part deals with each of the major forms of cancer treatment—surgery, radiation therapy, and chemotherapy. Each chapter should provide a solid background in language and concepts used in these fields.

Immunotherapy is not yet considered a major form of cancer therapy. But, with recent research and technological advances (e.g., monoclonal antibodies), immunotherapy is quickly moving into that role. Immunotherapy is presented along with chemotherapy because, in fact, it is a form of chemotherapy. "Biological treatment" refers to a type of immunotherapy, but, in current use, is really a synonym for immunotherapy.

The concept of the team approach to cancer treatment includes more specialists than are listed above. Other members (e.g., social workers, nutritionists, and so on) are presented in Part 6 (Understanding Cancer—For the Patient).

Other aspects of cancer treatment are presented here, including the role of a tumor board, cancer registry, the rights of patients, and the fascinating phenomenon of spontaneous regression of cancer. Finally, unproven methods of cancer treatment, which generally means "quackery," are discussed. This is a complicated and controversial subject, one that requires both an open mind and rigorous objectivity.

46

Principles of Cancer Surgery

Mark Renneker, M.D.

Surgery is the major method of diagnosing and treating cancer, and compared to all of the other treatment modalities put together—radiation therapy, chemotherapy, and immunotherapy—it has cured far more cancers. This is not to downplay the role of other cancer treatment methods, but rather to underscore the longstanding importance of surgery in the treatment of cancer.

The basic principles of cancer surgery—relating to biopsing, staging, treatment, and palliation—involve more than the general public is aware of; this is true even for many patients who have been through it.

For more specific information on cancer surgery than is provided in this brief chapter, refer to the extraordinary book, *Fundamentals of Surgical Oncology,* By Robert McKenna, M.D. and Gerald Murphy, M.D. (Macmillan Publishing Company, 1988). Though written for physicians, it is surprisingly readable.

FIRST PRINCIPLE: UNDERSTAND THE CANCER SURGEON

The road to having a cancer diagnosed and treated usually begins with a visit to one's personal physician (family physician, general practitioner, internist, or other primary care physician). If it is suspected that a cancer may be present, an appointment with a surgeon is usually the next step.

A surgeon who specializes in cancer is called a surgical oncologist. Surgical oncology is further sub-specialized. For instance, there are surgical oncologists who specialize in head and neck cancers, breast cancers, gynecological cancers, and so on. The majority of cancer surgery, however, is fairly straightforward and is performed by general surgeons.

More than any other type of doctor, patients seem awed by surgeons and are reluctant to ask them questions. "He's obviously so busy and his time is so valuable" and "I don't want to be a bother" are the type of things some patients and their families say; and, unfortunately, some surgeons aren't good at breaking down those barriers. Most surgeons try to do a good job of communicating with their patients, but some are simply not good at it—a failing usually excused if their technical surgical skills are held in high enough regard. Another factor is that many surgeons maintain a heavy workload (usually by choice, not by circumstance), so they really are as busy and under as much pressure as they seem.

These considerations aside, patients and their families should insist that the surgeon provide them with a steady stream of information through every step of the cancer diagnosis and treatment process; the burden shouldn't be on the patient and family to have to corner the surgeon to get their questions answered.

If, upon the first consultation with a surgeon—at the beginning of the cancer diagnosis or treatment process—you suspect that the surgeon may not be the kind of person who will work out well with you, ask your personal physician to send you to a different surgeon. (This applies to any physician or health specialist you are referred to.)

SECOND PRINCIPLE: CANCER ISN'T CANCER UNTIL IT'S BIOPSIED

This is not to say that biopsing causes a tumor to become cancerous—it doesn't, though this is a common misconception. The point being made here is that correctly obtaining a biopsy is of crucial importance. Every physician can remember at least one case in which, after first examining a patient, he felt practically 100% certain that the patient had can-

cer—but then sending them for a biopsy and having it turn out to be something other than cancer.

Obtaining a biopsy is usually easy, and can often be done without going into the hospital. But sometimes a major operation is required just to obtain a biopsy, for instance with suspected cancers in the abdominal organs.

Beware of undertaking any form of cancer treatment until the diagnosis of cancer has been confirmed by microscopic examination of tissue by a qualified specialist (i.e., a pathologist). In most cases of "cancer cures" by unproven methods of cancer treatment, the "cancer" was never actually biopsied, and was only a benign lump that could well have gone away without any "treatment."

In exceptional cases, treatment can begin without a biopsy: when the cancer diagnosis is 99.9% certain, and the risk of obtaining the biopsy outweighs the probable benefit of treatment. One example would be for a wide-spread, deep-seated, hard-to biopsy brain tumor causing severe, potentially fatal symptoms, that fits every criteria for cancer, based on radiographic studies (CT and MRI scans). In that circumstance, radiation therapy could be initiated without biopsy proof of the cancer.

THIRD PRINCIPLE: CHOOSE THE BEST BIOPSY METHOD

Every case is different, and there are a variety of biopsy methods to choose from. The responsibility of the surgeon is to present these options, and recommend which method he thinks would be best. The major forms of biopsy include:

- incisional biopsy: to cut into a tumor and remove a sample from it. This should ideally be taken from the edge of the tumor, so that it includes both tumor and normal tissue for comparison. The incision is made either with a scalpel, or with an instrument that takes a punch of tissue (called a punch biopsy). Long, thin biopsy forceps (surgically sharp pincers) have been designed to extract tissue samples through narrow instruments that may be non-surgically inserted into the body, for instance endoscopes (to biopsy suspicious growths in the GI tract), bronchoscopes (for lesions in the respiratory tract), and so on.

- excisional biopsy: to attempt to remove a whole tumor. This is most often undertaken for what clearly appear to be benign tumors and for small, obviously non-melanoma skin tumors that have no apparent spread or metastasis, and for internal organs at the time of surgery that are obviously completely diseased and that clearly need to be removed (regardless of whether or not a cancer is present).

• aspiration biopsy: to insert a needle into a tumor and apply vacuum pressure to suck out enough single cells or clumps of cells to make a microscopic examination for cancer. However, if this form of biopsy doesn't affirmatively indicate cancer, it can't be relied on to say that cancer isn't present—the needle might have missed the tumor. Aspiration biopsy is sometimes used for tumors in the thyroid and breast—organs close to the body's surface.

• fine-needle biopsy: to insert a hollow needle wide enough to obtain a core of tissue. This is sometimes used with an aspiration device. This procedure is increasingly being used in conjunction with CT and other radiographic procedures to help guide the needle.

Cytological studies, such as the Pap test or sputum cytology, are not considered forms of biopsy. They are too general, and take cells from too wide an area. If cells that appear to be cancerous turn up from one of these tests, the growth should be located and biopsied. This may be done by a more directed cytological evaluation, called brush biopsy: using a small bristle-tipped tool to "brush" the lesion to obtain cells, and sometimes tissue. This is usually done while directly visualizing the growth, for instance, through a culposcope (in the vagina and cervix) or bronchoscope (in the lungs).

Multiple biopsy procedures are sometimes required, to arrive at a definite diagnosis. The rule of thumb in considering what biopsy method to use is that "more is better"—the more tissue obtained, the more definitive the findings, and the less likely the need for additional biopsy procedures. This must be balanced, however, by the potential for disfigurement from a biopsy taken too aggressively.

FOURTH PRINCIPLE: BIOPSY FIRST, SURGERY SECOND

In the past, biopsy procedures were often scheduled to take place as part of the actual surgery. In other words, the patient was taken to the operating room, given full anesthesia, biopsied (by a method called frozen-section tissue biopsy, which permits a pathologist to examine it at that moment), and then the complete operation was performed if the biopsy was positive for cancer. In the case of breast cancer surgery, this often had devastating emotional conse-

quences on the patient—to go under anesthesia not knowing whether she would awaken to find her breasts intact.

With the variety of surgical approaches presently available to treat cancers—especially breast cancer—it is generally better to first do the biopsy, discuss the results and possible treatments, and then, if necessary, schedule the surgery. A delay of days or even weeks will make little, if any, difference. Also, the frozen-section tissue biopsy method is not always accurate—sometimes the pathologist can't render a definite diagnosis on the basis of a frozen-section. The regular method of preparing and examining biopsy specimens usually requires three to five days, and is the most accurate.

Also, multidisciplinary approaches to cancer may be precluded by rushing into surgery. In other words, once a biopsy is positive, other tests may be appropriate (see Staging, below). The case might be best presented to a team of cancer specialists (tumor board), to discuss treatment strategies that may not have been considered by the surgeon—for instance, the use of radiation therapy, chemotherapy, and/or immunotherapy before or in conjunction with the operation.

Finally, the days between the biopsy and the actual operation permit time for psychological adjustment and physical preparation for an operation (e.g., improving one's nutritional state to be stronger for surgery).

One-step procedures (biopsy and surgery the same day) are, however, sometimes best for highly probable cancers of the internal organs, such as of the pancreas or kidney, sparing the patient from having more than one major operation. Also, for some patients it is better emotionally to have it all done at once, rather than having to prepare for the surgery separately.

FIFTH PRINCIPLE: PRECISE STAGING IS THE GOAL

Once a cancer diagnosis has been made by biopsy, a comprehensive battery of tests are usually necessary to determine whether the cancer has spread, and to what parts of the body. This is called "staging."

The staging process should begin with a thorough head-to-toe physical examination (which should also have been done prior to the biopsy), followed by whatever additional tests are indicated. This often includes scans of the liver, bones, brain, and chest, using x-ray, nuclear medicine, ultrasound, and other imaging methods.

Sometimes additional surgical tests are needed, such as biopsies from lymph nodes and bones.

Special studies of the biopsy tissue may be done (e.g., hormone receptor tests), and tumor specific antigens may be looked for in the blood (i.e., carcinoembryonic antigen).

The staging results will usually help clarify what kind of surgical techniques should be considered, and what kind of operation, if any, should be performed.

SIXTH PRINCIPLE: BIG OPERATIONS AREN'T ALWAYS BEST

Two adages that have long guided cancer surgeons are "a chance to cut is a chance to cure" and "big operations for little cancers." The advent of non-surgical treatments for such cancers as Hodgkin's disease has rendered the first saying obsolete, and carefully conducted studies verifying the effectiveness of less extensive surgery for breast cancer have disproved the second saying.

A more accurate statement is that the first operation on a cancer has more chance for success than later operations. In other words, try to get it all the first time. Again, thorough staging makes this more probable.

The dilemma for the surgeon isn't how much of a cancerous organ to remove—that's usually obvious (the cancer appears white, like cauliflower, and distinct from normal tissue). The tough question is apt to be how much of the healthy-appearing tissues and lymph nodes to remove. That's where the surgeon's knowledge and experience will make the difference.

SEVENTH PRINCIPLE: A SCALPEL ISN'T A SURGEON'S ONLY TOOL

There are many new surgical techniques (and concepts). The field of surgical oncology has grown beyond the idea of just taking a scalpel and cutting out a cancer. In fact, a scalpel may be used only to cut through the skin. After that, methods of electrosurgery are common: using an electrical needle or blade to cut through or coagulate tissue.

Liquid nitrogen and other freezing methods may be used for cancers of the mouth, brain, and prostate. The temperature of an organ may be altered (i.e., hyperthermia). Chemical pastes are used (as in Moh's technique) for some skin cancers. Highly sophisticated lasers are used as surgical instruments on some head and neck, and gynecological cancers.

Cytoreductive surgery is a method that involves incomplete removal of a large cancer, to reduce it to a size that permits effective treatment with radiation therapy and/or chemotherapy (for instance with cases of Burkitt's lymphoma or cancer of the ovary). Also, cosmetic surgery, implanting prostheses, skin and tissue grafting, and organ transplantation are becoming more common procedures.

Cancer surgeons may also be called upon to place special tubes into major blood vessels, to administer chemotherapy, provide nutritional support, perform "second-look" operations to assess the progress of chemotherapy, or perform a variety of other tasks.

EIGHTH PRINCIPLE: INCURABLE CANCERS CAN STILL BE OPERABLE

A patient with widespread, obviously incurable cancer may still benefit from cancer surgery. This would be classed as palliative treatment. For instance, debulking a large cancer may prevent discomfort and obstruction of vital organs. And operations on nerves can sometimes significantly relieve pain.

NINTH PRINCIPLE: "CURED" CANCERS SOMETIMES RETURN

Months, even years, after successful cancer surgery, it is important to keep having regular checkups with the surgeon to look for any signs of recurrence, and to monitor for any problems relating to the surgery.

TENTH PRINCIPLE: RECOVERING FROM SURGERY IS A FULL-TIME JOB

It takes time to recover from surgery—at least a month, sometimes a year or longer. That time may be shortened by early and aggressive actions on the part of the surgeon, other members of the treatment team (especially physical therapists), and the patient. For instance, nutrition and exercise should be at the top of every day's agenda.

The real advances in surgical oncology in recent years have not been in surgical technique, but rather in unifying pre- and post-operative care. Multidisciplinary treatment teams can truly work wonders. Specially trained surgical nurse oncologists and oncology social workers are especially important, providing caring and human continuity during a time that seems interminable.

Far more often than not, cancer patients outlive their surgery and are cured.

47

Radiation Oncology: Principles and Practice

Rollin Odell, Jr., M.D.

Medical Director, Department of Radiation Oncology,
Samuel Merritt Hospital, Oakland, California

Radiation Oncology is that specialty of medical practice which utilizes ionizing radiation as a therapeutic modality to treat cancer. By artfully applying the sciences of radiation physics and radiation biology to the practice of cancer medicine, the radiation oncologist adds an important dimension to the management of the cancer patient. It is estimated that 60 percent of all newly diagnosed cancer patients in the United States will require radiotherapy at some point in their clinical course.

The use of radiation in medicine began at the turn of the century with the discovery of radium and the experiments of Madame Curie, Pierre Curie, and Wilhelm von Roentgen. Early workers used radium to treat superficial cancers with success as early as 1901. By 1905, a substantial body of literature describing the effects of radiation on tumors was in existence.

It was not until the 1920s, however, that accurate measurements of radiation could be made. In 1923, the Coolidge tube was invented, allowing for the first time the artificial production of radiations under controlled conditions. More powerful machines followed, but the modern specialty of radiation oncology did not develop until Cobalt-60 machines became widely available in the early 1950s. An off-shoot of the Manhattan project of World War II (development of the atomic bomb), this unit was able for the first time to kill tumors deeply situated in body cavities without damaging the skin. This was a revolutionary step forward, and led directly to the development of the extremely sophisticated machines in use today.

DEFINITION AND MEASUREMENT

Ionizing radiation is produced when packets of electromagnetic energy (photons) cause ejection of orbital electrons in adjacent tissue. Common sources of electromagnetic energy are other electrons, gamma rays, protons, neutrons, atomic nuclei, cosmic rays from space, or sub-atomic particles.

When these ionizing events occur, additional energy is released in the tissue. The amount of energy absorbed per unit mass of tissue is called the absorbed dose, quantitatively described in joules per kilogram. One joule/kg is the Gray (one Gray = 100 rad), the standard unit of radiation dose used in medicine. Tumor doses can be expressed in rads, centiGrays (cGy) (one centiGray = 1 rad), or Grays (GY), depending on personal preference.

PRODUCTION OF RADIATION

Today the clinical linear accelerator is the most widely used instrument for treating cancer patients (see Figure 47-1). Depending on design, this machine is capable of producing a broad range of photon energies (4 to 24 million electron volts), and can also be used to generate electron beams of energies from 3 to 30 million electron volts.

The photon energy and type of radiation determine the deposition of energy in tissue, which in turn determines both the amount and the distribution of the radiation's biological effect. The control of these permits the accurate application of radiation for the treatment of malignant disease.

Cobalt machines are still in use. They produce photons from the radioisotope Nickel-60. Because the isotope is housed in a perfectly cast lead container weighing over two tons, the apparatus is sometimes referred to as a cobalt "bomb." The gamma rays produced are equivalent to 3 million electron-volt photons produced artificially, more than adequate to provide acceptable depth penetration, with skin-sparing characteristics, when deeply situated tumors are treated (see Figure 47-2).

The above units are called super or megavoltage machines because they produce photons above 800,000 electron-volts. They are well suited for the treatment of deeply situated tumors because they spare skin and do not absorb energy preferentially in bone. Orthovoltage radiation machines (150,000 to 800,000 electron-volts) are still used, but only to treat superficial cancers where depth of penetration is undesirable. These machines deposit their energy maximally in the superficial layers of the skin, and in adjacent bony structures.

Betatrons and neutron generators are also in clinical use. Betatrons emit pure beams of electrons of variable energies, depending on the depth of the tumor one desires to treat. Both units were originally thought to offer a theoretical advantage over conventional photon machines, but in practice this has not proven to be the case.

Accelerators using heavy particles and pimesons (subatomic particles) are at present only used in research settings, where their potential for clinical work is being explored.

The use of machines to treat patients is called teletherapy (tele, Gr. meaning far off). Modern radiation therapy also requires the use of brachytherapy (brachy, Gr. meaning short), in which radioactive isotopes are inserted into and around the tumor. This is also referred to as implant therapy or interstitial therapy. In recent years, techniques have been developed to "afterload" the implant's radioactive sources. Guides are surgically positioned under controlled conditions, avoiding radiation hazard to operator, assistants, or patient. After accurate placement is assured, the radioactive materials can then be inserted as needed. Brachytherapy can be used as sole treatment, but it is most often employed as an adjunct to surgery or external beam radiotherapy (teletherapy).

Figure 47-1 A Modern Linear Accelerator. The machine is mounted so that treatment can be given from any angle. Note the customized beam blocks placed between the machine and the patient to optimize the treatment. One of the technicians is holding a compensator to further improve the radiation distribution.

Figure 47-2 A Typical Cobalt Unit. Source of radioactivity is housed inside the "head" of the machine eighty centimeters (about 32 inches) from the patient.

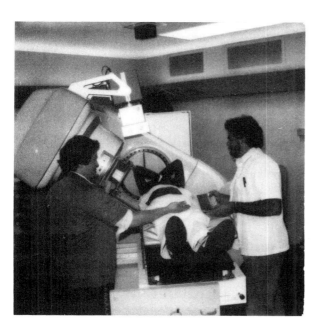

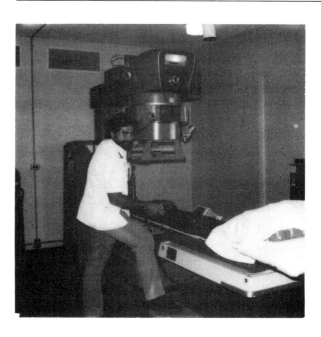

The skill of the radiotherapist in combining these sources of radiation determines in part how effective the treatment will be. Knowledge of the physical characteristics of the various radiations (radiation physics) and their effect on the multiple cellular, tissue, and organ systems of the human body (radiobiology), must be combined with an understanding of the biology of cancer in all its forms (oncology) in order for the proposed intervention to be maximally effective and at the same time least likely to produce severe side effects or long-term complications.

RADIOBIOLOGY

Radiobiology is the study of the interaction of ionizing radiation with biologic material. The most important fact to know is that radiation kills cells, and that it kills cells of malignant tumors more effectively than cells of normal tissue.

Cells are killed when the DNA, or chromosomes, are damaged beyond repair, or when cell processes are disrupted so that cell death is inevitable. Normal (non-malignant) cells can repair the damage caused by ionizing radiation more easily. This difference in response to radiation exposure between malignant and non-malignant cells is what makes radiation therapy successful.

There are more factors involved in the biology of tumors, however. Tumors are composed of various kinds of cells existing in a tumor bed. Some of the cells in the tumor are oxygen deprived, making them more resistant to radiation damage. In addition, some cells will be in a resistant phase of the mitotic cycle at the time of radiation exposure, and therefore less likely to be killed.

There are many other variables which affect radiocurability. By studying these phenomena, the radiobiologist may someday unravel enough of the puzzle to make radiation treatments even more effective.

Today's approach to the cancer patient often requires that combined modality therapy (surgery, radiation, and/or chemotherapy) be given concurrently or sequentially. Many chemotherapeutic agents have additive or synergistic effects with radiation. Surgery often interrupts blood flow, creates inflammation or scar tissue, or places tissue or organ systems in unaccustomed locations. All of these factors must be taken into consideration when planning a course of radiotherapy; every treatment is unique.

Some chemical agents have been found which either potentiate or suppress responses of tissue to radiation injury. Even though none are of clinical use at present, considerable research is being done in this area. If normal tissue, for instance, could be protected during radiation treatment, it would allow higher and presumably more effective doses to be delivered to the malignant tissue.

Heat is a cytotoxic agent, and combined with radiation has proven effective in destroying tumor growths. Hyperthermia, or the application of heat in a controlled fashion, is a recently developed modality, which adds a new dimension to our ability to destroy malignant disease.

Hyperthermia as an established cancer treatment is still evolving. If tumors can be heated evenly to between 42 and 45 degrees centigrade and the heat can be sustained for 45 to 60 minutes, many cells within that tumor will be destroyed. If radiation is also given immediately after or before the application of heat, the cell killing of the radiation is enhanced.

APPROACH TO THE PATIENT

The radiation oncologist must perform an independent and thorough evaluation of the patient's clinical condition to determine the appropriateness of using radiation in the management of each malignancy. This begins with a complete history and physical examination, and review of all laboratory and imaging studies. Additional studies may then be ordered. A psychosocial evaluation, dietary evaluation, and coordination with other treating physicians are necessary before a plan of treatment is presented to the patient and the family.

STAGING

Simply knowing the type of tumor is insufficient for the radiation oncologist. The location of the tumor in the body and its relationship to normal surrounding structures is equally important. By using the modern imaging techniques of bone, liver and brain scanning, computerized tomographic scanning, and magnetic resonance imaging, the oncologist can define with some precision the anatomic extent of disease. This process is referred to as "staging" the patient.

Having this information enables the radiotherapist to give more effective therapy with fewer side effects and complications. An accurate assessment of the extent of disease also provides the basis for giving the patient and family a better idea of the prognosis or probable outcome, and helps the treatment team and patient set appropriate goals.

PSYCHOSOCIAL ASPECTS

When confronted with a life-threatening illness, patients and family members may experience anger,

guilt, resentment, and anxiety at the very time they are being called upon to make important decisions regarding therapy. It is important that the oncologist recognize and honor the unique experience each patient/family is working through.

Often they have unrealistic expectations of success, or equally unrealistic expectations of failure. The radiation oncologist must evaluate these emotional aspects and allow for them in planning the treatment program. Where does the illness fit into the life-plan of the patient? Which ego defenses require bolstering, and which are already too strong?

The first task of the radiotherapist is to help the patient reestablish a sense of control. The best way to help is by presenting the patient a therapeutic program in a supportive way, in which the patient/family are involved in the decision-making.

As therapy proceeds, patients often become more open and able to talk about their illness. The treating physician can work to dispel some of the mystique surrounding cancer (too often perceived to be a "death sentence"), as well as the mystique surrounding radiation (widely feared because it cannot be seen, heard, felt, smelled, or tasted). To be the best possible help, the physician must try to get to know the patient. The fuller the physician's awareness of what the cancer experience means in the patient's life, the better.

Goal Setting

The radiation oncologist must be absolutely clear as to what the objectives of the proposed treatment are before presenting the program to the patient and family. This may include a realistic hope for "cure" (complete eradication of all cancer). But the experienced oncologist knows that factors other than those under his or her control will have a hand in the outcome.

If cure is not a realistic goal, then the oncologist will need to consider alternative goals, such as relief of pain, or relief of organ obstruction, or control of bleeding. These palliative benefits of treatment are often more gratefully received by patients than more extreme "curative" efforts.

THE RADIOTHERAPY TEAM

Radiation technologists, radiation physicists and dosimetrists (who measure the dosage), nurses, social workers, psychologists and supporting staff can all play an important role in helping the radiation patient. For many patients, the physician may only be a peripheral figure, and it is the secretary or nurse who greets them each day, offers encouragement, and provides psychological support.

TREATMENT PLANNING

After all the data has been collected, the general outline of the treatment program has been decided upon, and informed consent has been obtained, the radiation oncologist must decide the optimum dose/time over which the treatments are to be administered. This is called a fractionation scheme, and represents an achievable ideal or goal. Curative regimens usually require five to eight weeks of treatment, four to five days a week. Palliative courses are often shorter, and may be one to four weeks in length. Depending on the sensitivity of the normal tissue, daily treatments will vary between 150 cGy and 400 cGy.

The radiation oncologist strives to administer an effective dose, but at the same time must not create a situation in which the side effects are intolerable. In the vast majority of clinical situations encountered today, patients will be able to complete a planned course of therapy with only minimal to moderate side effects and no long-term complications.

The next step in the treatment planning phase is defining the tumor volume, a process referred to as "localization." Drawing on data from a combination of imaging techniques, his physical assessment of the disease, and his professional expertise, the radiation oncologist can determine exactly where in the body to deliver the radiation and how much is needed.

In all cases of curative treatment, a computer plan will be generated showing the dose distribution throughout the tumor and any dose-critical normal tissue within the treatment area.

The next step is a "simulation" of the treatment. Films of the patient in the treatment position are made for future reference, and marks are applied to the skin to insure the treatment will be administered identically each time. If special equipment is needed to facilitate treatment, specialized blocks or compensators to better direct the radiation beam, it is prepared.

CLINICAL APPLICATION

The theoretical basis for using radiation in the treatment of malignant disease has undergone considerable transformation in the last twenty-five years. Once thought of as an alternative to surgery, to be used only when surgery was not possible, it is now an independent treatment modality, appropriately utilized either alone, in combination with surgery, or as an adjunct to chemotherapy, depending on the disease process and its extent.

The limitations as well as the strengths of radiation therapy should be clearly understood. Radiocurability for most solid tumors (lung, bowel, breast, bladder, kidney, and head and neck cancers) for instance, is now perceived to be primarily a function of the volume of cells, which in turn is closely correlated with the size of the tumor mass. If the volume is too large (depending on tumor type), then no amount of radiation will be sufficient to destroy it.

In many cases, radiocurability is dose-dependent (within a certain range), and small tumors may require less radiation. Other variables to be considered, however, include degree of differentiation of the cells of the tumor, likelihood of metastases or spread to other parts of the body, and normal tissue tolerance to radiation.

Radiation therapy is used as the sole modality of treatment in many cancers arising in the oral cavity, the throat, the larynx, the tonsil, the palate, and the nasopharynx. If cure is to be achieved, both external beam and implant therapy must usually be employed, except when the tumor is quite small or excised grossly by an excisional biopsy.

Doses in the range of 6000 cGy to 7500 cGy over seven to eight weeks are necessary. Side effects can be severe, consisting of xerostomia (dry mouth), mucositis (inflammation of the mouth lining), anorexia (loss of appetite), and change in taste. Fortunately, most side effects diminish over time. If surgical excision of these tumors is possible, radiation can be given postoperatively in reduced amounts, to increase the likelihood of regional control of the disease.

Cancers of the uterine cervix are particularly radiocurable. The earliest tumors can best be eradicated surgically, but if the tumor has invaded more deeply, radiation therapy is often the treatment of choice. As with head and neck cancers, a combination of external beam therapy and implant therapy is necessary. The exact combination is dependent on extent of disease. If the disease is confined to the cervix, a heavier dose with implants is given. Disease extending beyond the cervix into the soft tissues of the pelvis requires greater emphasis on external beam therapy.

Hodgkin's disease, a lymphatic malignancy primarily affecting young adults, can be cured with radiotherapy alone in its early stages. Doses of 3500 to 4500 cGy given over five to seven weeks to involved lymph nodes are required. Large areas of the body covering many radiosensitive tissues must be exposed; therefore, the treatment must be carried out with the utmost care in order to prevent long-term complications.

Skin cancer is quite radiocurable. Radiation therapy is most useful where surgical deformity is undesirable, i.e., where involving eyelid, face, ear, nose, or forehead. If radiation is properly fractionated, cosmetic results are excellent.

Lung cancer, one of the most lethal of solid tumors, also can be radiocurable. While surgical resection is considered the optimum modality if a curative approach is realistic, the majority of lung cancers are not appropriate for curative surgical intervention. A small percentage of these patients are today cured with modern external beam radiotherapy. Doses of 6000 cGy given over seven to eight weeks can result in long-term local control that can translate into cure if the patient does not subsequently develop metastatic disease.

Carcinoma of the prostate, the second most common malignancy in men, is now radiocurable in early stages. High dose treatment (6500 to 7500 cGy) compared to radical prostatectomy (the most common curative cancer operation) gives equal long-term survival, and with fewer complications.

Carcinomas of the ano-rectum are now being treated curatively, using radiation alone or in combination with chemotherapy. These techniques preserve the anus, and early results show survival and local control equal to resectional surgery. Doses of 5500 cGy to 6500 cGy are required, depending on type and dosage of chemotherapy.

Certain rare childhood brain malignancies, such as medulloblastoma and retinoblastoma, are also potentially radiocurable. Surgical attempts at cure often produce unacceptable functional disabilities. By using optimum radiation techniques, many of these patients not only survive their malignancies, but avoid serious long-term complications.

A major breakthrough in cancer treatment has occurred with cancers of the breast. Cure rates remained constant over the many years when the only curative treatment offered was surgical. It has now been shown that for most early stage breast cancers, removing the lump surgically and treating the remaining breast, regional lymph nodes and underlying chest wall with radiation can offer equal survival and local control of disease. By using modern techniques with well controlled doses, cosmesis is excellent and long-term complications are minimal. 4500 to 5000 cGy is given throughout the remaining breast tissue over five to six weeks.

Adjuvant radiation (radiation given after surgery or chemotherapy) is used in the treatment of a wide variety of cancers. Radiation given after excision of sarcomas of the extremities, to both children and adults, has proven effective, preserving the limb and providing local control.

Advanced uterine endometrial cancers are given 4500 cGy over five weeks to the pelvis, improving survival rates and enhancing regional control of disease. Seminomatous testicular cancers, even if they have spread to abdominal lymph nodes, have improved survival rates if radiation is used along with surgical treatment. Radiation given to tumors of the rectum and colon, either preoperatively or postoperatively, show improved regional control of disease and may add to survival.

With many malignancies affecting children, such as Wilms' tumor of the kidney, Ewing's sarcoma of the bone, and neuroblastoma, radiation is employed as an integral part of the treatment program, contributing to the long-term survival and cure of many of these young patients.

Radiation therapy can also be a useful adjuvant for the chemotherapist in the treatment of lymphomas and leukemias. By treating local areas of involvement with radiation, the chemotherapist needs fewer drug interventions. Also, multiple myeloma, a malignancy of the bones causing local pain, can be given local radiation in low doses to give excellent pain relief.

The palliation of metastatic disease still makes up from forty to sixty percent of a radiation oncologist's practice. Solid tumors frequently spread to the brain, where they cause internal swelling leading to seizures, headaches, paralysis, mood changes, and loss of speech and a general deterioration of mental faculties. A brief course of radiation is often helpful in relieving these symptoms. Most patients tolerate the therapy well, but all will experience temporary epilation (loss of hair).

Malignancies also metastasize to bone, where they cause pain, weakness, and fractures (referred to as "pathologic fractures"). If spinal vertebrae are involved, in addition to back pain, pressure on the spinal cord can lead to lower extremity paralysis and loss of bowel and bladder control. A course of radiation therapy given early enough may prevent these complications, in addition to relief of pain for the majority of patients.

Soft tissue metastases can also be given palliation if the mass is blocking the bowel, ulcerating through skin surface, or causing bleeding, pain, intractable cough or respiratory obstruction. The fractionation scheme is variable, depending to a great extent on the prognosis of the patient and the location of the tumor.

Side Effects and Complications

In recent years, better administered radiotherapy has reduced the incidence of both short-term side effects and long-term complications. Aggressive, curative treatment, however, is associated with some risk of serious debility that may or may not be correctible.

The nature of the radiation damage depends on the site. Spinal cord damage may occur with neck and chest radiation. Brain and eye damage is associated with treatment to those areas. Lung scarring to some degree is always present following tumoricidal doses to the chest. Scarring in and about the membranes of the heart may occur following treatment to the chest or breast. Kidney damage, bowel damage, and liver injury can result from treatment of the abdomen. Bladder, rectal, and bowel damage can occur with treatment of the pelvis. Soft tissue and bone necrosis has been observed with excessive radiation of the extremities. Radiation carcinogenesis (cancers caused by radiation) has occurred, though infrequently, many years after therapeutic radiation treatment.

For the most part, the risk of these complications is low, and is outweighed by the risks of not being treated with radiation.

Future Prospects

Based on the twin disciplines of radiological physics and radiobiology, radiation oncology has come of age as a full-fledged member of the cancer treatment team. Over 2000 physicians in the United States devote full time to this specialty. Every major cancer center offers the full spectrum of radiation modalities.

How might radiation treatment be performed in the year 2000? Monoclonal antibody technology and better imaging techniques, will make it possible to target radiation more precisely, either by tagging the antibodies with radiation to serve as markers, or through more accurate radiation equipment. Cancer detection will be improved, so more tumors will be diagnosed earlier, when they are small and more often radiocurable. Drugs will be developed that will preferentially sensitize malignant tissue and/or protect normal tissue from the damaging effects of radiation.

ADDITIONAL READING

1. Perez C, Bradley L, *Principle and Practice of Radiation Oncology.* J.B. Lippincott, 1987. (Comprehensive, technical, but possible to read.)
2. Phillips T, Wara W, *Radiation Oncology, Volume 2,* Raven Press, 1982. (For radiation oncologists, but can be understood if you are patient.)

48

Chemotherapy, Immunotherapy, and Biological Treatments of Cancer

David S. McWaters, Pharm.D. and Mark Renneker, M.D.

At present, four modes of therapy are generally recognized as being effective in the treatment of cancer: surgery, radiation therapy, chemotherapy, and the use of anti-cancer biological agents. Surgical treatment of cancer has been with us since antiquity, and is still the major method of treating cancer. Radiation therapy had its beginnings in the early 1900s after Wilhelm Roentgen discovered the X-ray. Today, X-rays and other radiation-emitting sources are commonly used to treat cancer.

Cancer chemotherapy didn't begin until the 1940s. Despite initial optimism that cancer chemotherapy would be the "magic bullet" that would "cure cancer," today it cures only about 10% of cancers. This may not sound like a high percentage, but it adds up to over 50,000 people who are alive today, cured of their cancers, solely because of chemotherapy.

Physicians who specialize in cancer chemotherapy are called medical oncologists. Although the word "chemotherapy" literally means the "treatment of disease by means of chemical substances or drugs," its general use refers to the drug treatment of cancer.

Cancer chemotherapy is used for basically four reasons: to cure a patient, to palliate (reduce the severity of symptoms when cure isn't possible), to shrink a cancer so that less surgery or radiation therapy is needed, or as an additional treatment after surgery or radiation therapy to eliminate microscopic metastasis (called "adjuvant chemotherapy").

The biological treatment of cancer takes advantage of naturally occurring cellular processes to kill cancer cells. These agents, such as interferons, interleukins, or monoclonal antibodies, are called *biological response modifiers*. Biological therapy is the most recent addition to the anticancer arsenal. Only since the late 1970s have advances in molecular biology and genetic engineering made these innovative approaches possible. This newest form of cancer therapy was initially seen as separate from the chemotherapy field, but it is apparent that both are based on using anticancer drugs—natural or manufactured.

THE HISTORY OF CANCER CHEMOTHERAPY

The development of cancer chemotherapeutic drugs dates back thousands of years. The ancient Egyptians, and later Hippocrates, attempted to use escharotics (caustic agents) to treat cancers. Preparations of mercury, silver, and zinc were applied to tumors at least five hundred years ago. The first known attempt at systemic therapy occurred in 1865 when Heinrich Lissauer tried giving potassium arsenate to a patient with leukemia.

True success with cancer chemotherapy waited until the 1940s (see Figure 48-1). As is the case with many medical discoveries, a serendipitous observation led to a scientific breakthrough. During the First World War, it was noticed that soldiers exposed to mustard gas developed a profound leukopenia (decrease in the number of white blood cells in the blood), due to destruction of the bone marrow (where white blood cells are made). Then, during the

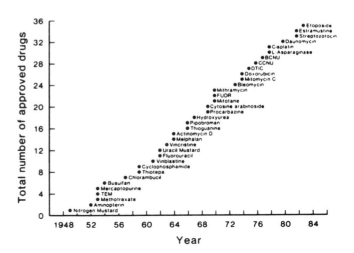

Figure 48-1 The Rate of FDA Approval of New Chemotherapy Drugs (excluding hormones). Table does not include drugs still in the experimental stage. *Source: DeVita VT, Hellman S, Rosenberg SA, eds.* Cancer—Principles and Practice of Oncology. *2nd ed. Philadelphia: J.B. Lippincott Co., 1985 p. 277.*

next World War, an American ship laden with mustard gas was bombed in an Italian harbor and many of the survivors later died of infection and internal bleeding, both signs of bone marrow failure due to exposure to the gas.

Scientists reasoned that perhaps mustard gas could be used to treat patients with too many white blood cells (i.e., lymphoma or leukemia). Unfortunately, mustard gas was found to be too toxic for medical use. A similar compound, called nitrogen mustard, was then tested and found safe and effective. Nitrogen mustard is now a mainstay in the treatment of lymphoma.

The period after the Second World War saw the development of many new classes of anticancer drugs. The first were the antimetabolites. Sidney Farber found that folic acid (a dietary biochemical necessary for amino acid synthesis and other vital functions) accelerated the growth of leukemia, and that chemicals which blocked (antagonized) folic acid, decreased abnormal white blood cell production in the bone marrow. In 1949, methotrexate, a folic acid antagonist, was first used with cancer patients. It is credited with the first chemotherapy cure, a young woman with gestational choriocarcinoma (a pregnancy-related cancer originating in cells associated with early embryonic development).

Today, about fifty different drugs have been found effective against cancer. Some are in widespread use and others are in various stages of development. Research now focuses both on the development of new drugs and how best to use those already discovered.

Perhaps nothing is so terrifying to a cancer patient as the thought of enduring the agony of unremitting pain. That many of the terminally ill do suffer so is a largely preventable medical tragedy. With today's understanding of the causes and nature of pain, and given the vast arsenals of medications and non-drug treatments, no patient should suffer needlessly.

Who gets pain:

It is a common misconception that all cancer patients suffer pain. In reality, about a third of all cancer patients complain of pain. Only about one-sixth of persons with localized cancer (i.e., nonmetastatic) have pain. However, closer to two-thirds of terminally ill patients have pain. The likelihood of pain is related to the type and site of cancer. About 85% of those with primary bone cancer will have pain, while only 5% of patients with leukemia complain of pain.

The most common causes of cancer pain are tumor invasion of bone, nerves and nerve roots, organs such as the liver or bladder, and infection or inflammation of the mouth's mucous membranes. About one-fifth of cancer pain is caused by the cancer treatment, and the rest by the effects of the tumor itself.

What is pain?

The word pain derives from the Latin *poena,* meaning punishment. Everyone intuitively knows what pain is, but finding an adequate definition is difficult. The International Association for the Study of Pain defines it as: "an unpleasant sensory and emotional experience associated with actual or potential tissue damage or described in terms of such damage." Perhaps a more meaningful definition of pain is that it is whatever the patient says it is.

If we accept the latter definition, then the patient becomes a partner with the physician and other health care workers in diagnosing and treating pain. Since medical science has yet to invent a "pain-o-meter," the patient is the only person able to assess the success or failure of treatment.

Acute pain is a biological alarm. It tells us when we're too close to a fire or when we step on a sharp object. Chronic pain, on the other hand, has no apparent biological purpose, especially for the terminally ill. Unremitting pain causes anxiety, depression, fatigue, emotional disturbances and insomnia, continually exacerbating the pain in a vicious cycle. Breaking this cycle begins by treating the pain.

The addiction myth

Patients and physicians alike share the myth that long-term use of narcotic drugs leads to addiction. Social prejudice has labelled morphine and other "strong" narcotics as abused drugs; patients are unwilling to take them and physicians are unwilling to prescribe them until all else has failed. This misconception often results in the undertreatment of pain.

Long-term use of narcotic analgesics does lead to physical dependence and tolerance. Physical dependence is characterized by a withdrawal reaction when the drug is stopped. Tolerance is the need for increasing doses of the medication to maintain pain relief. Neither of these effects has any relevance for a terminally ill patient.

First, there is no reason to stop taking the medication if it is relieving pain. Even if the drug is stopped and the patient has withdrawal, the symptoms resemble a mild flu rather than the raving psychosis portrayed in the movies. Second, if increasing doses of a narcotic analgesic are needed to alleviate pain, the dose should simply be increased.

Addiction is a physical need for a drug, often coupled with an overwhelming psychological obsession for obtaining it. It is virtually impossible to turn a terminally ill cancer patient into an addict.

Assessing and treating pain—eight crucial concepts

1. Accurate diagnosis of the cause(s) of pain is essential.

2. No two patients are alike. What works for one patient might not work for another. An effective treatment plan should be tailored to the individual.

3. What works today might not work tomorrow. Patients change and their responses to medication change. Adequate treatment necessitates a constant reevaluation of the patient's needs.

4. A "pain diary," kept by the patient, is enormously useful in assessing and treating pain. Where does it hurt? How does it feel? (e.g. sharp, dull, achy, burning, etc.) When does it hurt? What brings relief? What makes it worse?

5. Consider non-drug pain relieving strategies. Examples are meditation, relaxation training, biofeedback, hypnosis, and anything else that might work. Keep an open mind.

6. The treatment plan must be consistent with the patient's belief systems, and must have his or her enthusiastic cooperation.

7. The treatment should not be worse than the disease.

8. Minor or occasional pain may be treated on an "as needed" (prn) basis. More severe or continuous pain should *NEVER* be treated on an "as needed" basis. Instead, drugs should be given on a scheduled, around-the-clock basis, whether or not the patient is experiencing severe pain. It is much easier to prevent pain than to treat it.

CLASSES OF CHEMOTHERAPEUTIC AGENTS

The National Cancer Institute (NCI) has screened more than 250,000 substances for potential anticancer activity. Although the rate has slowed somewhat in recent years, about 15,000 compounds are screened in this country annually. For every 40,000 substances tested in animals, approximately 10 are deemed of significant interest to be studied in humans. Of these ten, only one drug will eventually prove truly useful. Despite years of such screening, only about 34 agents are currently approved by the federal Food and Drug Administration for use in human cancers. At this writing, more than sixty new drugs have investigational status with the NCI.

Those drugs in current use may be categorized into eight main classes, as follows:

1. Alkylating agents: one of the largest categories of cancer chemotherapeutic agents, they bind directly and irreversibly to important compounds (primarily DNA) to disrupt cell division. An example, mentioned previously, is nitrogen mustard.

2. Antimetabolites: another category that contains many different drugs, antimetabolites interfere with the action of crucial enzymes to inhibit nucleic acid synthesis necessary for DNA and protein production. Examples are 5-FU (5-fluorouracil) and methotrexate.

3. Antitumor antibiotics: like many antibacterial antibiotics, they are primarily derived from various species of fungi. They insert themselves into DNA strands, causing chromosomal breaks or inhibiting DNA-directed RNA synthesis. The most commonly used member of this class, doxorubicin (Adriamycin) is active against many types of cancer.

4. Plant alkaloids: derived from naturally-occurring plant materials, they prevent the mitotic spindle formation necessary for cell duplication and separation. Vinblastine and vincristine are derived from the periwinkle plant and etoposide (VP-16) comes from the May apple (American mandrake).

5. Hormones and hormone inhibitors: although their mechanisms of action are unclear, they are useful in a number of different cancers. Examples are estrogen, progesterone, and tamoxifen (an antagonist to the actions of estrogen).

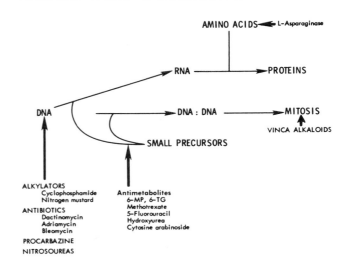

Figure 48-2 The Sites of Action of Chemotherapy Drugs.
Source: Martin J. Cline and Charles M. Haskell, Cancer Chemotherapy (Philadelphia: W.B. Saunders Co., 1975), p.3.

6. Enzymes: certain tumor cells have a unique requirement for asparagine, an amino acid necessary for protein synthesis. L-asparaginase is an enzyme that effectively starves these cells of asparagine, causing the death of the cell. Unfortunately, its usefulness is limited to acute lymphocytic leukemia; it has little effect on other tumors.

7. Miscellaneous chemotherapeutic agents: this category includes drugs with many different actions, but most inhibit DNA synthesis by directly binding to DNA. Cis-platinum is in this class.

8. Biological response modifiers: these substances, such as interleukin-2 and interferon, enhance the body's natural protective response against cancer. Most are derivatives of naturally-occurring compounds produced by the immune system. This is the newest class of anticancer agents.

The sites of action of the main classes of chemotherapeutic agents are diagrammed in Figure 48-2.

SIX BASIC PRINCIPLES OF CHEMOTHERAPY

1. Log Kill Hypothesis

Anticancer drugs are rarely able to kill every cancer cell in a single treatment. Maximum effectiveness seems to be a 99.9% kill. A large tumor mass or a disseminated cancer like acute leukemia consists of as many as one trillion (10^{12}) cancer cells. A trillion cancer cells weigh about 1 kilogram, or 2.2 pounds. A cancer of that size will almost surely be fatal. A chemotherapeutic drug given to a patient with a tumor of that size will kill 99.9% of the cancer cells, but still leave one billion (10^9) cancer cells. This fractional (logarithmic) killing ability of cancer chemotherapeutic agents is called the *log kill hypothesis*. The term means that the drug kills a constant fraction of cells, not a constant number, regardless of the number of cells present at the time of therapy.

To better understand the log kill hypothesis, consider this hypothetical example:

A 22-year-old college student has recently noticed a swollen lymph node in her neck. She goes to the student health service who refers her to a specialist. A biopsy shows that it is a lymphoma. After further evaluation, it is evident that other lymph nodes, although smaller and less noticeable than the first one, may be involved. Chemotherapy is chosen as the best treatment. Under idealized circumstances, the steps below show how the therapy would theoretically work:

1. The enlarged cancerous lymph node in her neck measures approximately 3 cm in diameter (slightly larger than 1 inch) and can be estimated to contain about 10^{10} cells (10 billion, or 10,000,000,000).

2. She is given a chemotherapeutic drug which, according to the log kill hypothesis, kills 99.9%, or 999 out of every 1,000 of her tumor cells. This leaves 10^7 cells (10 million, or 10,000,000) still alive.

3. Her tumor now measures less than $\frac{1}{8}$ inch in diameter. The other cancerous lymph nodes would be even smaller.

4. The drug is given once more, again killing 99.9% of the cancer cells. 10^4 (10 thousand, or 10,000) cells still remain.

5. Although 10,000 cells remain, the tumor is now so small that it cannot be felt or detected by X-ray.

6. Additional courses of chemotherapy are given to reduce the number of remaining cancer cells even further. Since only a fraction of cancer cells are killed each time, there will always be some left.

7. The immune system is relied upon to mop up the remaining cancer cells after the final course of chemotherapy has been given.

The clinical implications of the log kill hypothesis are obvious:

1. Treatment must be repeated many times in order to be sure of killing the maximum number of cancer cells possible.

2. A greater log kill may be achieved by using a number of anti-tumor drugs at the same time (combination chemotherapy).

3. It is best to start treatment when the number of cells is small enough to allow more complete tumor destruction. The benefits of early cancer detection are obvious here. Prior to chemotherapy, a tumor is often "debulked" by radiotherapy or surgery.

2. The Role of the Immune System

It is generally believed that once a tumor is reduced to fewer than about 10^5 (100 thousand) cells, the immune system begins taking over for the final kill. Chemotherapy needs a healthy immune system to be effective, and cancer recurrences are frequently because of a suppressed immune system. Factors known to decrease immune response include: surgery (although transiently), radiation therapy, poor nutrition, depression, stress, other disease states (e.g., AIDS), and even cancer chemotherapeutic agents themselves. Healthy immune function is required for all forms of cancer therapy to be maximally successful. Even in the best of circumstances, a few cancer cells will likely remain behind after radiation therapy or surgery. It is the immune system's responsibility to find and kill them.

3. The Cell Cycle

Any cell, normal or malignant, passes through a number of phases during its lifetime (see Figure 48-3). By convention, scientists refer to these phases as follows: Gap$_1$ (designated by "G$_1$") is the period prior to DNA synthesis during which active RNA and protein synthesis takes place. It is the time when the cell prepares for the next event, the Synthesis ("S") phase. During the S phase, which constitutes about one-third to one-half of the total cell cycle, DNA is synthesized. Cells in this phase are highly sensitive to many antitumor agents. Following Synthesis is another Gap phase ("G$_2$") during which the mitotic spindle apparatus is assembled and more RNA and protein synthesized. Then the cells undergo mitosis in the D ("Division") phase. It is also hypothesized that some cells enter a long resting state ("G$_0$") during which they may not be susceptible to drugs

Figure 48-3 The Cell Cycle.

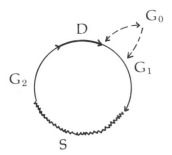

Figure 48-4 Growth Fraction.

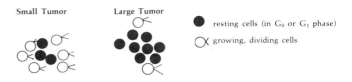

that are active only against cells that are dividing and growing.

Those drugs that are active during a specific phase of the cell cycle are called "cycle specific." Other drugs called "cycle non-specific," have an action that is prolonged and independent of DNA synthesis.

4. Tumor Growth

At any one time, the majority of cancer cells are likely to be non-dividing. Compared to large tumors, small tumors tend to have a higher "growth fraction"—a greater percentage of cells that are actively dividing (see Figure 48-4). They are therefore more likely to be susceptible to many anti-cancer drugs. As a cancer grows, more cells become non-dividing, forming most of the tumor mass.

It follows, then, that drugs which specifically affect DNA synthesis (cycle specific) are most effective against small tumors. Large tumors, on the other hand, respond better to cycle non-specific drugs. That is why, in general, cycle non-specific drugs are often prescribed for large tumors. Once a tumor is reduced in size, it becomes more effective to use cycle specific drugs.

Figure 48-5 neatly depicts the relationships between tumor growth, the immune system, and the log kill hypothesis. The scale on the verticle (y) axis represents the tumor cell burden and is expressed exponentially. The horizontal dashed line indicates a tumor of 10^9 cells (about 1 cm mass), the level at which a cancer generally becomes clinically detectable. If a tumor with 10^{12} cells (1 kg) could be debulked with radiation, surgery, or chemotherapy, to as few as 10^9 cells, an attempt at curative therapy could be made. If that curative attempt failed, and, as shown, the tumor again grew, another course of chemotherapy could perhaps effect a remission or cure. Finally, a tumor that is not curable may still be palliated, allowing the patient to live somewhat longer.

5. Solid Tumors Vs. Hematologic Tumors

In thinking about the uses of cancer chemotherapy, it is helpful to classify cancers as either hematologic or solid. Hematologic cancers include malignancies of the blood, bone marrow, and lymphatic system (leukemias and lymphomas). Solid tumors are everything else (e.g., lung, breast, colorectal, etc.).

Initially, solid tumors are confined to the tissue in which they started. If allowed to grow, cancer cells invade adjacent tissues and break off from the original tumor to enter the blood or lymph system, resulting in metastatic, disseminated disease. Hematologic cancers are, by their very nature, disseminated diseases; the blood and lymph systems run throughout the body.

This is an important distinction. Whereas surgery and radiation therapy are effective in localized cancers, chemotherapy has a systemic, whole-body effect and is sometimes the best treatment for disseminated cancers. Some clinicians consider solid tumors like breast cancer as systemic, already disseminated, and therefore use chemotherapeutic agents alongside surgery or radiation (adjuvant chemotherapy).

6. Tumor Resistance

Much like houseflies becoming resistant to the effects of DDT and bacteria becoming immune to antibiotics, tumor cells can develop resistance to chemotherapeutic drugs. Tumors contain many different kinds of cells, and some of these cells may be intrinsically resistant to the effects of one or more anti-tumor drugs. Also, cells that were formerly sensitive to a drug may mutate during treatment and become resistant. Even if only a tiny fraction of tumor cells is resistant, drug treatment "selects" them in the Darwinian sense, killing off the sensitive cells and allowing the resistant ones to multiply. This may be another reason for relapse after treatment. Treatment with the same drug after relapse usually has a poor chance for success.

Combinations of drugs are often used on the theory that cells are unlikely to be resistant to sev-

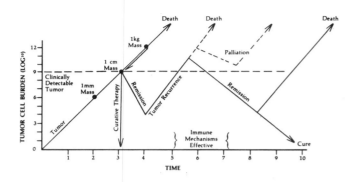

Figure 48-5 The Relationships Between Tumor Growth, the Immune System, and the Log Kill Hypothesis. *Source: Rubin P, ed. Clinical oncology for medical students and physicians, 5th ed (New York, American Cancer Society, 1978), p.43.*

eral dissimilar drugs. For most cancers, *combination chemotherapy* is more successful than single-agent treatment. Some chemotherapy "protocols" are designed to expose tumor cells to alternating cycles of "noncross-resistant" chemotherapy drugs.

CLINICAL CANCER CHEMOTHERAPY

Evaluating Response to Chemotherapy

When evaluating response to a particular chemotherapy regimen, oncologists frequently use words like "complete response" or "remission." Is this the same as "cure"? No. Oncologists use the following criteria to evaluate response to chemotherapy:

1.   Complete remission (or complete response): complete disappearance of all clinically detectable disease.

2.   Partial response: greater than 50% reduction in the size of discretely measurable tumors, with no evidence of progression elsewhere.

3.   No response: no change in the size of the tumor, either larger or smaller.

4.   Progression: tumor growth, usually an increase of 50% in measurable tumor diameter.

In general, the duration of a positive response must be at least one month to be considered truly positive. This minimum describes quite a different circumstance than a "cure." Using standardized criteria makes it possible to compare results of therapy. A "cure" from chemotherapy has to be defined individually for each patient and tumor. At a minimum,

it is a complete lack of measurable disease for several years.

While response rates are used by researchers and clinicians to evaluate short-term progress, to speak of survival rates is probably more meaningful. For example, in one study, 81% of patients with advanced Hodgkin's disease treated with chemotherapy had a complete remission, but only 58% survived 10 years.

Protocols

Crucial to research and to the rational use of chemotherapeutic agents is a system of prescribed doses, schedules, and drug combinations known as protocols. Clinicians follow protocols so that information can be easily collected and compared. It is through protocol studies that combination chemotherapy has become better understood, more effective, and more readily accepted. Adjuvant chemotherapy (the use of drugs in combination with surgery and/or radiotherapy), high-dose chemotherapy, and regional chemotherapy (applying chemotherapeutic agents directly to the tumor) are other approaches often used in protocols.

High-Dose Chemotherapy

In general, higher doses of a chemotherapeutic drug are more effective than lower doses, but intolerable side effects often limit the doses that can be used. An exception is the use of high-dose methotrexate. Methotrexate is most active against rapidly proliferating tumors with a high growth fraction, but is also toxic to normal tissues with a similar high growth fraction (e.g., bone marrow). A patient can be given a potentially fatal high dose of methotrexate that kills the cancer cells, and then, before the body's organs are permanently damaged, the effects of the methotrexate can be stopped by giving a folinic acid antidote called citrovorum factor (Leukovorin)—or simply, rescue factor. Some tumors, such as leukemias, respond very well to the combined use of high-dose methotrexate with rescue factor.

Combination Chemotherapy

With rare exceptions, the single, magic chemotherapeutic bullet has not been found. Instead, it has been found that the best way to approach treating a tumor with drugs is to develop a battle plan in which the cancer is attacked from all sides in a coordinated and sequential manner. Employing combinations of drugs takes advantage of their different sites of action (see Figure 48-2), different toxicities, and the varying time intervals in which they must be given.

Anti-tumor drugs are often given in cycles, to give time for the normal cells to recover and for the immune system to bounce back. However, if chemotherapeutic drugs are sequentially used which do not effect the same normal tissues, treatment need not be halted to allow time for recovery. Combination chemotherapy also reduces the chances of a tumor becoming resistant to treatment.

Combinations of drugs are often used to overcome the problem of resistance, on the theory that cells are unlikely to be resistant to several dissimilar drugs. Indeed, for most cancers, combination chemotherapy seems more successful than single-agent treatment. Some chemotherapy protocols are designed to expose tumor cells to alternating cycles of "noncross-resistant" chemotherapy drugs.

A good example of combination chemotherapy is the treatment of Hodgkin's disease (a tumor of the lymphatic system), with the "MOPP" regimen. MOPP is an acronym for *M*echlorethamine (nitrogen mustard), *O*ncovin (vincristine), *P*rocarbazine, and *P*rednisone. This protocol is given as follows: mechorethamine on days 1 and 8, Oncovin on days 1 and 8, procarbazine on days 1 through 14, and prednisone on days 1 through 14. The cycle is repeated every four weeks, for six courses. Thus, the entire treatment takes six months. The response rate to MOPP is spectacular, with up to 95% of patients responding, and 81% having a complete remission. These results are even more impressive when it is realized that chemotherapy is usually used in Hodgkin's patients with more widespread disease.

Perhaps the most complex use of combination chemotherapy is also found in the treatment of Hodgkin's disease. It was found that "ABVD" (*A*driamycin, *b*leomycin, *v*inblastine, *D*TIC) gave the same results as the MOPP regimen and could even induce remissions in those who had no response to MOPP. Because both ABVD and MOPP are combinations of drugs that are not cross-resistant and have different toxicities, they have recently been tested in alternating cycles. Using these eight drugs may be more effective than either MOPP or ABVD alone.

Recent advances in cancer chemotherapy have come both from the development of new drugs and a better understanding of how best to use those already developed. Choosing the appropriate time to administer a drug, or in which order to give a combination of drugs, is as important as which drugs are used.

Adjuvant Chemotherapy

Adjuvant chemotherapy is the use of anti-cancer drugs in conjunction with either surgery or radiation therapy. Such treatment holds the potential of increasing the cure rate of cancers with a high risk of recurrence after surgery or radiation therapy. For instance, complete removal of an osteogenic sarcoma (a cancer of the bone) by surgery cures only about 20% of patients. This low surgical cure rate indicates that these tumors generally have spread before surgery, although the metastases usually do not become apparent for six to eighteen months. Intensive chemotherapy given immediately following surgery seems to wipe out the distant (and clinically undetectable) pockets of tumor cells. Over half of patients treated with surgery and adjuvant chemotherapy are currently surviving more than two years.

Certain principles are important in defining treatment objectives for adjuvant chemotherapy:

1. Since smaller tumors are more easily cured by chemotherapeutic drugs than larger tumors, surgery or radiation therapy should first by used to reduce the size of a large solid tumor.

2. Patients should be identified who are at greatest risk for cancer recurrence and for whom chemotherapy may be of benefit. This assessment is based not only on the type of cancer, but on the size and location of the tumor at time of diagnosis, certain characteristics of the tumor cells themselves, the general condition of the patient, and the potential for an improvement in the patient's quality of life without undue hardships imposed by the drugs.

3. Drugs (usually in combination) should be used which are known to be active against that particular tumor. Treatment should be for an extended time period, and should use the highest drug doses that can be tolerated by the patient.

4. Treatment should be initiated as soon as possible after surgery or radiotherapy. The longer the delay in treatment with adjuvant chemotherapy, the less chance of cure.

Perhaps the best example of the current use of adjuvant chemotherapy is in the treatment of breast cancer. This is an area of active research, much controversy, and debate.

Fortunately, breast cancer, unlike many other solid tumors, is responsive to a number of chemotherapeutic agents. Surgery is the initial treatment of choice except for metastatic, advanced disease. However, even after all demonstrable tumor has been removed, there is still a significant risk of recurrence. The risk of recurrence is directly related to the number of lymph nodes (removed at surgery) that contain tumor cells. Women who are treated with mastectomy and who have no "positive nodes" have about a 25% risk of recurrence of their cancer within ten years. If one to three lymph nodes are positive, approximately two-thirds will recur within five years. Three-fourths will recur if four or more nodes are positive.

It is important to remember that these women have had all detectable tumor removed at surgery. The presence of tumor cells in the lymph nodes is an indication of clinically undetectable metastatic disease.

Despite initial optimism, the use of adjuvant chemotherapy in women with positive nodes has been somewhat disappointing. Only in premenopausal women, the minority of breast cancer cases, have researchers conclusively shown an increased survival. Although many drug combinations have been used, CMF (cyclophosphamide, methotrexate, and 5-fluorouracil) has been the most widely studied. Bonadonna and his colleagues in Milan, Italy, showed a 40% relapse-free rate, measured after five years, for CMF-treated premenopausal women with more than four positive nodes. This compared with 25% for women treated with surgery alone. The rates were 60% vs. 44% for women with one to three lymph nodes positive.

Unfortunately, this same positive trend wasn't seen with older postmenopausal women. A re-analysis of Bonadonna's data showed that these women didn't tolerate, or were thought unable to tolerate, the severe toxicities of the CMF regimen, and were given smaller doses of the drugs. Those postmenopausal women who received the full doses showed an improvement.

Thus, the use of adjuvant chemotherapy in older women is quite controversial. Should a series of drugs be given for up to a year, that causes hair loss, nausea and vomiting, and other severe side effects, in exchange for what may be only marginal benefit? On the other hand, recent research shows that older women are able to tolerate chemotherapy better than was previously appreciated.

Fortunately, recent advances in the use of hormonal agents offer another alternative. Breast cancer cells are now routinely studied for the presence of *estrogen receptors,* proteins on the cell's surface that interact with estrogen molecules. The results of these studies have important value to the patient. Tumors with positive estrogen receptors are less likely to recur and are more responsive to drugs that change the body's hormonal environment. Interestingly, postmenopausal women are more frequently estrogen receptor positive than premenopausal women. This may explain why breast cancer tends to be a less aggressive disease in older women. Progesterone receptors are also measured, and correlate with estrogen receptors in predicting recurrence and response to hormonal treatments.

Many drugs are available that either act as hormones or block the activity of naturally-occurring hormones. Tamoxifen is a drug that blocks the body's ability to use estrogen. Although the mechanisms are unclear, tamoxifen is effective as adjuvant therapy in reducing recurrence rates. It has the distinct advantage of having few side effects, so it may be the best drug for use in postmenopausal women with positive estrogen receptors.

Regional Chemotherapy

Along with developing new chemotherapy drugs, researchers are experimenting with different methods of administering chemotherapy. The theory with regional chemotherapy is that delivering the drug directly to the tumor will expose tumor cells to higher drug doses than the rest of the body, and side effects should then be less.

One such technique involves the use of a surgically implantable drug pump. The pump, about the size and shape of a hockey puck, is placed under the skin on the patient's abdomen. A catheter tube runs from the pump into the hepatic artery, the artery that supplies the liver with blood. The pump is filled with a chemotherapeutic drug and, over days, the drug is slowly infused through the catheter. The patient comes into the clinic about once a month to have the pump refilled, a relatively painless procedure. This particular arrangement is showing promise in treating colon cancer that has metastasized to the liver.

Another example of regional chemotherapy is intraperitoneal (inside the lining of the abdomen) administration. This may be useful for treating abdominal tumors, like ovarian cancer, that have spread throughout the body cavity.

Toxicity

The ideal cancer chemotherapy agent would be one that is 100% effective in killing cancer cells, but which leaves normal cells alone. Unfortunately, cancer cells are basically normal cells gone awry, so they share common metabolic pathways. Thus, chemotherapy is often toxic to normal cells as well.

Since many antitumor drugs act on dividing cells, normal tissues with a high growth fraction of dividing cells are at particular risk. Tissues with a high percentage of actively dividing cells are the bone marrow, the lining of the gastrointestinal tract, and the hair follicles. The overall toxic effects of chemotherapy are as follows:

Bone marrow suppression: anemia (low numbers of red blood cells), infection (due to low numbers of white blood cells), and bleeding (low numbers of platelets).

Gastrointestinal tract: ulcerations, dysphagia (trouble swallowing), and diarrhea.

Nervous system: nausea, vomiting, peripheral neuropathy (weakness, tingling or numbness in the extremities), and constipation (due to nerve damage).

Hair follicles: baldness (alopecia), and folliculitis (inflammation of the follicles).

Lungs: pneumonitis (an inflammation of the lungs) and pulmonary fibrosis (permanent lung damage due to fibrous tissue buildup).

Heart: congestive heart failure (due to heart muscle damage).

Blood vessels and surrounding tissues: extravasation (the drug leaking out or accidently being injected into tissue instead of a blood vessel) can cause severe local tissue damage, and phlebitis (inflammation of the blood vessels).

Many cancer chemotherapy drugs are themselves carcinogenic, and years after receiving them, new cancers may appear. Also, these drugs may be carcinogenic to health care workers who handle them. In addition, they may be teratogenic, causing malformations in the fetus of a pregnant woman.

For these reasons, special care must be taken when preparing and administering chemotherapeutic drugs. The preparation, administration, and disposal of these drugs should be done only by specially trained personnel using protective clothing and equipment.

Supportive Care

One of the major advances in chemotherapy has been the better use of supportive medical care in dealing with the unpleasant, and sometimes life-threatening, side-effects of anti-cancer drugs.

Patients undergoing intensive chemotherapy, such as that used in leukemias, are at high risk of serious infection, due to the disease itself and the drugs causing leukopenia (a decrease in the number of disease-fighting white blood cells). Modern multi-drug antibiotic treatment has greatly increased the survival rate of patients who become infected. These patients are also at greater risk of bleeding to death because of low levels of platelets, the blood component that helps in clotting. Transfusions with platelets are now commonplace and effective.

Supportive therapy includes attention to all adverse drug effects, such as the sometimes severe nausea and vomiting that often accompanies chemotherapy. One of the newest and most interesting medications for this problem is dronabinol, a derivative of marijuana. Patients have known for a long time that marijuana is effective for alleviating vomiting due to chemotherapy. Clinical research with marijuana cigarettes and THC (*tetrahydrocannabinol*), the active ingredient in marijuana, verified this observation and led to the development of this new medication.

Cancer patients often lose weight and are malnourished, so special attention to nutrition is critical. Recent advances in intravenous (by vein) feeding techniques make adequate nutritional support more of a reality than in past years. If food is thought of as medicine, then it may be the most important "chemotherapy" for cancer patients. Inventive and delicious recipes have been developed especially for those with cancer.

Most importantly, supportive care has come to include providing greater psychological and spiritual support for cancer patients and their families.

Risk-Benefit

The key concept underlying the use of all chemotherapy, as well as other modes of cancer treatment, is that the treatment should not be worse than the disease. Cancer chemotherapy can save lives and alleviate suffering. For many cancer patients, the benefits of chemotherapy may be well worth the risks. Other patients with cancer may be best helped by not being given drugs, certainly when they cause unpleasant adverse toxic effects and prolong hospitalization, without improving the length or quality of life. In many instances, whether or not to undergo chemotherapy is a tough decision, which must ultimately be left up to the patient.

THE BIOLOGICAL TREATMENT OF CANCER

With recent advances in molecular biology and a greater understanding of the immune system, has come the potential to boost the body's immune response and alter how cells mature and grow. *Biological response modifiers* are agents capable of manipulating biological control mechanisms, and include interferons, monoclonal antibodies, and other agents (see Figure 48-6). Although monoclonal antibodies, interleukins, and interferons are the only agents discussed here, it should be realized that many biologicals and biological response modifiers are being investigated for their anti-cancer effects. The next

Figure 48-6 Biologicals and Biological Response Modifiers. *Source: Oldham RK, Smalley RV: Biologicals and Biological Response Modifiers. IN: DeVita V, Hellman S., Rosenberg S. Cancer—Principles and Practice of Oncology, 2nd edition 1985 p. 2224. J.B. Lippincott. Used with permission.*

IMMUNOMODULATING AGENTS
Alkyl lysophospholipids (ALP)
Azimexon
BCG
Bestatin
Brucella abortus
Corynebacterium parvum
Cimetidine
Sodium diethyldithiocarbamate (DTC)
Endotoxin
Glucan
"Immune" RNAs
Krestin
Lentinan
Levamisole
Muramyldipeptide (MDP)
Maleic anhydride-divinyl ether (MVE-2)
Mixed bacterial vaccines
N-137
Nocardia rubra cell wall skeleton (CWS)
Picibanil (OK432)
Prostaglandin inhibitors (aspirin, indomethacin)
Thiobendazole
Tuftsin

INTERFERONS AND INTERFERON INDUCERS
Interferons (alpha, beta, and gamma)
Poly IC-LC
Poly A:U
Tilorone
Brucella abortus
Viruses
Pyrimidinones

THYMOSINS
Thymosin alpha-1
Other thymic factors
Thymosin fraction V

LYMPHOKINES AND CYTOKINES
Antigrowth factors
Chalones
Colony-stimulating factor (CSF)
Growth factors (transforming growth factor-TGF)
Lymphocyte activation factor [LAF-interleukin 1 (IL-1)]
Lymphotoxin
Macrophage activation factor (MAF)
Macrophage chemotactic factor
Macrophage cytotoxic factor (MCF)
Macrophage growth factor (MGF)
Migration inhibitory factor (MIF)
Maturation factors
T-cell growth factor [TCGF-interleukin 2 (IL-2)]
Interleukin 3 (IL-3)
T-cell replacing factor (TRF)
Thymocyte mitogenic factor (TMF)
Transfer factor
B-cell growth factor (BCGF)
Tumor necrosis factor (TNF)

ANTIGENS
Tumor-associated antigens
Vaccines

EFFECTOR CELLS
Macrophages
NK cells
Cytotoxic T-cell clones
T-helper cells

MISCELLANEOUS APPROACHES
Allogeneic immunization
Liposome-encapsulated biologicals
Bone-marrow transplantation and reconstitution
Plasmapheresis and ex vivo treatments (activation columns and immunoabsorbents)
Virus infection of cells (oncolysates)

several years should see the development of many new and novel biological treatments for cancer.

The biological treatment of cancer is not a new idea. It has long been recognized that the immune system plays a vital role in protecting the body from cancer and in helping to rid the body of cancer once it has been established. Ideally, if one could manipulate the immune system, a selective killing of cancer cells could be engineered that wouldn't damage normal tissues.

Biological response modifiers are not limited to their effects on the immune system. There are several mechanisms by which they can act:

1. By increasing the body's defense mechanisms (augmenting the immune response).

2. By suppressing those components of the immune system that inhibit tumor cell killing.

3. By increasing the cellular maturation of tumor cells (cells that are fully mature tend not to divide).

4. By inhibiting the growth of cancer cells.

Non-Specific Immunotherapy

Non-specific immunotherapy refers to attempts to increase the overall activity of the immune system. This is different than specific immunotherapy which is directed at cancer cells in particular.

The earliest use of non-specific immunotherapy began in the late 1960s when it was noticed that children who had been immunized against tuberculosis with the bacteria, *Bacillus Calmette-Guerin* (BCG), had a lower incidence of leukemia. Researchers found that, in addition to providing immunity against tuberculosis, BCG stimulated the entire immune system.

Studies using BCG were carried out throughout the 1970s in a number of different cancers. It now appears that BCG has very modest activity against some leukemias and lymphomas, advanced prostate cancer, and breast and lung cancers. It doesn't appear that it can be relied upon as a single therapy for cancer.

Extracts of the bacteria, *Cornybacterium parvum,* also stimulate the immune system, and have been widely studied. Results have been disappointing, with only sporadic effectiveness reported.

Levamisole, a drug used to treat protozoan infections, is also thought to have immunological effects. Like BCG, it may have moderate effectiveness with certain cancers.

In general, non-specific immunotherapy is of limited benefit.*

Specific Immunotherapy

The 1970s also saw research aimed at developing a tumor cell vaccine. The idea is not new. Antibacterial vaccines have been used throughout much of this century. In theory, if an antigenic substance like a bacteria or a cancer cell is injected into the bloodstream, the body's host defenses will manufacture antibodies and mobilize various white blood cells to destroy it. Researchers tested injections of both live and inactivated tumor cells in patients with various cancers. Despite encouraging preliminary results, long-term results were mostly negative.

Why didn't specific immunotherapy work? Many reasons have been offered: the difficulty in finding and purifying a tumor cell antigen; the complex nature of the immune system; and the wide variation in both cancers and cancer patients.

Interferons

Interferons are a group of small proteins produced by cells of the immune system. They are complex, and research in this area is a hotbed of activity. Interferons were first discovered in the late 1950s when it was noticed that certain white blood cells produced a protein, in minute amounts, after exposure to viruses. While some interferons have potent antiviral activity, it was later found that others inhibit cellular proliferation and modulate the effects of cells involved in the immune system. Interferons can be grouped into one of three classes: alpha, beta, and gamma interferons. Of these, the alpha interferons are the best understood.

It wasn't until the 1970s that appreciable amounts of interferon could be extracted and tested clinically. However, these early products were quite impure. Genetic engineering now provides ample quantities of pure interferon for testing and therapeutic purposes. Using recombinant DNA technology, a piece of DNA specific for the manufacture of interferon is inserted into the DNA of a bacteria or yeast cell. These bacteria (or yeasts) are then grown in culture. In the process of making their own proteins, they manufacture large amounts of interferon.

Interferons have been extensively tested against many cancers. In particular, alpha-2 interferon is active against some leukemias and lymphomas, Kaposi's sarcoma, mycosis fungoides (a T-cell cancer that affects the skin), and ovarian cancer. It has proven to be the most active agent tested against hairy cell leukemia, a rare cancer, named because of the leukemia cells' appearance. Over 90% of patients with hairy cell leukemia respond to alpha-2 interferon. In 1986, two preparations of alpha-2 interferon were approved by the Food and Drug Administration (FDA) for use in patients with hairy cell leukemia.

Interleukins

The interleukins are a group of proteins, related to interferons, that are produced by the immune system. The most widely studied is interleukin-2 (IL-2), discovered in 1976. In 1985, positive preliminary results using IL-2 in patients with advanced cancers were widely published in the lay press. The National Cancer Institute received over 1,000 telephone calls daily from patients requesting the drug.

Partly because of this publicity, controversy surrounds IL-2. Proponents say that IL-2 is a promising treatment and that several years will be needed to determine how best to use it. Critics claim that IL-2 treatments have unacceptably severe side-effects and that they are too expensive. At this point it is still too early to tell if IL-2 will be a safe and effective treatment for cancer.

Natural Products as Antitumor Agents

For a number of years, Bruce Ames at the University of California, Berkeley, has been urging

*Methods of non-specific immunotherapy will continue to be tried, particularly in combination with other treatment methods. An interesting example of this are attempts in the late 1980s to use malaria as a treatment method, (i.e., giving malaria to cancer patients). This combines the strategy of an infection non-specifically boosting the immune system with that of hyperthermia (malaria causes predictable high fevers). Supporting this approach is the fact that cancer incidence tends to be lower in areas infected with malaria.

the scientific community to devote greater attention to naturally occurring anti-cancer substances, particularly those that appear in plants. Some plants, he points out, are resistant to the kinds of tumors that affect most other plants.

The retinoids, from which vitamin A is derived, were the first such natural anti-tumor agents that gained recognition, and are being evaluated for their ability to prevent, reduce, and treat cancers—particularly those of the skin.

More recently, a large class of naturally occurring plant substances called flavonoids has come under study because of their remarkable effects. Flavonoids appear to augment immune function by stimulating NK (natural killer) cells, as well as inducing interferon and interleukin (via cytokines).

The future of cancer treatment and prevention holds tremendous promise in the area of naturally occurring antitumor biological substances.

Monoclonal Antibodies

Part of the problem with early immunological research can be explained by borrowing a term from computer programmers: "garbage in; garbage out." Antibodies, antigens, and other biological products were difficult to isolate and purify, and only available in minute quantities of low purity. That has changed in the last few years. Remarkable advances in genetic engineering now provide investigators with large quantities of highly purified biologicals.

Monoclonal antibodies are a good example. It is now possible to fuse a lymphocyte (producing an antibody specific for a cancer cell) with a mammalian cell (usually a mouse cell) in a package called a hybridoma. These hybridomas can be grown in large quantities in tissue cultures, and produce large amounts of specific antibody.

Monoclonal antibodies have a number of potential uses. Since they are specific for an antigen on the tumor cell's surface, when injected into the body they will travel through the bloodstream until they encounter a tumor cell and then attach themselves to it. If a radioactive molecule (a radioactive "label") is attached to the antibody, clinicians can trace the concentrations of radioactivity in the body and thus pinpoint the location of pockets of tumor cells that previously would have escaped detection. If a molecule of a chemotherapeutic drug or highly toxic substance (an "oncotoxin") is attached to the antibody, the tumor cell will be killed.

The use of monoclonal antibodies in basic research is blossoming. However, monoclonal antibodies as a therapy hasn't progressed to the point where it is clinically useful except in experimental centers. Monoclonal antibodies may go the way of the tumor cell vaccine, but more than likely they will lead to real advances in anti-cancer therapy.

ADDITIONAL READING—Chemotherapy

1. Hellmann K, Carter S, Fundamentals of Cancer Chemotherapy. McGraw-Hill, 1987. (Good general text, often technical, gives specifics per type of cancer.)

2. McGuire D, Yarbro C, Cancer Pain Management, Grune & Stratton, Inc., 1987. (A lot of good ideas and strategies.)

3. Oldham R, Principles of Cancer Biotherapy, Raven Press, 1987. (The first comprehensive text on the use of biological response modifiers to treat cancer.)

4. Pinedo H, Chabner B, Cancer Chemotherapy, Elsever Science Publishing Co., Inc. 1985. (Highly technical.)

5. Skeel R., Handbook of Cancer Chemotherapy—2nd edition. Little, Brown and Co., 1987. (Just that, a handbook.)

**A complete list of chemotherapeutic drugs, their uses and side-effects appears in the Appendix.

49

Spontaneous Regression of Cancer

An Interview with Warren H. Cole, M.D.

Reprinted with permission from "Spontaneous Regression of Cancer," Ca—A Cancer Journal 24(5): 274–9 (September, October, 1974).

In the following article, Arthur I. Holleb, MD, the editor of *Ca—A Cancer Journal for Clinicians* interviews Warren H. Cole, MD, Emeritus Professor of Surgery, University of Illinois, College of Medicine, Chicago, Illinois—*M.R.*

Editor: *Spontaneous regressions of cancer have baffled investigators since 1897 when Halsted reported the mysterious disappearance of breast cancer metastases. This strange phenomenon, once viewed with suspicion, is now regarded more seriously. Dr. Cole, what is meant by "spontaneous" regression?*

Dr. Cole: We define spontaneous regression as the complete or partial disappearance of cancer which cannot be attributed to treatment, if any was given. The phenomenon is not synonymous with cure. Actually, since all regressions must have a cause, the term "spontaneous" is a misnomer; idiopathic or biologic regression is a more accurate description.

Editor: *How frequently do cancers regress spontaneously?*

Dr. Cole: The phenomenon is extremely rare. Some investigators estimate the incidence is as low as one in 100,000 cancer patients. If we knew the exact incidence, it might be more frequent than that.

Editor: *Quite frankly, how do you account for the current interest in this phenomenon?*

Dr. Cole: Interest has increased over the years as more physicians are persuaded of the authenticity of the phenomenon. Many investigators now believe that studying documented cases and finding the cause or causes of spontaneous regression will bring us closer to better control of cancer.

Editor: *Have many examples of spontaneous regression been documented?*

Dr. Cole: Dr. Tilden Everson and I assembled 176 patients from the literature of the past 70 years and from colleagues. These reports fulfilled the qualifications of (1) a confirmed diagnosis of cancer and (2) a regression that could not be attributed solely to treatment. We excluded hundreds of unverified cases of spontaneous regression as well as patients with squamous cell epitheliomas, leukemias and lymphomas because of the marked fluctuation in growth rate.

The duration of spontaneous cancer regressions in these 176 patients varied from less than six months to more than 10 years.

Editor: *Did certain cancers regress spontaneously more often than others?*

Dr. Cole: Although spontaneous regressions were noted in tumors of 18 different anatomic sites, more than half occurred in carcinoma of the kidney (17.6 percent); neuroblastoma (16.5 percent); malignant melanoma (10.8 percent); and choriocarcinoma (10.8 percent). (Figure 49-1.)

Editor: *Are there any explanations for these regressions?*

Dr. Cole: I am convinced that there is no *single* explanation, but rather many causes. After careful analysis of our 176 patients, we were able to group all the incidents or factors that could be related to spontaneous regression of cancer into seven categories. They include: hormones; drugs; removal of carcinogen; immune reaction; irradiation; operative trauma; fever and/or infection. Although one or all of these might exert a role in the spontaneous regression of cancer, I have no conclusive proof.

Editor: *Could some of these seven factors have been coincidental to the regression of cancer?*

Dr. Cole: Yes, it is possible. For example, although 20 cases of spontaneous regression could be linked to hormonal factors, many regressions occurred in tumors that are not hormone-dependent or in women who are not postmenopausal. In three instances, adenocarcinomas of the kidney regressed after treatment with a progestational agent; in one patient, a sarcoma regressed during amenorrhea; and in three women, melanomas regressed following parturition. These data suggest that while a hormonal factor may be responsible for some spontaneous regressions, in others it may be pure coincidence.

Similarly, only two of the three examples of spontaneous regression attributed to drugs could plausibly be due to unusual drug sensitivity. In one patient, a neuroblastoma regressed after several courses of nitrogen mustard; in another, a neuroblastoma regressed after biopsy of the primary tumor and subsequent treatment with triethylenemelamine. In a third patient, however, it is unlikely that regression of a choriocarcinoma and presumptive pulmonary metastases was due to treatment with chlortetracycline, since evidence of metastases persisted for seven months after discontinuation of this drug.

Editor: *Is the removal of a carcinogen from the environment a logical explanation for some cases of spontaneous regression?*

Dr. Cole: One would expect that removal of a carcinogen might account for many examples of spontaneous regression. However, we found only 15 cases that could fit into this category. In 10 of 13 patients, bilateral transplantation of the ureters into the bowel,

Figure 49-1 Collected Cases of Spontaneous Regression of Cancer

Type or Location of Cancer	Number of Cases
Hypernephroma	31
Neuroblastoma	29
Malignant melanoma	19
Choriocarcinoma	19
Bladder	13
Soft-tissue sarcoma	11
Sarcoma of bone	8
Colon and rectum	7
Ovary	7
Testis	7
Breast	6
Metastatic cancer, primary unknown	4
Uterus	4
Stomach	4
Liver	2
Larynx	1
Lung	1
Pancreas	1
Thyroid	1
Tongue	1
Total	**176**

in preparation for a radical cystectomy, was followed by regression of bladder cancers. There thus appears to have been some factor in the urine responsible for either the development or the continuing growth of these tumors. In the other two patients, bladder cancers regressed after transplantation of only one ureter.

It is possible that these and other patients who experience spontaneous regression of cancer have accidentally avoided a yet unknown carcinogen. However, it is unusual to expect that removal of a carcinogen could reverse an already established cancer, and that it could do so in only a few weeks or months. Obviously, lung cancers do not quickly regress once a patient stops smoking cigarettes.

Editor: *Can you suggest other causes of these regressions?*

Dr. Cole: Perhaps the immune response was so intense in these patients that bladder cancers regressed once the carcinogen, or part of the carcinogen, was eliminated. In fact, I believe that increased immunologic resistance, either temporary or permanent, is the most significant explanation for most spontaneous regressions of cancer.

Editor: *How many of the 176 cases of spontaneous regression could be attributed to immunologic factors?*

Dr. Cole: The question should really be answered in two parts. First, we documented only 14 cases of spontaneous regression that were linked to possible immunologic factors. The most dramatic examples occurred in three patients with malignant melanomas. In one patient, the tumor regressed after a blood transfusion from a patient who previously had a spontaneous regression of melanoma; in another, the regression followed a transfusion from a patient who had a 10-year cure after radical excision of a melanoma; and in a third patient, regression followed three transfusions from the blood bank, the last of which was blood group A, Rh-negative.

In addition to these few examples, however, I believe that many other cases of spontaneous regression associated with operative trauma, irradiation and infection are more adequately explained by an immunologic mechanism.

Editor: *Are you suggesting that operative trauma plays no role in the spontaneous regression of cancer?*

Dr. Cole: Absolutely not. Based on present knowledge of the behavior of tumors, certain cases of spontaneous regression are difficult to explain solely in terms of operative trauma. For instance, in one group of 10 patients, regressions occurred after only partial removal of the tumor, a procedure which may sometimes increase growth. In another 41 patients, metastases regressed after excision of the primary. Surprisingly, 22 of these patients had adenocarcinomas of the kidney and presumptive pulmonary metastases which regressed after nephrectomy.

I am convinced that in these more than 50 cases, operative trauma, due either to partial or complete excision, triggered an intense immune response which caused the tumor to regress. . . .

50

What Is a Tumor Board?

Mark Renneker, M.D.

A tumor board is a panel of cancer specialists composed primarily of surgeons, chemotherapists, pathologists, diagnostic radiologists, and radiotherapists who meet on a regular basis to review cancer cases jointly and to make recommendations regarding further diagnostic procedures and suitable up-to-date treatment plans. These cases are presented to the tumor board by physicians in the community served by the hospital in which the board meets. In this era of of multimodality therapy whereby, for example, a breast cancer patient may be treated by a surgeon, radiotherapist, and chemotherapist, it is important to have all of these treatment activities carefully considered and well-coordinated so that the patient receives the best possible care.

To sit in on a tumor board meeting is to have the unique experience of seeing physicians admit to the limits of their knowledge, saying "Frankly, I don't know what is the best thing to do"—and to witness the often heated discussion that ensues. One realizes that cancer treatment is not always done in a cookbook fashion—new recipes are often called for. Invaluable to the tumor board is the tumor registry (see the following article) which can provide pivotal information by showing which treatment approaches have worked and which have failed in the past. Tumor boards and cancer registries are required of a hospital cancer program by the American College of Surgeons.

Every cancer patient should ask their physicians to consider presenting their case to the tumor board. No matter how straightforward, every case is unique—and no doctor knows everything there is to know about cancer.

51

Cancer Registries

Calvin Zippin, Sc.D.

*Professor of Epidemiology, School of Medicine,
University of California, San Francisco.*

A cancer registry can provide information on the most common forms of cancer, which cancers are on the increase or decline, who are high and low risk individuals for various forms of cancer, how cancer is being treated, and what percent of patients are alive at, say, five years after diagnosis. From clues provided by registry data on high and low risk groups we can gain some insight into possible causative agents. Similarly, data entering a registry system can help us determine whether screening programs for cancer of the breast, for example, are followed by an increased proportion of early diagnoses of breast cancer. Registries may also dispel incorrect impressions regarding patterns of cancer morbidity. Thus, data from cancer registries show that the frequency of cancer of the uterine cervix in women fifty years of age and older was on the decline for some years prior to the widespread use of cervical cytology in the diagnosis of this disease.[1]

By knowing the stage of a patient's disease at the time of diagnosis, the physician, using statistics compiled by tumor registries, will have some information on the likelihood of a cure and will therefore be guided in determining his approach to management. Only by means of a system for summarizing our cancer experience can we assess changes in the types of problems requiring our attention, or facilities required for diagnosis and management. Similarly, such systems aid us in assessing our progress or lack of progress in disease prevention, control, and management.

Cancer registries have been in operation in individual hospitals in the United States in large numbers since the 1950s when the American College of Surgeons[2] required a hospital to maintain a registry for approval of the hospital's cancer program. The hospital registry records basic information on each diagnosis of cancer seen in that institution and provides for the continued medical supervision of each patient through a system of annual patient follow-up. Most registries record for each diagnosis identifying information on the patient, the site and morphology of the tumor, how it was diagnosed (histologically, radiologically, clinically), the extent of disease, and how it was treated. From this, tabulations can be made by which to summarize the hospital's cancer experience. Approximately 800 hospi-

tal cancer programs are currently approved by the American College of Surgeons.

Centralized programs bring together data from a number of institutions and help provide a broader picture of cancer diagnosis, treatment, and survival.[3] A number of centralized programs encompass all institutions within defined geographic bounds and offer a means of obtaining cancer incidence rates for the populations and sub-populations residing within the county, regional, or statewide boundaries of the registry area. The National Cancer Institute conducts a still broader reporting system[4] that brings together data from five statewide registries (Connecticut, Iowa, Utah, New Mexico, Hawaii), five metropolitan areas (Detroit, Atlanta, New Orleans, Seattle-Tacoma, San Francisco) plus the Commonwealth of Puerto Rico. This program not only provides for an overall assessment of cancer risk throughout the United States but also enables comparison of risks from one geographic area to another. It also allows studies of survival results for all cancer patients in defined geographic areas.

Although registries have major roles to play in our struggle against cancer, there are limitations to be noted. Ordinarily registries cannot provide definitive evidence of the superiority of one mode of therapy compared with another unless the data are obtained exclusively from controlled clinical trials programs providing for randomization to assure comparability of treatment groups. On the other hand, evidence from cancer registries *suggesting* the superiority of a specific modality of treatment can serve as an indicator of the need to carry out a clinical trial.

Before undertaking the development of a registry program, it is essential that the purposes to be served are clearly defined, that provision is made for complete collection of the data that is regarded as essential to meet those objectives, and that adequate staff and facilities will be available to provide for quality control of the data collected and for regular summarization of the data and for distribution of reports. From this it is hoped that continuing education of the medical community will be enhanced, that the level of care of the cancer patient will benefit, and that our understanding of the causation of cancer and its natural history will be augmented.

[1]C. Zippin and D. A. Wood, "Special Problems in Cancer Control, Cancer Registries," *Continued Education Series No. 106* (Cancer Control, University of Michigan, 1962), pp. 250–272.
[2]*Cancer Program Manual,* Commission on Cancer, American College of Surgeons, 55 East Erie Street, Chicago, Illinois 60611, 1974.

[3]*Cancer Patient Survival Report No. 5,* U.S. Department of Health, Education and Welfare, Public Health Service, National Institutes of Health, 1976.
[4]The Cancer Surveillance, Epidemiology and End Results (SEER) Program; Biometry Branch, National Cancer Institute, U.S. Department of Health, Education and Welfare, Bethesda, Maryland, 10 pages, April 1976.

52

Rights of the Cancer Patient

Melvin J. Krant, M.D.

Reprinted with permission from "Rights of the Cancer Patient," Ca—A Cancer Journal for Clinicians *25(2): 98–100 (March/April, 1975).*

The following editorial is written by a physician and is directed towards other physicians.—*M.R.*

What cancer means to the patient is different, frequently, from what cancer means to a doctor or health care worker.

It is much within our education, of course, to look upon the processes which dislodge people from normality as being diseases, those things indeed which take them away from any normal stance, and which our education prepares us to correct. So, we spend much of our energy processing thoughts which have to do with the biologic nature of disease. But frequently the patient's concerns are quite different. To a sick person having a disease is part of something larger. With long-term, chronic, and especially fatal disease, there is a search for meaning: Why am I sick, what is my life now to me and to others? What does it mean now to be becoming unto death? For that cancer patient who is not cured, the thought is constantly there as to what this all means, as he must now live his life through becoming unto death. It is one of the great paradoxes of modern American medicine that we offer a patient many ways to extend his living, but at the same time, we extend his dying. The imposition of both phenomena simultaneously presents the sick individual and his family with a confusing signal. Physicians appear to act as if only treatments for life are permissible, and that helping people to adjust to their dying is not. But even this is not always true, adding to confusing signals that are given.

At one end of the medical behavioral spectrum for the advanced cancer patient, for example, is the notion that there's nothing more that can be done. This attitude is frequently seen in large centers, not so much in research centers. The message is that there is a limited technology available, at the end of which the patient is to be discharged someplace else, since there's nothing else that can be done. Exactly what is to happen to such a patient and his family is left unclear, and unstated.

At the other end of the spectrum is what we see in research centers, namely, that the patient is always to be under treatment until he dies. In this latter implication are two things, I think. One is that the patient owes the researcher something. He owes something by giving up his disease to be manipulated by one experimental form or another. Even though he's not profited by it, somebody in the future may profit. Therefore, as a member of the human race, we insist, he owes us his illness to be researched.

I'd like to warn about this latter avenue, which is never really discussed, namely, the powerful seductiveness of medicine, to offer something to patients which has little to do with their particular benefit but has much to do with this research design.

We have to be consistently careful in our eagerness to pursue some righteous task, which may be related to elucidation of a disease process, or which may have some implication for the future as far as eradication is concerned, that we do not act as if the patient was a particular sacrificial lamb. A fatal disease may induce a regressive state in one's ego, that is, in the capacity to maturely handle most major problems. Patients indeed do frequently fantasize of being rescued. This process occurs often as an effort to deny the implication of fatal disease. However, these same patients are often also quite realistic in their recognition that being cured, or getting over their illness, is not to be their province. The point is that through such agencies as fantasy, which we sometimes call hope, patients place themselves in a position to hand over control of their lives and destinies to the physician. Our power and our authority can seduce them to go on into one magical effort after another seeking cure or seeking betterment. I use the word seduce in the sense that the physician or researcher does not truly expect an improvement in the patient's condition to take place with the particular treatment employed but instead wishes to gain information or feels impelled to do something for psychological purposes. The treatment is preferred because patients supposedly want to be treated. Many patients offer themselves for experimental procedures willingly, recognizing its limitations. But many do so because they feel powerless to say "no."

We must be very cautious when we look at the cancer patient in the light of experimental chemotherapy, because seduction plays against the best of what men are. Patients desire life. If we continue to offer patients one treatment after another, especially one failing treatment after another, they may not be able to say "no"—indeed they may appear to say "yes" each time, but we force them into despair and disbelief. Such patients become very isolated and alone, with deep feelings of resignation, rather than hope. We have not helped them in their search for meaning, in their efforts to find peace and order. Secondly, we physicians frequently feel that unless we are doing something active therapeutically, we are not doing anything. New physicians have great authority. We have stupendous power. We are, and can be looked upon as the great rescuers, as the great fathers and mothers, whether we are doing something active or not. Just our "being there" is powerful. We can easily abuse such power. We can abuse it by reducing people to disease states, instead of magnifying their capacity to be truly human. We can confuse ourselves by equating our impotence in preventing death with our power to help our advanced cancer patients. In supporting patients and families to cope with the dimensions of the dying period as a real effort, we can be powerfully therapeutic. The physician can be highly influential in arranging those supports that can be helpful in dying, and not just treating disease. Such efforts should allow the patient to stay in control of his limited resources, rather than be forced into submission to our systematic, observational attitudes which look only at the disease and not at him.

Operationally, we can examine such questions as: how often do we use the hospital to incarcerate somebody, or how often do we use our clinics to have people coming back for our sakes and not for theirs?

All this is not to say that we are evil, or selfish and certainly I'm not stating that if given an opportunity, most patients would not prefer to have life rather than death. This is obviously so. But, in fact, the world of advanced cancer is today a world of many experimental procedures and treatments in which the main temptation is to treat the patient as if he must acquiesce to our suggestions because he thinks only of life. The physician may force a patient into feelings of isolation and into regressive behavior if the patients feel that they must say "yes" to each therapeutic suggestion for fear that they would be otherwise abandoned by their doctors. Even patients who say, "Don't tell me anything; just take care of me, that's what I want," are most frequently asking not only to be saved, but to feel that they will not be abandoned. But with such patients especially, we must not reject them even further. We must not make them regress even further to satisfy our own narcissistic needs and our refusal to allow death a dignified moment.

It is important for a patient to be able to say no and feel safe in so doing. It is important that somebody can say, "I don't want to do that," and feel that he can come back because he'll still be loved and he'll be looked after. And it is important to recognize that in this safekeeping a physician exercises his best clinical caring. James Jackson raised this issue some hundred years ago when addressing a fourth-year class at Harvard, he said there were four major jobs that a physician must accomplish. First, of course, is to make a diagnosis; secondly, to institute a treatment appropriate to that diagnosis; thirdly, to try and make somebody more comfortable by alleviating his symptoms; and fourthly, to give patients a feeling of safe conduct. Whatever the problem, the physician should offer trust. In this regard, then, my plea is simply that we make an arena where people can safely stay in control of their lives and feel secure in rejecting what we want to do, but not being rejected because they have to do so. We can encourage patients to exert the best of their decision making, and help them to get to the end of their life in a gratifying way, rather than feeling that the only way they can have our comfort, the only way they can have medical care, is to say yes to every procedure that is offered to them.

53

Cancer Quackery

It is estimated that from $10 to $25 billion is spent yearly on unproven health cures in the U.S., and of that amount, approximately fifty percent is spent on "quack" cures for cancer. In California alone, cancer patients spend over $500 million per year. Practically every cancer patient will, at one time or another, give serious consideration to trying one of these methods; or, at least one friend or family member will urge them to consider it.

The tremendous sums of money involved, and the harm that can come to patients, makes cancer quackery an enormous problem in the cancer field. Complicating the matter is an ideological and political quagmire that separates traditional, or conventional medicine, from alternative, or holistic, medicine. To align yourself with one side or the other is to risk not truly understanding the problem. It has little to do with the worthiness or righteousness of one type of medicine over another (there are probably just as many quacks in traditional medicine as there are in alternative medicine); cancer quackery has to do with fear and misunderstanding of cancer.—*M.R.*

Unproven Methods of Cancer Management

RONALD N. GRANT, M.D. and IRENE BARTLETT, B.S.

Excerpted with permission from "Unproven Methods of Cancer Management—1976,"
American Cancer Society, pp. 1–18.

Unproven methods of cancer management are as much a part of the cancer problem as is the disease's capacity to kill. Fear of cancer is nearly universal and becomes increasingly more acute the closer one comes to the disease, either as a patient or as a member of the family of the patient. Standard management with surgery, radiotherapy and/or chemotherapy, unfortunately, may be so fearsome in itself that many people are strongly tempted to seek unproven methods of treatment. The stakes are high.

FEAR AND UNPROVEN CANCER REMEDIES

In light of these alarming facts, it is not surprising that the public is afraid of cancer and that enthusiastic claims for unproven remedies have appeared in increasing numbers to exploit these fears.

For more than any other reason, people go to proponents of unproven methods because they are afraid. What are their specific fears? (1) They fear that all cancers are incurable. Many people do not know that localized and even some moderately advanced cancer *is* curable. (2) They fear the expense. Many think it is less expensive to procure and use unproven methods than to place themselves under the care of a reputable physician. (3) They fear surgery, radiation or chemotherapy. Many prefer the illusion of painless, prompt medical "miracles." (4) They fear that their own doctor has given up hope and they are ready to clutch at any straw. . . .

PROPONENTS OF UNPROVEN METHODS OF CANCER MANAGEMENT

Proponents of unproven methods are encouraged by the nature of the disease itself. Statistics indicate that cancer is on the increase; the disease is often fatal; it is expensive; and has a psychological impact on the family that is difficult to bear.

The cancer quack is the beneficiary of the overworked, the incompetent, the disinterested, the brusque professional and orthodoxy's misuse and overuse of drugs, the "no time to listen or explain" syndrome, therapy that is often prolonged and unpleasant, the fear of mental or physical incapacity, and the "what have I got to lose attitude."

Proponents of unproven methods of cancer management range from ignorant, uneducated, misguided persons to highly educated scientists with advanced degrees who are out of their area of competency. Some proponents hold Ph.D. or M.D. degrees. Their false promises and exaggerated claims lead patients and their families to believe that cure can be achieved or at least that marked improvement is possible. The hope they offer is sometimes considered worth the large sums of money that the "treatment" may cost. Unfortunately, many patients with curable cancer leave the care of competent physicians to be treated with a worthless, unproven remedy until a cure by accepted methods becomes impossible; thus, they have effectively been killed instead of cured. Proponents of unorthodox methods often seek out cancer patients and their families as the prime targets of their propaganda, playing not only on fear and ignorance, but on the natural desire to make suffering loved ones as comfortable as possible.

Certain common features are noted among those with some scientific background or degrees:

- They tend to be isolated from established scientific facilities or associates.

- They do not use regular channels of communication (current, reputable, scientific journals) for reporting scientific information. Physicians of this type tend to publish articles in journals which are not read by cancer specialists.

- They claim that prejudice of organized medicine hinders their efforts.

- They are prone to challenge established theories and attack prominent scientists with bitter criticism.

- They are quick to cite examples of physicians and scientists of the past who were forced to fight the rigid dogma of their day.

• They are often inclined to use complex jargon and unusual phraseology to embellish their writing.

• Their records are scanty or nonexistent.

• They often discourage, or even refuse, consultation with reputable physicians. If a scientific evaluation of their methods is made, they generally decline to accept the results, claiming that the "medical trust" is against them.

• Their method of treatment is often secret and is available only from them. Or, the mode of administration depends on special judgment which can be learned only from them.

• They discount biopsy verification in cancer diagnosis, sometimes by saying that it "spreads" the cancer. They may accept patients who have already been cured of cancer by orthodox means but fear they have not.

• They may use proven drugs or other methods of treatment as adjuvants to the unproven therapy, and if a favorable effect on cancer is shown, claim that it is the result of their unproven remedy.

• They may have multiple unusual degrees such as N.D. (Doctor of Naturopathy), Ph.N. (Philosopher of Naturopathy), or Ms.D. (Doctor of Metaphysics.) These degrees may have been received from correspondence schools.

• Their chief supporters tend to be prominent statesmen, actors, writers, lawyers, even members of state or national legislatures—persons not trained or experienced in the natural history of cancer, the care of patients with cancer, or in scientific methodology.

A common pattern is that of the proponent who has tried a remedy in several people with what seem to be good results. These are often based entirely on the subjective response of the patient, which may result from the false hope instilled in him. The proponent claims the results as "research," which in turn provides the basis for testimonials—the earmark of this type of treatment.

Some proponents do not claim to have a cancer cure, and treat only advanced cases for palliation, charging only the cost of the materials used. On investigation, it is usually discovered that there is no documentation to support their claimed results. Careful objective records are not available. Diag-

noses are not confirmed by biopsy. Treatment used is not made freely available to other investigators for independent trial under controlled conditions.

HOW CANCER PATIENTS BECOME INVOLVED WITH UNPROVEN METHODS

Personal Contact

Proponents of unorthodox methods seek out cancer patients and their families as the prime targets of their propaganda. In some areas, the traffic in unorthodox medicine is so well organized that proponents of unproven methods have been able to infiltrate hospitals in order to tout their remedies in waiting rooms; patients have been persuaded to forego conventional treatment by apparently "chance" acquaintances who have "inside" information about the alleged success of an unorthodox treatment. Their typical arguments include: "This is non-toxic and therefore harmless; the patient has nothing to lose and everything to gain." "Nobody claims that this will cure cancer, but it *controls* cancer and relieves the patient's pain." "The patient has a right to the treatment of his choice, and it's evil to deprive him of that choice." . . .

Books—Magazines— Advertisements

An important factor in the promotion of unproven methods of cancer management is our free press, making it possible for books, magazines, newspapers and the mass media to present seemingly favorable information on unproven methods. Books on medical science, especially if they are so-called controversial medical problems, are quite appealing to the reading public. This type of book is often so skillfully written that the average reader concludes that he himself can make a valid judgment on the merits of the treatment in question, usually in favor of its use. By distributing pro and con information throughout the book, the author may give the reader the impression that he is impartial and therefore factual, although the argument is heavily weighted in favor of the method. The reader, once convinced, then becomes a promoter of the treatment, recommending it to his associates and friends.

Unproven cancer remedies get additional support from sensational mass circulation magazines which are anxious to publish the latest "pseudo-scientific theories" and "advances," especially if they are controversial.

In addition to sporadic articles in mass circulation magazines, there are a variety of "health" magazines which are especially interested

Figure 53-1 Scientifically Unproven Methods of Cancer Management (Diagnosis and Treatment)—Partial Listing. The American Cancer Society—National Office, has information available on all of the methods listed here. New methods (often *old* methods, just renamed) appear each year. Also, realize that this listing is primarily for the United States and Western Europe—other parts of the world would have an equally long list.

Alklyzing punch
Almonds
Aloe vera plant
Anticancergen Z50-zuccalaytic test
Antineol
Antineoplastons
Asparagus oil
Bacteria enema
Bamfolin (S.N.K.)
H. H. Beard methods
Biomedical detoxification therapy
Bonifacio anticancer goat serum
Cancer lipid concentrate and the malignancy index
Carcalon
Carcin
Carrot/celery juice
Carzodelan
Cedar cones
CH-23
Chamoruls
Chaparrel tea
Chase dietary method
C.N.T.
Coffee enemas
Coley's mixed toxins
Collodanrum and bichloracetic acid— Kahlenberg
Compound X
Contreras method
Crofton immunization
Diamond carbon compound
DMSO (haematoxylin dissolved in dimethyl sulfoxide)
Esterlit
Ferguson plant products
Fresh cell therapy
Fresh defatted bile capsules
Frost method
Ganner Petroleum
Gerson method
Glover serum
Goat's milk
Grape diet
Greek cure
H-11
Hadley vaccine and blood and skin tests
Hemacytology index (HCL)
Hendricks natural immunity therapy

Hoxsey method
Hubbard E meter and Hubbard electrometer
Hydrozine sulfate
Immunoaugmentative therapy (IAT)
Iscador-mistletoe
Issels combination therapy
Javaro head-shrinking compound
Kanfer neuromuscular handwriting test
KC555
Kelly maignancy index (ecology therapy)
Kallzyne
Koch treatment
Krebiozen
Laetrile
Lewis methods
Livingston vaccine
Macrobiotic diet
Makar: intradermal cancer tests (ICT)
M-P virus
Marijuana
Mercenene
Millet bread
Milluve
Mucorhicin
Multiple enzyme therapy
Naessens
Olive oil
Oncon juice
Orgone energy devices
Polonine
Psychic surgery
Rand vaccine
Revici cancer control
Samuels casal therapy/ endogenous endocrinotherapy/Daussets method
Sanders treatment
Simonton method
Snake meat
Snake oil capsules
Staphylococcus phage lysate
Sunflower seeds
Ultraviolet blood irradiation—intravenous treatment
Unpolished brown rice
Unsulfured raisins
Vitamin B-15 pangamic acid

in unproven treatment regimens. Most are issued monthly and reflect an opposition to the "medical monopoly" and accepted forms of treatment. Such magazines are the forum for proponents of unproven remedies and non-medical approaches to health in this country, and many individuals get information on these unproven methods from them. A favorite ploy is to send a gift subscription to the family of someone under treatment for cancer.

One of the most popular "health" magazines is *Prevention*, published by Rodale Press. This magazine carries articles on unproven methods and developments in the health field. Articles are generally well written and often include features on worthless methods of cancer management, sometimes by the chief proponent of the method. *Prevention* magazine also publishes advertisements of unproven methods of cancer treatment and/or books which describe them.

Radio and Television

With the interest in cancer so general and the desire to find an effective treatment for cancer so widespread, any unproven remedy which becomes well known and controversial is likely to be discussed on television and radio. Personalities and issues associated with unorthodoxy often appeal to the "show business" instincts of broadcasters. Attempts are made to set up pro and con confrontations in the hope of starting lively debates. If the representatives of conventional treatment refuse to participate, pointed references to their refusal are made on the air. When only the proponents are interviewed, some moderators attempt to even things up by playing the devil's advocate, but the proponents almost always get the last word. . . .

"Health" Organizations

As mentioned previously, much information on unproven methods reaches the public through meetings and other activities of "health" organizations which are in opposition to the "medical monopoly." Such organizations adopt high-sounding purposes and purport to be concerned about freedom of choice for the patient, the costs of medical therapy and the protection of the public; they play on fear and rely on testimonials and personal experience. These organizations have strong fund-raising campaigns through sales, dues and fees. They hold revivalist-type meetings and feature highly emotional appeals. Laetrile, Krebiozen, Hoxsey and the Gerson dietary method are some of their widely promoted unproven remedies.

One such organization is the International Association of Cancer Victims and Friends (I.A.C.V.F.), founded in 1963 by Cecile Hoffman, a cancer patient who believed her life had been saved by the use of Laetrile. Mrs. Hoffman died in 1969 of metastatic cancer. . . .

Sponsorship by Prominent Individuals

In addition to support or promotion by organized "health" groups and various types of publications, unproven remedies are often championed by prominent citizens.

Entertainers, socially prominent persons, celebrities and others in the public eye may be persuaded to promote various unproven methods of cancer management. These individuals, while they are often sincere, do not have the scientific training or background to judge the merit of the method they are promoting, and are unaware of the strict criteria for scientific investigation necessary before a drug or method of diagnosis or treatment is acceptable for medical use. They are uninformed of the proven effective medical treatments available and the danger of delay in not using them.

STANDARDS OF SCIENTIFIC INVESTIGATION OF UNPROVEN METHODS

If the investigation is to be conclusive, scientific standards must be established. These should be the normal scientific criteria required to substantiate any claim for a product and must be capable of confirmation by others.

Standards of investigation in cancer should include at least the following criteria: complete evaluation of all clinical and laboratory data presented by the proponent including case histories, X-rays, and microscopic slides; reproducible analysis of the drug and laboratory results; observations on the effects of the therapy under study in a sufficient number of patients with biopsy-proven cancer; assessment of treatment results for each case compared to other previous or concomitant therapy; examiniation of autopsy data and; consultation with other investigating groups.

PROBLEMS CONNECTED WITH INVESTIGATION OF UNPROVEN METHODS

The history of medicine reveals numerous instances in which important advances came from rather humble beginnings. Leads must be followed if there is the slightest possibility of gain. Numerous letters are received by various government and private agencies from people deeply anxious to help provide a cure. So, in many instances, some preliminary investigation by a qualified agency is required. However, it would be physically impossible and scientifically absurd to investigate every suggestion, no matter how well-meaning, that is offered by the lay public.

With most unproven methods of cancer management it is difficult if not impossible to secure the cooperation of the involved proponents. Difficulties may develop in several ways:

- The amount of supporting evidence is extremely scant.

- Frequently, biopsy proof is lacking; when available, it is sometimes found that the entire tumor has been removed surgically or destroyed radiologically prior to initiation of the treatment in question.

- Patient interviews are hard to obtain.

- Case histories are incomplete.

- No patient follow-up information is available.

- Autopsy data is usually not provided.

- A sample of the product is unobtainable for analysis and trial.

In addition to the difficulty of initiating and carrying out such a scientific evaluation of unproven cancer remedies, an unfavorable result is seldom accepted by the proponent or causes any reduction in his efforts and promotions.

Because of the medical profession's insistence on reliable standards of proof of efficacy and safety, the proponents of unproven remedies are prone to charge that they are being persecuted by the "medical trust" or "organized medicine."

MAJOR SOURCES OF INFORMATION REGARDING CANCER AND ITS MANAGEMENT

Various agencies and organizations participate in reporting and investigating claims made for new methods of cancer management. They include: The American Cancer Society, American Medical Association, Federal Food and Drug Administration, National Cancer Institute, U.S. Postal Service, U.S. Public Health Services, State Cancer Commissions and Advisory Councils, certain reliable cancer research centers and independent, scientifically trained cancer investigators willing to cooperate.

The American Medical Association

The American Medical Association's Department of Investigation, an educational activity of the A.M.A., has since 1906 maintained extensive files on all aspects of unproven methods, as well as on cultism, faddism, imposters, and pseudo-medicine. It actively cooperates with other agencies in the investigation of unproven methods of cancer management.

The Food and Drug Administration

The Food and Drug Administration under the mandate of the Food, Drug and Cosmetic Act has regulatory control of food, drugs and devices in interstate commerce.

Under the 1962 Amendments to the FD&C Act, "New Drug" sections of the law, proof of efficacy and safety of drugs (including cancer remedies) are the responsibility of the sponsor of the drug. Devices and drugs are subject to other sections of the Act pertaining to labeling, misbranding, hazards to health and advertising of prescription products. Advertising of over-the-counter products is under the legal control of the Federal Trade Commission.

Field districts of the F.D.A. are located throughout the country. Each division has its own chemists, inspectors and testing laboratories. When necessary, reports are made to the Department of Justice with recommendations for seizure, criminal prosecution or injunction actions in the Federal Courts.

The National Cancer Institute

The National Cancer Institute, at the request of proponents or other interested agencies or individuals, conducts scientific investigations of new cancer remedies. One of its major efforts involves a national cancer program to enhance the development of major Comprehensive Cancer Centers throughout the country.

The U.S. Customs Service

The U.S. Customs Service is actively engaged in anti-smuggling activity to suppress cancer quackery.

The U.S. Postal Service

The Fraud Division of the U.S. Postal Service actively engages in the investigation of worthless cancer tests and remedies promoted through the mails. These investigations have resulted in the conviction and sentencing of individuals who use the mails to defraud the public. . . .

EDUCATION

The American Cancer Society's Program on Unproven Methods of Cancer Management

The American Cancer Society, in its efforts to control unproven remedies, has adopted the following objectives:

• To develop more effective means of dealing with claims made for the diagnosis and/or treatment of cancer that are advanced without acceptable evidence of value.

• To encourage investigation through scientific or other qualified organizations of unestablished claims for cancer diagnosis and treatment.

• To develop and encourage educational programs, providing the public with information on specific cases as well as a better understanding of the criteria for assessing the merits of claims made for cancer tests and remedies.

• To encourage physicians to provide adequate care of patients with far advanced cancer because it is, in the main, these individuals who unwittingly fall prey to "cures" which have no proven merit.

• To encourage physicians to maintain well documented case histories to include data on subjective and/or objective improvement or progression of disease while under treatment.

The National office of the American Cancer Society stands ready to assist reporters, editors, science writers, program directors and others in checking the validity of claims made for cancer tests and remedies from information contained in its files on unproven methods of cancer management. Early diagnosis and prompt, proper treatment is a life and death matter. An informed press and public are the best safeguards against the hazards of cancer quackery.

Material concerning unproven methods of cancer management, is obtainable on request to the National office. . . .

CONCLUSION

Unproven methods of cancer management cannot be completely eliminated until all cancer is brought under control. As long as some forms of cancer remain curable, promotion of unproven methods will continue.

Control of unproven method of cancer management lies on three fronts:

Investigation . . . Legislation . . . Education.

In an attempt to combat unproven methods, the following measures are recommended: Development of more effective means of dealing with exaggerated and unfounded claims for cancer diagnosis and treatment by encouraging investigation by scientific or other qualified organizations; promotion of state anti-quackery legislation; formation of state cancer commissions and other state and federal programs to prevent exploitable treatment of the public, and lastly; encouragement of educational programs. The public must be provided with information regarding specific cases, and offered a better understanding of the standards of investigation which must be met before any new drug or device is approved for use by the medical profession. Education also alerts the patient to his responsibility in seeking treatment from a qualified specialist in cancer. In addition, professional education programs are necessary to provide better and more concerned understanding of the patient's needs and his family's fears, thus dispelling the tendency to seek unproven methods of cancer management.

The reader may also want to refer to Jarvis, W., Helping Your Patients Deal with Questionnable Cancer Treatments. *CA—A Cancer Journal,* 1986, 36:5. It is an excellent article for both physicians and non-physicians.

6

Understanding Cancer
—For the Patient

54

Persons Who Have Had Cancer

"Ultimately the importance of cancer lies in its effect on people."
Stanley L. Robbins, 1976

To have a life-threatening disease such as cancer can teach one a great deal about how to live. Akira Kurosawa, the master Japanese film director, made an extraordinary movie in 1952 entitled *Ikiru* (translated "to live"). *Ikiru* is about a man who discovers he has a terminal cancer and then sets out to finally *live*.

It is a unique experience to be able to listen to a cancer patient discuss his experiences with the disease and how it has changed his life perceptions. Stephen Bray agreed to record his experience with cancer for the purposes of this book. Mr. Bray is a baseball writer and political journalist, living in Olympia, Washington.—*M.R.*

An Essay

Stephen Bray

The often overlooked side of cancer is the ultimate psychological impact on those who survive the disease. How does living with cancer and preparing to die from it alter one's ability to live later without cancer? In my case, understanding this question has become a primary concern. My experience with cancer has been the most significant factor in my personal development. That experience has led me to study American history and culture as a way of explaining the context for the conflict between personally- and socially-determined values. From this perspective I continue to analyze and interpret the meaning of my response, a response that was shaped by the circumstances surrounding my illness.

My illness was discovered inadvertently by a student health doctor three weeks after the beginning of my freshman year of college. Within a week I was re-examined by a specialist and underwent an operation during which a malignant testicular tumor was removed. For the following two months I received daily radiation therapy as a precautionary procedure. When I was released, I felt physically exhausted, but assumed that I was healthy.

The illness had been discovered at an impressionable period—during my transition from family to school. I was at school in Connecticut, my home was in Indiana, and my family was spending the year in England where my father was teaching. Entering college, I was in a vacuum socially, but I was introspective and intellectually eager. If the period of radiation therapy had concluded my encounter with cancer, I doubt that the long-term reaction would have been so influential. The recurrence of disease, and accompanying it, a new intensity of treatment and increasing alarm molded my lasting impressions.

During a routine spring checkup, several new lesions were discovered in my lungs. This produced a whole new ball game. I embarked on a strenuous program of chemotherapy. I viewed the program then as exceedingly unpleasant and inconvenient, but without worry for its possibly fatal implications. Studies provided a major source of distraction. The nausea accompanying each treatment drained my energy, and the growing lethargy shielded me from fears. As I still had no identity as a sick person, I couldn't confront directly the image of cancer. My moods fluctuated wildly, but I associated the discom-

fort with the therapy and not with the disease. Only when the tumor stopped responding to treatment, which frightened both the doctor and my parents, did I begin to worry.

I had managed to remain oblivious to the seriousness of my illness until the prognosis worsened. Now, unbeknownst to me, my chances for living were only a few percent. My own understanding derived not from statistics but from the devastating side effects induced by a new experimental drug. At the same moment I was becoming highly self-conscious of my own illness, I realized that I was residing on the hospital's equivalent of Death Row. When I heard through my wall the final unconscious cries of a young woman in the adjacent room, my introduction to the reality of cancer was completed.

Throughout this period I had kept a journal. After a long stretch of seeming indifference, the journal began recording signs of distress, and also an effort to find meaning in the experience. One day I wrote, "It is to my advantage to get more treatments. It seems paradoxical to wish pain and nausea upon yourself." In order to rationalize the paradox, I made a contract with my future: "I am choosing and being forced to live. With this choice I expect something. Is it just life? No! I'm purchasing freedom. Released from traditional bonds and expectations, I will now define how and under what conditions I'll live." This was the positive theme, promising myself an open future in return for enduring the present. It represented a measure of hope. On the other side, the negative theme was the awareness of and preparation for the idea of death. In the same week that I appealed to a future freedom, I wrote, "Death has become an obsession with me. It surrounds me, haunts me and forces me to acknowledge it." The two themes were not distinct voices, but interrelated. The intensity of feeling which informed the latter sparked the former. I concluded one entry with the declaration, "Consciousness of death offers consciousness of life."

My metaphysical debates were largely private matters between me and my journal. On the surface, a cheerful exterior maintained warm relations with the many hospital personnel. I was too immersed in momentary pain or pleasure to reveal more complicated responses. But with neither close friends nor nearby family for support, my hidden meditations dominated my outlook. Life became seen as a deferred mixture of pleasure and pain, a series of good and bad moments, and the idea of death as a source for creative thinking. The fear of death, therefore, gradually subsided. As accommodation with death proceeded, I became increasingly estranged from the activities, concerns and values of daily life of which I was only an observer, and in turn, the unpleasantness of treatment became less tolerable. Ironically, in other words, the successful coming-to-terms with the likelihood of death mitigated the initial fears, reduced the attachment of life at any cost, and made acceptance of difficult treatment more unbearable. I had achieved a state of peace with myself. As a result of this experience, my identity was realized and I felt content. The values I increasingly recognized fell outside the conventional challenges and rewards of life. I had attained completeness independently, and life was now viewed not as an arena for fulfillment but as slow, agonizing, self-destruction. I wanted out. That didn't require an active gesture, simply a decision to stop treatment.

Before I could act on these beliefs, the doctors decided on their own to change strategy, and elected lung surgery instead of continued chemotherapy. Nobody was ever more delighted to undergo such an operation. I didn't desire death as much as I desired to relieve myself of the infliction induced by prolonged chemotherapy with uncertain results. The extended treatment was weakening not only my body but my mind. Fortunately, surgery introduced the last stage of therapy.

Upon recovering, I felt obligated to live with the commands which pushed me along. I refused to lose the sense of completeness I had recently and painfully obtained. Cancer had become an excuse, albeit an extreme one, for confronting and evaluating myself. It served as a stimulus for accelerated personal growth, reducing to several months a process of self-realization and affirmation which often takes a normal lifetime. It left me with a new self-image and an altered perception of society. With new priorities and expectations, I refused to assimilate on former terms. I sought satisfaction, but in doing things for their intrinsic value. In personal relationships I needed to express myself honestly and intensely. Whether in work or play, my new identity was too secure and valuable to risk compromising through false commitments. While, formerly competitive, I no longer enjoyed participating in competitive situations. For example, although sports had previously played a major role in my life, I now rejected athletics. I felt uncomfortable playing games where the outcome could influence my self-worth. The same perspective helped shape my changing attitude toward the purposes of school and careers. If I still desired to be successful, it was now based on a personal definition of "success."

The experience with cancer provided a base from which to better understand myself and society. The experience with cancer was too subjective and instrumental ever to be forgotten. It was a state of intensity which can never be recaptured, and offered insights which cannot be denied. My reconciliation with death became ingrained in my new perspective toward life. As a result, it also imposed a permanent mode of detachment. In order to protect the fragile sense of wholeness created by that experience, I feel obligated to maintain a distance between myself and the world. But perhaps that's a small price to pay for the privilege of being able to look back and remember.

Suggested Reading

Testicular cancer is the most common cancer of young men. Two excellent books written by young men, like Stephen Bray, describe the experience of having testicular cancer.

1. *The Road Back to Health—Coping with the Emotional Side of Cancer,* by Neil A. Fiore, Ph.D. (Foreword by Norman Cousins). Bantam Books, 1984.

2. *Vital Signs—A Young Doctor's Struggle with Cancer,* by Fitzhugh Mullan, M.D. Farrar, Straus and Giroux, Inc., New York, 1985.

55

Everything You Ever Wanted to Ask or Tell Your Physician But Were Afraid to, Lying on Your Back in a Hospital Bed, Tied to an IV Pole, Feeling Helpless, Vulnerable, and Dependent

Steven Leib, M.D.

How has cancer affected your sexuality? What was it like the moment you were told you had cancer? How could the doctor have said it better? What made you give up chemotherapy and opt for Laetrile? As your wife's best friend and supporter, what was it like to be treated by the doctors as a nonentity just at a time when your participation in the health care team seemed most critical? Once you discovered the lump in your breast what made you delay in seeking out your physician? Could you share your feelings about what it was like to have cancer?

These are just a few of the questions that were asked of an intimate group of people with cancer, their family and friends, in a seminar called "Understanding Cancer," designed by Mark Renneker and myself when we were still medical students. What these very special people with cancer were able to share with us students could never be taught in a medical school or learned from a textbook.

The seminar had two expressed purposes and one implied:

1. to have cancer patients teach us as future health professionals about their experiences with a life-threatening disease;

2. to attempt to teach cancer patients something about the biological, clinical, and psychosocial aspects of their disease;

3. by providing this forum for the free exchange of information, attitudes, feelings, and experiences, to build a support group for all participants. Since we students in the health professions were perceived to be in a nonthreatening, advocacy role, we were in a unique position to achieve these goals.

Who were the people involved in this seminar and why would anyone want to participate in such a revealing experiment? Basically, these people were like you and me. They had a common desire to learn more about cancer and to share their own knowledge of it, a special knowledge that comes from personal experience. The group included people with cancer at all stages of the disease, from veterans who for twenty years have been free of all symptoms, to those just recently diagnosed, to those facing imminent death. They ranged in age from eighteen to eighty years and were sick with cancers of the breast, lung, testicles, larynx, nasopharynx, and colon-rectal area as well as with Hodgkin's disease, leukemia, and others. The participants were by no means representative of all cancer patients. All were volunteers and so were probably more open about their disease and better able to communicate about it. Nevertheless, perhaps they were able to articulate some of the feelings that other cancer patients have left unspoken. At the very least, what they had to say was true for them.

At the beginning of the seminar, we challenged them to come up with ten "pointers" they always wanted to tell their health care provider. The list below describes the advice they wanted us to take back to our fellow students and to anyone involved in the fight against cancer. This is what they wanted *you* to know, the distillation of their experiences:

1. Involve the family from the very beginning . . . patients belong to families not to us . . . cancer is a family disease and affects all members . . . it's important that everybody knows that everybody knows.

2. Dare to be vulnerable and show it . . . don't be afraid to share your feelings—it allows patients to do the same . . . believe in your patient's right to question, make suggestions, and be critical when appropriate . . . respect your patients for their knowledge.

3. Be there . . . make your presence felt at the bedside.

4. Don't lie or withhold information . . . be honest and open . . . keep patients fully informed . . . you owe it to patients to at least give them a chance to take a stand against their disease . . . you can never say too much because patients hear when they are ready.

5. Treatment should be no worse than the disease it tries to cure or ameliorate . . . consider carefully the benefits of medical technology versus its tendency to lead to overtreatment; to isolate individuals from their families, homes, and all that gives meaning to their lives; to take away decision-making power and dignity.

6. Tend to other needs . . . don't let a person's cancer blind you to the fact that he or she is still a person who wants to play sports or make love despite an amputation or colostomy.

7. Help give meaning to their disease . . . consider involving an individual in a patient panel or "Reach to Recovery" program.

8. "Treat me like a person who happens to have cancer, not like a child or diseased organ."

9. There is no virtue in dying a painful death—control the pain.

10. Never allow the patient to give up hope . . . there's always something that can be done to improve the quality of a person's life—or death.

This then is your challenge—to take these directives and make them a part of your fight against cancer.

56

Understanding Cancer: Personal, Interpersonal and Social Considerations

Laura E. Nathan, Ph.D.

Laura Nathan has been actively involved with the American Cancer Society and the Biology of Cancer courses for over a decade—beginning at UCLA as a student, then as a student coordinator, and now as a professor and faculty sponsor at Mills College. As a sociologist, she has developed a unique cancer course: "The Social Aspects of Cancer"—which is one of the most popular classes on the Mills campus. She has also chaired the Biology of Cancer Sub-Committee of the American Cancer Society, California Division.—*M.R.*

When dealing with cancer, you are not alone. Since nearly one million new cases of cancer are diagnosed each year, many other patients, friends, and families are having experiences that are similar to yours. This article covers subjects that I have presented in my courses, which students have found valuable. I hope you will too.

THE CONTEXT OF HUMAN ILLNESS

Although few things seem as individual or as personal as illness, all illnesses have social aspects as well. When you are sick, you experience the pain and discomfort associated with your disease. Once your problem has been diagnosed, you then experience not only the physical consequences of the disease, but also the effects of treatment.

As a sick person, you face potential social repercussions from being ill. If your illness is acute and mild, such as a sore throat or cold, there is virtually no stigma attached to being ill; in contrast, there is often considerable benefit, in the form of release from typical responsibilities and being taken care of and pampered. However, if your condition is chronic and/or life-threatening, the negative consequences can be considerable. For example, people may no longer want to spend time with you, and you may become socially isolated. Further, health care is extremely costly (to both individuals and nations), and loss of job productivity due to illness can be enormous. Finally, some diseases, such as cancer, AIDS, Alzheimer's disease, and heart disease, due to their prevalence and the impact they have on society, are considered major social problems.

Actually, these three realms—personal, interpersonal, and social dimensions—have impact from the beginning, back where attempts are made to identify the causes or origins of illness. On the personal level, there are a number of choices that people can make and activities in which they can engage which make it more or less likely that they will get certain diseases. On the interpersonal level, being a member of a family or having friends who favor certain habits may influence behavior in ways that will affect overall health: if the habits of the group promote health, the individual will benefit; on the other hand, if the lifestyle shared by the group is unhealthy, members of the group will be at high risk for those illnesses related to the group's bad habits.

On a societal level, the degree to which policy and legislation act to reduce risk will influence illness rates. For instance, continued emphasis on disease treatment and cure at the expense of prevention will limit opportunities to reduce disease incidence. Societal priorities and health-related laws often reflect the political and economic interests of powerful self-interest groups in our society as much or more than the interests of the general public.

Peoples' lives reflect the overall fabric of social history. The kinds of problems that individuals confront will be shaped largely by the historical moment, and by the political, economic, and social system in which they live. Yet, because we are human, we experience our lives in a personal way, without paying too much attention to the larger social forces. But whether we think about it or not, what we as individuals experience is typically part of a larger picture.

With respect to illness, the kinds of diseases that people get and die from today are quite different, in the aggregate, than those which threatened people a century ago. As a consequence, the kinds of issues that are raised by modern diseases, and the kinds of challenges that patients and their families must confront are, in a very real sense, problems confronting nations as a "sign of the times."

When thinking about cancer, we know that there is a greater incidence of cancer today than in the past and we wonder why. We can find some reasons when we look at the changed context of our lives. The current prevalence of cancer can be understood in light of widespread control of yesterday's killer afflictions, people living longer and thus extending the time in which they can develop cancer, and the increased number of environmental hazards present in industrialized society. Increases in some types of cancers among some groups must also be understood in relation to contemporary social attitudes and associated behaviors. For example, the increase in lung cancer noted for American women, is undoubtedly associated with women's liberation and a relaxation of sex roles, leading to increased cigarette smoking among this group.

CANCER AS A MODEL ILLNESS

Because of its far-reaching effects on individuals and society, cancer has an impact on us all. Given the kinds of problems, questions, and emotions raised by this disease, it can be used as a model for looking at all chronic and terminal illness. If we are able to understand the major behavioral and social issues as they relate to cancer, we then have a better handle on these aspects of all major illnesses. There are many human issues that are common to all life-threatening diseases, and by looking at the personal, interpersonal, and social aspects of cancer, we can begin to see the connections between the physical and non-physical aspects of serious, chronic, and life-threatening illnesses.

Through epidemiologic studies we have learned quite a bit about human relationships to cancer. We know that certain ethnic groups have a much higher incidence of certain kinds of cancer than others. While some elevated risk among certain groups may be linked to genetic predisposition, a fair amount of increased risk is often related to the life-style shared by the group.

Cultural factors also have an impact on response to cancer symptoms. There is tremendous variation between ethnic groups in how typical members of each group respond to symptoms of illness. Some groups, such as Jews and Italians, tend to investigate symptoms immediately, while other groups downplay the meaning of symptoms and encourage denial for as long as possible. In all disease processes, the earlier a disease is diagnosed the better the chance of health. With cancer perhaps more than any other illness, a delay in following up on symptoms can mean the difference between life and death.

Another factor related to delay behavior is fear. Fear is a common reaction to the unknown, and it is a response that many people have to life-threatening illnesses. Until recently, cancer was the disease category most feared by the American population. For years, people would have trouble even mentioning the word. But there have been tremendous cancer education efforts over the past several years, and these have helped to calm some of the public trepidation. Currently, the public response to the AIDS epidemic is more intense than the response to cancer. AIDS is now the disease most dreaded by our citizens, and the fear of AIDS that permeates our nation is similar to our earlier fear of cancer.

Delays in seeking medical attention can also be related to the way in which the health care system is organized. Knowing when and how to gain access to formal organizational settings such as hospitals and health centers requires certain skills and/or knowledge that some individuals do not have. Furthermore, people may have a hard time seeking help from medical professionals, because these are people with whom they have little in common. The perceived ease with which one can use the health care system will influence both the frequency of periodic check-ups and the lag time between evidence of symptoms and seeking medical attention for those symptoms. The more comfortable individuals are with the system, the greater the chance they have for finding cancer early and receiving effective treatment. It is often important that you, as an individual, promote your own wellness by seeking recommended routine health exams, even when you may be uneasy around health settings and health workers.

As implied above, if patients feel comfortable with their physicians, they will be less likely to delay in seeking diagnosis and treatment for disease. Thus, it is important to focus at least some attention on the relationship between patient and physician. There are three models for the doctor-patient relationship that are relevant to cancer (and other serious illnesses).

The first type of relationship, and that which is considered most traditional, is one of <u>activity</u> on the part of the physician and <u>passivity</u> from the patient. This is a situation where the doctor takes control, and in some instances there may not be a practical alternative. In cancer treatment, when surgery, chemotherapy, or radiation therapy is being administered, it is often necessary for the patient to sit back and let the physician be in charge.

The second type of doctor-patient relationship involves guidance and cooperation. In this doctor-patient model the physician tells the patient what needs to be done, and the patient is called upon to comply with the physician's instructions.—such as <u>compliance</u> in following a prescribed diet or taking medications.

The third doctor-patient model is less traditional, and difficult for many patients, but it is particularly important; and it has an impact on the other styles of interaction as well. This is the model of <u>mutual participation</u>. Mutual participation implies a partnership between physician and patient, and involves patients drawing upon physicians for knowledge and support so that they (the patients) may help themselves.

This is particularly important in cases of chronic illness, where patients are called upon to look after their health a substantial part of the time. Mutual participation is also critical when decisions must be made. Without the good doctor-patient communication implied in mutual participation, it can be difficult to get patients to comply with instructions and allow physicians to administer treatment. Also, of critical importance in many cancer cases, good communication and mutual participation play an important role in early detection of disease.

PERSONAL, INTERPERSONAL, AND SOCIETAL CONTRIBUTIONS TO CANCER

We see then, that what we do as individuals and as a society can and will have an impact on our health. While the state of knowledge about cancer is far from complete, the evidence that we do have allows us to begin to evaluate the human role in the struggle against cancer. Although some people are more prone to cancer than others, certain steps taken by individuals can reduce cancer risk. Similarly, while it is unlikely that all cancer could be entirely eliminated, specific measures, if adopted by society, would lower overall cancer rates.

Factors associated with lifestyle do play a role in cancer incidence. In the United States, the most common sites of cancer are lung, colon-rectum, and breast. Epidemiological evidence suggests that all three of these cancers are related to basic habits. Diet has been implicated in many cancers, with high intakes of fat associated with both colo-rectal, and breast cancer, and low fiber intake being associated with colon cancer. Tobacco use is related to a number of different cancers, and cigarette smoking is a major risk factor for lung cancer.

Other cancers have also been found to be related to behavior. For example, aspects of sexual history, particularly early sexual activity and multiple partners, place women at increased risk for cervical cancer. In general, while there is no guarantee that cancer can be avoided by following all lifestyle/behavior guidelines for preventing cancer, doing so does minimize your risk.

Our relationships with people we care about, particular family and friends, can, at least indirectly, influence our risk for cancer. As suggested earlier, the habit of the groups to which we belong tend to become our habits. If you grew up in a family that had a high-fat diet, for example, it would be natural for you to continue eating these same types of foods. Even if you learn about the importance of reducing fat intake, changing personal habits can be difficult. Similarly, if your friends are all smokers, it is more likely not only that you will try cigarettes, but that you, too, will be a regular smoker. Of course it is much easier to never begin smoking than to stop once you are a smoker.

There are a number of interpersonal factors that will influence early detection of cancer. While these factors may not directly contribute to cancer incidence, they do have an impact on cancer death rates, since early detection of cancer is associated with increased survival. Family and friends tend to have a strong influence on whether you regularly practice breast or testicular self-examinations. They are also in an excellent position to urge and assist you in use of the health care system—both for routine check-ups and for follow-up on symptoms when there is a suspected problem.

Within the society at large, both public policy and social attitudes play a role in cancer causation. Chemical carcinogens are widespread in our environment. Unless our society establishes policies that strictly control carcinogens and suspected carcinogens, we, as individuals, will be at risk for exposure to cancer causing agents. This is even more true in certain occupational settings, where exposures are stronger, and last over a prolonged period of time.

The Federal government has enacted some legislation to control carcinogenic substances, but opposition from special interest groups has generally made it difficult to establish effective prevention programs. For the most part, governmental efforts to regulate exposure to carcinogens have been disorganized and ineffective.

Other policies established by the government work directly against cancer prevention. The best example of this is the subsidies given to tobacco growers.

Social attitudes affect individual behavior, and in this way prevailing opinions can influence cancer incidence. For example, lying out in the sun is currently popular in our society. Suntans suggest a life of leisure, and healthy outdoor life. In fact, suntans have falsely come to be associated with good health, and tanning salons have become thriving businesses throughout the United States. We know that unprotected exposure to ultraviolet light is a major risk factor for skin cancer. Yet, despite this knowledge, millions of people strive for the perfect suntan—each year planning outings and holidays focused around getting a tan, and employing sunlamps when natural sunlight is not available.

Prevailing views of health and illness also have an impact on cancer rates. The American public generally, and the American medical profession more specifically, concentrate on illness rather than on health. Time, effort, and money are disproportionately spent on finding treatments for diseases *after* they are diagnosed. If we could refocus our resources on the promotion of health, chances are great that cancer and other illness rates would decline considerably.

The point that I am making here is that basic values, both those held personally and those shared by the majority in society, do have an impact on health and illness.

THE IMPACT OF CANCER ON SOCIETY

Cancer is an expensive proposition for those who have it. There are both direct and indirect costs associated with diagnosis and treatment. Additionally, nearly all cancer patients are unable to participate in their normal work and family roles for at least some period of time. Treatment costs and loss of productivity are issues that go beyond individual hardships—they are public problems that have an impact on the entire society.

Cancer accounts for about ten percent of the total cost of disease in the United States. A National Center for Health Statistics study revealed that in 1985, overall costs for cancer exceeded $71 billion dollars. Of those, nearly $22 billion were in direct costs, and an additional $8.6 billion were related to loss of productivity. The remainder of the costs were identified as mortality costs—the costs to society related to premature death as a result of cancer. Given the enormous drain on society that results from cancer, in terms of health care dollars, production, and family functioning, a greater emphasis on prevention must become a national priority.

PERSONAL AND INTERPERSONAL CONSEQUENCES OF CANCER: THE IMPACT ON PEOPLE'S LIVES

People respond to news of cancer in a variety of ways. Fear and thoughts of death are typical responses, but shock, denial, anxiety, anger, and depression are also common. With long-term and terminal illness, both patients and those close to them typically go through several stages, and experience a number of different reactions—sometimes experiencing two or more emotions simultaneously. While the range of emotions is in itself often difficult to handle, on an interpersonal level there can be further complications. It is not reasonable for any of us to expect that our responses to the diagnosis and subsequent treatment will be the same as anybody else's. Each person, whether patient, family member, or friend, must respond to the situation in his or her own way, and allow others their personal responses as well.

Another fairly common response to cancer and other illnesses, and one that can operate on both personal and interpersonal levels, is guilt. Often people diagnosed with cancer believe that if they had engaged in specific behaviors or had refrained from certain activities, they would not have gotten cancer. Further, those who had knowledge about the importance of early detection for treating cancer may feel guilty that they delayed seeking medical attention when symptoms first surfaced.

Similarly, family members and friends of cancer patients may even blame them for not taking better care of themselves. The process of feeling guilty about being sick is a throwback to the Moral Decay Theory of disease, which suggests that illness is punishment for having done something bad. According to this theory, sick people were evil and were paying for their sins; those who were well were morally righteous. While individuals do have some control over their risk for cancer and other diseases, there is no foolproof way to insure that a particular person will remain free from cancer. Once a person is ill, it does not do anybody any good to blame the victim.

Some people, out of fear and ignorance, are afraid to be around cancer patients. And even when this barrier is overcome, many people are still unsure about how much exposure to the cancer patient is "safe." Although the tendency to ostracize cancer patients has diminished over time, it is still not uncommon for some people to behave as if cancer is highly contagious. Unfortunately, cancer patients are sometimes treated differently, and less considerately, than other people. One example I have heard involved a physician whose cancer had been in remission for several months. At a friend's birthday celebration, champagne was being served in fine crystal. When he—the former cancer patient—was served his champagne, it came in a styrofoam cup.

Incidences such as this can be painful. So can having people that you once thought of as friends seemingly abandon you because you are ill. Such experiences can be profoundly painful for cancer patients, but it can help to understand the source of the rejection. We need more education so that fears can be directly confronted and worked through.

Not all of the personal and interpersonal problems resulting from life-threatening illness are a direct consequence of the disease. Sometimes cancer treatments bring their own complications. Treatments that affect normal social interaction, such as surgery for cancer of the larynx, can act to further isolate patients, by making them self-conscious and unwilling or unable to engage in conversation. Treatments for head and neck cancers, which can result in dramatically altered appearance, can be particularly devastating to social interaction in a society that places a high value on attractiveness. Other treatment side effects, such as hair loss or the loss of a limb, also alter appearance and may inhibit social interaction. Cancers of the sex organs and their treatments may result in impaired sexual function. Both altered appearance and impaired functioning are potential by-products of cancer treatment, and either can be devastating to social functioning and self-esteem.

Diminished self-esteem is also often related to a loss of social roles. When people are ill, they typically take on what sociologists call "the sick role," one feature of which is exemption from normal expectations. People who are disabled over a long period of time (because of disease, treatment, or both) must transfer responsibilities to others. For example, if a family's main income earner is unable to work, someone else has to provide an income for the family. Similarly, if the person who is ill is the family's primary caretaker, somebody must take on the caretaking role.

If the person taking on the additional tasks is a family member (as is usually the case), there is potential for strain in interfamilial relations. The person who takes on the additional role is at high risk for suffering overload and burnout, and yet may experience guilt for resenting the additional demands.

The patient sometimes feels guilty for burdening the family members, while at the same time resenting them for taking over what was his or her domain. On a personal level, in transferring previously held responsibilities to others, the patient may experience a deep sense of loss, wholly in addition to the loss of health. Social roles are central to personal identity, and when they are relinquished, it is often difficult to maintain self-esteem.

At every stage of the cancer experience, at diagnosis, during treatment, and, if the disease is terminal, throughout the dying process, communication is important. Although it is often difficult, patients, friends and family members, and health care workers need to be able to discuss the situation and their feelings with one another. Physicians may sometimes behave in a paternalistic fashion, and tell patients only what they think their patients should know. Family members, too, often attempt to shield the patient and each other from upsetting information. Sometimes, with cancer, people shy away from talking about the reality of the situation. Often everyone, patient included, knows that the patient has cancer and/or that the condition is terminal. Yet, all those involved participate in a kind of collusion, the assumption generally being that it is easier to bypass sensitive issues.

This is typically done with the best of intentions to protect patients, but withholding information is often no kindness in the long run. Ultimately, not talking about the concerns that are troubling everyone can set up barriers rather than help relationships proceed normally.

Since cancer is often terminal, personal, interpersonal, and social issues related to death and dying also come into play. It is crucial to remember that whether or not a person's cancer is terminal, living as normal a life as possible is important for everyone involved. Therefore, patients should be encouraged to do as much as they can, while at the same time knowing that they can rely on others for help when help is needed.

CONCLUSION

The human mind has a tremendous capacity for reason. When we are faced with traumatic illnesses like cancer, the causes of which are complex and still not entirely understood, we have a tendency to seek simple explanations for the disease, and in some cases to assign blame.

We may find comfort, even, in accusing the person who has the illness, in identifying habits or attitudes that we feel may have led to the cancer. There are certainly behaviors that increase one's risk of getting cancer, behaviors that can be controlled, but these don't tell the whole story—what may be a very dangerous behavior for some may pose little risk for others. While we feel more comfortable with an explanation, any explanation, than with a maze of mysterious origins, once a cancer occurs, finding fault benefits no one.

Cancer patients themselves can take comfort in the fact that they aren't alone in their fight with the disease—others face the same situation. Patients may learn a great deal about how to cope successfully with illness by making contact with people engaged in the same struggle. At the same time, we should all realize that each person is a unique individual, and that responses to diagnosis and treatment will vary. In a crisis, you will find your own path, and you should not feel that you must react as others have.

Major health threats—such as cancer and AIDS—usually emerge as catastrophes for patients, for those who care about them, and for all of society. Catastrophe has a way of pushing human beings to their limits. Some people behave heroically, offering love and support in abundance. Others, typically out of ignorance, will fail to react at all—or worse, will respond with hostility and rejection. People who are ill, and those who care about them, must gather strength where they find it, and must recognize the fear that prevents others from bringing their courage to forcefully meet the challenge of life-threatening illness.

57

For You, the Patient

Ernest Rosenbaum, M.D.

*Dr. Rosenbaum is Associate Chief of Medicine, Mount Zion Hospital, San Francisco,
California; Clinical Professor of Medicine, University of California, San Francisco,
California; Chief of Oncology, French Hospital Medical Center, San Francisco, California;
and Medical Director, Better Health Programs, Regional Cancer Foundation. Chapters 57
through 62 are excerpted from* A Comprehensive Guide for Cancer Patients and Their
Families *by Dr. Rosenbaum and the listed individual authors.*

Cancer, like other chronic diseases, has important psychological and
social, as well as medical, dimensions, and the cancer patient's needs
go beyond basic medical treatment. In the healing arts, an artificial
division has existed between the mind and body—the clergy, psychologists, and psychiatrists have worked to heal the mind and spirit, while
the clinical physician and medical team have treated the body. As medicine has become more specialized, the division between mind and body
therapy has tended to be further exaggerated; but in order to heal the
whole patient, the idea of ***total patient care*** must be coordinated with
specialization.

When you are ill, you have one overriding goal: health and a
return to an active, fulfilling life. An integrated, organized program of
overall care facilitates getting well faster. Rehabilitation should be a
multidisciplinary effort involving physicians, nurses, paramedical personnel, social workers, family, friends, clergy, *and—most importantly—
you, the patient.* A well-organized, structured program coordinated by
the health care team can be tremendously effective. It can make the
difference between continued good health and illness and between
chronic debility and recovery.

The purpose is to provide rehabilitation programs to complement the standard forms of cancer therapy (surgery, radiation therapy, and chemotherapy). These programs involve the physician, the patient, and the health care team: the physician is responsible for directing and implementing the programs; the patient is responsible for understanding and utilizing these programs; and the health team—clergy, educators, L.V.N.'s, nurses, dietitians, social workers, therapists (occupational, physical, and recreational)—is responsible for helping in the areas of their specialties. The total team approach offers the best form of therapy; to use less or only part of the team means the patient will only be receiving partial care.

When you are an active participant in your medical care and rehabilitation, you can maintain a sense of control over your disease and your therapy. Only you can take responsibility for your state of mind, nutritional status, and physical fitness. The act of taking responsibility is in itself an important factor in maintaining self-esteem, a feeling of independence, and faith in your ability to cope. It is a critical part of therapy.

COMPREHENSIVE CARE AND REHABILITATION

The Mind

Interest is growing in the mind's role in causing disease. Evidence indicates, for instance, that stress may depress the body's immune response to cancer. We are most interested here, however, in the mind's influence on the course and outcome of therapy. Medical histories record many so-called "hopeless" cases in which patients rallied or regained their health. Often when we have witnessed unexpected remissions or cures, we have felt the added crucial factor was the will to live. Your attitude and will to live are critical elements of survival. We therefore seek to encourage a positive attitude of hope and a strong will to live.

To deal with the common problems of alienation, loss of self-esteem, depression, helplessness, and hopelessness, you will need to call on all of your resources. How you eventually do it, only you can decide; there is no right way and no wrong way. We encourage the pursuit of any supportive discipline that appeals—from traditional psychiatry to less traditional methods, such as biofeedback, meditation, visualization, and yoga. There is no proof that these practices can cure cancer, but in supporting your mental attitude, they will help you play the positive role needed to support your prescribed medical treatment.

It is important to recognize psychological problems early. You can be overwhelmed by the impact of your disease and lose your ability to cope. Once you are able to participate actively, your health care team can help strengthen your will to live by their own positive attitude, by supportive counseling, by projecting realistic goals, and by helping you become involved in an organized program of recovery. Active involvement will give you a feeling of control and ability to cope that will result in increased hope and a strengthened will to live.

The Body

Nutrition. Many cancer patients die not of cancer itself, but of progressive malnutrition. Calorie and protein deficits initiate a vicious cycle: decreased appetite and weight loss result in fatigue and weakness; with progressive weakness patients become less active and remain in bed, inviting skin breakdown, pressure sores, and reduced immune resistance to infection.

Good nutrition is critical to healing after surgery, to the body's tolerance of radiation therapy and chemotherapy, and to general mental and physical well-being. Every effort must be made at the time of diagnosis or initiation of therapy to prevent malnutrition. The longer the delay, the longer the convalescence and the slower the recovery and healing process.

Exercise. Physical therapy is not routinely prescribed for the cancer patient, yet convalescing patients who undertake little or no exercise experience a continual loss of muscle strength and suffer prolonged physical debilitation. In order to combat this debilitation, and the mental depression that accompanies prolonged inactivity, muscles and joints should be limbered and strengthened by regular, gentle exercise. You can begin to exercise even while you are still confined to your bed; and if you do, you will be in much better condition to start moving about when you are able to get out of bed. Massage is also a form of exercise and is good for muscle tone and circulation.

Physical rehabilitation is, of course, important for its own sake, keeping muscles active and encouraging mobility and physical independence. But it is also important in terms of "total person" therapy—for better mental health, as well as for the physical resources needed in the struggle to get well.

Sexuality. Your sexuality can sometimes be affected by a serious illness such as cancer. Often the combination of physical changes and emotional stress can place a strain on the expression of sexuality, and can create concerns about sexual desirability.

These problems are not unique, and they can be solved. They need to be approached with patience—through communication between you and your partner, sometimes through learning to alter the nature of your sexual expression, and sometimes through professional counseling.

If you were comfortable with and enjoyed your sexuality prior to your illness, the chances are excellent that you will be able to keep or regain your sexuality despite the changes brought about by cancer. You may, indeed, find that your illness brings about an increased closeness between you and your sexual partner.

Supportive Services

The Patient-Support Teams. Too few patients are really aware of the patient-support teams that function in the hospital, the doctor's office, and the home. In order to interact to best advantage with those who share in your care, you must understand their roles in the total medical support system. Your awareness of specific mutual responsibilities will help them do the most for you and enable you to fulfill your role as the most important member of your health care team.

Social Services. Many social services are available to patients and their families, both in the hospital and in the community: hospital medical social workers, home health care agencies, national organizations like the American Cancer Society, and various rehabilitation services offered by trained volunteers who have had cancer themselves.

The medical social worker in the hospital can help as someone to talk to during crisis periods, as well as to provide assistance in practical matters, such as financial aid, transportation, job-related assistance, home care planning, and referral to community services. Community services, whether local or a branch of a national organization, can provide practical aid, help in rehabilitation, and often bring the experience and emotional support of recovered cancer patients.

58

The Will to Live

Ernest H. Rosenbaum, M.D.
Isadora R. Rosenbaum

The will to live is a natural instinct in all of us—the instinct to fight for our lives when challenged by a life-threatening crisis. Your will to live can be a critical element affecting the quality and sometimes even the length of your life.

Often when patients have enjoyed prolonged or unexpected remissions or cures, we have felt that the added critical factor was the will to live. We have often seen how two patients, similar in age, diagnosis, degree of illness, and treated with the same program, can experience widely different therapeutic results. The only discernible difference was the pessimism of one and the optimistic determination of the other.

How the will to live can be nurtured varies with each person. Positive feelings like hope, love, courage, effort, endurance, and faith are all important in supporting the will to live, but there are times when you will be exhausted by continued problems and ready to give up the struggle to survive. Yet for many reasons you will continue to fight—perhaps because of encouragement from family, friends, or a member of your health care team, or perhaps because you have heard of how others have prevailed after despair and multiple failures. The will to live is also sustained by the innate character and personality of the individual: your talent and desire may help you succeed where others might give up.

> When I speak of the will to live, I don't mean some kind of simple, blind faith or optimism. To me it has more to do with the kind of stance or posture that one adopts toward the disease, namely an aggressive fighting posture. Having an attitude of doing battle with the disease and having some knowledge of the drugs, the program, and so on makes it easier to cope with the discomfort because one then understands what is going on.—*A 22-year-old man with acute leukemia*

We have found that the best thing we can do to strengthen the will to live is to involve you as an active and aggressive participant in combating your disease. When patients approach their disease in "an aggressive fighting posture," they are no longer helpless victims. Instead, they become active partners with their medical support team in the fight for improvement, remission, or cure.

This partnership must be based on honesty; communication; education about the nature of disease, therapy, and rehabilitation; and on *shared responsibility*. Your health care team gives therapy and support: you, for your part, assume responsibility for continuing work in such areas as nutrition, physical exercise (most particularly), and mental attitude. The result of this partnership is an increased ability to cope; this, in turn, nurtures the will to live.

Just as the will to live can be nurtured by positive attitude, so can it be undermined by fear, anger, loss of self-esteem, and alienation—the "Four Horsemen"* of doom. These are common responses to the diagnosis of cancer; if allowed to go unresolved, they can lead to feelings of helplessness, futility, resignation, and loss of the will to live.

FEAR

Cancer is the most feared of all diseases. In fact, the word "cancer" is the most feared word in the English language. After questioning many newly diagnosed cancer patients, we have found that much of the disproportionate fear associated with this disease is due to the anticipation of prolonged periods of suffering and disability and to the belief that little can be done to control the malignancy or relieve its symptoms—although nothing could be further from the truth. Some patients react to the diagnosis of cancer in much the same manner that people in primitive societies react to a witch doctor's curse—as a sentence to an inevitable and ghastly death.

The phrase "frightened to death" is more than a figure of speech. In primitive societies people have been literally frightened to death by the imposition of a curse or spell, known as "bone pointing." When a person who believed in the phenomenon was "boned," he withdrew from the world, stopped eating, and waited to die. Death could take place in a few weeks. Such deaths have not been explained medically, even with an autopsy, but it seems apparent that the paralytic effect of fear played an important role. The victim's fear stems from ignorance and superstition; he has been encouraged to believe in the power of the curse and, in effect, to carry it out on himself.

In modern medical practice, a similar phenomenon may occur when a patient, out of ignorance or superstition, believes the diagnosis of cancer to be a death sentence. For instance, a physician may tell a patient that the surgery or other treatment has been unsuccessful and that nothing more can be done. She may simply accept the idea that she is going to die, and extinguish the will to live. Such patients can die quite rapidly, long before their disease has progressed enough to cause death by itself.

The diagnosis of cancer is not a death sentence. The first question patients ask is usually: "How long have I got?" Unfortunately some physicians will answer, "six months," "a year," "two years," without qualifying their answer. What the physician is doing is quoting a published average for patients with a specific type of cancer. He may fail to tell the patient

---

*The biblical Four Horsemen of the Apocalypse—conquest, war, famine, and death—were sent to ravage the earth in preparation for its final destruction.

that the average is made up of survival figures from a number of patients, some of whom lived much shorter and some much longer than the projected time.

It is impossible to predict longevity for an individual patient prior to therapy. Even after therapy has begun, an interval of time is necessary to assess response. Until the response to therapy has been established, *no* projection is feasible. Furthermore, even if one therapy is not successful, another may still be possible. There is *always* hope that you may outlive any average projection by many months or years.

> I was given a prediction of one year. Actually, what happened was my surgeon told me on Thanksgiving Day, "I am sorry, but the surgery did not help." He did not say much else. I asked him how long long and he said, "About a year." My thoughts have been around my year being up this November. I am just not going to make it, so I think I will make my plans now for when it happens.—*A 52-year-old woman*

Specific predictions of when a patient is going to die are not valid. Such misinformation can only stifle hope and the will to live. It engenders feelings of futility, that nothing can be done to extend life beyond the predicted time—and that come that time, death will come. As in primitive societies, ignorance and superstition can give fear an extraordinary power to induce a self-fulfilling prophecy.

Knowledge and understanding are the only keys for freeing yourself from unreasonable fear. If you want the truth about cancer, don't listen to what your well-meaning friend has to say about his Uncle George. The best source of reliable knowledge about your cancer is your physician, preferably one who specializes in the treatment of cancer, and other members of your health care team. They should also be people with whom you can establish a firm rapport and to whom you can communicate your fears. Make sure they will take the time to communicate with you.

When a physician makes the effort to explain carefully the nature of cancer, anticipated problems, and future tests, most patients are surprised to learn that their ideas about the disease were considerably more pessimistic than the facts warrant. They find that most of their fears can be resolved by understanding the problems to be faced, the treatments and other supportive measures, and by having a reasonable estimate of the discomfort and inconvenience to be expected. Then they are in a position to adopt a positive attitude and to accept the compromises that the disease and the planned treatment impose upon their lifestyle.

You will probably have to deal with the fears of others. One patient whom we have been treating for advanced cancer for the past six years has taken meticulous precautions to ensure that most of her closest friends do not discover her illness in order to protect herself from their potentially negative reactions. Your own fears may be under control, but having to deal with the fears of well-meaning friends can drain emotional energy reserves and cause depression. However, rather than hide your disease, you may feel better including close friends, as well as family, in consultations with the doctor so that they may be able to function as part of your informed support team.

> Every patient runs the risk of encountering fear, pessimism, or other destructive attitudes on the part of doctors, nurses, family, friends, or acquaintances. Patients will also be overwhelmed at times by their own fears, discouragement, or sadness. This is normal. Nevertheless, the patient who is willing to fight and to accept guidance and support in his fight for life will have the basic confidence and equanimity with which to confront the ignorant and the fearful. Although fears and fantasies don't disappear, they are put into a manageable perspective. The individual is free to do more than engage in solitary battle with self-made phantoms.—*A 42-year-old patient-physician*

ANGER

Much of your reaction to the diagnosis of cancer depends on your personality and how well you have adapted to life's problems in the past. Some people have difficulty coping with any adversity. Every time they meet a problem they ask, "Why me?" When such a person develops cancer, he may spend all his emotional energy being angry that the disease is happening to him. To the person with a positive attitude toward adversity, cancer is a problem that can be attacked in the same way as other problems—with the determination to make the best of it.

Anger is a normal reaction and a way of grieving during the initial shock period following the diagnosis of cancer. In fact, if anger cannot be felt or expressed, it may turn into depression. However, if anger remains unresolved, it takes away energy that could be channeled into coping with the disease and living life as fruitfully as possible.

In order to resolve anger, you must first recognize why you are angry. Often the anger and bitterness about one's disease is displaced. One makes major issues out of minor events—like complaining about someone being late or the dinner not being satisfactory, or finding fault with a friend or mate. This displaced anger may be self-defeating; it can alienate people when you need friends most.

By recognizing your anger for what it is, you will be setting your mental attitude to cope with it. Letting the anger out by talking about it—even screaming, punching a pillow, or throwing things—can further help release its hold on you. Finally, you can direct the energy of your anger and try to apply it in a positive direction by putting it to work to fight against your disease and to get as much out of life as possible.

> Cancer is devastating. At first you can't even think about it. You're smacked hard and all the wind goes out of you. You don't begin to think about yourself and your family and your reasons for living. I have seen people destroy themselves with their attitude in all kinds of situations, and, although I don't believe your attitude can cure your disease, I do believe it can help you. Therefore, I reject my negative thoughts. It sounds insane, but it keeps me healthy. Negative thinking breaks down my energy level. Although my drive and my will and my pace are basically the same as they were before, I have changed in one way. I no longer fly off the handle over unimportant matters. My priorities are being alive and loving my family. I've always loved life, and the biggest pain is that I didn't have enough of it when this thing happened. So I said, "Screw you, world! I just ain't leaving."—*A 40-year-old woman*

LOSS OF SELF-ESTEEM

The very idea of having cancer may itself threaten your self-esteem. Old superstitions still cling to the word cancer—that it is a disgrace that would not have happened if you were really a whole human being, or that it is a supernatural punishment. These are only superstitions; having cancer does not mean that you are bad or less worthy, physiologically or otherwise, or that you are guilty of some terrible past wrongdoing. The disease can happen to anyone; in fact, one out of every four people in the United States will have cancer.

> When people ask me, "How could God let it happen to me? What justice is there from such a God?" I tell them that God is not doing something to hurt them. Illness or death before one's time is a malfunction of nature just as much as an earthquake or a hurricane.—*Rabbi Joseph Asher*

Cancer can take away or change the particular things that have given you your sense of self-esteem—body image, independence, the ability to accomplish and produce, the ability to contribute to society through work and responsibility, and the ability to provide for your family.

Changes in body image due to surgery, radiation therapy, or chemotherapy may have a devastating effect on your self-esteem, particularly if the changes are visible to others. You may experience the loss of body parts, voice changes, scars or skin changes, hair loss, or weight loss. Patients undergoing ostomy surgery (the creation of an artificial opening connecting the bowel to the skin) may feel humiliated because they must wear a bag to collect body wastes. Surgery affecting the genitals or reproductive organs may cause loss of self-esteem because one thinks that one is not "really a man" or "really a woman" any longer.

The body is not the self. Communicating with other cancer patients who have undergone similar body changes will help to remind you that, as you can relate to them for who they are, so others can relate to you for who you are, with or without any physical abnormalities. Volunteers from various organizations made up of cancer patients can also help you to adjust emotionally, and, in turn, you may be able to be of value to others.

A major problem affecting self-esteem is the loss of independence and control that are inevitable, to some extent, for every cancer patient. At the outset, disease and therapy make you dependent on the medical system for your very life. In the hospital you are dominated by the medical system; tests are carried out, therapy is given. When you eat, bathe, eliminate, walk, or even sleep may all be determined by others. You may feel humiliated by having to use a bedpan or by having your body exposed to doctors and nurses. You may not be able to return to work or to carry out former responsibilities at home. You may have to be dependent on family, friends, or social service agencies for personal care, household help, or financial needs. You may feel guilt at being a burden and feel that you are of no value to others. Until illness deprives us of normal responsibilities, we may not realize how much our sense of self-esteem is related to accomplishment, productivity, and the ability to "pull our weight" and care for others.

Your sense of independence and self-esteem can be increased by taking responsibility in areas that you *can* handle. You can speed up your rehabilitation by eating a nutritionally adequate diet, exercising regularly to increase your strength and mobility, and performing as many self-care tasks as possible. Keeping progress charts will bolster your sense of accomplishment.

Involve yourself in supportive programs for your rehabilitation, such as patient support groups, special group counseling for cancer patients, or biofeedback training. If no support groups exist in your community, enlist the aid of a social worker, counselor, or clergyman, or find other cancer patients and begin one yourself. Choose the tasks you can do in your home. Caring for a pet, growing plants, or giving to family members in thoughtfulness and attention what you may not be able to give in physical effort can be outlets for your ability to nurture and will give you a sense of self-esteem.

If work and former interests must be put aside, you can find new ways of being productive: try writing, art, music, sewing, knitting, crocheting, or crafts. You may find talents that you have not had the time to explore before.

ALIENATION

Nothing can be as destructive to the will to live as alienation—the feeling of being cut off from life. Isolation and loneliness can cause some patients to lose their will to live and to give up and die very rapidly because they have lost their connection with other human beings. Cancer patients may experience isolation due to physical circumstances—hospitalization, loss of employment, or confinement to the home; social isolation may be felt because of the attitudes of other people; and you may also experience alienation from within because of your own attitudes.

While our society espouses rehabilitation of the disabled, in reality we tend to shut people with chronic diseases out of employment. A patient who has had cancer but who is able to work may not be able to return to her former job because her employer is afraid that she may not be able to carry out her responsibilities or that she may relapse. If she does return to work, she may be avoided by fellow workers because they are afraid cancer may be contagious, or because they do not know how to relate to her.

Family and friends sometimes inadvertently isolate the cancer patient. They may be initially sympathetic and attentive, but with time they may drift away; they have their own problems and their own lives to live. They may also find it difficult to carry on normal conversation with someone who is actually ill or dying, and they may not know how to relate to you. You then feel you're being abandoned by those you thought cared most.

Loneliness and alienation may exist for the cancer patient even when he is not physically or socially isolated. The uncertainty and the life-threatening nature of the disease put one in touch with the essential aloneness with which one must face death. Even the patient who is surrounded with family and friends may feel alone, and perhaps lonely, in this awareness.

In fighting their disease, some patients may turn so much of their energy and attention inward upon themselves that they lose contact with the rest of life and create an isolation and loneliness that they may not recognize is self-inflicted. Other patients may withdraw from their connections with the outer world because their focus is on grieving and feeling sorry for themselves. The patient who regards cancer as an automatic death sentence may unconsciously cut his ties with life and live as if he already belongs to the dead.

When isolation is thrust upon you from the outside, when old connections to life are broken, you must learn to make new bridges. Loss of independence may encourage you to wait for "things to happen." You may feel frightened or pessimistic about taking any steps toward making a new life; yet we all have the capacity to alter our direction, make changes, and rearrange our strategies.

ATTITUDE

Some people are destroyed by the mental and physical effects of illness, while others call on their inner reserve to sustain themselves in such a crisis. What makes the difference? Why do some people respond positively to suffering, while others are unable to endure?

> There is no medicine like hope
> No incentive so great
> And no tonic so powerful
> As the expectation
> Of something better tomorrow
> *Orison Swett Marden*

Hope is an essential part of your will to live. Hope can be maintained as long as there is even a remote chance for survival. It is kindled and nurtured by even minor improvements, and maintained when crises or reversals persist, by the positive attitude of family, friends, and the health support team. But primarily hope will come from yourself, if you are willing to do everything you can to improve your health and if you are willing to fight for your life.

Even when you are very ill, you have untapped physical and emotional reserves that you can command. If utilized, these reserves will help you to survive yet another day and will become the foundation of your recovery program. When exhausted soldiers march home after a rigorous day, they sometimes begin to march and sing in cadence. They have a revival of mood and spirit, and find new energies and strength. So can you, even when exhausted by disease and illness; you too can muster reserve energies.

59

Nutrition for the Cancer Patient

Ernest H. Rosenbaum, M.D.
Carol A. Stitt, R.D.
Harry Drasin, M.D.
Isadora R. Rosenbaum

Good nutrition—the right foods in the right amounts—is needed for general good health and is particularly important when you are ill. The nutrients in food provide energy and the building blocks your body needs for proper functioning and tissue repair. Illness creates an even greater need for essential nutrients, as the body must fight disease and repair damage caused by disease. Food is therefore far more than something to delight the tastebuds—it is an essential ingredient in the fight against disease. It can be as important as your medicine.

Maintaining good nutrition is a particular problem for cancer patients because cancer and cancer therapy, whether it be surgery, radiation therapy, or chemotherapy, often cause a loss of appetite or otherwise make it difficult to eat an adequate amount of food. Many cancer patients lose great amounts of weight, fifteen to thirty pounds, or even more. They become malnourished almost to the point of starvation, setting up a vicious cycle: decreased appetite and weight loss result in fatigue and depression; with progressive weakness comes less activity and even less appetite; further weight loss and weakness bring reduced resistance to disease and a poorer outlook for survival.

However, with good nutrition you will heal better after surgery; you will experience fewer unpleasant side effects—such as nausea or vomiting—from radiation therapy and chemotherapy; radiation therapy will not need to be interrupted as often; you may be able to tolerate more chemotherapy; and your immune system will be better able to resist infection. You will feel better, physically and mentally, and you will be able to be more active.

You should not wait until you have lost weight to begin thinking about good nutrition, for once weight loss begins, it is difficult to reverse the trend and to achieve adequate nutrition.

The lining cells of the intestine, which are responsible for absorbing nutrients from digested food, are changed when a person is malnourished—resulting in cramping, bloating, and diarrhea after eating. This in turn makes it more difficult to maintain a proper level of nutrition. Therapy becomes more difficult to tolerate, often leading to further nutritional deterioration. Thus you want to do everything you can to *prevent* malnutrition from occurring, *beginning at the time of diagnosis or initiation of therapy.*

CAUSES OF NUTRITIONAL PROBLEMS

There are numerous reasons why maintaining adequate nutrition is exceptionally difficult for patients with cancer. Many problems—most commonly, loss of appetite—often occur as side effects of cancer and cancer therapy. The foods you eat can affect the problem—they can aggravate it, or they can help reduce it.

Loss of Appetite

Cancer therapy or the cancer itself may cause changes in your body chemistry that result in a loss of appetite. Pain, nausea, vomiting, diarrhea, or a sore or dry mouth may make eating difficult and cause you to lose interest in food. These chemical processes are not subject to any form of voluntary mental control. You may also lose your appetite because of anxiety or depression about your disease. Often patients who have been informed of the possible diagnosis of cancer lose five to ten pounds while awaiting test results.

A totally different approach to eating is required when appetite is no longer an adequate signal to begin or to stop eating. You will need to learn to eat even when you do not feel like eating and to approach eating as an important part of your therapy program.

Malabsorption

Adequate nutrition is diminished by malabsorption. For a number of reasons, food may not be absorbed normally from the intestines into the bloodstream. A decrease in the digestive juices that regulate absorption may be caused by cancer of the pancreas, the body organ that produces many of these juices. Abnormal connections may occur between loops of the intestine, thus causing food to bypass important parts of the intestine where nutrients are normally absorbed into the bloodstream.

Physical Problems

Physical problems may also interfere with food intake and proper nutrition. Patients with tumors in the mouth and neck area and patients receiving radiation therapy to these areas or the esophagus may have significant mouth or throat pain or difficulty in swallowing. Those who have undergone surgical removal of part of the stomach or gastrointestinal tract or who have had abdominal irradiation may have problems of early filling, diarrhea, cramps, and decreased absorption.

Radiation Therapy and Chemotherapy

Radiation therapy and chemotherapy can also cause nutritional problems. Radiation therapy to the head and neck area frequently results in a loss of taste perception and decreased production of saliva, along with inflammation and pain. Radiation to the abdomen may cause some damage to the bowel, resulting in cramps, diarrhea, malabsorption, or obstruction. Chemotherapy can inhibit appetite and affect the mouth and esophagus.

Abnormalities in Smell and Taste Perception

Abnormalities in smell and taste perception are common, especially for those who have received radiation therapy to the neck and mouth area. A loss of taste perception will make it more difficult to avoid weight loss.

Taste loss tends to be greater in proportion to the extent of tumor. You may develop an aversion to meat. These forms of "taste blindness" make it critical that the smell, appearance, and texture of food be given increased importance.

Early Filling

A common problem is early filling—a feeling of being full after having taken only a few bites of food. For many, this problem of eating can be eased by taking smaller portions more frequently throughout the day.

Depression, Anxiety, and Fear

People eat less when they are depressed. Seeing their bodies waste away may further serve to convince depressed patients of the hopelessness of their situation—an often unfounded fear. Anxiety and fear can also take away appetite. The best treatment here is a positive approach toward therapy at all stages.

Suggested Reading

For detailed suggestions, menus and recipes consult *A Comprehensive Guide for Cancer Patients and Their Families,* by Ernest H. Rosenbaum, M.D. and Isadora R. Rosenbaum, Bull Publishing Co., Palo Alto, CA 1980.

60

Rehabilitation Exercises for the Cancer Patient

Ernest H. Rosenbaum, M.D.
Francine Manuel, R.P.T.
Judith Bray, O.T.R.
Isadora R. Rosenbaum
Arthur Z. Cerf, M.D.

Physical fitness is a matter of movement. In the normal process of everyday life we undertake many activities that involve the use and maintenance of normal muscle tone. When we are healthy, walking, making the bed, shopping, climbing stairs, jogging, and other common activities are accepted as a matter of course and do not require special training or assistance.

In acute or chronic illness, however, when prolonged bed rest is essential, if no attempt is made to exercise, muscular weakness, tissue breakdown, and poor function of vital organs may ensue. In order to preserve these vital functions it is crucial that physical activity—i.e., supplemental exercises aimed at maintaining *muscle tone, normal joint motion,* and *physical strength*—be instituted and performed regularly, beginning as early as possible.

Many forms of exercise can play a role in improving your fitness—isotonic, isometric, rhythmic repetitive movements, and activities of daily living—all of which can improve your stamina, muscle strength, and endurance. Massage therapy is also a valuable aid in improving your physical fitness, since it improves circulation and relaxes your mind and body.

When you have been ill and bedridden or inactive for a long time, you may have a difficult time regaining your strength. Your joints may seem stiff and your muscles weak. Your body is suffering from *disuse*. The longer you remain inactive, the longer it will take to regain your lost strength and return to active living. To get back on your feet again, you need to gradually put your muscles and joints to *use* by exercises that limber and strengthen them.

You should begin to exercise even while you are still confined to your bed. That way your muscle strength will not deteriorate, your joints will not get stiff, and when you are able to get out of bed you will be in much better condition to start moving about. Exercising while bedridden minimizes complications such as bone deterioration, muscle weakness, bed sores, and blood clots. Exercising will also help increase your appetite and help you achieve a feeling of well-being.

Exercise can be fun and by its invigorating nature may help in working through depression and reducing boredom. With regular exercise your level of physical ability and fitness will gradually improve. You will find you have more energy and stamina, and you will also receive the additional benefits of improved mental status, appetite, relaxation, and sleep at night.

Suggested Reading

A complete set of rehabilitation exercises (demonstrated by Jack LaLanne) is shown in Chapter 5 of *A Comprehensive Guide for Cancer Patients and Their Families,* by Ernest H. Rosenbaum, M.D. and Isadora Rosenbaum, Bull Publishing Co., Palo Alto, CA, 1980.

61

Sexuality and Cancer

Jean M. Stoklosa, R.N., M.S.
David G. Bullard, Ph.D.
Ernest H. Rosenbaum, M.D.
Isadora R. Rosenbaum

Sexuality in its many aspects can sometimes be affected by a serious illness, such as cancer, and by its treatment. By "sexuality" we mean the feelings we have about ourselves as sexual beings, the ways in which we choose to express these feelings with ourselves and others, and the physical capability each of us has to give and experience sexual pleasure. Sexuality can be expressed in many ways—in how we dress, move, and speak, as well as by kissing, touching, masturbation, and intercourse. Changes in body image, activity tolerance, and anxieties about survival, family, or finances can place strain on expression of sexuality and can create concerns about sexual desirability.

If you were comfortable with and enjoyed your sexuality prior to your illness, the chances are excellent that you will be able to keep or regain a good sexual self-image despite the changes brought about by cancer. Many people who have cancer or who are the partners of persons with cancer may not experience any change in sexual feelings or behavior. Others may find that increased closeness and communication resulting from the experience of illness enhances their sexuality. Still others may never have considered sexuality to be of great importance in their lives, or may consider it less important now than previously.

Many people with serious illnesses find that the circumstances they need to enjoy their sexuality have been altered in some way because of the illness and its treatment. Under the stress and worry of a life-threatening illness, expression of sexuality frequently takes a back seat. It is difficult to feel sexual when you are fighting to survive, are in pain, or are constantly tired. Treatment for cancer may involve lengthy hospitalizations and separations from those you love. Hospitals or convalescent facilities usually do not provide much privacy, and hence there may be little opportunity for sexual expression.

During illness, the control you usually experience over your body may be lost, and you may feel inadequate and helpless. Often, serious illness may change the way you experience your body, or actually change the way you look, through surgery, amputation, scarring, weight loss, or other events. These changes may create painful anxiety about whether you will be able to function in your accustomed social, sexual, and career roles or about what people will think of you. This anxiety, the depression and fatigue that may accompany it, and the numerous other worries that can occur with serious illness understandably make sexuality assume less importance.

Once the immediate crisis of serious illness has passed, however, sexual feelings and how to express them may become important to you. Feeling anxious about resuming sexual activity is normal and natural. It is easy to "get out of practice" when you are away from any activity, sexual or otherwise. You may have questions about whether sexual activity will hurt you in any way or how you will be able to experience sexual pleasure. Your partner may share the same worries and may be especially concerned about tiring you out or causing you pain.

Once you begin to resume sexual relations, your comfort and confidence should gradually increase. If not, sexual counseling may help you to discover ways to deal with problems you are having. For many people, a "new start," by themselves or through counseling, is refreshing and may create opportunities for greater intimacy and sharing.

Starting new relationships is a task we all face at one time or another, but it can be made more difficult by worries about our worth and attractiveness. If your body has undergone changes as a result of your illness and treatment, you may have questions about whether you are still desirable, how to please your partner, or what dating will now be like. Whether you are looking for a new relationship or already have a regular partner, you may find yourself in the position of having to share your feelings about these changes with someone, perhaps for the first time.

This sharing may feel awkward at first and learning how and when to start talking about sexual issues may not come easily. You may feel shy or nervous about exploring new and different ways of experiencing sexual pleasure. You may wait for your partner to make the first move toward sexual activity while your partner waits for you to make the advances. This waiting game is often misunderstood as rejection by both people. To think of breaking the silence yourself may be frightening. Yet a good move is to make the first move. The payoff—greater understanding of each other's needs and concerns—is usually worth it.

Survival Overshadows Sexuality. Remember that stress, depression, worry, and fatigue may temporarily lower your interest in sex. It is normal and natural for someone who loses good health to experience such feelings. When you are ill, just coping with basic everyday decisions may seem like a burden. Taking one day at a time and being patient with yourself is important. Sexual interest and feelings will no doubt return when the immediate crisis of illness has passed.

Expect the Unexpected. The first time you have post-illness sexual relations may be a new and different experience. Physical limitations or fears about performance, appearance, or rejection may initially prevent you from focusing on the pleasure of your sexual contact. On the other hand, you may instead be surprised by enjoying unfamiliar pleasurable sensations. Such new experiences are often reported by people who have recently divorced, lost a job, or weathered a family crisis, as well as by people recovering from an illness. If you expect some changes as part of the natural recovery process, they will be less apt to distract you from sexual pleasure if they do occur.

Give Yourself Time. It can be natural at first for you or your partner to be frightened of, perhaps even repulsed by, physical changes such as scars or unfamiliar appliances. Such feelings are usually temporary, and talking about them, frightening as they may be, is usually the first step to mutual support and acceptance. Becoming comfortable with changes in yourself and your sexuality will probably not happen overnight. Take the pressure off yourself about having to "work on sex." Reaching a satisfactory and enjoyable sex life will happen one step at a time. At first you may want to spend some time by yourself exploring your body, becoming familiar with any body changes that have occurred and rediscovering your unique body texture and sensations. Once you feel relaxed doing this, move on to mutual body exploration with a partner, if you wish.

Communication Is All-important. The more talking and sharing you can do, the more your awareness of what feels good to you sexually will probably increase. It is rarely easy for anyone to begin talking about sex. You might try initially by sharing with your partner some of the myths or expectations you grew up with about sexuality. Often this is humorous and may break the ice in starting a frank discussion about your sexual needs and concerns. Make "I . . ." statements about what is important for you and how you feel. Rather than general statements, try something like: "I would really like to experiment with different positions that would be more comfortable for me. How would you feel about that?" Then ask your partner to try these "I . . ." statements also.

Take the Pressure Off Intercourse. When you first begin to resume sexual activity, try spending some time in pleasurable activities such as touching, fondling, kissing, and being close without having intercourse. Reexperience the pleasure of playing, holding, and being held without having to worry about erections and orgasms. Once you feel comfortable with this, you can proceed at your own pace to other ways of being sexual, including intercourse if you wish. Intercourse is only one of many routes to sexual satisfaction. Your own experimentation and exploration can help you discover what feels best and what is acceptable to you.

Don't Let Your Diagnosis Dictate What You Can Do Sexually. Your sexuality cannot be "diagnosed." You will never know what you are capable of experiencing in terms of sexual pleasure if you don't explore being sexual—new positions, new touches, and above all, new attitudes. You are the sexual expert about yourself; your brain is your best sex organ, and its ability to experience sensation is virtually limitless.

You Are Loved for Your Total Worth, Not Just for the Appearance of Your Body. If you were considered lovable or sexually desirable before your illness, chances are you will be afterward as well. Don't make the mistake of placing so much importance on the way you used to look or feel that you can no longer appreciate your unique worth. Your partner and friends will continue to love and value you as long as you let them. The crisis of illness often brings people who love each other even closer together and enriches their relationships in ways they never expected.

You Don't Have to Do It All Yourself. Don't hesitate to seek counseling or information if problems arise. Help is available from a wide range of sources. If you do have questions about sexuality or are experiencing some difficulties you wish to discuss further, we would strongly urge you to bring them up with your health care providers or to ask them to recommend competent sex counselors or therapists in your area. Other resources that may be available near your home include persons or groups of people who themselves have had cancer and who have had experience in talking about sexual concerns with others.

62

Stress and Cancer

Mark J. Doolittle, Ph.D.

> The cure of many diseases is unknown to physicians . . . because they are ignorant of the whole. For the part can never be well unless the whole is well.
>
> *Plato*

In recent times there has been a substantial shift in health care toward a recognition of the wisdom of Plato's creed—namely, that mental and physical are not separate, isolated, and unrelated, but are instead vitally linked elements of a total system. Health is becoming increasingly recognized as a balance of many inputs—physical and environmental factors, emotional and psychological states, nutritional habits, and exercise patterns.

As a part of that balance, the role of stress is well established as the cause of a broad range of disorders. For example, it is now generally acknowledged that for heart disease—still the nation's leading cause of death—emotional stress is a major risk factor equal in importance to such other recognized risk factors as hypertension, cigarette smoking, elevated serum cholesterol level, obesity, and diabetes. Stress also has been recognized as an important risk factor in high blood pressure, ulcers, colitis, asthma, pain syndromes (e.g., migraine, cluster and tension headaches, backache), skin diseases, insomnia, and psychological disorders. Most standard medical textbooks attribute anywhere from 50% to 80% of all disease to stress-related origins.

THE NATURE OF STRESS

We often speak casually of "stress" as if its meaning were well established; but scientific study has continued to provide new meaning for the concept and new importance for its role in health and disease. While the word may imply a purely mental reaction, research has shown that virtually every part of the body is involved. Most research has focused on the so-called fight-or-flight response that the body exhibits in situations of threat and on the long-term effects of chronic stress, in which the body is subjected to repeated arousal.

The fight-or-flight response has been shown to produce a wide variety of mental and physical changes. For instance, when a car swerves toward us on the highway, we may consciously feel afraid, anxious, and angry. Internally our body is literally reverberating from head to toe with all the aspects of the stress response: a part of the brain called the hypothalamus stimulates the pituitary gland, which in turn activates the thyroid and adrenal glands, which quickly flood the bloodstream with adrenalin, cortisone, and other stress hormones. The entire body is affected: heart rate increases; blood pressure rises; breathing becomes faster; body muscles tighten; facial muscles constrict; eye pupils dilate; hearing becomes sharper; sugar is secreted into the bloodstream for energy; blood flows to the brain and muscles and away from the stomach and intestines; bowel and bladder relax, readying for discharge of unneeded waste; brain wave activity quickens; palms of the hands sweat; and hands and feet become colder as blood flows away from the skin to the brain and muscles.

This complex fight-or-flight response was well designed as a survival mechanism for a caveman, warrior, or pioneer. Danger would arise suddenly, be either fought or fled from, and life would return to its previous level. In addition to its usefulness for physical survival, the fight-or-flight response carried with it an emotional safety valve: by discharging the internal tension, either in physical struggle or escape, the body first released the built-up pressure, then eventually went to a counter-stress, let-down phase, and finally returned to a state of equilibrium. The pendulum swung first to fight-or-flight, then back to post-stress let-down, then finally worked its way back to the neutral non-stress state.

What worked in other societies often does not work in ours. Recent research has shown that the fight-or-flight response can, ironically, become a threat to our health and survival.

It is not difficult to understand how modern cultural changes increase the chances for arousal of the stress syndrome: living conditions become more crowded, noisy, and polluted; the pace and intensity of life increases; mass media remind us constantly of the deaths, injuries, and threats residing all around us. When the total environment is itself increasingly and chronically stressful, the tendency is for the fight-or-flight response to be chronically activated. If the body is unable to let down on a regular basis, the pendulum tends not to swing back to its midpoint, but to be pulled more and more toward a chronic stress response. The result is a slowly rising level of internal pressure.

This prolonged buildup of tension and excessive arousal can lead to a host of disorders. In addition, many researchers have found that chronic stress can wear down our body's defenses, thereby lowering our immune response and making us more vulnerable to all sickness, including cancer.

Against the background of increasing cultural pace and pressure, some researchers have attempted to clarify just how stressful life events are related to sickness. After long research, Drs. Thomas Holmes and Richard Rahe developed a scale based on forty-three common stressful experiences, in the order they were found to be related to illness (see Figure 62-1). By checking the items that have occurred in the last year, you will arrive at a total score that indicates your supposed level of vulnerability to illness.

This scale clearly reflects the fact that *change*, whether positive or negative, tests our ability to *adapt*. However, the scale needs to be interpreted cautiously; the higher the score, the higher the *probability* that a person will become sick. But high scores (above 300) do not necessarily mean a person *will* get sick, only that the risk is greater.

When difficult and threatening events occur, it is how we perceive and respond to them that determines the intensity of the stress. As any sailor knows, it is not the direction of the wind that determines our course so much as how we set the sails—in sailing parlance, known significantly as the "attitude" of the sails. Our attitude about what we feel we *should* be and the imagined punishment if we fail determine how we see and react to events.

In a classic study of heart disease patients Dr. Flanders Dunbar noted the recurring trait of compulsive striving; the patients would rather die than fail. The study showed clearly how attitude can create a chronic life-threatening situation where no real threat exists.

Failure is not death, and it is certainly not worse than death. But as long as we believe that it is, our bodies will respond with the fight-or-flight response just as if we were being attacked. Given such a set of beliefs, events that might be handled with relative ease instead create the constant bur-

Figure 62-1 Social Readjustment Rating Scale

Rank	Event	Value	Your Score	Rank	Event	Value	Your Score
1	Death of spouse	100	_____	23	Son or daughter leaving home	29	_____
2	Divorce	73	_____	24	Trouble with in-laws	29	_____
3	Marital separation	65	_____	25	Outstanding personal achievement	28	_____
4	Jail term	63	_____	26	Spouse begins or stops work	26	_____
5	Death of close family member	63	_____	27	Starting or finishing school	26	_____
6	Personal injury or illness	52	_____	28	Change in living conditions	25	_____
7	Marriage	50	_____	29	Revision of personal habits	24	_____
8	Fired from work	47	_____	30	Trouble with boss	23	_____
9	Marital reconciliation	45	_____	31	Change in work hours, conditions	20	_____
10	Retirement	45	_____	32	Change in residence	20	_____
11	Change in family member's health	44	_____	33	Change in schools	19	_____
12	Pregnancy	40	_____	34	Change in recreational habits	19	_____
13	Sex difficulties	39	_____	35	Change in church activities	19	_____
14	Addition to family	39	_____	36	Change in social activities	18	_____
15	Business readjustment	39	_____	37	Mortgage or loan under $10,000	17	_____
16	Change in financial status	38	_____	38	Change in sleeping habits	16	_____
17	Death of a close friend	37	_____	39	Change in number of family gatherings	15	_____
18	Change to different line of work	36	_____	40	Change in eating habits	15	_____
19	Change in number of marital arguments	35	_____	41	Vacation	13	_____
20	Mortgage or loan over $10,000	31	_____	42	Christmas season	12	_____
21	Foreclosure of mortgage or loan	30	_____	43	Minor violation of the law	11	_____
22	Change in work responsibilities	29	_____		**Total**		_____

Source: Holmes, T. H. and Rahe, R. H.: "The Social Readjustment Rating Scale." *Journal of Psychosomatic Research,* 11 (1967): 213–18. Used with permission.

den of chronic stress—with the ironic possibility of creating an actual life-threatening illness if the pressure is not removed.

On the positive side, it is equally true that by altering our attitudes and tension-producing habits, we may tip the scales in a more healthful direction. Recent research in areas such as biofeedback and meditation has shown that we can become aware of our stress responses and can influence them.

STRESS AND CANCER

The idea that stress-related factors play a role in the onset and course of cancer, though controversial, is certainly not a new or radical notion. As far back as the second century A.D., the Greek physician Galen noted that melancholy women appeared more likely to develop cancer than cheerful ones. Eighteenth-

and nineteenth-century physicians frequently noted that severe life disruptions and resulting emotional turmoil, despair, and loss of hope seemed to occur prior to the onset of cancer. In 1870, Paget emphasized that emotional disturbance was related to cancer:

> The cases are so frequent in which deep anxiety, deferred hope, and disappointment are quickly followed by the growth and increase of cancer that we can hardly doubt that mental depression is a weighty additive to the other influences favoring the development of the cancerous constitution.

In 1885, Parker made the mind-body connection in a prophetic way by emphasizing the *physical* results of emotion:

> There are the strongest physiological reasons for believing that great mental depression, par-

ticularly grief, induces a predisposition to such disease as cancer, or becomes an existing cause under circumstances where the predisposition had already been acquired.

Despite the consistent trend of these observations, the interest in more physical interventions—such as radiation, surgery, and chemotherapy—seemed to draw the main body of medical attention away from the emotional contribution. Furthermore, the lack of tools for dealing with stress understandably has led to a reliance on these medical interventions.

Emotional Life History Pattern of Cancer Patients

Recently, exploration of the role of stress and emotions in cancer, led by the work of Lawrence LeShan, has aroused new interest. Over the past quarter century, LeShan has studied the lives of over five hundred cancer patients, many of whom he worked with in psychotherapy. Overall, he found a distinct emotional life-history pattern appearing in 76% of the cancer patients studied, but in only 10% of a control group of non-cancer patients. This pattern had four distinctive features:

• The person's childhood was marked by extreme difficulty in establishing warm, satisfying relationships. Usually because of parental death, divorce, chronic conflict, or prolonged separation from one or both parents, the child developed a deep sense of isolation and loneliness, with a hopeless view of ever gaining lasting, fulfilling relationships. To compensate for these fears, the child tried to please others first in order to win affection.

• In adulthood, the person found strength and meaning in a relationship or career and poured a great deal of energy into this vital source of support.

• This key source was removed—through death, divorce, disillusionment, or retirement—and the childhood wound reopened, leaving the person with a repeated sense of loss, despair, hopelessness, and helplessness.

• Feelings, especially the negative ones like anger, hurt, and disappointment, were constantly bottled up; in fact, others viewed the person as "too good to be true." But the superficial saint-like quality was a reflection of a deeper inability to express hostility and an overcompensation for feelings of unworthiness.

The pattern described by LeShan has been found with remarkable consistency by other researchers. However, it is most important to understand that this research identifies emotions as *one possible factor* in the development of cancer—*not the only one.*

Positive Role of the Emotions

This research can also be seen as suggesting a *positive* role for the emotions in cancer. For, as an attitude of hopelessness and helplessness may hurt a person's chances for health or recovery, so can an attitude of determination, hope, and fighting back help lead to a positive outcome. If bottling up emotional expression and holding a reservoir of tension inside can create a dangerous load of chronic stress, so can learning to let go reduce that burden and its risk.

This perspective has led many physicians and patients to recognize that a comprehensive approach to cancer includes dealing with the emotional and stress-related aspects of cancer. Even physicians who are skeptical of the role of stress in the onset of cancer generally speak of the will to live as an important element in the treatment process. Adding counseling and stress reduction techniques to traditional medical care is becoming more common. Cancer treatment is beginning to focus on the "whole" person, as Plato put it, and on how the patient may actively join in the rehabilitation effort.

COPING WITH STRESS

> It is much more important to know what sort of patient has a disease than what sort of disease a patient has.
>
> Sir William Osler

The importance of attitudes, feelings, and beliefs has been evident in various types of research inquiry.

The Placebo Effect

First, it is well known, though perhaps not well understood, that if a person has faith in the treatment and believes that it will work, the chances are greatly increased that the treatment will work—even if the treatment has no known therapeutic value. In science this is described as the placebo effect, and it is one of the most powerful tools available to the health practitioner. The power appears to rest solely on the strength of positive beliefs and expectations on the part of both the patient and the doctor; the placebo effect is stronger if the doctor also believes that the treatment is effective.

This phenomenon, which might better be described as the effect of positive expectations, is remarkable. As Freese states:

> The cold hard facts are there: In the severe pain following surgery, in the pain of angina pectoris, in headache, cough, seasickness, the common cold, the placebo, in studies covering more than a thousand patients, relieved some 35 percent.

The more severe the pain, the more effective the placebo. And the placebo effect goes beyond pain relief to effecting actual changes in the state of disease.

For example, two groups of patients with bleeding ulcers were given the same medication, but one group was told by a physician that the drug would undoubtedly produce relief, while the second group was told by a nurse that the drug was experimental and of unknown effectiveness. In the first group 70% showed significant improvement; in the second group 25% had improvement. The sole difference was the positive expectation created in the first group.

In another intriguing study, 150 patients were divided into three groups. The first group was the control group and received no medication. The other two groups were told they were going to receive a new drug that would increase health and longevity. One of these groups received a placebo, and the other group the actual drug. After years of follow-up, the first group showed a normal amount of illness and mortality; the experience of the placebo group was significantly better than the first group; and the third group displayed about the same amount of additional improvement over the placebo group. Thus, while the drug was effective in reducing illness and prolonging life, so also was the placebo.

How the power of belief affects the body remains a mystery. Recent research suggests that the placebo may relieve pain by releasing the body's own natural painkilling chemicals. But whatever the mechanism, the fact remains that attitude and belief can play a vital role in the success or failure of any treatment. To ignore or neglect the power of positive expectations and beliefs is to abandon one of the most valuable tools known to medicine.

Biofeedback

Another area that confirms the influence of mind on body is the recently emerging field of biofeedback. Basically, biofeedback involves showing a person, through the use of sensitive electronic devices, activities of the body that used to be considered involuntary and beyond conscious influence—for example, heart rate, brain wave activity, and skin temperature. The startling finding has been that if a person can "see" his internal biological activity (through reflecting displays of lights and sounds), he can generally learn to exercise some conscious influence over that activity.

While the study of biofeedback is still in its early stages, it has already proved effective for a broad range of stress-related problems, including heart disorders, high blood pressure, migraine and tension headaches, asthma, ulcers, and chronic pain. The range of effective use keeps expanding. Biofeedback has even taught epileptics to reduce seizures by controlling brain wave activity.

Meditation

In addition to these areas, recent research in the previously "unscientific" realm of meditation has shown that simple periods of daily deep relaxation can have important and lasting effects on a wide variety of stress disorders, perhaps most notably high blood pressure.

Change

Given the research described earlier and these additional facts, the conclusion seems inescapable: for a person facing cancer, learning to cope with stress in a different, self-nourishing way can be an important factor in aiding the treatment process, increasing chances for recovery, helping to prevent or minimize future flare-ups, and maximizing the quality and length of life. Coping with stress is only part of a comprehensive treatment program, but it is a part perhaps most susceptible to influence by the individual patient.

POSITIVE ATTITUDE

Perhaps the most noted and controversial proponents of the importance of stress in cancer have been Carl and Stephanie Simonton. In addition to providing traditional medical care, they have emphasized a full-scale treatment of the psychological aspects of cancer. Their perspective emphasizes mobilizing the positive attitude of the patient as part of the treatment. If chronic stress increases the probability of cancer, they reason that reducing stress and encouraging the will to live should improve the chances of recovery and enhance the quality of life. To that end, they employ relaxation, imagery techniques, and intensive counseling in addition to usual medical treatments. As they have described this aspect of their approach.

Essentially, the visual imagery process involved a period of relaxation, during which the patient would mentally picture a desired goal or result. With the cancer patient, this would mean his attempting to visualize the cancer, the treatment destroying it and, most importantly, his body's natural defenses helping him recover.

The Simontons believe that a positive attitude toward treatment is a better predictor of response to treatment than the severity of the disease. Although the extent of "mind over matter" is not known, dealing with stress and encouraging the will to live are undoubtedly important in extending the length of life and enhancing its quality. To what extent a person can actually influence his immune system and help it fight cancer remains to be explored. To have suggested twenty years ago that people with epilepsy would today be stopping their seizures through control of their own brain waves would have been considered sheer nonsense; yet that, and much more, is now a reality.

The importance of mobilizing the mind as a positive ally cannot be questioned, whatever the ultimate limits of its curing force. Cancer is a dreaded disease, perhaps the most frightening diagnosis a person can face. Helping the person facing it to cope with that fear is clearly an essential element of any complete treatment.

The perspective emphasizing the relationship between stress and cancer carries with it a new role, not only for doctors and other health practitioners, but for patients as well. No longer can patients be seen, or see themselves, as passive recipients of treatment, helpless bystanders awaiting the outcome. In many ways the patient's motivation, attitude, and behavior can be the key elements in shifting the scales from a poor outcome to a good one.

Suggested Reading

Anatomy of an Illness, by Norman Cousins. W. W. Norton & Company, Inc., New York, 1981.

Biofeedback and Self-Control, An Aldine Annual on the Regulation of Bodily Processes and Consciousness. Chicago: Aldine. Published annually. Annual highlights of scientific research in the field of self-regulation.

Getting Well Again, by Carl and Stephanie Simonton. Los Angeles: J. P. Tarcher, 1978. Discussion of scientific basis for comprehensive cancer treatment and for encouraging and developing "the will to live."

Love, Medicine, and Miracles: Lessons Learned About Self-Healing from a Surgeon's Experience with Exceptional Patients, by Bernie S. Siegel. Harper & Row, 1987.

Mind as Healer, Mind as Slayer, by Kenneth Pelletier. New York: Delacorte Press, 1977. Summary of scientific research on stress and major illness, and description of treatment modes available.

Pain, by Arthur S. Freese. New York: Penguin Books, 1975. Summary of all aspects of the pain problem—disorders, causation, and treatment.

The Relaxation Response, by Herbert Benson. New York: William Morrow & Company, 1975. Report on a simple relaxation procedure Harvard researchers found to significantly reduce high blood pressure.

The Stress of Life, by Hans Selye. New York: McGraw-Hill, 1978. Original work by the leading figure in the field of stress. Discusses the impact of stress upon the body.

The Wisdom of the Body, by Walter B. Cannon. New York: Norton, 1963. Original description of the "emergency" or "fight or flight" response and its relation to health and body functioning.

You Can Fight for Your Life, by Lawrence L. LeShan. New York: Harcourt Brace Jovanovich, Inc., 1978. Describes psychotherapeutic experiences with cancer patients and how attitude appears related to outcome, both positively and negatively.

63

What is an Ostomy?

Barbara Dorr Mullen
Kerry Anne McGinn, R. N.

from *The Ostomy Book—Living Comfortably with Colostomies, Ileostomies, and
Urostomies* by Barbara Dorr Mullen and Kerry Anne McGinn, RN. Bull Publishing
Company, 1980.

Most people have never heard of ostomies, yet they are relatively common. There are no precise statistics, though it has been estimated that roughly three times as many ostomies are performed as mastectomies. But like mastectomies a generation ago, people don't talk about them.

The reason for the silence is understandable: Many are cancer-related, and people are not generally anxious to discuss a rearrangement of their plumbing. On the other hand, ignorance breeds fear, and a little knowledge can go a long way toward helping ostomy patients, as well as those who support them.

Barbara Mullen was a reporter, and when she found herself faced with this frightening procedure, she decided to learn all she could about it, so she could provide for others the information that would have been so helpful for her. Kerry McGinn, her daughter, offered to help, and brought her professional training and experience as a nurse to the project.—*D.C.B.*

An *ostomy* is a man-made opening into the body. An *abdominal ostomy* (the kind we're interested in) is the passageway a surgeon constructs through the abdominal wall as an exit for body waste—feces or urine. Such a change becomes necessary when the normal channel of elimination can not be used because of illness, accident or birth defect. A new outlet must be developed.

Ostomy refers to the total change the surgeon makes. *Ostomate* is one common term for a person who undergoes this change in personal plumbing. The new opening one can see on the abdomen is called a *stoma*.

There are three general categories of ostomies. A *colostomy* is the rerouting (permanent or temporary) of the colon (large intestine). *Ileostomy* describes such a detour in the ileum (the last section of the small intestine). *Urostomy* is a general term covering a number of different surgical procedures to redirect urine to the outside of the body when the bladder (or occasionally another part of the urinary tract) must be bypassed or removed, or when nerves do not control the discharge of urine.

More than a million and a half North Americans, ranging from infants to great grandparents, know what an ostomy really means—because they have one.

The most common ostomies—colostomies and ileostomies—involve the digestive tract and depend for their success on its amazing ability to adapt to change.

Everything we eat, from apple pie and steak to pizza, yams, and zucchini, must be broken down into tiny particles and changed to simpler chemical substances which can be absorbed into the blood stream. The resulting nutrients make their way to cells throughout the body, thus providing constant fuel and materials for energy, growth, and rebuilding. This complex process of digestion takes place in the long (26 feet or longer in an adult) twisting internal canal known as the digestive tract, alimentary canal, or gut.

Digestion starts in the mouth, where food is chewed and enzymes in the saliva begin the process. From there, food goes via the esophagus to the stomach where churning action, different enzymes, and weak acid continue mechanical and chemical changes.

Becoming more liquid at each stage, the food proceeds into the small intestine, where substances from the liver and the pancreas further the process, breaking down even the most exotic foods into simple sugars, amino acids, and fatty acids. To be used by the body, the digested food must pass through the walls of the small intestine by way of countless tiny fingerlike projections (villi) which line the small intestine.

By the time food reaches the colon (large intestine or large bowel), most of the nourishment has been absorbed. Here the major tasks are absorbing water and some mineral salts, and transporting and storing the indigestible remains of the food in the lower part of the colon and the rectum. At the far end of the versatile winding digestive tract, the anus is a ring-like *sphincter* which opens to release feces.

The digestive tract is surrounded by smooth muscles which contract and expand, thus helping food move from one end of the tract to the other by the rhythmic waves known as *peristalsis*. These waves are almost constant; there are also stronger contractions, known as mass reflexes, which occur at the time of bowel movements.

Usually, the whole process of digestion is so automatic and so efficient that we forget its marvelous complexity (the liver alone has over 300 functions). As Thomas Fuller said, "Eaten bread is forgotten."

Occasionally, there is a massive breakdown in the system. The intestine may be blocked, completely or partially, by cancer, injury, or birth defect. Or food may rush through the digestive tract so quickly that there is little chance for nutrients to be absorbed; in severe inflammatory bowel disease, the person may be starving. In all these cases, an ostomy may become necessary.

The body adjusts quite nicely to a shortened digestive tract. If the ostomy occurs near the end of the digestive tract, as in most colostomies, the person has lost only a storage area, and a sphincter to release feces. If the ostomy is farther up in the digestive tract, as it is in a few colostomies and in ileostomies, the ostomate has also lost part of the ability to absorb water and mineral salts; thus the discharge tends to be less formed. But the remaining intestine eventually takes over some of this water-absorbing function, and the kidneys, the major regulators of water and mineral salts for all people, with or without ostomies, handle the rest of the adjustment.

Colostomies account for 65 to 75% of all abdominal ostomies. Since colo-rectal cancer, the most common cause for a colostomy, usually occurs in people over 50, and since it causes little or no distress in its early stages, most colostomates are over 50, and are surprised and shocked by what's being done. There's been no warning, or only such subtle hints as a change in bowel pattern, excessive gas, or a trace of blood in the stool.

In contrast, people who have ileostomies (which account for perhaps 10 to 15% of all ostomies) tend to be teenagers or young adults, and they've often had plenty of warning. Most have had a long or unusually severe bout with a fiery dragon of a bowel. Inflammatory bowel disease has laid them low with severe diarrhea (often bloody), cramps, and weight loss. In many of these cases, an ileostomy represents an instant cure. The colon has been a battle field; without it, peace is probable.

The final 10% of ostomies are urinary diversions, urostomies of one kind or another. After the kidneys have filtered wastes out of the blood, they flush excess fluid and wastes as urine through narrow tubes to an expandable storage area (the bladder) and then out of the body. At least some kidney function is essential for life, but any other part of the urinary tract can be removed or bypassed. Because reasons for urostomies vary from birth defects to cancer of the bladder, the age range here is wide, and many different surgical techniques are used.

In any abdominal ostomy, the damaged, diseased, or useless section of intestine or urinary tract is removed (or disconnected). To provide for the essential elimination of feces or urine, a new exit must be made.

In a colostomy or a standard ileostomy, the surgeon brings the end of the remaining intestine through the muscle, fat, and skin of the abdominal wall, forming a tunnel which folds back on itself like a turtleneck, and stitches it in place.

One variation on the ileostomy is the *continent ileostomy,* or Kock pouch, in which part of the small intestine is fashioned into a reservoir which is then attached to the inside of the abdominal wall. A slender tube, also made from the small intestine, leads from the reservoir out through the abdominal wall to become a stoma.

To construct an *ileal conduit,* the commonest kind of urostomy, the surgeon cuts a short section of small intestine away from the rest of the intestine, closes it at one end, and connects to it the narrow tubes leading from the kidneys; the open end of the disconnected segment of intestine is then brought through the abdominal wall as a conduit, or passageway, for urine to the outside of the body.

The stoma which results from any of these ostomies could be described as a soft valve. It stretches to permit waste to be expelled. During inactive periods, the tissue pulls together, rather like puckered lips (stoma, in fact, means "mouth"). Although it expands and contracts, the stoma does not have the firm muscle control of the anal or urinary sphincter; voluntary control of bowel movements or urination must be replaced by something else.

For many ostomates, an appliance is that "something else." An appliance is a man-made pouch, usually of thin flexible plastic or rubber, which is adhered to the skin over the stoma to hold feces or urine until a convenient time for disposal. An alternative chosen by many colostomates is *irrigation,* a kind of enema through the stoma, which permits them to empty the bowel at their convenience. They

wear only a soft pad or a very small appliance over the stoma.

Since people with a continent ileostomy still have an internal storage area, they need no appliance; instead, they insert a plastic tube into the reservoir at regular intervals to drain feces.

Even though the view through a temporary post-op pouch may be a bit foggy, that first look at a new stoma in full, living color can be a real shocker.

Although the stoma usually shrinks slightly in diameter as post-operative swelling goes away and normal diet and exercise resume, the red color remains. This is logical, since this new exit is still a part of the intestine, lined with essentially the same kind of soft velvety mucous membrane as the mouth.

Unlike an incision, a stoma requires little healing. The stitches used are often the kind that don't need to be removed. A urostomy stoma starts to expel urine immediately, even before the new urostomate has left the operating room; the other types of stomas start discharging feces in a few days.

Stomas come in many shapes and sizes, depending on the kind of ostomy—and the person who owns it. Some are smaller than a dime in diameter; others are several inches or more across.

Shape varies as much as size. Some are round, some oval, and others are a bit irregular in shape. Most colostomies have the stoma raised slightly above the abdominal wall, perhaps $\frac{1}{4}$ to $\frac{1}{2}$ inch. Where drainage is more constant, as is the case with urostomies and ileostomies, the stoma is usually longer. From $\frac{3}{4}$ to one inch is said to be the ideal length. This length helps discharge waste directly into an appliance, instead of letting it pool on the skin.

At first, it's a temptation to feel over-protective about one's stoma, feeling it's so fragile it might be damaged by a draft of wind in the shower. While reasonable protection is essential, the stoma is surprisingly tough. It's not harmed by water, during sexual contact, or even by gentle bumps against furniture. It does bleed easily, even from as little cause as an overzealous swipe with a wash cloth, because many tiny blood vessels are very close to the surface of the stoma. An appliance or a soft pad will protect it from the friction of clothes.

Some stomas are constructed in the best possible location; others are not. Ideally, the ET or the surgeon (singly or together) spends time with the ostomate-to-be before surgery, watching how the shape of the abdomen changes when the person is sitting, standing, or walking—where the waistline is, where valleys and bulges occur. Then the probable site is marked.

If possible, the stoma is centered on a smooth and relatively flat plane, away from old scars or bones that protrude. Not all abdomens are ideal, however.

Sometimes, because of fat or scars, there isn't any really good location for the stoma. And even with advance planning, the surgeon may change the site because of conditions discovered during the operation.

Within a few months after surgery, the stoma should settle down to a fairly consistent size, shape, and color. The shape may vary a little with change of position or activity, even coughing. Weight loss or gain (pregnancy, for example) may alter the contour of the stoma. But, different as stomas are from person to person, an individual stoma should look about the same from day to day, year to year. If the color or the shape changes much without an obvious reason (a too-tight appliance, for instance), it's time to check with a professional.

All intestinal stomas secrete some mucus, a thick liquid which helps lubricate and protect the intestine. As surplus mucus is discharged, it serves as a natural cleaning agent for the stoma. In addition, the skin around the stoma thrives on showers and baths, free of an appliance. However, scrubbing is not necessary and may hurt a stoma. A gentle sponge bath is another alternative.

In the 18th and 19th centuries, ostomies carried very high risks. With no anesthetics or antibiotics, patients clenched their fists and recited the 23rd Psalm. Mortality was high. With new techniques, surgical and postopertive risks are greatly reduced, especially when surgery is done promptly.

Although grouped under common headings, no two ostomies (and no two stomas) are exactly alike—each is a very personal thing. There are some new habits to learn but that's a small enough price to pay for an improved or extended life.

Figure 63-1 Ostomies of the Digestive and Urinary Tracts.
To make the relationships clearer, the artist has left out most of the small intestine, which twists and winds for 20 feet or more around the abdomen from the end of the stomach until the ileum, the last section of the small intestine, joins the large intestine (colon).

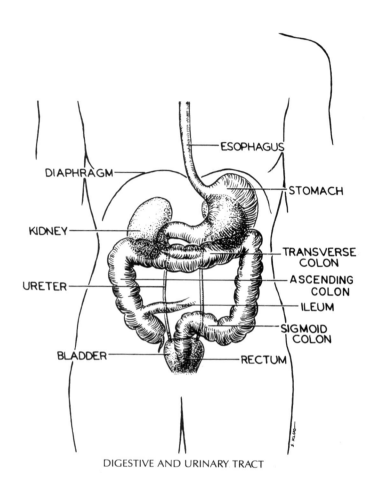

DIGESTIVE AND URINARY TRACT

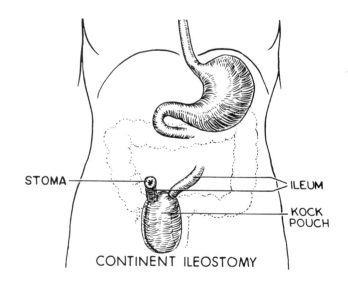

CONTINENT ILEOSTOMY

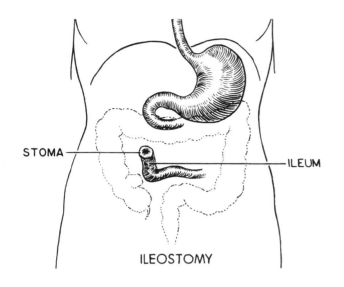

ILEOSTOMY

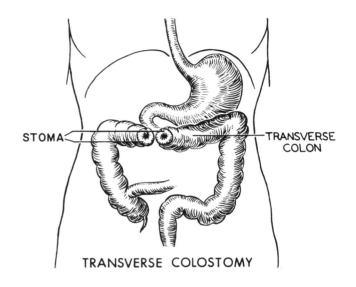

TRANSVERSE COLOSTOMY

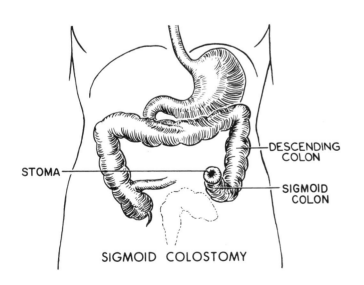

SIGMOID COLOSTOMY

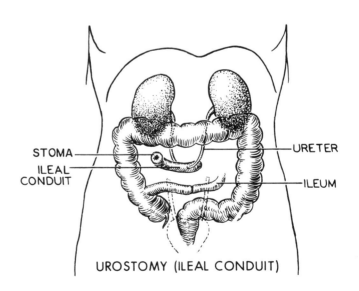

UROSTOMY (ILEAL CONDUIT)

64

Job Discrimination

American Cancer Society

Reprinted with permission from the American Cancer Society, California Division, "Job Discrimination," The ACS Volunteer, 22(2): 1-5 (1976).

"A job is more than my profession; it's my connection with life."

This is the assertion and the plea of a woman who lost her job following successful breast surgery. "When the third place turned down my application as 'not suitable' I began running around tearing my hair and screaming, though only I could hear it, "My God, what am I going to do?' "

Is this an isolated case? Or is it a problem, even a nightmare, faced by countless cancer patients?

A landmark study of the work experiences of cancer patients has shown that cancer patients do face job discrimination not only in hiring and firing, but also in attitudes, job assignments and benefits.

The recently completed study—the first factual, systematic look at the problem—was made for the American Cancer Society's California Division by Professor Frances L. Feldman of the University of Southern California School of Social Work.

The study shows that . . .

• More than half (54 percent) of the persons interviewed described at least one work problem related to their illness.

• Nearly one-fourth (22 percent) reported being rejected for jobs because of previous cancer treatment.

• Over one-third (39 percent) said they feared future job discrimination.

• Of the 29 percent who were no longer working for the same employer as before their cancer diagnosis, 40 percent left for cancer-related reasons and 8 percent said they had been dismissed or "pressured" into leaving because of their cancer treatment. The seven persons in this latter group had worked for their employers from one month to 20 years.

• Nearly one-fourth said they were the targets of negative attitudes or discrimination in their jobs.

• Nineteen percent of the persons in the survey thought their working conditions or salary levels had been adversely affected.

• Almost two-thirds of those working part-time and 40 percent of the unemployed were unable to find full-time work. They blame their failure on their cancer history.

• A small group (5 percent) reported reduction in health benefits or exclusion from group health plans and 8 percent were ineligible for any or for increased group life insurance coverage.

Not all the results of the study are negative. In fact, nearly half (46 percent) of the persons said they had never had work problems because of their cancer.

In addition . . .

• Over three-quarters of the group reported salary increases, many because of promotions or increased job responsibilties.

• Most persons still working for the same employer said their health and insurance benefits were the same as other employees.

• Five persons who had changed jobs had been recruited by their current employers after their illnesses.

Since this study there has been legislation passed in some states to eliminate discrimination because of a medical condition, such as cancer, but the problem is still widespread.

65

Death and Dying

"Thanatology" is the science dealing with death and dying. In the late 1960s, the health field began to take notice of the special needs of the dying and that interest has continued to grow. Accompanying this awareness has been a better understanding of the meaning of life and living.

Laurens P. White, M.D. from the University of California, San Francisco, School of Medicine was one of the early supporters of the Biology of Cancer Program, sponsored my studies in medical school on developing cancer education programs (and this book), is a specialist in medical oncology and thanatology, and is the President of the California Medical Association (1988).—*M.R.*

. . . Mortuis Vivos Docent

Laurens P. White, M.D.

Death will affect you, and although it seems unbelievable, it may well affect me. My attitude toward your death will never be quite the same as it is toward my own, but it will be affected by the context in which I view my own death. The degree to which I have incorporated death into my life will directly affect the way I handle my dying, and if I am a physician, nurse, clergyman, friend, or lover, it will affect the way I deal with you when I am involved in your dying. Many have thought and written about this problem, perhaps none more directly and usefully than Seneca in letters to Lucilius:

> Rehearse death. To say this is to tell a person to rehearse freedom. A person who has learned how to die has unlearned how to be a slave. He is above and beyond the reach of all political power. What are prisons or bars or warders to him? He has an open door. There is but one chain binding us in fetters and that is our love of life. There is no need to cast this love out altogether, but it does need to be lessened somewhat so that in the event of circumstances ever demanding this, nothing may stand in the way of our being prepared to do at once what we must do sometime [p. 72].

A. E. Housman (1936) put a similar thought in more poetic, if less forceful, language:

> *I to my perils of cheat and charmer*
> *Came clad in armour by stars benign.*
> *Hope lies to mortals, and most believe her,*
> *But man's deceiver was never mine.*
> *The thoughts of others were light and fleeting*
> *Of lovers meeting or luck, or fame.*
> *Mine were of trouble and mine were steady*
> *So I was ready when trouble came [pp. 15-16].*

A good deal of our problem in dealing with death must be related to its unknown, and perhaps unknowable, quality. Our fear of our own death may be exacerbated by our reaction to and fear of the death of someone for whom we care. Professor Jacob Needleman (1969) went to the heart of the matter when he wrote:

> The first step in regarding another as mortal is to acknowledge with all of our being that we do not know what a person is or what death is, but that we have fears about these things and a contradictory view of reality that goes hand in glove with those fears. This awareness of our own ignorance and fear would be, if we are to believe Socrates, the beginning of wisdom. The hasty flight from this awareness either into philosophical presumption, religious sentimentality, or dogmatic faith in the Cartesian natural science would be the reversion to ignorance. And what good can come from ignorance? [p. 736]

Caring for a patient who is going to die has all the elements of threat, failure, and helplessness which we so often associate with the process of dying itself. It is not surprising that this should be so, because in the process of caring for a person there is, to a greater or lesser degree, some identification with his problem as well as with his personality. To the physician engaged in such a dyad the impending or threatened death of a patient may be even more of a threat than it might be to someone else, for the physician tends to have a greater fear of death than does the ordinary individual. It is the purpose of this essay to look at some of the things which are involved in patient care, including some of the fantasies which contribute to the difficulty, and to propose some changes in the physician's concept of his or her role which might go some distance toward resolving them.

PHYSICIAN-PATIENT RELATIONSHIP

There are probably very few relationships as satisfying to all those involved as the relationship between a competent surgeon and a patient with acute appendicitis who is in pain and threatened with serious illness. To the surgeon the role of rapid intervention, diagnostic astuteness, reassurance, and then curative action reassures his need for a sense of mastery, a sense of involvement, and a need for validation of his success. To a patient who is in pain, with considerable apprehension, and an awareness that things have gone very wrong indeed, a most important need is for someone to make things right. He can't do it alone, and the patient is aware that he depends on someone else. When a brief and definitive operation is done, the patient's dependence is short-lived, although no less real, and he is rapidly restored to the ranks of those who are able to maintain an independent life and make their own decisions. The patient's need for action is met by equal need on the part of the physician to act, and ordinarily there are no complications involved in this sort of a relationship. Each participant has a defined role, and each one's conception of that role can be validated in a short time.

In contrast, the doctor treating a patient who is not going to get well and the patient with a fatal illness have changes in their roles which may be difficult either to acknowledge or to accept. This is probably especially true for the physician who, from his training and from his need, may still consider his role to be that of curing the patient, but who, by the current definitino of dealing with the patient with incurable disease, is not going to have his efforts climaxed by cure, or the survival of the patient. It is, therefore, clear that if physicians cannot change their ideas about their roles as physicians, they are going to feel frustrated and on many levels a failure because of their inability to cure dying patients. This sense of failure on the part of physicians is very real, and I cannot think of any way in which the death of a patient can be regarded by physicians as a reassurance of their sense of mastery. The death of a patient not only affects their human feelings, but also magnifies their feelings of impotence, ineptness, and even guilt. If the physician makes a negligent mistake in treating a patient, and is aware of the mistake, he should feel guilty. (It is, perhaps, fortunate in one sense that we probably don't recognize most of our medical mistakes.) Ironically, however, the physician may feel guilty and incompetent upon the death of a patient even when performance and judgment, viewed by himself and others, have been of the first order. As I will discuss further, this sense of guilt and incompetence appear to be related to the fantasy that the physician should be able to cure all diseases and endow all patients with eternal life.

It is obvious that one immediate solution to this problem, which would delight us all, is for a new cure to be found for some specific disease that could make us feel successful and could avoid a lot of suffering. Short of that happy outcome, a more practical approach to the problem is to change in some way our concept of what our job as physicians may be. I will get back to this point later.

A QUESTION OF SEMANTICS

Words are toys of the mind, but like toys they may condition the way in which we think about things. Years ago, the Ford Foundation published a series of records on semantics and the extent to which the words we use condition our feelings and understanding of things. This record pointed out that, in the United States and to a great extent in England and the Anglo-Saxon countries, when children misbehave, they are admonished to "be good, don't be bad." In France, in contrast, when children misbehave, they are admonished to "soi sage," be intelligent. In Germany, the admonition is to "get in line." In Scandanavian countries, the warning is "var shnell," be kind. In Southwestern America, in the Hopi Indian tradition, the child is told "that is not the Hopi way." One can imagine that this sort of use of words conditions the way in which people growing up in these backgrounds think of their misbehavior. In San Quentin prison, when death row existed and prisoners sentenced to death had to be moved for any reason, the prisoner was shackled and conducted by two guards down the endless corridors of the prison, and the word went in front of him "dead man coming." There can be little question that such a shout would condition the reactions of those hearing it, whether they be guards, inmates, or the "dead man" himself.

To an extent which I can't calculate, the use of the word *terminal* to describe a patient must have a great role to play in the way in which we regard such a patient, as does, of course, the word *patient* itself. In your home you are a human being with whatever that implies to you and me, whereas in my office you are a patient. To some extent this defines you in my mind and me in yours. Hopefully, your role as a patient can be as little restrictive as possible, but, obviously, if you are seriously ill, you are more of a patient and have given up more of your independence than somebody who requires no medical care at all. Add to this the notation *terminal,* and not only does your condition become further defined in my mind but so do some of my feelings about what can be done for you and what can be done by me. Now, it is obvious that if I die today, I am terminal at this minute. The fact that I don't feel terminal has nothing to do with my terminality, and it can be seen in this rather simpleminded way that terminal as applied to an individual really means someone who dies shortly. Terminal really doesn't mean someone who I say is going to die, because I am so often wrong. Therefore, it seems important to me to make this distinction and for physicians to avoid the loose use of the word *terminal*, with all of the implications it has on an emotional level both for the doctor and for the patient.

THE PHYSICIAN'S ATTITUDE

Since so much that happens in the relationship between doctor and patient depends on the doctor's attitude, it is worth spending some time examining this. At the outset, it seems important to emphasize that we are all going to die. Even if a cure for cancer of the lung appeared tomorrow, this would simply mean that one reason for death had been eliminated, not that death itself had disappeared. It was no more than 100 years ago that medicine could accomplish so little that there would have been no need to emphasize that the role of the physician was not to cure patients; this was often a goal, and when it occurred, always a pleasure, but it, by no means, defined what the role of the physician was. As medical skills have increased and the medical armamentarium has been considerably enlarged, the cure of some diseases has become a reality. It's probably worth emphasizing that the prolongation of life which has occurred in the last 2000 years has come mostly from preventive medicine, not from curative medicine, from preventing illness, not from curing it. It is, however, our ability to cure some diseases that has created the problem for physicians which is so acute at the moment, namely, the inability to cope effectively with one's role as a physician when the patient does not get well.

It is argued by those of a trivial turn of mind that if the goal of a physician is not the cure of the patient, then the physician isn't trying very hard. Nothing could be further from the truth, assuming that we are speaking of physicians of good character and good will. When the goal of the physician is not cure, but rather care, more attention may be paid to what the patient really needs, rather than what the physician really needs. I am by no means unconcerned about the physician's needs, but want to set them in a frame of reference where they make some sort of sense in terms of what is possible with the patient. If the physician's main need is to care and to exert his best professional skills to provide the patient with optimum care, this may obviously be accompanied by the patient improving, or even getting completely well, and such a result is a delight to both participants. It may, in the event that the patient fails to get well, allow the physician to continue to give that concerned and loving care which ought to be every patient's right, without feeling that

he is a failure, and without a feeling of complete loss of mastery in a complicated situation. It is the sense of mastery which appears to be at the heart of the problem.

A physician who feels that he can cure lung cancer . . . has simply had too little experience with patients with lung cancer to be considered an expert. For a physician confronted with a patient with lung cancer, to state to the patient that nothing can be done is really to acknowledge a loss of the sense of mastery, because what he is really saying is that nothing can be done to cure the patient, and what the patient is hearing is that nothing can be done at all. It is from this sense of frustration and defeat on the part of many physicians that patients, faced with a complex and life-threatening illness, and given no support from their physicians, seek out magic and quack remedies offered by those unscrupulous or merely ignorant "healers" who recognize the importance of offering something to a desperate person. It is a profound fault on the part of medical professionals that so much of the time their feeling of impotence leads them to reject the patient, who in desperation then turns to these unscrupulous practitioners for the emotional, and often magical, support that seems to be needed. In such a situation, if a physician can acknowledge that the patient can't be cured, but that his job goes far beyond curing a patient to caring for him or her, and that caring for a dying patient can be important, rewarding emotionally, and helpful in a variety of ways, then he has done a great deal to support a patient in this difficult time. It is a curious anomaly that in this relationship it appears to be the doctor who is unable to accept his real role, rather than the patient who is unable to accept his fatal diagnosis.

I am convinced that one of the main reasons why most doctors are doctors is that they are convinced that in any relationship with doctor and patient it's the patient who is going to do the dying. There must be some level of resentment of this situation on the part of many patients, and I have heard often enough a patient saying, "I just wish you had my disease, not I." Nonetheless, the patient seems to have less trouble accepting the potential outcome of his or her illness than the doctor does accepting his or her inability to change that outcome. Therefore, the obvious suggestion is that physicians change their concepts of their role, particularly with patients with what are currently fatal diseases. The role of physicians should, therefore, be one of caring for patients, providing both expert technical care and the involved, concerned human care for another individual. This means helping them through the process of dying when that becomes inevitable. It means not abandoning patients because they are dying, not abandoning them because we conceive of them as terminal, or conceive of them as being already dead.

TECHNOLOGY AND DEATH

Curiously, our technology has allowed us to become trapped in a dilemma about prolonging life. This concerns the ability of physicians to maintain certain physiologic parameters of life after an individual has reached a point in illness or injury where useful or enjoyable life appears to be over. We are all aware of patients who have been kept "alive" by the use of respirators, IV fluids, and repeated cardiac defibrillation or massage. There is no question of the value of these heroic measures in certain cases of cardiac arrest, chest injury, or shock. It is the application of these life-prolonging methods to someone whose life seems to be over which raises difficult, but proper, questions. Our lack of clear-cut answers may be related to at least four problems: (1) Our technology is so recent that we have had only a brief time to try to think out, and even to feel out, answers. (2) Our definition of death is in the process of changing, in part because of our technology, and increasingly is being thought to center on "brain death" and not on the former parameters of absent heart beat and respiration. (3) No definition of death is going to satisfy everyone, and we can all share the awareness of the difficulty of being absolutely certain as to when a person is really dead. We accept our fallibility and shudder at the responsibility of working within its strictures. (4) The responsibility for making the life-death decisions we now face is very harsh.

When I listen to lay groups discussing this issue, I am struck with the frequency with which physicians are blamed for "keeping people alive," or for "using people as guinea pigs." This blame we must accept, because our technology has created the problem, and created the real fear in many minds that after all chance for meaningful life has passed, people may be kept indefinitely "alive" at the hands of the medical profession. Perhaps we should appreciate the compliment implicit in this appraisal of the power we physicians have, with so much work, recently acquired. Most physicians are, however, deeply concerned with ways of making appropriate decisions as to the use of this power. Its use involves very difficult decisions about life, about when a patient is beyond recovery, about when a brain is truly dead. These decisions are to be made by people who are usually quite aware of their fallibility and their weakness. We must also admit that many physicians do regard their role as being able to prolong life, any life, for as long as possible and with whatever means are available. I cannot condemn any person dedicated to that goal, and it is within that framework, and at the hands of those workers, that our dilemma is created. It is vital, however, to be absolutely clear about the distinction between prolonging life and prolonging the process of dying, when the latter means simply the temporary postponement of the cessation of heartbeat and respiration by mechanical means after the brain, the essence of the individual, has ceased to function. Perhaps we might leave it that this is an area which requires much open thought, an area in which many points of view have merit, and which is too important to be resolved solely by physicians.

In California the recent passage (1976) of the Keene Bill (AB 3060) has directly tackled this problem. This measure provides an individual with the legal right to leave written instructions for his family and physicians that, in the event of illness preventing him from expressing his wishes or illness which makes recovery unlikely, he does not wish to allow or to undergo extraordinary measures to prolong his life. We, in California, are waiting to see the effect of this bill. It clearly represents a response to the nightmare of the Quinlan case, as well as an effort to assure the patient of some control over his dignity and destiny.

DISCUSSING DIAGNOSIS WITH PATIENTS

One of the ways in which physicians may help patients is by treating them as individuals of unique worth to whom we owe not only our best efforts but our honesty. By this I mean that all patients should be told in as direct and open a way as possible our conception of the facts as they relate to their illness. By facts, I mean diagnosis by name, and discussion of prospects in detail. By in detail, I do not mean in the most frightening or antagonistic or ominous way possible, but in as straightforward a way as possible. I also think this should probably be done on more than one occasion, because so often patients hear selectively, and they should probably have the opportunity to discuss our idea of reality as it relates to them as often as they want to. Some patients won't want to even once, but these are definitely in the minority. Other patients, of whom it might be said that such a discussion would hurt them irreparably, would probably not hear anything they didn't want to hear. All of us who are involved in this practice are aware of numbers of patients who, after extensive discussions of diagnosis and its implications, appear to be completely unaware of their diagnosis. By the same token, we are also aware of patients whose doctors have told them nothing, who are intimately aware of their diagnosis and its implications, and who in kindly fashion do not trouble the physician who seems unable to talk to them about these unhappy details. It appears to be almost an axiom that patients may know either much more than we have told them or much less, and that the only thing they can't stand to hear from us is a lie. When we are unable to talk to them about their disease, just as when their families are unable to talk to them, they really have nowhere to turn. The isolation of illness is then compounded by our clear instructions that it is not to be talked about. Our unwillingness to talk about someone's disease and his or her feelings about it is not consistent with giving good care.

Another important element in discussing diagnosis with patients is making sure that the family is involved in such a discussion. If a patient knows one thing and the family another, communication is diminished by at least that amount. Discussions with the family are vital, but I make it a point to try not to discuss diagnosis and prognosis with the family without the patient being present. In this way everybody knows at the same time what everybody else knows, but, more importantly, everybody knows that everybody knows, and that different stories are not being given to different people. There probably are a few people who don't like, or perhaps can't tolerate, this sort of discussion, but they are certainly a tiny minority, and in my experience, and that of many others, if they can't tolerate it they will quickly forget that such a discussion ever took place.

THE ROLE OF DENIAL

It is important to discuss the role of denial in patients with serious or fatal illnesses. It is equally important to recognize that denial exists in the professionals of the helping professions as well. We are all aware of moments in our lives when we have refused to admit the reality of something displeasing. There must be many more moments when our denial of reality blanks it completely from our awareness. Some people seem to have more of this tendency or capacity than others, and a few, who deny our form of reality, have various psychiatric diagnoses attached to their problems and their lives. In general, it would seem that denial is not adaptive or helpful as a way of dealing with problems. Most of us have come to view denial as a bad thing, and to see those persons who use denial as making some sort of error. A long series of patients, who have taught me so very much else, have also convinced me that denial is not necessarily a mistake, particularly in patients who face certain grim realities. This is probably true because denial is so variable, both in its degree and in the time span it occupies.

Many years ago a patient gave me a phrase, an understanding, and a gift which have been central in my life for 25 years. His name was Charles Young, and the gift beyond my repaying. He was dying of melanoma, early in middle life, riddled with metastases which were apparent to him, and not responding to the ineffective drugs then available. He was concerned about the effect upon American life of the then Senator Joseph McCarthy, and one day told me he thought he'd fly to Washington and assassinate McCarthy, saying, "Before they could even get me on trial, I'd be dead." Then, with an enigmatic smile, he added, "You know, Laurie, I know I'm dying, but I don't really believe I'm dying." In these simple words he gave me an answer to the engima of denial, and in truth, a solution for dealing with it. Since then, I haven't felt any great need to "deal with it" in most cases. I can deal with the patient, being as truthful as I know how to be, and the denial which is built into the patient will enable him or her to deal with the truth. A very few people seem to look disease and death steady in the eye, using little denial. For them, withholding the truth would seem to be an obscene trickery, unlikely to deceive for long. At the other extreme are those few individuals who may follow a detailed discussion of their diagnosis and prognosis by asking if someone could tell them what is wrong with them. In short, it appears that the great majority of humans have a degree of denial which is appropriate to them; that this denial is consistent with the ways in which they have dealt with other problems and realities in their lives; and that it forms an integral, if occasionally variable, part of the way they deal with illness, and if necessary, with impending death. From the point of view of the medical professional, therefore, denial on the part of the patient can often be used as an ally or a strength. It allows some of our errors of commission or omission to escape too much notice.

Hackett and Weisman (1969) have studied the knowledge held by groups of patients about their diagnosis and prognosis. They found interesting differences in their sample, with almost all patients with heart disease having been given detailed information about both factors, but with only 7 of 20 cancer patients so fully informed, although 10 others had been given some information. Of even more interest, however, was their observation that only 9 of 20 patients with heart disease were fully aware of diagnosis and prognosis, even though nearly all had been told, and that 10 of 20 patients with cancer, not all of whom had been told, were aware of diagnosis and prognosis. A similar study has been done with children with leukemia, where a massive effort to screen the children from awareness of the facts of their cases was carried out, without any apparent effect on the children, 96 percent of whom were aware of what was happening and what it could mean to them.

And what of denial on the part of the health professional? How many hundreds of times have women found lumps in their breasts, and asked their physicians to do something, only to be told it was nothing serious. In San Francisco only 60 percent of internists and family physicians will perform Pap tests on their female patients, although this test can be lifesaving in detecting cervix cancer at a curable stage. Similar refusal to perform sigmoidoscopy can be cited. It is clear that a great deal which can be done for early diagnosis of cancer is not being done. It is my view that laziness is not the reason, but rather an unwillingness to find something unpleasant. It may be a vestige of the old fear of the herald bringing bad news to the emperor. It may relate to our identification with the patients, and our fear that similar tests might produce bad news in ourselves. Certainly very few physicians and nurses get checkups, annual physical examinations, or other routine measures which might help in early diagnosis or lead to preventive steps. And this unwillingness, in the light of what we know, largely stems from denial. In opposition to this I must cite the very large number of physicians who have stopped smoking, which is certainly a lifesaving step. I recently, however, had a call from a man who smoked heavily, and who had asked his physician if he should stop. The physician said there was no need, since by having a chest film every 6 months, an early cancer of the lung could be picked up and cured, in the event it occurred. Such is clearly not the case in a disease with an overall cure rate of less than 5 percent, even in so-called "early cases," and it turned out that the particular physician was also a heavy smoker. I advised the man to quit both cigarettes and that physician, because denial on the part of the professional was affecting the advice he gave. I'm sure there must be times when this is true for us all.

One of the main reasons for having these matters openly discussed is encompassed in what I'll loosely call "the will of the patient to resist his illness." No one has been able really to define this well, or to produce any data that confirm this view, but many have the impression that patients who fight their disease may outlive those who give in easily. Ignorance of what one has, even assuming that it will persist, is certainly no basis for fighting it. A well-informed patient might be expected to be in a better frame of mind to fight than one who does not recognize the realities that he or she is facing.

This recognition of "reality" is a complex, and probably central, issue for those threatened with early death. Denial certainly operates at any level of such awareness, but an ability to acknowledge, if not to accept, the reality of one's condition, may be of great importance in dealing with it.

During the great slaughter of people in the German concentration camps, the German technicians developed and carried out an ingenious series of deceptions to screen the victims from the reality of their impending execution. Speed was essential, calmness and ruthless efficiency important, but the main ingredient in the success of so much killing was an unwillingness on the part of the victims to imagine, or to accept, their fate. Starved, beaten, terrified, dehumanized, in strange surroundings, the victims can hardly be criticized for their failure to resist. The same behavior was seen in Russian soldiers, Dutch Jews, American pilots. No resistance was ever offered during the entrance into the camps, when so many were immediately gassed and cremated. All the resistance, when it happened, came from groups within the camps who had discovered what their fate would be and who had decided to fight for their lives. One will never know whether such a fight ever took place in the pure death camps, such as Belsec, for no one survived to tell of it. At Treblinka, Sobibor, and Auschwitz, groups did organize, did plot, and eventually did fight. At Treblinka, where over 800,000 were slaughtered, 400 fought, and 45 survived.

Elie Cohen, a physician who survived Auschwitz and has written about it in Eric Boehm's *We Survived*, described his delusional thinking upon entering the camp. Knowing of its purpose, and of his likely death, he convinced himself that, as a physician, he was likely to be spared because the Germans might need physicians. Rabbi Leo Baeck, the chief rabbi of Berlin, was a prisoner at Theresienstadt in the so-called "privileged" camp/ghetto. When the decision to move the Jews to Auschwitz for gassing was made, he found out what was in store. He decided to withhold the information from the others, reasoning that "to live in the expectation of death by gassing would only be the harder." Although the Germans deported most of the ghetto, about 4000 stayed in Theresienstadt, and most survived the war. Of the nearly 50,000 deported to Auschwitz, Baeck was one of the few who survived. One might wonder what thoughts this man had for the remainder of his life about his decision not to warn his fellow prisoners.

Some of the survivors of the holocaust have written about themselves, their experiences, and their feelings. They all seem to share an overwhelming sense of guilt at having survived, when so many of their friends and families did not. This guilt seems inevitable and sad. Many have attributed some of their guilt to what they did in an effort to survive: their daily fight for food, shelter, and better work gangs, their stealing from their fellows and even denouncing others to obtain rations or favors. They rather uniformly describe themselves as grimly fighting to escape a fate which was claiming others, and which they recognized clearly. It appears from their testimony that the survivors of the holocaust came from the group which saw clearly that they were doomed to die, and fought endlessly to escape that fate. The majority of this group died, too, but some survived. In the group which either denied the reality of what was happening, or which, having recognized their doom, chose not to resist, survival was, apparently, almost nil. It must also be admitted that the will to resist could not have been a constant thing, and must have fluctuated and been affected by many chance and intentional factors.

HONESTY BETWEEN PHYSICIAN AND PATIENT

It seems to me that this lesson from the holocaust, and from their epicenter, the Polish killing camps, if I am interpreting it correctly, has a great deal to say to us about how we deal with people facing death from disease. If we deny them the relevant information about diagnosis, prognosis, and available remedies, we deprive them of even the choice of whether to fight for their lives. If, from their own denial, or unwillingness to fight, they decline to fight for themselves, it is another matter, but I deeply believe we are obliged, in honor and good faith, to acquaint them, and not just a family member, with the relevant facts about their situation.

In addition, patients who know that physicians will be honest with them about something as important as diagnosis and outlook may expect physicians to be honest about other details as well. In contrast, patients whose physicians lie to them usually are found out because patients are at least as smart as physicians, and can quickly pick up obvious lies. It is an imprudent patient indeed who, after being lied to, will believe other elements of what the doctor chooses or refuses to tell him. By being truthful, I do not mean that I advocate the rather sorry practice that some physicians have of telling a patient how long he has to live. I regard this as an effort on the part of the physician to pretend to a mastery that he doesn't possess, to pretend to a certainty of the future that would make a fortune teller blush. I have often heard patients say, "Well, the doctor gave me 6 months to live," and shared their amusement as we discussed this proffered gift several years later. This sort of imperial soothsaying does not dignify either the practice of medicine or the physician who does it. Nonetheless, patients and their families often ask how long they have to live, and it has seemed to many that this question concerns itself more with whether the physician is going to stick it out however long it takes than with knowing exactly the date on which the patient is expected to expire. Therefore, a reasonable response is "I don't know how long you are going to live, but I do know that we will go through it together, with whatever it takes, and for as long as it takes."

ANGER AND DEATH

One of the sad things that often happens while we are caring for a dying patient is that the frustration of the experience and the difficulty of dealing with the feelings that it engenders may lead us all to anger. If depression is perhaps the most common of the unpleasant feelings, anxiety is probably the least tolerable, and most of us substitute anger for anxiety. If we are anxious because of a patient's illness, and our inability to control it, it may be easier for us to be angry with the patient, to be angry with a family member who may have called once too often, or to be angry with another physician who has been involved in the patient's care. It is important to recognize that much of this anger very likely represents our expression of a general feeling of frustration rather than an appropriate reaction to someone's misdeeds. It is also worth remembering that both the physician involved in the care of a dying patient and the patient himself need all the support they can get. This support can most appropriately come from the family, but also in great measure, when the patient is hospitalized, from the nursing staff, from social workers, from ward attendants, and in a curious and delightful way, from other patients themselves. I have often thought that a good deal more therapy goes on in my waiting room than I am aware of, and at times, a good deal more than goes on in my treatment rooms.

ACCEPTANCE AND DEATH

Religious conviction is a great source of strength for those who believe. The threat of death represents a real test of the depth of belief and of the support it brings. Only yesterday I again saw the strength which profound belief in God brought to a young physician very close to death, but I have also recently seen deep disbelief appear in a dying woman, whose last words were "don't pray over me."

For many who face death the clergy are traditional, and occasionally helpful, members of the health care team. For those to whom religion is a source of strength, the clergy can be of great help in mobilizing this strength and in sustaining contact with the living. Many clerics are sources of strength themselves, and their humanity may make this help as available to those without specific religious feelings as to members of their own church. Like all of us, the clergy often have problems about death, problems which need to be worked through before they can become more comfortable with a dying person or his family. Like all of us the clergy have ways to achieve distance, to defend themselves against too much feeling. Where a physician may retreat behind a supposed life-sustaining machine, a clergyman may retreat behind prayer to prevent more personal involvement. Awareness of his own feelings and weaknesses is as important to the priest or rabbi as it is to a physician or nurse, and as uncommon.

What a human needs as he faces death is no different from what he needs in life, and love best expresses what he needs to receive and to give. Those of us in the helping/caring professions need the same in no less a sense, and profoundly need to be able to give love at the same time that we use our scientific and technical expertise. For all of us, whether with or without religion, the future involves accepting a common mortality. We all seem to seek "meaning" in life and in death, and in our personal and professional relationships. Peter deVries (1961), in his masterpiece *The Blood of the Lamb,* described this dilemma better than I can.

> I believe that man must learn to live without those consolations called religious, which his own intelligence must by now have told him belong to the childhood of the race. Philosophy can really give us nothing permanent to believe, either: it is too rich in answers, each canceling out the rest. The quest for meaning is foredoomed. Human life "means" nothing. But that is not to say it is not worth living. What does a Debussy Arabesque "mean," or a rainbow, or a rose? A man delights in all these, knowing himself to be no more—a wisp of music and a haze of dreams dissolve against the sun. Man has only his two feet to stand on, his own human trinity to see him through: Reason, Courage and Grace. And the first plus the second equals the third [p. 241].

References

Boehm, E. (ed.) *We Survived.* New Haven: Yale, 1949.

deVries, Peter. *The Blood of the Lamb.* Boston: Little, Brown, 1961.

Hackett, T., and Weisman, A. Denial as a factor in patients with heart disease and cancer. In *Care of patients with fatal illness, Annals of the New York Academy of Sciences,* 1969, 164, 802.

Housman, A. E. *More poems.* New York: Knopf, 1936.

Needleman, J. The perception of mortality. In *Care of patients with fatal illness, Annals of the New York Academy of Sciences,* 1969, 164, 733.

Seneca. *Letters from a Stoic.* R. Campbell (ed. and trans.). Harmondsworth, Maryland: Penguin, 1969.

66

Questions and Answers on Death and Dying

Elisabeth Kübler-Ross

Excerpted with permission from Questions and Answers on Death and Dying (New York: Macmillan Publishing Company, 1974), pp. 1–2, 3–4, 7, 9, 12–13, 16, 18, 21–22, 33, 35, 38, 88, 89–90.

One of the pioneers in the field of death and dying is Elisabeth Kübler-Ross. She is well known for her work with dying patients, and her 1969 book *On Death and Dying*. In it she describes five stages most people go through in dealing with a fatal illness: denial and isolation, anger, bargaining, depression and finally, acceptance. Kübler-Ross' work in recent years has focussed on understanding and helping AIDS patients.—*M.R.*

The dying patient has to pass through many stages in his struggle to come to grips with his illness and his ultimate death. He may deny the bad news for a while and continue to work "as if he were as well and strong as before." He may wish to shield his family (or his family may want to shield him) from the truth.

Sooner or later he will have to face the grim reality, and he often reacts with an angry "why me" to his illness. If we learn to assist this angry patient rather than to judge him—if we learn not to take his anguish as a personal insult—he will then be able to pass to the third stage, the stage of bargaining. He may bargain with God for an extension of life, or he may promise good behavior and religious dedication if he is spared more suffering. He will try to "put his house in order" and "finish unfinished business" before he really admits, "This is happening to me."

In the depression stage he mourns past losses first and then begins to lose interest in the outside world. He reduces his interests in people and affairs, wishes to see fewer and fewer people and silently passes through preparatory grief. If he is allowed to grieve, if his life is not artificially prolonged and if his family has learned "to let go," he will be able to die with peace and in a stage of acceptance. (Examples of these stages are described in detail in my book, *On Death and Dying*, (Macmillan, 1969). . . .

TELLING THE PATIENT

When is the time for an attending physician to tell his terminally ill patient of his diagnosis?

As soon as the diagnosis is confirmed a patient should be informed that he is seriously ill. He should then be given hope immediately, and by this I mean he should be told of all the treatment possibilities. We usually then wait until the patient asks for more details. If he asks for specifics I would give him an honest, straightforward answer. I do not tell the patient that he is dying or that he is terminally ill. I simply tell him that he is seriously ill and that we are trying to do everything humanly possible to help him to function as well as he can. . . .

When does the patient begin to die and when, then, does our relationship begin to be one with a dying patient?

In our interdisciplinary workshops on death and dying our relationships started with the hospi-

talization of the patients who had a potentially terminal illness. I believe, however, that such preparation should start much earlier and that we should teach our children and our young people to face the reality of death. They would then not have to go through all the stages when they are terminally ill and have so little time to deal with unfinished business. You live a different quality of life, as you do when you have faced your finiteness. . . .

DIFFICULTIES IN COMMUNICATION

I am concerned about physicians who cannot answer questions in a straightforward way. When a patient asks if he has cancer and the doctor does not say no, there is only one option: "I do not know yet." A refusal to say one or the other will be interpreted by the patient as a tacit yes, and with no indication of how serious his condition is he may suspect he is in pretty terrible shape and this may hasten his demise.

I don't think it will hasten the patient's demise. It may give him some sleepless nights, it may make him worry and wonder, it may give him more anxieties, perhaps, but sooner or later he will again ask the physician a straightforward question. If he still does not receive an answer, he will try to find out through his family, his minister, nurse, or social worker about the true state of his health. Hopefully, one of his friends or a member of the hospital staff will then answer his questions. . . .

Can you say more about deciding where to put your help when the family and patient are present and the need of the family is greater?

You always help the ones who need the help the most. . . .

Since you do not believe in telling a patient a concrete number of months or years of life expectancy, would you agree that it is good to tell him the chances of survival at specific periods of time such as three months, or one year, or two years, or five years?

We have found that patients who have been given a specific number of months of life expectancy, do not do well. Our prognosis is not that accurate that we can tell a patient how much time he has to live. If we tell a man that he has six months to live and he survives the six months, he is often in a very difficult predicament in that he is no longer living and not able to die. I think it is much more honest to say that we do not know, the chances look very slim at this time. If he insists on specifics, the physician should then give him some statistical approximations so that he has some idea of how long he has to put his house in order. . . .

DENIAL AS A FIRST LINE OF DEFENSE

. . . Why is it that many doctors still refuse to tell patients that they have terminal illnesses? Is this trend changing?

There are many physicians who are uncomfortable about telling their patients they are seriously ill, but the trend is changing. More and more physicians are beginning to be comfortable about this. We now have more medical schools who include the care of the dying patient in their curriculum. With medical students having had some instruction, some lectures or workshops, and some assistance during their formative years, there is a good chance that there will be more physicians in the near future who will be comfortable with dying patients. . . .

A patient with a history of cancer (surgery two years previously) is advised readmission for symptoms, but instead goes to Florida for the winter. Is this denial? His wife goes along with his decision and goes on this journey.

A patient who has had cancer two years before and has a readmission for similar symptoms probably senses that this is now a recurrence of his cancer. He also probably knows that the months, perhaps the years ahead, will be filled with hospitalizations and less and less functioning. It may be his way of saying, "Let's live it up once more. Let's get this trip to Florida in so that we can at least have a memory of having been together in Florida, a dream that we were always dreaming about but were never able to fulfill." After he has completed this unfinished business he will most likely return to the hospital and be a much better patient than if he always nostalgically thinks, "If I had only gone to Florida with my wife." It is, again, important that we do not judge these patients because they do not gratify our needs for an immediate hospitalization and that we do not necessarily label them as "denial." All that it means is that this man has made a choice; it is his choice and his right to make it. . . .

WHY ME?

Can you give a few more suggestions of how to handle a patient when he asks, "Why me?"

I tell them, "I don't know why you," but you may ask the question the other way around, "Why not you?" Since all of us have to face death and dying it has to happen to any one of us sooner or later. He is really asking, "Why is it happening to me now?" I would let him raise this question so that he will then be able to express his anger and anguish and ventilate all his feelings of dismay and other concerns. This will give you cues as to how to help him.

I am a terminally ill patient. When I first found out about my conditon I realized that my future had been taken away from me. I was very angry. Have you seen similar feelings?

Most of my patients react the same way. They are shocked and they are angry that their future has been taken away, but gradually they realize that they are still living today, that they still have a tomorrow. Because they have a limited time to live, very often they live with more intensity, with different values, and enjoy life more because they do not always plan for tomorrow and next year, the way healthy people do. . . .

THE END OF LIFE
—HOPEFULLY ACCEPTANCE

Have we really been talking about death and dying or about life and living before death occurs? I suspect that reflection on the difference will be rewarding.

When I give lectures on death and dying and share with you what we have learned from our dying patients, it is very clear to me that these are lessons for the living. It is from our dying patients that we learn the true values of life, and if we could reach the stage of acceptance in our young age, we would live a much more meaningful life, appreciate small things, and have different values. . . .

I have heard that at the end of a dying person's life, a summary of their whole life flashes before their eyes. Have you heard of this, too?

Many of my dying patients have relived experiences from their past life. I think this is a period of time when the patient has switched off all external input, when he begins to wean off, when he becomes very introspective, when he tries to remember incidents and people important to him, and when he ruminates once more about his past life in an attempt to, perhaps, summarize the value of his life and to search for meaning. We found that little significant memories and moments with loved ones help the patient most in the very final stage of his life. . . .

My parents are over sixty years of age. All their good friends seem to be dying or dead. When I visit home, my mother talks about not wanting to get old and feeble. She receives gifts and says that I should have the gifts when she is dead. I don't know what to say to my parents about such matters.

I think you should understand that it is not very pleasant to be getting old and to be losing one's friends and relatives one by one. It is understandable that many people in our society do not want to get old because they do not have large families who can care for them when they are unable to attend to their own needs. It is not very enjoyable to spend the last years of your life in a nursing home. You can empathize with your mother and try to think now of what you would do if she reaches an old age. If you hear your mother's wishes now while she can still think clearly and while you can talk about it at a rather lengthy distance from her anticipated death, things will be much easier later on. . . .

WHERE DO WE BEST CARE FOR OUR DYING PATIENTS?

A woman whose husband is dying of cancer wants him to die in the hospital so her two children will "not have to face his death." The man has made it very clear he never wants to go back to the hospital. How can I work with the wife to change her feelings about this? She will not even acknowledge his diagnosis or impending death with the children.

I do not know how old the children are, but I am a strong believer that patients should be allowed to die at home and the children should share these last few weeks or days with the father. It is important that you are not angry with his wife, who is obviously not ready for the impending death of her husband. If you really care for her, if you can spend time with her, if you can help her to express her anguish about "her husband deserting her and the children," then you may be able to help her face the reality and with some additional help of perhaps a visiting nurse and some house calls on the part of the physician, you may be able to convince this woman to help her husband to die at home. . . .

Would terminal patients be able to adjust better to impending death if they were allowed to die in their homes surrounded by the family rather than in an institution?

Most patients prefer to die at home, but there are a few who prefer to die in a hospital. Mothers, for example, who do not want to expose their children to the final crisis, or people who have been very lonely and have had poor family relationships, sometimes prefer to die in an institution. You have to evaluate each case, and if a patient prefers to die in an institution, you should not push for discharge. The majority of our patients have preferred to die at home and we make every possible arrangement to make this wish come true.

Should dying patients be segregated? By this I mean should we have special hospices or wards for dying patients?

It does not matter a great deal whether dying patients are put together on the same ward or intermixed with other patients who can get well. It is much more important how the staff feels about these patients. The general atmosphere is more important than the location of the patient. We have found special units for critically ill patients, and especially the hospice idea, extremely helpful, not so much because the patients are segregated, but because you can hand-pick a staff who is comfortable in the face of dying patients and you therefore have an environment of love, acceptance, care, and hope. Also, they eventually become specialists in terminal care, who can keep the patients physically and emotionally as well as spiritually comfortable.

67

Hospice Care

Edward J. Larschan, J.D., Ph.D.
Richard J. Larschan, Ph.D.

Source: The Diagnosis is Cancer *by Edward J. Larschan, J.D, Ph.D. with Richard J. Larschan, Ph.D., Bull Publishing Company, 1986.*

This segment is in some ways the hardest for me to write. But the reality is that for many cancer patients, including me, no cure yet exists. For us the day may come when we again must choose—not this time among different doctors and treatment centers, but between alternative settings in which to die.

In medieval times hospices were way stations generally run by religious orders which welcomed, fed and cared for travelers and pilgrims. Today that original sense of a safe refuge has a special meaning for cancer patients. The first modern hospice, St. Christopher's, was established in London in 1967 by Dr. Cicely Saunders as a humane alternative to hospitalization for those in the final stages of terminal illness. The first hospice in the United States was started along similar principles in 1974 in New Haven, Connecticut, and by 1984 there were more than 1,000 hospice programs nationwide.

As we use the term today, hospice no longer refers just to a place, but to a philosophy of care for patients for whom curative treatment is no longer possible. The Hospice of Fort Wayne, Indiana, describes it as a "special way of caring for people whose time is measured. The emphasis is on living each day as fully and comfortably as possible, surrounded by home and family." By providing physical, psychological, social and spiritual support to patients and their families, hospice strives to "control and relieve the emotional, spiritual, and physical suffering that sometimes accompanies the parting stage of life." Here is the National Hospice Organization's philosophy, as expressed by the Fort Wayne group:

> Hospice affirms life. It does not attempt to either hasten or postpone death as a natural process. The last stage of life can be a time for growing and sharing. It can be a time for cherishing, savoring and letting go. Hospice exists in the hope and belief that through education, care and sensitivity to needs, patients and families may be free to attain a degree of mental and spiritual preparation for death that is satisfactory to them. Hospice is there to support the family so that the patient can be at home in his or her familiar surroundings as much as possible.

The hospice team, comprised of physicians, nurses, social workers, psychologists, clergy and specially trained volunteers, provides most care in the patient's own home, although approximately 5 percent of the hospices are located in separate, nonhospital facilities; short hospital admissions are arranged if medically necessary. Management of pain and other symptoms of terminal illness is the primary focus of the medical treatment. Hospice physicians are not concerned about addiction and therefore supply narcotic medication regularly, without waiting for the patient to undergo extreme discomfort before doing so. No longer worried about pain,

the patient enjoys improved quality of life and increased well-being; that, in turn, permits him to concentrate on family and friends, often making acceptance of death much easier.

Emotional support to patients and their families is central to the hospice concept. A nun at a New York hospice described a form of support she found important: "Dying people often just can't let go of life . . . they hang on if something is not quite right . . . usually there's one thing that allows them to release. During the final moments, I sit with them, stroking their arm, talking, hoping to find it." Once, at the side of a man she sensed was feeling guilty, she recalls saying, "I want you to know there is a heavenly Father who loves His children, even if they sometimes get dirty hands and faces." He then relaxed visibly and a few mintes later died in peace. Religion is not the only form of comfort supplied by the hospice team, but this example, from a *New York Magazine* article by Marilyn Webb (August 1, 1983) well illustrates the kind of support provided by hospice team members.*

The team evaluates each family individually and devises a plan of care suited to the particular circumstances. Team members are available in person or by telephone 24 hours a day, 7 days a week—Helping care for and comfort the patient, sometimes staying with him so the family can attend to obligations outside the home, or else simply permitting them to get out of the house for rest and recuperation. They arrange child care, offer sympathetic understanding and companionship, and after the patient's death, help the family through bereavement.

Hospice programs exist in every state. More than half belong to the *National Hospice Organization* which has established standards to assure the highest quality of hospice care, as well as become a national clearing house for locating hospice programs. During 1984 the NHO published a directory of more than 1,000 programs, entitled *Hospice Coast to Coast,* available through NHO headquarters.

Increasingly, expenses of hospice care are being covered by private insurance carriers. Medicare has paid for hospice care since November, 1983, under Part A, the hospital insurance program. Covered services under Medicare include physician and nursing services, medical appliances and supplies (including outpatient drugs for symptom management and pain relief), home health aide and home-

---

*Excerpts from "The Hospice Way of Death," by Marilyn Webb, reprinted with the permission of New York Magazine.

maker services, therapies, medical social services, counseling, and required short-term in-hospital care. These benefits extend for two 90-day periods and one 30-day period (a lifetime maximum of 210 days) for patients who qualify under Medicare Part A, are certified by their doctor and the director of the Medicare certified hospice program to be terminally ill, and who elect hospice care. These and additional matters regarding Medicare coverage, individual, group, and disability insurance, taxes, and other practical considerations are discussed at greater length in *The Diagnosis is Cancer* by Edward J. Larschan, JD, Ph.D.

68

The Living Will

Edward J. Larschan, J.D., Ph.D.
Richard J. Larschan, Ph.D.

Source: The Diagnosis is Cancer *by Edward J. Larschan, J.D, Ph.D. with Richard J. Larschan, Ph.D., Bull Publishing Company, 1986.*

As we all know, recent 'advances' in medical technology have made it possible for the heart and lungs to be kept going even after disease or accident has caused the brain to stop functioning. As a result, more and more people are concerned about the question of how they will die. Documents called *Living Wills* have therefore been developed to let people decide, while they are still healthy, or at least mentally competent, the extent to which drugs or equipment should be used to prolong their lives artificially once recovery is no longer really possible.

Living Wills are based on the right to privacy found in the U.S. Constitution, and the right to bodily self-determination as found in the common law (previous court decisions). For example, as early as 1891, the U.S. Supreme Court stated that, "No right is held more sacred, or is more carefully guarded, by the common law, than the right of every individual to the possession and control of his own person." In another instance, the highest court in New York held that, "a competent adult has a right to determine whether or not to undergo medical treatment." The right of patients to refuse medical treatment, even when life-sustaining, was emphasized by the President's Commission for the Study of Ethical Problems in Medicine and Biomedical and Behavioral Research in 1983.

So widespread is concern among Americans on this issue that, as of August 1985, 36 jurisdictions (including Washington, D.C.) have "Right to Die" legislation in effect. Approximately 9 of the remaining 15 states have laws pending—namely, Hawaii, Massachusetts, Minnesota, New Jersey, New York, Ohio, Pennsylvania, Rhode Island and South Carolina. The only hold-outs are: Alaska, Kentucky, Michigan, Nevada, North Dakota and South Dakota.

According to the *Society for the Right to Die,* Virginia's 1983 "Natural Death Act" "is one of the best living will laws to be enacted to date" (except that it imposes no penalty upon a doctor who refuses to comply with the patient's wishes, or to transfer the patient to another doctor). I have chosen it to illustrate efforts by one state to grant to its citizens the right to a natural death. Quoted are only those parts of the statute that give an idea of its scope and intent:

It declares that "all competent adults have the fundamental right to control the decisions relating to their own medical care, including the decision to have medical or surgical means or procedures calculated to prolong their lives provided, withheld or withdrawn." And specifically, it asserts that "the artificial prolongation of life for persons with a ter-

minal condition may cause loss of individual dignity and secure only a precarious and burdensome existence, while providing nothing medically necessary or beneficial to the patient." For which reasons, the statute provides that "a competent adult" has the right "to make an oral or written declaration instructing his physician to withhold or withdraw life prolonging procedures or to designate another to make the treatment decision for him, in the event such person is diagnosed as suffering from a terminal condition."

If such a declaration is in writing, it must "be signed by the declarant in the presence of two subscribing witnesses. An oral declaration may be made . . . in the presence of a physician and two witnesses." The declaration is fully revocable at any time "when communicated to the attending physician." And also quite significant, a *Living Will* declaration "shall not, for any purpose, constitute a suicide. Nor . . . affect . . . the terms of . . . life insurance."

A few states define "Brain Death," which is important in decisions regarding discontinuance of artificial life-support systems. Virginia does not define brain death, but North Carolina, for instance, does—as indicated in the following excerpt from the North Carolina Right to Natural Death Act:

The determination that a person is dead shall be made by a physician . . . applying ordinary and accepted standards of medical practice. Brain death, defined as irreversible cessation of total brain function, may be used as a sole basis for the determination that a person has died, particularly when brain death occurs in the presence of artificially maintained respiratory and circulatory functions. This specific recognition of brain death as a criterion of death of the person shall not preclude the use of other medically recognized criteria for determining whether and when a person has died.

Concern For Dying: An Educational Council, has been exploring the complex moral, religious, medical, legal and humanitarian aspects of the "Right to Die" issue. They will send, free of charge, a model "Living Will" for use in jurisdictions which don't have "Right to Die" laws. They also provide model "Living Wills" that meet the requirements where such legislation does exist. Their literature includes, along with the model "Living Will," supportive opinions from Popes John Paul II and Pius XII, as well as Protestant and Jewish leaders.

Concern for Dying has established a Living Will Registry—a computerized system where a copy

My Living Will
To My Family, My Physician, My Lawyer and All Others Whom It May Concern

Death is as much a reality as birth, growth, maturity and old age—it is the one certainty of life. If the time comes when I can no longer take part in decisions for my own future, let this statement stand as an expression of my wishes and directions, while I am still of sound mind.

If at such a time the situation should arise in which there is no reasonable expectation of my recovery from extreme physical or mental disability, I direct that I be allowed to die and not be kept alive by medications, artificial means or "heroic measures". I do, however, ask that medication be mercifully administered to me to alleviate suffering even though this may shorten my remaining life.

This statement is made after careful consideration and is in accordance with my strong convictions and beliefs. I want the wishes and directions here expressed carried out to the extent permitted by law. Insofar as they are not legally enforceable, I hope that those to whom this Will is addressed will regard themselves as morally bound by these provisions.

(Optional specific provisions to be made in this space — see other side)

DURABLE POWER OF ATTORNEY (optional)

I hereby designate _____ to serve as my attorney-in-fact for the purpose of making medical treatment decisions. This power of attorney shall remain effective in the event that I become incompetent or otherwise unable to make such decisions for myself.

Optional Notarization:

"Sworn and subscribed to

before me this _____ day

of _____, 19_____."

_____
Notary Public
(seal)

Signed_____

Date _____

Witness _____

_____
Address

Witness _____

_____
Address

Copies of this request have been given to _____

_____   _____

(Optional)   My Living Will is registered with Concern for Dying (No. _____)

TO MAKE BEST USE OF YOUR LIVING WILL

You may wish to add specific statements to the Living Will *in the space provided for that purpose above your signature.* Possible additional provisions are:

1. "Measures of artificial life-support in the face of impending death that I specifically refuse are:

   a) Electrical or mechanical resuscitation of my heart when it has stopped beating.

   b) Nasogastric tube feeding when I am paralyzed or unable to take nourishment by mouth.

   c) Mechanical respiration when I am no longer able to sustain my own breathing.

   d) _____

2. "I would like to live out my last days at home rather than in a hospital if it does not jeopardize the chance of my recovery to a meaningful and sentient life or does not impose an undue burden on my family."

3. "If any of my tissues are sound and would be of value as transplants to other people, I freely give my permission for such donation."

The optional Durable Power of Attorney feature allows you to name someone else to serve as your proxy in case you are unable to communicate your wishes. Should you choose to fill in this portion of the document, you must have your signature notarized.

If you choose more than one proxy for decision-making on your behalf, please give order of priority (1, 2, 3, etc.).

Space is provided at the bottom of the Living Will for notarization should you choose to have your Living Will witnessed by a Notary Public.

Reprinted with permission of Concern for Dying, 250 West 57th Street, Room 831, New York, NY 10107, (212) 246-6962.

---

of your Living Will is kept on file in their New York office. They review your Living Will to see it is filled out correctly, assign a Registry Number and retain a copy. *Concern for Dying* can answer questions you may have about procedures and options, offering the latest information about laws in your state. (Remember, every state has different legal requirements!) For a one-time enrollment fee of $25, in addition to the Registry and information services, you also receive a credit-card-size plastic mini-Will containing your address, *Concern for Dying*'s address, a short version of the Living Will and the fact that you have already prepared a full-sized and witnessed Living Will. Of course, like other important aspects of your treatment, it makes sense to discuss the entire matter with your doctor.

The *Society for the Right to Die* also provides Living Will Declarations for jurisdictions both with and without Right to Die statutes. Copies may be obtained at no charge by writing to them at 250 West 57th Street, New York, NY 10107; telephone: (212) 246-6973. This thoroughly professional organization is well worth contacting if you're in any way concerned about the 'dying with dignity' issue.

7

Cancer Prevention and Early Detection

69

Practicing Cancer Prevention

Mark Renneker, M.D.

This chapter focuses on how to actually prevent cancer. As presented earlier in this book (see Chapter 2—Principles of Cancer Prevention), cancer prevention is easiest to understand if thought of in terms of primary cancer prevention (to prevent cancer from ever developing) and secondary cancer prevention (early detection of cancer—finding it before symptoms have developed, when it is most curable).

PRACTICING PRIMARY CANCER PREVENTION

Some people don't believe that cancer can be prevented. Could you convince a skeptic? What would be your answer to the question, "What cancers can be completely prevented (i.e., with primary prevention)? What examples would you use?

Let's practice—these are things you should know.

Start by choosing a factor that is known to cause cancer, for instance smoking, and then list the types of cancer associated with that factor. Do that for every cancer-causing factor you can think of and soon you'll have a list of cancers that can be largely prevented—that you can substantially lower your risk of developing.

If you've read the parts of this book on the causes of cancer, and on the major sites of cancer, this is what your list should look like:

1. SMOKING: cancers of the mouth (lip, tongue, gums, cheek, floor, roof), throat, larynx, lung, kidney, bladder, esophagus, stomach, pancreas, and possibly cervix and some leukemias.

2. SMOKELESS TOBACCO: cancers of the mouth, and possibly esophagus and stomach.

3. OBESITY: cancers of the colon and rectum, breast, prostate, gallbladder, ovary, and uterus.

4. HIGH-FAT DIET: cancers of the colon and rectum, breast, gallbladder, uterus, prostate, and testes.

5. LOW-FIBER DIET: cancers of the colon and rectum.

6. LOW INTAKE OF VITAMIN A (beta carotene) & VITAMIN C: cancers of the larynx, esophagus, stomach, colon-rectum, prostate, bladder, lung, and possibly cervix.

7. PRESERVED FOODS (nitrate-cured, salt-cured, smoked): cancers of the esophagus and stomach.

8. ALCOHOL: cancers of the mouth, throat, larynx, esophagus, liver, and probably breast.

9. VIRUSES (human papilloma/venereal warts, hepatitis B, Epstein Barr, HIV, and others): cancers of the cervix, liver, naso-pharynx, some lymphomas and leukemias, and the AIDS-related cancers.

10. PARASITES: cancers of the liver and bladder.

11. SEXUAL PRACTICES: cancers of the cervix, penis, anus, and the AIDS-related cancers.

12. REPRODUCTIVE FACTORS: cancers of the breast and ovary.

13. OCCUPATIONAL: cancers of the skin, lung, liver, and kidney.

14. ULTRAVIOLET RADIATION (i.e., the sun): cancers of the skin, including melanomas.

15. IONIZING RADIATION (i.e., medical radiation): cancers of the thyroid, skin, and possibly the testes, ovary, breast, and some leukemias.

16. MEDICAL PRACTICE (i.e., iatrogenesis): cancers of the uterus and vagina (estrogens), and those that are medical radiation-related.

The list could also include factors that are chiefly protective, such as a high-intake of cruciferous vegetables and of fiber, and possibly exercise. Also not on the list are less agreed upon causative factors, like coffee.

PRACTICING SECONDARY CANCER PREVENTION

If you do have a cancer developing, it will take conscious effort on your part to find it early. You will need to correctly examine yourself for those cancers you are at risk for, and be sure to have a physician or other health professional double-check your self-examinations, as well as provide examinations that you can't perform on yourself.

The potential self- (and maternal) examinations include:

1. Skin self-examination

2. Lymph node self-examination

3. Mouth self-examination

4. Thyroid self-examination

5. Breast self-examination

6. Testicular self-examination

7. Vulvar and vaginal self-examination

8. Anal and rectal self-examination

9. Prostate self-examination

10. Self-testing for blood in the stool

11. Infant exam by mother

Each of these methods will be described in detail in the following chapter(s).

The components of a physician's standard checkup that may result in the detection of early, asymptomatic cancers include direct inspection and/or palpation of the:

skin	vulva, vagina, cervix (including Pap smear and pelvic)
lymph nodes	
oral cavity	
thyroid	testes
breast	anus, rectum
	prostate

Depending upon age, sex, and medical history, other procedures that may be recommended include:

mammography

sigmoidoscopy

sputum cytology

endometrial biopsy

There is little agreement from specialty to specialty, and country to country, on cancer screening tests. For the Pap smear, for example, the recommendation of the Canadian Task Force on the Periodic Health Examination (1979) is for Pap smears to be done every three years from the age of sexual activity until age 35, and every five years thereafter. On the other hand, the American College of Obstetrics and Gynecology recommends annual Pap smears for all women.

The American Cancer Society issues its own recommendations. The most recent set of American Cancer Society guidelines for cancer checkups were issued in 1980, refined somewhat in 1984-85 and 1987, and may be modified in the future—but they are likely to remain the "gold standard" for our country for some years to come. This book supports the American Cancer Society cancer checkup recommendations.

PRACTICING CANCER PREVENTION

A Personal, Family, and Community Cancer Prevention Plan

Awareness is only the beginning; it's what you do with that awareness that makes a difference. It's time to take what you've learned about cancer and its prevention and apply it to yourself and those around you.

Each person should have a personal cancer prevention plan. You should know which cancers you are at risk for. Are any of the cancers in your family (even back to your grandparents) the genetic or familial type? At anytime in your life, have you had significant exposure to cancer-causing substances? What are your present health habits? Do you use tobacco? How does your diet compare to the cancer-risk reducing diet described in this book? Do you examine yourself, or have the necessary tests done, for those cancers you are at risk for? A personal cancer prevention plan is a personal action plan.

Develop a cancer prevention plan for your family. Does anyone in the family smoke? If so, they are jeopardizing the health of the rest of the family. Whoever prepares the food should become particularly knowledgeable about cancer risk lowering through diet and nutrition. If you have a choice about where your family will live, choosing a clean, nonpolluted location should be a priority.

Finally, be aware of the fact that many solutions to the cancer problem depend on a community cancer prevention plan. Consider volunteering with the American Cancer Society. With what you've learned from this book alone, you could help develop (or give) educational programs for schools, businesses, and other community organizations. Political awareness and action is a large part of a community cancer prevention plan.

Do you worry that the factory just down the road from you is spewing cancer-causing chemicals into the river, or contaminating the ground water? Is your worksite safe? Is your child's school asbestos-free? Find out—for your own benefit, for your family, and for the people around you. Take action if it is needed. That's practicing cancer prevention.

In 1981, after studying at length all available research data on cancer screening, the American Cancer Society released the following guidelines. Significantly, chest x-rays were no longer recommended, Pap smears were no longer automatically recommended yearly, and mammography was recommended with greater frequency.

The guidelines were modified in 1985, 1987 and 1989, and will no doubt require future modifications.

Bear in mind that these guidelines are for the screening of asymptomatic people, and do not account for possible significant factors in a person's medical history.

Test or Procedure	Sex	Age	Frequency
Chest x-ray		—not recommended—	
Sputum cytology		—not recommended—	
Sigmoid-oscopy	M&F	over 50	after 2 neg. exams 1 year apart
Stool hidden blood slide test	M&F	over 50	every year
Digital rectal examination	M&F	over 40	every year
Pap test	F	all women 18 or older; all women who are sexually active	yearly, after 3 negative exams, may be less frequent
Pelvic examination	F	20–40 over 40	every 3 years every year
Endometrial tissue sample (biopsy)	F	at menopause women at high risk[1]	at menopause
Breast self examination	F	over 20	every month
Breast physical examination	F	20–40 over 40	every 3 years every year
Mammography	F	between 35–39 40–49 over 50	baseline every 1–2 years every year
Health counseling and cancer checkup[2]	M&F M&F	over 20 over 40	every 3 years every year

[1] history of infertility, obesity, failure of ovulation, abnormal uterine bleeding, or estrogen therapy.
[2] to include examination for cancers of the thyroid, testicles, prostate, ovaries, lymph nodes, oral region, and skin.

70

Self-Examination
for Cancer

Mark Renneker, M.D.

This chapter presents a complete set of cancer self-examination procedures, some better known than others. With the exception of breast
self-examination, none have had extensive study as to effectiveness.
But the fact remains that patients—not doctors—more often find their
own cancers. Until that situation changes, knowledge and practice of
cancer self-examination will remain the cornerstone of a personal cancer prevention and early detection plan.

Decide on your use of the following self-examination procedures
on the basis of your age, sex, risk factors, and the American Cancer
Society guidelines for cancer checkups (listed in the previous chapter).

SKIN SELF-EXAMINATION

For Men and Women of All Ages, Particularly if Light-Skinned and Over 30

Cancer of the skin is the easiest to detect of all cancers, the simplest to treat, and has the highest overall cure rate. Most physicians do not examine their patients' skin very thoroughly—you can do a much better job.

Skin self-examination involves examining 100% of your skin, head-to-toe. You should particularly focus on sun-exposed areas like the forehead, nose, lips, cheeks, tops of the ears, back of the neck, upper chest, shoulders, arms, and backs of the hands.*

As with any self-examination method, you are looking for a change—and to know if there has been a change, you need to know what's normal for you.

General skin changes to look for include loss of normal skin markings, change in color, or toughening of the skin. Later signs include rough areas and small pits (ulcers) that may scab and crust, and fail to heal in less than a month.

All skin cancers begin as small, painless growths. With time, some skin cancers become hard, raised, red or red-gray, pearly or shiny, and may have faint red or purplish veins on or around them (basal cell skin cancer); others become ulcerated, with scaling, crusting, oozing, or bleeding, with a rolled, irregular border (squamous cell skin cancer); and still others may begin as a small mole which is asymmetric, has an irregular border, multiple colors (e.g., black, red, pink, orange, blue, brown, tan, and white), and quickly grows larger (malignant melanoma).

1. To properly perform skin self-examination you need to be in a well-lighted room (usually the bathroom or bedroom) that has a large mirror (full-length is best). You will need a small hand-mirror and, if available, a magnifying glass. Undress completely. Plan to spend about five minutes.

2. Get to know what your skin generally looks like. First scan your skin, overall. Use the mirrors to assist you in places you can't directly see. Notice the different tones and color of your skin. What areas seem to be receiving the most sun? What areas seem to be aging faster than others? Where are your most prominent moles—and how many moles do you have?

*Additional information on how to spot a skin cancer is in Chapter 21—Skin Cancer.

3. Then begin a systematic examination, starting with your hands. Slowly work your way up your arms to your shoulders. Turn your hands and arms so that you can see every side. Use the magnifying glass to examine any suspicious moles or spots. Run your hands up and down your arms, and over your shoulders—sometimes you'll feel rough areas that you can't see. These are usually keratoses, which may be harmless seborrheic keratoses (greasy feeling, often dark in color, they seem to be stuck-on), pre-cancerous actinic keratoses (red, scaling rough patches), or both.

4. Now move in front of the mirror—get the light right—and closely look at your face and neck. This is the most important part of skin self-examination—you're examining the part of the body where the most skin cancers and pre-skin cancers are found. Start at the hairline. Begin scanning back-and-forth horizontally, and slowly work your way down over the forehead, eyes, temples, cheeks, nose, lips, and mouth. Men should be sure to check the skin under their side-burns and any facial hair. Finally, gently run your fingers over your face, feeling for rough areas. And don't forget to look and feel over the ears, under the chin, and across the neck.

5. Do you have any bumps or rough spots on your scalp, that you perhaps notice when you wash or brush your hair? Any bald spots? To see much of your scalp you'll need one or both of the mirrors. Also, you may want to use a hair dryer on a cool setting to lift the hair from the scalp so you can more closely examine it.

6. Use both mirrors to examine the back of the neck and shoulders. This is also a high-risk area, because of the beating it takes from the sun.

7. Use both mirrors to examine the entire length of your back, your buttocks, and down the back of your legs. Ask your partner or a friend to assist you in looking at any suspicious areas.

8. Directly examine the fronts of your legs and feet. If necessary, use a mirror to see the bottom of your feet and between your toes. Look for any dark spots under the toenails (and fingernails), which could be the first sign of a malignant melanoma. Also, run your hands over your lower legs to feel for any rough areas (as with the arms).

9. Consider choosing your ten largest or most peculiar moles to specially check. If you think a mole may be growing larger, measure it with a good ruler, and take comparison measurements in

a month. Consider making a "mole map" to remember which ones you've chosen to follow, and as a place to record your measurements. You could even photograph your moles. [Note: If a mole appears for the first time when you are an adult, it deserves close attention—however small it is.]

10.   Examine your skin with your memory— are there areas where you had a blistering sunburn or radiation? Always be sure to check those areas. Especially watch for new moles or rough spots.

LYMPH NODE SELF-EXAMINATION

For All Men and Women, Particularly Between 20 and 40, or At Risk For AIDS

Lymph nodes (sometimes referred to as "glands") are small bean-shaped structures located throughout the body. As part of the immune system, they usually swell in reaction to bacteria, viruses, or cancer. Painless enlargement of lymph nodes is often the first sign of blood-borne cancers like leukemia, cancer of the lymph nodes (lymphoma, including Hodgkin's Disease), and of infection by the human immunodeficiency virus. Lymph node enlargement from most of the major cancers, like lung and breast, is not an early sign, and represents advanced disease.*

Exploring for lymph nodes can be difficult. Most nodes will probably be too small to be detected by your examining fingers. Of those that can be felt, most will be bean-sized (less than one centimeter in diameter) and represent old or recent infection, and only rarely cancer.

The head and neck is where the most lymph nodes are accessible to self-examination. People with a history of severe ear or throat infections (i.e., from childhood) will often have permanently enlarged neck nodes. The other major areas to examine are the axilla (armpits), and groin.

Lymph node self-examination should be done monthly. Do it standing or lying. Try to spend about three minutes on the head-and-neck region, and one minute for each armpit (and arm) and each side of the groin (and leg). Use visual inspection, as well as feeling with the pads of your fingers.

*For additional information, read the chapters on the immune system, lymphoma, and AIDS.

To find a lymph node you need to "trap" it. Concentrate on moving the skin over the underlying tissues, rather than moving your fingers over the skin. Again, you are seeking to notice a change from what your lymph nodes normally feel like.

In sequence, check for the following nodes (see Figures 70-1, 70-2, 70-3):

1.   Pre-auricular—in front of the ear.

2.   Posterior auricular—in back of the ear.

3.   Occipital—at each side of the base of the skull. These nodes are hard to find.

4.   Tonsillar—at the angle of the jawbone (mandible).

5.   Submaxillary—half-way between the ear and chin. (Note: to feel the tonsillar and submaxillary nodes you may need to cock your head to the side, as if you were trying to hold a telephone to your shoulder, and run your fingers out from under the tucked-in jawbone and try to trap the node against it.)

6.   Submental—in midline, an inch or so back from the tip of the chin.

7.   Superficial cervical chain—overlying the strong, frontal neck muscles (sternocleidomastoids) and the easy-to-feel pulsating carotid artery. This

Figure 70-1 The lymph nodes of the neck. *Illustration reprinted with permission from Barbara Bates, M.D.,* A Guide to Physical Examination, *J.B. Lippincott Company, Philadelphia, PA. 1974.*

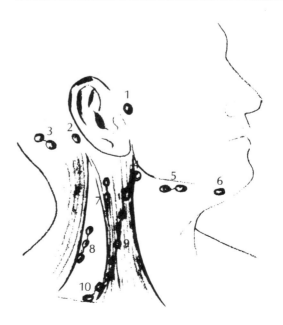

Figure 70-2 Lymph nodes of the breast, axillae, and clavicular region. *Illustration reprinted with permission from Barbara Bates, M.D., A Guide to Physical Examination, J.B. Lippincott Company, Philadelphia, PA. 1974.*

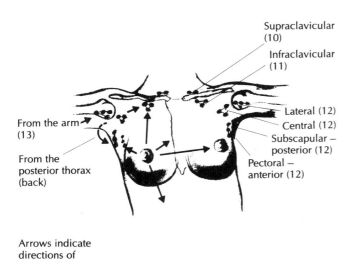

Supraclavicular (10)
Infraclavicular (11)
From the arm (13)
From the posterior thorax (back)
Lateral (12)
Central (12)
Subscapular – posterior (12)
Pectoral – anterior (12)

Arrows indicate directions of lymph flow

Figure 70-3 The inguinal (groin) lymph nodes. *Illustration reprinted with permission from Barbara Bates, M.D., A Guide to Physical Examination, J.B. Lippincott Company, Philadelphia, PA. 1974. Used with permission.*

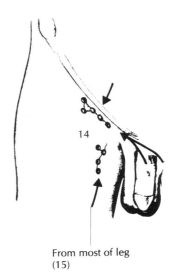

14

From most of leg (15)

is a long chain of nodes, running from below the ear down to the collarbone. Note: if equal masses can be felt on both sides of the neck, they are probably not lymph nodes—they may be the hard, movable cartilage and bones surrounding the Adam's apple.

8. Posterior cervical chain—along the front edge of the trapezius muscle (the back-of-the-neck muscle that is often sore from work and stress) is a three to four-inch chain of nodes. Most people can feel at least one node in this area.

9. Deep cervical chain—under the sternocleidomastoid muscle, these nodes are inaccessible to examination unless you hook your thumb and fingers around the muscle to find them.

10. Supraclavicular—running along the top of the collar bone.

11. Infraclavicular—running just under the collar bone.

12. Axillary—with one arm relaxed at your side, or resting on a desk or counter (if sitting), and using your opposite hand, cup together your fingers and reach high into the arm pit and slowly and gently slide your fingers down under the pectoralis muscle, and along the edge of your breast. Lotion or cream may help give you a finer touch. Women sometimes have permanently enlarged nodes (or scar tissue) here from previous infections of the axillary sweat glands.

13. Elbow—nestled in a pocket just above the inner knob of the elbow. These nodes are rarely felt.

14. Inguinal—to each side of the hard pubic bone (above your genitalia) are a chain of nodes that run diagonally four inches or so up each side of your groin and down the inner side of your leg. If you've had herpes, your inguinal nodes may be permanently hard and enlarged. An infection in the foot or leg may cause swollen, tender inguinal nodes.

15. Popliteal fossa—at the back of the knee (where it bends, alongside the tendons of the hamstring muscles). Only rarely can nodes be felt in this area.

MOUTH SELF-EXAMINATION

For Men and Women, Especially Tobacco Users and Drinkers

It's easy to examine your oral cavity—all you need is a good light and a mirror. Do it monthly—it only takes about a minute.

Early changes in the mouth suggestive of cancer or pre-cancer are painless white patches (leukoplakia) or red patches (erythroplasia). Signs of irritation in the mouth, for instance from tobacco or alcohol, are generalized inflammation (redness). Check for irritation from dentures or dental bridges (if present) or sharp or broken teeth. Also, the early signs of Kaposi's sarcoma (i.e., AIDS) are purplish spots on the roof of the mouth.

1. Position yourself in front of your bathroom mirror. Shine light into your mouth (either directly or reflected off the mirror). You may want to purchase and use a small dental mirror (found in most drug stores)—keep it from fogging by heating it or by applying a thin coat of soap, and then wiping it off.

2. First look at your mouth. How do your lips look? Are there any sores that you've gotten used to—that have been there for some weeks?

3. Use your thumb and index finger to take hold of the middle of your lower lip from the inside and outside. You want to be pinching it between your fingers, as you would an earring. Then, slide your fingers down the length of your lip towards your left cheek, then sweep over the entire area of the cheek up to the upper lip. Then sweep back down to the lower lip again, and start up the opposite cheek to the upper lip on that side. You are feeling for any lumps, unusual thicknesses, or sore spots in your lips.

4. Now use your fingers to roll out the lips and cheeks to look at the mucosal lining of the mouth. This is where you are looking for red or white patches. You'll probably see whitish ridges along the inside of the cheek where your teeth sometimes bite it.

5. Raise your tongue to the roof of your mouth (or lift it with the end of your toothbrush) so you can see under it. It's common to have small purplish bumps there, and some people have paired midline bony knobs there and on the roof of the mouth (called torus palatinus).

6. Inspect the roof of the mouth by holding your head back, and then get a look down the back of your throat. Your tonsils are mid-way back, and are at the base of each side of the arch that divides your mouth and throat. They are commonly red, swollen, and scarred from prior infection. The uvula is the little thing that hangs down from the back of the throat that waves around when you breath in and out.

7. Finally, inspect your tongue—the top, sides, and underside. Use your two fingers again to examine its entire thickness.

Do lymph node self-examination (described above) with your mouth self-examination. Read Chapter 31—Cancer of the Mouth and Throat for additional information.

THYROID SELF-EXAM

For All Men and Women, Particularly With a History of Irradiation

The thyroid gland is located in the neck, just below the Adam's apple (thyroid cartilage) and just above the notch formed by the joining of the collarbones (clavicles) and the top of the breast bone (sternum). The thyroid gland is shaped like a butterfly, measures only about three inches across, and feels like tender, pounded-thin veal. (See Figure 70-4).

You can easily learn how to check your thyroid gland. Do it monthly. It only takes about a minute.*

1. Stand in front of your bathroom mirror and watch the thyroid area when you take a swallow of water. A slight bulge can usually be seen to rise up from the sternal notch when you swallow. Get the lighting just right, so you can best see, and do it again. Is the bulge more to one side, or does it seem particularly prominent? If so, that may be abnormal. Check by feeling it with your fingers.

2. Using either hand, place your fingers in the area of the thyroid and gently press backwards, against the windpipe. You're feeling for the isthmus of your thyroid (see Figure 70-4). If you are pressing too hard, you'll feel like gagging or coughing. You can only feel the thyroid if you press gently.

*For additional information, read Chapter 38—Thyroid and Other Endocrine Gland Cancers.

Figure 70-4 Anatomy of the neck, showing structure around the thyroid. *Illustration reprinted with permission from Barbara Bates, M.D., A Guide to Physical Examination, J.B. Lippincott Company, Philadelphia, PA. 1974.*

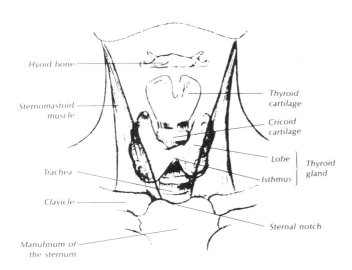

Hyoid bone

Sternomastoid muscle

Thyroid cartilage

Cricoid cartilage

Lobe

Isthmus } *Thyroid gland*

Trachea

Clavicle

Sternal notch

Manubrium of the sternum

3. Let your fingers slide to the side of the windpipe, under the front edge of the sternocleido-mastoid muscle. That's where the lobes of the thyroid lie. They'll be harder to feel than the isthmus.

4. You shouldn't feel any lumps in the thyroid, but if you do, and there are many oatmeal-like lumps, that's probably only a type of goiter. A hard, single lump is of concern. Have it checked out.

[Note: the next time you see your health provider, ask them to double-check your thyroid exam.]

BREAST SELF-EXAMINATION (BSE)

For Women of All Ages, Particularly if Over 30

In late 1987, the American Cancer Society began teaching a new, more effective breast self-examination procedure. The procedure described below combines the new ACS method with pointers that have proven useful in teaching women BSE at the Cancer Education and Prevention Center of Merritt Hospital, Oakland, California.

If you have a regular menstrual cycle, examine your breasts at the end of your menstrual period—when they will be less tender and swollen. If you do not have menstrual periods, choose one day of the month to be your BSE day, for example, the first day of the month or the day of your birthday.

The important thing is to develop a habit of BSE—the same day each month, lying in the same position, using the same starting point, and so on.

1. At least once per month, stand in front of a mirror and inspect your breasts. Spend about one minute. Begin with your arms at your sides (Figure 70-5), then elevate your arms and turn side-to-side so you can see all of your breast (fig. 70-6). Finish by leaning forward and pressing into your hips with your hands (fig. 70-7). You are looking for any changes in the skin (dimpling, puckering, redness, rash) or changes in the size or shape of the breast or nipple.

2. Lie down somewhere comfortable and where you won't be disturbed, for instance in or on your bed, or on the bathroom floor. Some women may be able to perform BSE in the bath, if they can position their breasts correctly. (Note: it is no longer recommended that BSE be done standing in the shower.) This part of the exam can be done right after your visual inspection, or separately.

3. Let's arbitrarily start with the left breast. Position the left breast so that it is maximally flattened and spread out over your chest. Placing your left arm behind your head will help, and so will turning your body to the right (Figure 70-8).

Figures 70-5 to 70-12 Steps in doing breast self-examinations. Illustrations by Ken Miller.

Figure 70-5

Figure 70-6

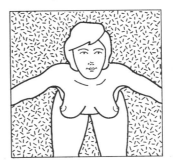

Figure 70-7

Figure 70-8

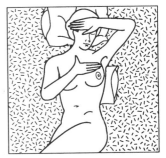

Area to be examined

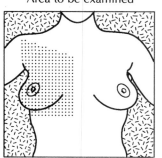

Verticle strip examination method

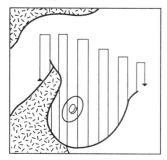

Circular examination method

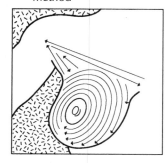

Wedge examination method

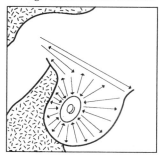

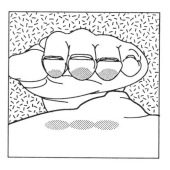

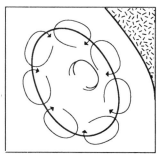

Large-breasted women may need to use their right hand to hold up the side of their left breast, or need to place a pillow under their left shoulder.

4. Choose where to start your exam based on the pattern of search you think will work best for you. All are effective if 100% of the breast is examined (Figure 70-9).

5. Place the pads of the middle three fingers of your left hand (Figure 70-10) on your left breast. Many breast specialists recommend using body lotion or oil to allow your fingers to slide more easily. Soapy water works well if you are in the bath.

6. Move your fingers in small dime-sized circles or in a careful sliding motion if you are using lotion or soapy water. Just be sure that every inch of tissue is examined. Use varying pressures to feel: (1) just under the skin (light-pressure); (2) into the breast gland tissue (firmer pressure); and (3) down to the chest wall (deep pressure). But don't press so hard that it hurts—that might discourage you from doing BSE in the future (Figure 70-11).

7. The last step (with each breast) is to check for any discharge from your nipple. Many women have a scant amount of whitish discharge that col-

lects on their nipple—and that's probably normal for them. But if there is a bloody or foul-smelling discharge, that's abnormal. To do the A+ breast self-exam, you'll milk your breast to check for discharge. Women who have breast-fed will know what this means: to ring your hand around your breast, and slowly squeeze out towards the nipple (Figure 70-12).

8. Reverse position to check your right breast. Spend at least two minutes per breast. Do it by the clock, or set a timer if necessary. Spend longer if you have large breasts.

9. When you are getting started in learning BSE, repeat your exam as often as necessary— daily or weekly—to find out what is normal for you. Is one breast just naturally larger, or more sensitive in some places? Do you have lumpy breasts? (Note: breasts are made of gland, muscle, fiberous tissue, and fat, and they are naturally lumpy—but most women don't know that, having probably never felt another woman's breasts.) You need to memorize the feel of your lumpiness. If you find a lump or groups of lumps in one breast, you'll probably find nearly the same lumpiness in the same area of the other breast. Some women draw a map or write down their findings.

10. After learning what's normal for you, do your breast self-exam monthly. Changes will be harder to notice if you do your BSE more frequently than once-a-month. Report any problems or changes to your health professional without delay. Also, have them periodically evaluate your BSE technique to be sure you are doing it correctly.*

---

*For additional information, read Chapter 24—Breast Cancer.

Figure 70-12

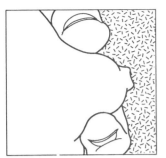

TESTICULAR SELF-EXAMINATION (TSE)

For All Men, Particularly if Caucasian and Between 20 and 40

While cancer of the testes is relatively uncommon, accounting for less than 1% of cancers in men, it is one of the most common cancers in young men in the 20 to 35 age group. There are also a number of relatively common benign swellings and tumors in and around the testes which must be differentiated from cancer, making TSE an especially important procedure to do.

As is the case with women and breast cancer, most testicular cancers are first discovered by the patient rather than the physician. Since testicular cancers found early and treated promptly have excellent chances for cure, learning how to examine your testes properly can help save your life. It really doesn't take much effort to search for those small lumps, and you only have to do it once a month. Use the simple TSE procedure shown below:

1.   The best time to examine your testes is right after a hot bath or shower. The scrotal skin is most relaxed at this time, and the contents can be felt more easily. Do it while standing or lying down.

2.   Each testicle should be examined separately. Use your right hand to check your right testicle and vice versa. Place your index and middle fingers on the underside of the testicle and your thumb on top. Gently roll your testicle between your thumb and fingers, being sure to examine the entire area of each testicle. (See Figure 70-13.)

Figure 70-13 Testicular Self-Examination. *Illustration reprinted with permission from Barbara Bates, M.D., A Guide to Physical Examination, J.B. Lippincott Company, Philadelphia, PA. 1974.*

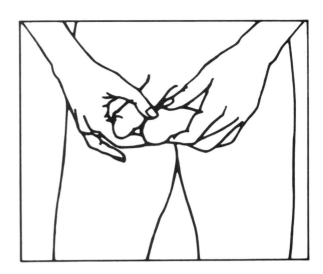

3.   What you are feeling for is any change or difference in your testicles—particularly by comparing one testicle to the other. Testicular size varies in males. And there may be a natural difference in size between the right and left testicle. Also, the left usually hangs lower than the right. You need to know the normal state of your testicles before you can notice abnormal changes.

4.   Feel for size, shape, consistency, sensitivity to pressure, and compare the left to the right testes.

5.   Do this once a month, or more frequently if you like. It should only take 30 seconds to 1 minute per testicle. There are not significant cyclic hormonal changes (size, cysts, sensitivity, etc.) in testes as there are with breasts. (See Figure 70-14.)

6.   A cancer of the testes most often begins as a painless, isolated, pea-like bump on one testicle. It would feel like a small pebble embedded in the surface of the testicle. Or, if you imagine the testicle as a grape, you are delicately feeling over its surface as if to find the stem—if it were still in place (and that would be the cancerous nodule). You shouldn't be pressing so hard that it hurts—cancer grows on the surface of the testicle, and less so inside of it, and it is easily felt. Occasionally, a person with testicular cancer may have a dragging or aching sensation in the groin or scrotum. Pain is a late symptom.

Figure 70-14 Testicular Anatomy.

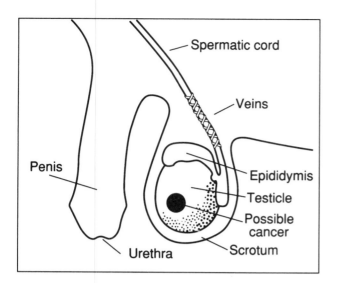

Figure 70-15 Vaginal Self-Examination. *Source:* "Doing your Own Vaginal Self-Exam," by Carol Berry. *Medical Self-Care—Access to Medical Tools, #3 Winter 1977/78,* Box 717, Inverness, Calif. 94937. Used with permission.

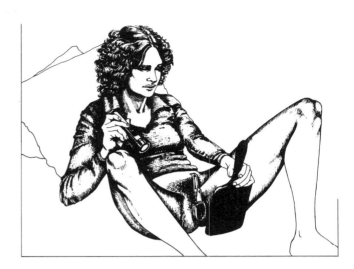

7.   Please be aware that the majority of testicular changes are not cancer; for instance, a recent painful swelling is likely to be an acute inflammatory or infectious process such as orchitis (often seen with mumps) or an epididymitis. The epididymis is a collecting structure for sperm on their way from where they are made in the testis to the vas deferens to the prostate. You should be able to feel the epididymis on each testicle. It's cupped over the inward and upper pole of the testes. Inside of it are firm structures such as the collecting ducts and vessels. Medial, or midline, to the epididymis is a hard cord—the vas deferens (spermatic cord). Clustered atop the epididymis are veins, which in some men will feel like a small bag of worms (called a varicocele).

8.   If you detect any change in your testes, see a doctor—don't fool around.*

VULVAR AND VAGINAL SELF-EXAMINATION

For All Women, Particularly Young Women with Multiple Partners

Though you won't find pamphlets on this form of self-examination in the offices of the American Cancer Society, it has long been advocated in the women's health field.

*For additional information, read Chapter 29—Testicular and Male Genitalia Cancers.

You are looking for any sores, spots, or growths on any part of the genitalia. Once again, you need to know what is normal for you to recognize subtle abnormalities. Especially be watchful for venereal warts, which can appear on the skin around the genitalia, on the vulva, in the vagina, or on the cervix. They are flat, raised, warty growths that don't hurt, and often appear in groups.

Vulvar self-examination should be done monthly. You only need a good light and a comfortable place to sit. With your legs apart, visually examine and palpate the external genitalia: the skin under the pubic hair (mons pubis), the outer and inner labia (the rounded folds around the vagina), and the outer mucosal lining of the vagina, including the clitoris and urethra.

Vaginal self-examination requires that you have a speculum, hand-mirror, and flashlight. The speculum is inserted into the vagina so you can direct light inside to see the inner walls of the vagina and the cervix (Figure 70-15). To find out where to get a speculum, call a women's health center or ask your health provider for one. Also, ask your health provider to show you the best way to insert the speculum, so that the cervix is brought clearly into view—and have him or her point out what to look for on the cervix (bring a hand-mirror when you go for your next pelvic exam). Vaginal self-examination is well-described by Carol Berry, R.N., N.P., in *Medical Self-Care,* edited by Tom Ferguson, Summit Books, NY. 1986.

ANAL, RECTAL, AND PROSTATE SELF-EXAMINATION

For Men (Include Prostate) and Women, Particularly if Over 40

As with vulvar and vaginal self-examination, examining your own anus, rectum, and (for men) prostate gland isn't commonly recommended in traditional medical circles, but it is presented in the self-care literature. It really isn't very difficult to do if you can get past any squeamishness you may have about examining these parts of your body.

This exam would be especially important if you have (or think you have) hemorrhoids, rectal bleeding (which may or may not be from hemorrhoids), venereal warts (they are often in or around the anus), and if you practice anal intercourse.

1.   Anal Self-Exam: sit on the floor, and use a good light (flashlight or, to free up your hands, a goose-neck lamp). Reflect light off a hand-mirror that you've positioned so that you can see your anal area. With your hand(s), spread the buttocks to completely expose the anus (the mucosal lining from the anal canal should be visible). Look for any sores, shallow fissures or abrasions, tags of skin (from past fissures or healed hemorrhoids), or swollen, bluish bumps (hemorrhoids).

2.   Rectal self-exam: do this as part of the anal self-exam, or while lying on your side in a knees-up fetal position, standing in the shower, or lying back in the bathtub. Men will probably find it more difficult than women—most physicians will confirm that their male patients have tighter anal sphinctors, and complain louder during a rectal exam. If you're doing it yourself, you can go at your own pace, and it will be easier. It shouldn't cause pain. (Figure 70-16.)

Do this exam after having a bowel movement, so the rectum is free of stool. Use some kind of lubricant (petroleum jelly or vaseline), and a plastic glove if you want. Insert whichever finger is easiest. If you have internal hemorrhoids, you'll feel an engorged area about one inch up the anal canal. You'll know you're in the rectum when you feel a shelf all around your finger tip. Rotate your finger and run it over as wide an area of the rectum as possible.

You are checking to be sure you don't have a rectal polyp (a slippery feeling bump that may freely slide around) or cancer (hard, rubbery). If there is blood on your finger after removing it from the rectum, it is not probably due to your exam—it represents a problem, and you should see your doctor promptly, for an examination to

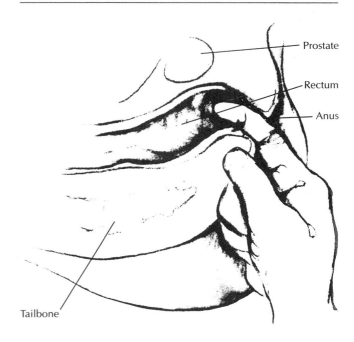

Figure 70-16 Anal, Rectal and Prostate Self-Examination. *Illustration reprinted with permission from Barbara Bates, M.D., A Guide to Physical Examination, J.B. Lippincott Company, Philadelphia, PA. 1974. Used with permission.*

Prostate

Rectum

Anus

Tailbone

learn the origin of the bleeding.*

3.   Prostate self-exam: for men, during the rectal self-exam you will notice that you can easily feel the prostate gland. It is on the side of the rectum closest to your penis. The lower part of the prostate gland begins about one-and-a-half inches up from the anal opening. The entire gland is normally about the size of a small apricot, and has the consistency of almost-ripe-enough fruit. You'll feel a central groove (called the raphe) down the middle of the prostate, and a domed lobe to each side. (It is normal to feel that you need to urinate when the prostate is examined.)

If the entire gland is bulging, and feels squishy and soft like over-ripe fruit, that may represent the condition known as benign prostatic hyperplasia (BPH). With BPH the prostate may feel lumpy. If the prostate feels swollen and hurts when you press on it, it's probably harboring an infection. If you feel a hard bump in the prostate (hard like your knuckle), or if the entire prostate feels hard like a rock, that may be cancer. Be sure to review the chapter on prostate cancer.

*For additional information, read Chapter 23—Cancer of the Colon and Rectum.

SELF-TESTING FOR BLOOD IN THE STOOL

For Men and Women, Annually After 50

Colorectal cancers and large polyps frequently bleed. But the blood often becomes mixed in with the stool, and is hard to see.

Various kits are available from pharmacies to test yourself for hidden (occult) blood in your stool. Most require that you collect samples from two areas of a stool, from three consecutive bowel movements (because even large colorectal cancers only bleed intermittently), and then have the six slides developed. This is usually done by your physician's office staff, the pharmacy, or, if the developer came with the kit, by you at home. When a drop of the developer is placed on the stool specimen, a blue color will appear within thirty seconds if blood is present. The blue should emanate from the specimen; if, instead, a faint blue line seems to ring the wettened paper, it is not indicative of blood.

A different type of kit requires that you place a specially designed card in the toilet with a bowel movement, and notice the color changes on the card.

All home stool blood testing systems recommend that for one to two days before starting the test you should:

(1)   avoid taking any medications that upset your stomach and cause bleeding (e.g., aspirin, ibuprofen, naproxen, prednisone);

(2)   avoid taking vitamin C or other chemicals that can block the chemical reaction that would tell you if blood were present (a false negative result);

(3)   avoid eating raw or rare meat (animal blood can cause a false positive result);

(4)   eat lots of fiber and fresh vegetables, nuts, and popcorn, which will lead to a bulkier stool with "buzz-saw" husks hanging from it—causing a polyp or cancer (if present) to bleed when the stool passes by.

After each bowel movement, use the small spatula/stick that comes with the kit to take a sample directly from the stool. Do not take the sample from toilet paper after wiping.

Do not do the test if you see actual blood in the toilet water, on a stool, or on the toilet paper. Instead, report to your physician, you're bleeding!*

*For additional information, read Chapter 23—Cancer of the Colon and Rectum.

INFANT EXAM BY MOTHER

Every mother's fear is that her baby or young child will develop cancer. However, these cancers are extremely rare. Also, mothers can check their children for cancers almost as well as a doctor.

The type of cancer you are checking for is named after each part of the exam. For further information, review the chapter on childhood cancers.

1.   Skin exam: while bathing or dressing your child, pay special attention to notice any bruises, discolorations, or swellings under the skin. If present it may just be a place where the child was bumped, but if the abnormality persists for a number of days, it should be examined by a physician. [leukemia]

2.   Lymph nodes: read the lymph node self-examination section of this chapter. Check your child using the same method. [lymphoma]

3.   Eye exam: in a darkened room, shine a light into each eye to check for the normal red reflex. [retinoblastoma]

4.   Mouth exam: carefully look inside the mouth and throat for any masses or abnormalities. [rhabdomyosarcoma]

5.   Bone exam: run your fingers over the leg and arm bones, feeling for any lumps or tender areas. [bone cancer]

6.   Abdominal exam: start at the edge of the rib cage and use one or two fingers to gently probe the entire abdomen for any masses. [Wilms' tumor of the kidney]

71

Breast Cancer Detection— Mammography and Other Methods

Kerry Anne McGinn, RN, BSN, MA

Excerpted from Keeping Abreast—Breast Changes that Are Not Cancer, *by Kerry Anne McGinn, RN, BSN, MA, Bull Publishing Company, Palo Alto, CA, 1987.*

When Dr. Virginia Griswold, radiologist, first told the surgeons at her hospital what she expected of them, they were dumbfounded.

"Surgeons trust their fingers and what they can *feel*. But here was I, the new radiologist, reading mammograms and recommending breast biopsies on the basis of something that could be seen on an X-ray but not felt. They'd say, 'You want me to do a biopsy because of some tiny white specks on a film? You're kidding, aren't you?'

"I won't say we almost came to blows, but there was a *lot* of conflict at first. Now most of them have become true believers!"

MAMMOGRAPHY

By the time a cancerous lump can be felt in the breast, it usually contains more than a billion cells. It has been growing for several years, doubling from one cell to two, from two cells to four and, in time, from one billion cells to two billion.

Originally, doctors used mammograms—the special X-rays which show the internal structures of the breast—primarily to confirm a lump they could feel. During the 1960s, however, mammography matured into a screening technique for large groups of women without disease symptoms. As radiologists saw more and more breast films, they noticed that at times certain features in a mammogram (particularly calcium deposits) which often accompanied cancerous lumps could be seen even when there was no lump to be seen or felt. Could these changes, they wondered, be early signs of cancer?

Joining forces with surgeons and pathologists, the radiologists discovered that while these X-ray changes most often signaled benign breast processes, in many cases they revealed cancer or carcinoma in situ. (Mammography only *detects* signs that *might* be cancer; *diagnosis* requires a biopsy or other test.)

The radiologists were jubilant. When cancer is detected and diagnosed this early, before there is a lump to palpate, it is almost always curable, often with minimal treatment.

What Mammography Shows

What clues is the radiologist searching for on a mammogram (see Figure 71-1)? Dr. Frederick Margolin, chief radiologist at Children's Hospital of San Francisco, summarizes: "If this is a woman's first mammogram, and I don't have anything to compare it to, I look for several things.

"I check for *symmetry*: In most women, the right breast isn't too different from the left. I check the amount and kind of tissue. Are there any abnormal-appearing *lumps or localized densities*? What about the *architecture of the breast*? (The lacy network of fibers in the breast can be distorted by a cancer even before we can see the cancer itself.) I observe the *skin* for thickening or irregularity. I check the *axilla* (armpit) for anything unusual.

"Finally, I use a magnifying glass to see if there are any *clusters of calcifications*. That's probably our most helpful early sign that there might be a cancer developing—or an area of duct carcinoma in situ.

"Of course, if I have an earlier mammogram for comparison, I look for any *changes* that have occurred since the last examination."

Obviously, radiologists are curious about any large "lump" appearing on a mammogram. Each lump has characteristics—like shape, regularity of outline, density and the presence or absence of a "halo" (or lighter area) around it—which are clues to whether it is benign or cancerous. But radiologists are especially interested in the subtle changes that can't be seen or felt during physical examination of the breast: lumps too small to palpate, calcifications (also called microcalcifications), and architectural distortions.

It is sometimes difficult to tell if abnormalities seen in a mammogram mean benign disease or cancer. Calcifications, for instance, those tiny white specks of calcium salts left as cellular debris, can appear in a cluster with ductal cancer—or as benign changes after inflammation or injury of the breast, or when the ducts become plugged with debris which can calcify. Radiologists look at the size and shape of each individual speck, and at the number and pattern of calcifications, for clues as to whether the cluster is benign or cancerous. A small number of round calcifications is less worrisome than a large number of long, branching calcifications.

Similarly, architectural distortions sometimes mean cancer, but often don't. Radiologists look with special care at stellate (star-shaped) gatherings of fibers; an unseen cancer can be pulling the fibers into this unusual conformation.

If there's something questionable on the mammogram, the radiologist may recommend either immediate biopsy or a follow-up mammogram in a few months, depending on *how* suspicious the find-

Figure 71-1 This is a mammogram of a normal breast with no mass or calcifications.
Source: Courtesy of the American Cancer Society—California Division.

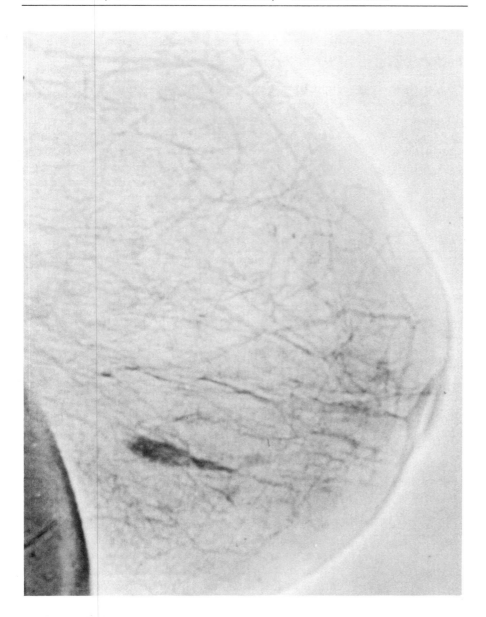

ing is. No radiologist wants to put a woman through the anxiety, discomfort, and expense of a biopsy without sufficient reason; on the other hand, no radiologist—or patient—wants to miss a cancer if it's there (see Figure 71-2).

Dr. Margolin considers mammography an art rather than an exact science. Some findings on a mammogram are clear-cut. Others require a judgment call, based on a radiologist's training and experience. We depend on the radiologist's expertise, sensitivity, and even hunches, and it makes sense to ask questions: Does the radiologist deal with mammograms every day or, at least, quite often? Any special training in mammography?

Mammography complements physical examination. Some abnormalities show up on one, some on the other, and some on both. If there's a palpable lump which doesn't appear on the mammogram, most radiologists would defer to a surgeon's judgment about whether it needs aspiration or biopsy.

Machines and Techniques

What about the machines? Both mammography and Xeromammography (or Xeroradiography, pronounced "Zero...") use X-rays to visualize the breast. The differences between the two lie in the recording devices and the final product. A mam-

Figure 71-2 The mammogram at left shows areas of cysts filled with fluid which often produce lumps. Fortunately, this kind of lump can be treated easily in a physician's office. The mammogram at right shows a large breast cancer that could have been detected much earlier. Mammograms are most valuable in detecting very small cancers that are easier to treat and cure. *Source:* Courtesy of the American Cancer Society—California Division.

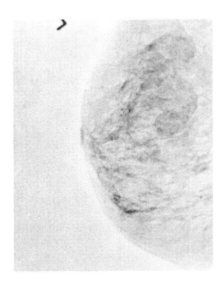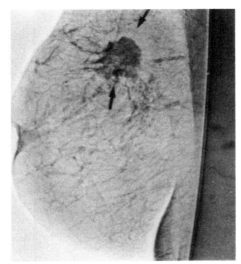

mogram is an X-ray *film*, with breast structures in black and white, like a large photographic negative. In contrast, a Xeromammogram (or Xeroradiograph) uses electrostatic energy to produce a blue and white picture on *paper;* the technique was developed by the Xerox Corporation—hence the name.

The two techniques provide pictures of comparable quality. Some radiologists prefer one technique over the other, largely because their training and experience have made them more familiar with that one.

Getting a Mammogram

What happens when a woman is scheduled for a mammogram?

Each X-ray department issues its own preliminary instructions. Most recommend that the woman wear a blouse or other easily removable clothing above the waist. Deodorant, perfume, powder, and even poorly rinsed soap on the breast and armpit area can cause misleading findings on the mammogram, and should be washed off before the examination. The woman may be asked to complete a form detailing her breast and reproductive history, risk factors, and any breast symptoms. If there is any possibility that the woman is pregnant, mammography is postponed if possible; if the mammogram is urgent, the woman will need special protection (usually a lead apron below the breasts).

For the exam, a technician flattens the entire breast between two hard plastic layers, appropriately called a *compressor* (see Figure 71-3). (There are other kinds of breast-compressing devices, but this is the most common type.) To produce the picture, the X-rays pass through an opening in the machine and then through the breast, exposing the film beneath.

Ordinarily, the technician takes two or three pictures of each breast from different angles, repositioning machine, breast, and the woman's arms for each image. For each mammogram, the technician steps away from the machine, tells the woman to stop breathing for a few seconds, and takes the picture. The technician develops the films, and the radiologist checks them to be sure the quality is adequate and that no additional views are needed before the woman leaves. Later, the radiologist's written report is sent to the woman's doctor.

Sometimes, the radiologist wants *magnification views* of a questionable area. These pictures enlarge a small area one-and-a-half to two times, and show it in much greater detail. This may either calm the radiologist's suspicions or confirm them. From the patient's point of view, the process is the same, except that the breast is positioned with special care so that the questionable area is at the center of the picture.

In case of a suspicious breast discharge or other nipple/areola irregularity, the doctor may want more detail of that area than the routine mammo-

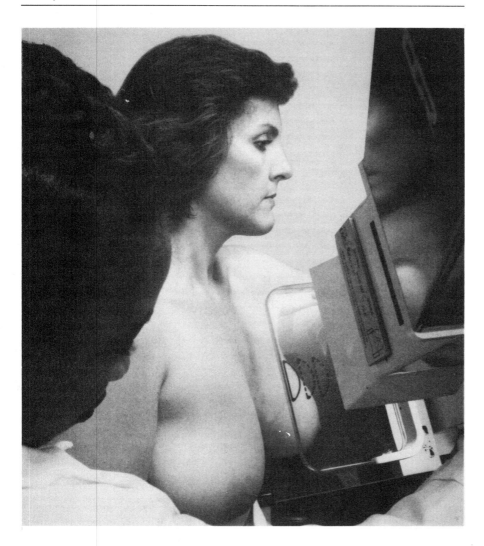

gram captures, and may arrange for a *duct X-ray.* For this, the radiologist gently enlarges one (or more) of the pores at the end of the nipple and carefully injects a small amount of special fluid until the woman experiences a sensation of fullness. This fluid shows up clearly on the X-ray to outline the suspect duct(s). This procedure is seldom necessary, however, and is used only rarely.

Why Don't More Women Get Mammograms?

The technique is simple and life-saving. Why do so many women hesitate?

1. "I'm scared of what they'll find." It's a normal reaction to be afraid of the unknown. However, most screening mammograms show normal breasts, without a hint of cancer—and are reassur-

ing. In the unlikely case of cancer, the scary part is *not* finding it early.

Of course, mammography doesn't change what's happening inside the breast; it simply detects it. If there is anything suspicious going on inside there, I, for one, want to find it as early as possible so that it can be cured with the least possible disruption in my life. That's what regular screening mammograms offer.

2. "It hurts." When Ann Landers printed a letter from "N.Y. Victim" complaining about pain from a mammogram, she was inundated with letters. Women called for revenge on the "male [who] invented that diabolical machine."

Yes, it can be uncomfortable—but it should *not* be painful and should not cause bruising. That's a lesson I've had to learn the hard way, as a veteran of frequent mammograms (as follow-up for calcifications), which usually include repeat and magnification views. (Once, after a painful session with an over-zealous student technician, I discovered that one large and prominent cyst had disappeared, presumably popped by a very forceful compression!)

It's much more comfortable for women who menstruate to have mammograms taken during the first half of the menstrual cycle, when the breasts are softer and less likely to be tender; the pictures may be a little clearer, too, with the breasts at relative rest. (I have friends who swear by eliminating caffeine from the diet for two weeks before mammography: coffee, tea, cola, and chocolate. Some X-ray departments recommend this in their preliminary instructions.)

And I've learned that the technician makes a big difference, and that I can speak up, if necessary. The breasts do need to be flattened somewhat for a clear picture with the newer "low-dose" techniques, which deliver smaller amounts of radiation than older processes. However, the primary elements of the "low-dose" technology are the sensitivity of the film and the improved focusing of the X-rays themselves, rather than the compression of the breast.

Squeezing the breasts more to get good pictures of difficult-to-visualize breasts is like shouting at a person with impaired hearing: It doesn't work. Accurate films can be taken with *reasonable* compression. Many experienced technicians compress the breasts to the point of discomfort, then release the pressure a tiny bit. Also, the compression lasts only a few seconds.

"Sure, it's uncomfortable," agrees Dr. Griswold, "but any woman who would refuse to have mammograms for that reason needs to do a lot more thinking."

Dr. Griswold should know. As a radiologist, she reads mammograms all the time. As a woman, she undergoes periodic mammography. And as a daughter, she saw her mother's early and minimal cancer detected by mammography, long before there was a lump to feel.

3. "Is it safe?" There is *no* evidence that mammography has ever induced a breast cancer, even with older, higher-dose techniques.

Dr. Margolin believes that, "Like everything else, it's a risk-benefit ratio. We know that large doses of radiation, like at Hiroshima (100 rads or more in a single exposure) are associated with increased numbers of breast cancers 15 years or more down the road. This is especially true if the radiation was received by a very young woman, with rapidly growing tissue that is more susceptible to radiation damage.

"But mammography delivers 1000 times less radiation than that, and many experts believe such tiny doses are harmless. With newer mammogram machines, it is estimated that the risk of developing a breast cancer from the radiation exposure of a mammogram is equivalent to the lung cancer risk of smoking half of one cigarette. Even if such a cancer did develop after 10-20 years, it would most probably be detected by the mammogram while it was early and curable.

"We have the proven benefit of early detection of breast cancer when it's curable versus a theoretical risk. *It's no contest!*"

For our maximum safety, what questions do we need to ask? Is this a *dedicated* mammography unit, one intended and used only for mammography? Is this *low-dose* radiation equipment? (The total dose of radiation for all views of each breast should be one rad or less.) How old is this equipment? (Machines less than five years old are preferred, because they incorporate the safest new technology and have fewer chances of equipment malfunction.) Does the technician have special training in mammography?

4. "It's expensive." Some insurance policies and most health maintenance organizations pay all or part of the costs of mammography. In addition, prices vary considerably from facility to facility. In my community, there's a mobile van which provides screening mammograms (read by a radiologist simply as "normal," "abnormal," or "questionable"), at about one-quarter the cost of those done in an office or hospital with direct radiologist supervision. Or we might decide to put aside a few dollars each month to pay for periodic mammograms.

False-Positives and False-Negatives

Mammography is an effective tool for detecting cancer—but it is not perfect. On the average, the mammogram will find nine out of 10 breast cancers. It is more accurate for some women than for others. Breasts containing moderately large amounts of fat are ideal for mammography, as even the smallest abnormality is easily detected. On the other end of the spectrum is the very dense breast with little or no fat. As the fat acts as a background on which the silhouette of breast structures is portrayed, its absence makes the mammogram more difficult to interpret.

Viewing the mammograms of a woman with very dense breasts is like looking through a thick fog. Density comes from normal working breast tissue in young women, from individual variations in the numbers and arrangement of ducts and glands, and from benign breast changes, such as cysts and overgrown fibrous tissue.

Breast changes *may* show up distinctly in even the most dense breasts. However, radiologists are much less confident that they will see a lump, thickening or change in the breast architecture of dense breasts, although calcifications sometimes show up quite clearly.

If our breasts are especially dense, we need to know about it. "Very dense breasts," as mentioned on a mammography report, refers to a visual finding, but it also means that we must rely more on our fingers and eyes and on our doctor's breast examinations—and less on mammograms—than we would otherwise. The doctor may recommend ultrasound or another imaging technique, or a diagnostic test if there's a question about a specific area. As the years pass, the dense breast tissue is replaced by fatty tissue, which makes the breasts easier to visualize on mammograms.

Because of their shape, with most of the breast tissue right at the chest wall, very small breasts can be a challenge to compress and mammograph accurately. Dr. Margolin claims, however, that even quite small as well as very large breasts can usually be examined adequately with careful technique.

Since about one of every ten breast cancers will not be found by X-ray, mammography has approximately a 10% *false negative* rate even when performed and interpreted very carefully. This reinforces the importance of BSE and professional physical examination of the breasts.

False positive results occur too. The mammogram may show worrisome calcifications which are not associated with a cancer, a lump which may be a benign tumor, or changes due to old inflammation or injury. As all of these may be suspicious findings to the radiologist, biopsy may be suggested. Two out of three times, when a mammogram prompts a biopsy, no cancer or duct carcinoma in situ is found.

Mammograms—When?

How often should women have mammograms? Baseline mammography between ages 35 and 40 gives the radiologist comparison films for later years when cancerous changes would be more likely to occur. (Before age 35, breast tissue tends to be too dense to visualize well, and is particularly sensitive to the effects of radiation.)

Current American Cancer Society guidelines call for mammography every one to two years between ages 40 and 50, depending on a woman's risk factors and symptoms, and every year after that. Both Dr. Margolin and Dr. Griswold believe that these guidelines will be reversed eventually, to recommend mammograms yearly between ages 40 and 50, and every two years after that. Their rationale is that breast cancers which appear before menopause tend to grow faster than those which occur later in life; thus, surveillance every two years after age 50 should

be adequate to detect cancerous changes at an early, curable stage.

Not everyone agrees that mammograms are advisable for a woman before menopause. Critics question both the effectiveness and the safety of mammography for women in the 40-to-50 age group. Awaiting results of large-scale studies currently in progress, the US Preventive Services Task Force, for instance, states: "Presently, no completed study has demonstrated that screening for breast cancer in a woman under the age of 50 years decreases mortality."*

Periodic mammograms are appropriate to follow up certain X-ray findings (when the appearance is not sufficiently suspicious for an immediate biopsy), or to check something newly discovered during physical examination. The frequency of such follow-up examinations varies with what's being evaluated, but is seldom more often than every four to six months.

OTHER IMAGING TECHNIQUES

Mammography is currently the workhorse of breast-imaging techniques. Nothing approaches it for all-around accuracy, both for screening breasts without symptoms and for imaging breasts where a problem is suspected.

But it's not a perfect technique, and some day another procedure—either one already available or one not yet imagined—may challenge mammography. Currently, other processes are used in tandem with mammography and/or in a few specific situations where they are better. None has demonstrated the ability of mammography to detect duct carcinoma in situ and early invasive breast cancer, however.

Ultrasound projects high-frequency sound waves into the breast. The sound waves bounce off different kinds of tissue in characteristic ways. A computer then reads the pattern of echoes and produces a visual representation of the breast.

The technique works best in showing whether a particular mass is solid or fluid-filled, especially in very dense breasts. It also shows the area close to the chest wall, an area often difficult to image with mammography. It may be safer than mammography early in pregnancy, or for women under 30 if

*US Preventive Services Task Force, "Recommendations for Breast Cancer Screening," *JAMA: The Journal of the American Medical Association*, Vol. 257, No. 16 (April 24, 1987), p. 2196. For a more complete discussion of the arguments against mammography for women before menopause, see Boston Women's Health Book Collective, *The New Our Bodies, Ourselves*, Simon & Schuster, Inc., New York, 1984, pp. 493–6.

a suspicious lump is found by palpation. However, ultrasound doesn't show calcifications, changes in breast architecture, or some small lumps that mammography would detect, and is thus at a disadvantage in finding in situ carcinoma or very early invasive breast cancer.

For an ultrasound examination using an automated water path scanner, the woman lies on her stomach and immerses her breasts in a tank of warm water; alternatively, she positions the breasts in a special water cushion. Another technique, which many radiologists prefer, is to use a hand-held instrument placed directly on the breast.

Ultrasound examination is a painless procedure which takes 15 to 30 minutes.

Thermography and other heat-sensing techniques capitalize on the fact that the body radiates, or throws off, heat—more of it in areas with greater blood flow. In theory, if a rapidly-growing tumor demands more nutrition from an increased blood supply, a detectable "hot spot" may develop. Each technique uses a different kind of material (heat-sensitive crystals, for instance, or a probe) to sense temperature changes.

Heat-sensing processes show cancers that are fairly large and/or near the surface of the breast which produce marked temperature changes at skin level. They do not detect deep tumors well, and don't give the information about in situ carcinoma or early signs of cancer that mammography can.

Before a thermogram, the woman sits in a cool room until her skin temperature lowers. Then her breasts are placed against the sensitive material, which registers any temperature variations, often with different colors.

In *diaphanography* (transillumination), light shining through the breast shows the breast interior. A fiberoptic device (a tube containing special light-sending fibers) directs infrared light through the breast; the transmitted light is then photographed with infrared film. Healthy breast tissue, a cyst, a benign tumor, or a cancerous tumor have a characteristic color and appearance, to the trained examiner.

Diaphanography does not show calcifications or changes in breast architecture. It cannot accurately distinguish cancer from mastitis (inflammation of the breast) or bleeding.

There is no known risk from diaphanography.

Computed tomography (CT) can find some cancers in small, very dense breasts, but it is a poor screening technique because it uses relatively large doses of X-rays, requires an injection into the vein, and is quite expensive. *Magnetic resonance imaging* (MRI; it used to be called nuclear magnetic resonance or NMR) uses an interaction of magnetism and radiowaves to image the breast structures. It appears to be safe, though expensive, but has not yet proven if it can detect small tumors or distinguish malignant tumors from benign ones.

A new imaging technique still being researched uses *monoclonal antibodies:* perfect, laboratory-produced copies (clones) of cancer antibodies. Experimenters add a dye or other marker to these antibodies, inject them into the body where they find and cling to any cancer cells, and then use special X-rays to take pictures. This works best as a follow-up procedure for a woman who has undergone treatment for breast cancer; her own antibodies to her particular cancer are cloned. It is *not* a general screening technique. As the test moves out of the experimental stage, it should become less expensive and more readily available.

Someday, we'll learn how to prevent breast cancer. Until that day, we rely on the earliest possible detection, diagnosis, and treatment of any breast cancer that does occur. We want a test that detects any and every breast cancer in any woman dependably, accurately, early, safely, and inexpensively.

Right now, mammography is the best we have—but maybe tomorrow. . . . ?

Mammography Recommendations for All Women*

35–40 years	One baseline mammogram
40–50 years	A mammogram every 1 to 2 years
After 50	A mammogram every year

*The recommendation are for well, asymptomatic women. Women with a personal or family history of breast disease may require different recommendations.

72

Flexible Sigmoidoscopy

Mark Renneker, M.D.

WHAT IS IT?

Flexible sigmoidoscopy is a visual examination of the lower part of the large bowel (the rectum and the colon) with a narrow (about one-half inch wide), short (about two feet long), flexible, rubber tube. (Figure 72-1 and 72-2)

The flexible sigmoidoscope was invented in the 1970s, but only came into widespread use in the 1980s. It is different from the old, rigid sigmoidoscopes which for many patients were uncomfortable. Flexible sigmoidoscopes use fiberoptics—tiny light-carrying, bendable fibers—to see around corners and into small places. It is a very safe procedure that causes little or no discomfort. (Figure 72-3)

WHY HAVE FLEXIBLE SIGMOIDOSCOPY?

Sigmoidoscopy is so important and safe that the American Cancer Society recommends that ALL people over the age of 50 have it done on a regular basis. This includes both men and women. It is recommended that it be routinely done every three to five years.

Flexible sigmoidoscopy helps make sure that your colon and rectum are healthy. In addition to flexible sigmoidoscopy, two other colon and rectum health tests are recommended by the American Cancer Society: (1) yearly (after age 40) digital (finger) rectal examination, and (2) yearly (after age 50) home stool testing for hidden blood. All three of these tests should be done; no one of the tests can take the place of another.

Also, flexible sigmoidoscopy may be recommended to you for other than "routine" reasons—for instance, if (1) blood has been found in your stool, (2) you've had a change in your stool or bowel habits, or (3) you have a family history of diseases of the colon and rectum, (family members should be screened beginning at an age ten years younger than when the family member was diagnosed or by age 50).

WHO PERFORMS FLEXIBLE SIGMOIDOSCOPY?

More and more family physicians and internists are providing this procedure for their patients. Virtually all gastroenterologists (an internist specializing in

Figure 72-1 The Large Intestine *Source:* Illustration courtesy of The Procter & Gamble Company.

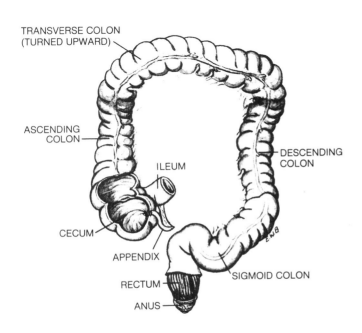

Figure 72-2 Rectum and Anus *Source:* Illustration courtesy of The Procter & Gamble Company.

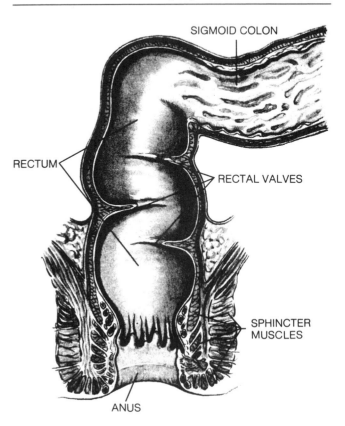

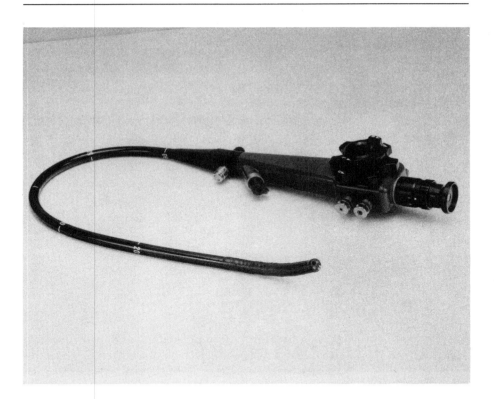

diseases of the GI tract) perform flexible sigmoidoscopy (as well as colonoscopy), and so do many proctologists (surgeons specializing in diseases of the anus and rectum). Not many gynecologists know how to do flexible sigmoidoscopy, but it is hoped that more will learn.

Many other physicians, however, know how to perform rigid sigmoidoscopy. If rigid sigmoidoscopy is all that is available to you, it's better than not having sigmoidoscopy at all (but tell your doctor you'd prefer having flexible sigmoidoscopy—if it can be arranged.)

WHAT CAN FLEXIBLE SIGMOIDOSCOPY DETECT?

With the sigmoidoscope the physician can look at the lining of the bowel. Of course the best result of such an examination is that everything is found to be normal. However, up to half of all people over the age of 50 have been shown to have small growths in their intestines (small and large) called "polyps." Over 90% of these are benign. (Figure 72-4.)

President Reagan had many polyps in his large bowel, and helped educate the American public about this condition by his openness in disclosing the results of his examinations.

A polyp is like a bump or a berry that grows out from the lining of the intestine. Usually they are less than half-an-inch in size and are harmless. But sometimes they bleed because they get pushed around by the stool coming down the bowel, and a small percentage of them will over time, usually years, slowly get bigger and become cancers. Almost all cancers of the colon or rectum began as one of these small polyps. The smaller a polyp is, the less likely it will contain cancer. Small polyps can easily be removed. That is the main reason why sigmoidoscopy is done: to find these little polyps and remove them and in doing so to prevent cancer or find it early.

Other diseases of the bowel can also be detected with sigmoidoscopy. These include: inflammation of the rectum (proctitis) or colon (colitis), outpouchings of the bowel (diverticulosis), and other conditions.

PREPARING FOR FLEXIBLE SIGMOIDOSCOPY

Physicians vary as to the amount and type of bowel preparation they recommend for flexible sigmoidoscopy. Many recommend only minimal preparation—for instance, a single enema given an hour or so before the procedure. A Fleet's brand Enema®, for instance, can be bought over-the-counter (without prescription) in any drug store, or your health provider may provide you with one beforehand. It should be given by yourself at home one to two hours before coming in for your appointment. It involves inserting a small amount of cleansing fluid into your rectum with a special applicator. (Lying on your left-side is probably the best position, and try to keep it in for at least five minutes—Don't worry, your bowels won't move that suddenly). If your returns are not clear, repeat the enema.

More aggressive cleansing of the bowel may be recommended, particularly if you've had problems with constipation. This may include following a special diet (i.e., clear liquids) for one to two days, taking tablets or drinking a special laxative solution the night before, not eating the day of the exam, and using enemas until you are completely cleaned out the morning of the exam.

GIVING PERMISSION

You should be asked to give written or verbal permission (informed consent) before performing the test. This is a requirement that applies to any test or procedure that involves placing any tube into the body. Requiring your permission ensures that you have been informed why you need the test, how the test will be performed, and what are the risks from having such a test done.

HOW THE PROCEDURE IS DONE

The procedure will almost certainly be performed with you in a lying position (on your left-side on a regular office examining table), but some physicians still prefer a specially designed table that tilts forward (putting your head down, and your buttocks up). You can expect that the outside of your rectum (the anus) will be inspected, first visually, then with an examining finger. Some physicians will then use a small anoscope (about four inches long) to mainly look for hemorrhoids. Then the flexible sigmoidoscope will be inserted (see Figure 72-3).

Attached to the sigmoidoscope are hoses that allow air to be put in and taken out. Without stool in it, the bowel is like a balloon that isn't inflated—so air must be put in to open things up for inspection. This may make you feel like you need to move your bowels. Speak up, because the air can be easily suctioned out, and adjusted to your comfort level. Also, bear in mind that your bowels are not accustomed to anything going "upstream," so that you will need to physically and mentally adjust to that sensation.

Figure 72-4 A benign polyp found by flexible sigmoidoscopy. As is sometimes the case, it is attached to the bowel wall by a stalk. A polyp like this will usually cause no symptoms for many months or years. It is only about half-an-inch in size. The small opening on the lower left represents a condition known as diverticulosis—outpouchings in the bowel wall. *Source: Primary Care and Cancer,* December 1986. Dominus Publishing Co., Inc., Williston Park, NY. Used with permission.

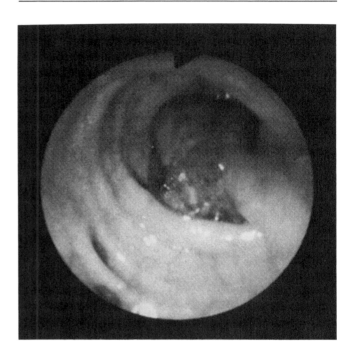

The entire examination may take anywhere from five to fifty minutes, depending upon how easy it is to negotiate the many curves in your colon and the skill of the examiner. The average amount of time for just the flexible sigmoidoscopy part of the exam is ten to fifteen minutes. The length of scopes used varies from about 30 to 70 centimeters, which also has some bearing on how long it will take.

RISKS OF FLEXIBLE SIGMOIDOSCOPY

The risks of this procedure are minimal but can include discomfort and bleeding, and very rarely infection or perforation of the bowel. This almost never happens. The rare times that perforation has occurred has usually been in people who are already acutely sick in the abdomen or bowel and who are already patients in the hospital.

Also, let it be known before the examination if any of the following conditions apply to you: blood clotting abnormalities, hepatitis/liver disease, heart conditions, pregnancy, intestinal parasites, or being at risk for AIDS.

AFTER SIGMOIDOSCOPY

1. Diet: Eat as you would normally. Occasionally, people will feel thirsty because of fluid loss from the enema and the procedure itself.

2. Gas: Some patients experience mild amounts of gas or the sensation of being bloated. This should pass within hours.

3. Biopsy: If a biopsy was performed, a small amount of blood may appear in your stool with your next bowel movement. Call or be seen if this continues or if bleeding is severe.

4. Polyp: If a polyp was detected, this may or may not be biopsied, but usually you will be referred to a gastroenterologist for removal of the polyp. A full colonoscopy is also done at that time to be sure no other polyps are higher up in the colon. A barium enema may also be advised.

Remember, though, the smaller the polyp, the greater the chance that it will be benign. You will be advised if your polyp or growth is thought to have a strong possibility of containing cancer.

5. Diverticula: If diverticula were found, you will probably be advised to go on a high-fiber diet. Diverticula are small outpockets in the bowel wall that are extremely common in people over 50 who eat a Western diet. They can sometimes become infected (a condition called diverticulitis; when they are present but not infected, it is called diverticulosis.)

6. Follow-up: As stated above, the American Cancer Society recommends that all people, men and women alike, have sigmoidoscopy beginning at age 50, every three to five years. Discuss these guidelines with your physician to determine when your next exam should be.

73

Diet and Cancer Prevention

Lorelei K. DiSogra, Ed.D., R.D. and
Charles A. DiSogra, M.P.H., Ph.D.

CANCER CONTROL OBJECTIVES FOR THE YEAR 2000

In 1985, the National Cancer Institute set as its national goal the reduction of cancer mortality by 50% by the year 2000. Achievement of this goal depends more on screening and prevention, and less on advances in research and treatment. Adoption of a low-fat, high-fiber diet by all Americans is a critical component of NCI's prevention strategy.

The NCI has estimated that a minimum of 30,000 lives, and as many as 150,000 lives, could be saved annually through dietary changes. With regard to specific cancer incidence, the NCI estimates that the suggested dietary modifications could result in a 50% reduction in cancer of the colon and rectum, a 25% reduction in cancer of the breast, a 15% reduction in cancers of the prostate, endometrium, and gall bladder, and an unquantifiable reduction in cancers of the stomach, esophagus, pancreas, ovaries, liver, lung, and bladder (1).

TYPES OF DIET AND CANCER RESEARCH

Before reviewing the individual dietary components associated with cancer, it is important to understand the criteria behind the judgments about what recommendations to make. Rather than depending on any single study to provide conclusive evidence, the ideal judgment is based on the results of several different types of studies. These are: epidemiological studies; tests on experimental animals; *in vitro* tests for genetic toxicity; and clinical intervention trials.

A variety of epidemiological investigations provide information about the occurrence of cancer in people and the foods consumed by those people. In case-control studies, the diets of persons who have a specific cancer are compared with diets of a control population of cancer-free persons. In cohort studies, epidemiologists follow a population of cancer-free persons over time, observing who develops the disease and investigating how they differ from those that remain free of cancer.

Other epidemiological studies look at the populations of different countries, as well as cultural, or religious groups to compare cancer mortality rates with unique dietary practices. An important extension of this is the use of migration studies which examine the cancer incidence or mortality rates of people who move from one country to another. For example, in Japan there is a low rate of breast and colon cancer. However, among descendants (3rd generation) of Japanese who have migrated to the United States, the rates of breast and colon cancer are much closer to the higher American rates. A change to the high-fat American diet from the traditional low-fat diet in Japan is one of the suspected causes of this change in cancer rates.

In addition to epidemiological studies, research with laboratory animals provides well-controlled experiments for testing dietary hypotheses and exploring the related biological mechanisms of function and causation. Rats and mice are the most commonly used laboratory animals for testing the effects of different diets on the development of cancer.

The *in vitro* tests are studies which use bacteria or tissue cultures to identify chemical substances (natural or synthetic) that are carcinogens and/or mutagens, or that promote or inhibit cancer growth.

Another type of investigation is a "clinical trial," in which persons at high risk for a specific type of cancer are asked to adopt a diet hypothesized to lower that risk. After a number of years, the cancer rate of this experimental group is compared to a control group that was not following a special diet.

CRITERIA FOR ASSOCIATION

Concordance of findings from several types of studies allows some conclusions to be drawn about the role of dietary components in the development of cancer. Standards at the NCI ideally require that criteria of consistency, temporality, strength, specificity, and coherence be met when drawing conclusions about diet and cancer studies (6). *Consistency* means many studies with similar conclusions. *Temporality* requires that the observed relationship is relevant within the time-frame of the study (i.e., did the differences in diet exist long enough before the appearance of any cancer?). *Strength* refers to the magnitude of significant differences observed in the study's statistical findings. The criterion of *specificity* relates to the absence of alternative hypotheses regarding observations (i.e., is the factor being studied reasonably responsible for the results?). And finally, a biological plausibility, or *coherence* of explanatory biomechanisms should exist for the diet and cancer connection being proposed. It is insistence that these criteria be met that generally justifies the current judgments about the role of diet in the development or prevention of cancer.

DIETARY RESEARCH ISSUES

A key difficulty in conducting studies on what people eat is the less than perfect methodology for collecting dietary data. Obtaining information on what people are currently eating by record keeping, recall, or reporting the frequency of consumption of specific food items is clearly problematic (7–12).

A concern about some cancer studies arises when subjects are asked to recall their diet of some period 10 or 20 years earlier. Such questions are valid, because of the belief that a particular dietary pattern over many years may have contributed to the presence or absence of a certain cancer. However, individual memories of such practices are notoriously unreliable. And there are a number of other factors. Were they following various weight-loss diets? Was their weight going up and down? Did they have medical conditions, such as a cancer in its early stages, that may have affected their nutritional state? These are the types of uncertainties that cause many an investigator sleepless nights. In most cases, the methods employed are the most practical possible and are chosen because of the lack of a more precise alternative. Nevertheless, results must always be interpreted with caution and good judgment.

It should be noted that the data for almost all studies are (disease) site specific. For example, it would be more common to conduct a study on diet and breast cancer, as opposed to a general study of diet and "cancer." Thus, when one speaks of increasing or decreasing the risk of cancer by dietary manipulation, the data that support those judgments are for specific sites only.

It is therefore clear that generalizations to cover all cancers, or unstudied sites, should be made with due caution, if at all. Also, association is not the same as causation. For example, while it may be increasingly evident that high-fat diets are associated with breast cancer, the data would not warrant the conclusion that dietary fat caused breast cancer. Issues of causation and the role of dietary components in the mechanisms of carcinogenesis have not yet been settled by laboratory investigators.

DIETARY FACTORS AND RISK OF CANCER

Dietary Fat

Of all the dietary components studied to date, scientists have the largest and most compelling body of scientific evidence for an association between dietary fat and certain cancers. Excessive dietary fat has been linked to an increased risk for cancer of the breast, colon, prostate, testes, uterus, and ovary. Although saturated and unsaturated fats have been examined separately in epidemiological studies and in various combinations in animal studies, it appears that total fat consumption is the real influencing factor (127).

Breast cancer is the leading cause of cancer mortality and morbidity among U.S. women (2). Since 1942, studies with experimental animals have demonstrated a relationship between dietary fat and breast cancer. Diets high in fat increase both the incidence and multiplicity (occurring in more than one breast) of mammary tumors in animals. Laboratory animal studies indicate that dietary fat impacts on cancer incidence when the manipulation of diet occurs during the promotional phase of carcinogenesis. Reduction in dietary fat, even if done late in the promotional phase, has resulted in a reduction in incidence of breast cancer in animal models (13–18).

Epidemiological studies have shown a positive correlation between the level of dietary fat and the incidence of breast cancer (19–26). In studies of migrants, the incidence of breast cancer increases coincident with increases in dietary fat (27–31). Case-control and cohort studies have also associated high dietary fat intake with elevated risk for breast cancer (32–38).

One recent study (Willet's 1987 cohort study), showed no clear relationship between increasing levels of fat intake and the risk of breast cancer (39). However, the fact that this study's lowest category of fat intake was not below 30% of calories (the current recommendation) limits the force of the conclusions (and underscores the difficulty of doing this type of research in a society where fat consumption is almost universally too high). In countries such as Japan where the rate of breast cancer is very low, fat intake is closer to 22% of calories. Based on the majority of the laboratory and epidemiological research to date, a high degree of concordance exists which links high fat diets with breast cancer.

Among both men and women, colon cancer is second only to lung cancer as a cause of cancer deaths (2). Colon cancer is primarily a problem of Western industrialized countries whose diets can be broadly characterized as being both high in fat and low in fiber. Low-fiber diets have, therefore, also been associated with colon and rectal cancer. Thus it is strongly suspected that the risk for colon cancer, and to a lesser extent rectal cancer, may involve both of these dietary components.

When different countries are compared both for their consumption of fat, and for mortality due to colon cancer, a strong positive association is observed (39). Some studies, including case-control studies, have suggested that saturated fat from meat consumption, particularly beef, may be the most important factor (40–42). However, a number of animal studies have suggested a promotional effect of bile acids on tumorigenesis (43–44). Increases in

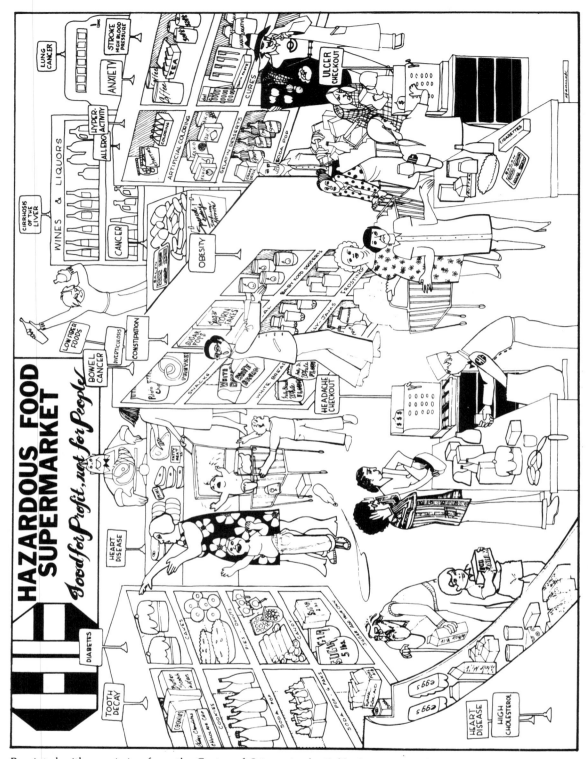

Reprinted with permission from the Center of Science in the Public Interest, Washington, D.C.

the consumption of dietary fat result in increased bile acid production. High concentrations of bile acids greatly enhance the appearance of tumors in animal colons subjected to known carcinogens (45–47).

Although a variety of international and case-control studies have associated high-fat diets with cancer of the testes (38), uterus (38, 48), ovary (49), pancreas (50–51), and prostate (52–55), colon cancer and breast cancer have received the most study relating to dietary fat.

All of this research strongly suggests that a reduction in total dietary fat intake would be a prudent recommendation. It has been variously estimated that the American population currently consumes 36% and 41% of total calories from fat. The two different estimates are derived from the National Food Consumption survey (NFCS), 1977–78, and the Second National Health and Nutrition examination survey (NHANES–II), 1976–80, respectively. Much of the difference between these two survey estimations is rooted in their methodologies (56). The true figure probably lies somewhere between the two figures. The U.S. Dietary Goals, issued in 1977, recommended a diet with 30% of the calories from fat (57). This reduction is considered minimal. However, NCI recommends a diet that contains 30% or less of total calories from fat for maximum benefit. For many Americans, achieving this NCI goal would mean cutting their dietary fat intake almost in half. Such low-fat diets are not known to be in any way injurious to health, and, as part of a balanced diet with adequate total calories, would reduce the risk for both cancer and heart disease.

Reducing dietary fat to 30% of total calories can be accomplished by *choosing less* fatty meats, whole milk and full-fat dairy products, fats and oils, and bakery and snack foods. The NCI booklet, *Nutrition and Cancer Prevention: A Guide to Food Choices,* provides detailed consumer information on how to reduce total dietary fat. Figure 73-1 provides information on the fat content of many common foods (128).

For the average adult who consumes 2,000 calories per day, fat from all foods should not exceed 67 grams in order to achieve the recommendation of 30% of total calories from fat. A small inactive adult who consumes 1500 calories per day should limit fat intake to 50 grams per day; a large physically active adult who consumes 2500 calories per day should limit total fat to 83 grams per day.

Fiber

It is widely accepted that a diet high in fat and low in fiber increases risk for colon cancer. While high amounts of dietary fat are considered to be a cancer promoter, adequate amounts of dietary fiber is thought to play a protective role. Fiber is the structural component of plant cell walls and is not digested by enzymes in the digestive tract. The beneficial role of fiber results from the fact that fiber enters the large intestine virtually intact.

The term, fiber, actually includes a variety of complex carbohydrate substances, i.e., cellulose, hemicellulose, pectins, gums and mucilages. Each has different properties and physiological effects. These various fiber substances are grouped into two categories or types: water-soluble and water-insoluble (58). Soluble fibers are found in fruits, vegetables, dried beans and peas, and oats, whereas, insoluble fibers are found in whole grain products, wheat bran, and the skin of vegetables and fruits.

The beneficial effects attributed to dietary fiber are the sum of the properties and actions of both soluble and insoluble fibers. In fact, much of fiber's popularity and support is based on the theory proposed for how fiber protects the large bowel: In the colon, insoluble fibers act to increase the weight of the stool by holding water, thus increasing fecal bulk and diluting the concentration of fecal bile acids and other possible co-carcinogens. Insoluble fibers also interact with intestinal bacteria, creating a laxative effect, which results in shortening stool transit time, thereby reducing the time that fecal bile acids and secondary bile acids are in contact with the walls of the colon. Research suggests that soluble fibers act to bind fecal bile acids and secondary bile acids in the large intestine (6).

For more than a decade before the theory gained acceptance, Burkitt hypothesized that dietary fiber played a role in protecting against colon cancer (59). He observed that Western industrialized countries with low-fiber diets have high mortality rates of colon cancer. However, those same diets are also high in fat. It is therefore difficult to separate the effect of fiber alone and attempts to do so have been inconclusive. (60).

Case-control studies have demonstrated an inverse relationship between dietary fiber and colon cancer (61–64). Some laboratory studies suggest a protective effect for bran and cellulose from chemically induced carcinogens in rats and mice (65, 66). In human populations, it has been suggested that the pentosan fraction of whole wheat may be a specific fiber component offering some protection from colon cancer (67). Recently, Greenwald and Lanza reviewed the role of dietary fiber in the prevention of cancer (8).

Both ACS and NCI recommend an increase in the consumption of dietary fiber by the general population. With the average American now consuming 11 grams of dietary fiber each day, NCI recommended that this amount be doubled to a range

Figure 73-1 Fat and Calories From Some Foods*

If you choose to reduce the fat in your diet to 30 percent of your daily calories, for a 2,000 calorie diet that is about 67 grams of fat.

Food	Serving	Calories	Grams of Fat
Dairy Products			
Cheese:			
American, pasteurized process	1 oz	105	9
Cheddar	1 oz	115	9
Cottage:			
Creamed	½ cup	115	5
Low-fat (2%)	½ cup	100	2
Cream	1 oz	100	10
Mozzarella, part skim	1 oz	80	5
Parmesan	1 tbsp	25	2
Swiss	1 oz	105	8
Cream:			
Half and half	2 tbsp	40	3
Light, coffee, or table	2 tbsp	60	6
Sour	2 tbsp	50	5
Ice Cream	1 cup	270	14
Ice Milk	1 cup	185	6
Milk:			
Whole	1 cup	150	8
Low-fat (2%)	1 cup	125	5
Nonfat, skim	1 cup	85	trace
Yogurt, low-fat, fruit-flavored	8 oz	230	2
Meats			
Beef, cooked:			
Braised or pot-roasted:			
Less lean cuts, such as chuck blade, lean only	3 oz	255	16
Leaner cuts, such as bottom round, lean only	3 oz	190	8
Ground beef, broiled:			
Lean	3 oz	230	15
Regular	3 oz	245	17
Roast, oven cooked:			
Less lean cuts, such as rib, lean only	3 oz	225	15
Leaner cuts, such as eye of round, lean only	3 oz	155	6
Steak, sirloin, broiled:			
Lean and fat	3 oz.	250	17
Lean only	3 oz	185	8
Lamb, cooked:			
Chops, loin, broiled:			
Lean and fat	3 oz	250	17
Lean only	3 oz	185	8
Leg, roasted, lean only	3 oz	160	7
Pork, cured, cooked:			
Bacon, fried	3 slices	110	9
Ham, roasted:			
Lean and fat	3 oz	205	14
Lean only	3 oz	135	5
Pork, fresh, cooked:			
Chop, center loin:			
Broiled:			
Lean and fat	3 oz	270	19
Lean only	3 oz	195	9
Pan-fried:			
Lean and fat	3 oz	320	26
Lean only	3 oz	225	14

Food	Serving	Calories	Grams of Fat
Rib, roasted, lean only	3 oz	210	12
Shoulder, braised, lean only	3 oz	210	10
Spareribs, braised, lean and fat	3 oz	340	26
Veal cutlet, braised or broiled	3 oz	185	9
Sausages:			
Bologna	2 oz	180	16
Frankfurters (1 frank)	2 oz	185	17
Pork, link or patty, cooked (4 links)	2 oz	210	18
Salami, cooked type	2 oz	145	11
Poultry Products			
Chicken:			
Fried, flour-coated:			
Dark meat with skin	3 oz	240	14
Light meat with skin	3 oz	210	10
Chicken, roasted:			
Dark meat without skin	3 oz	175	8
Light meat without skin	3 oz	145	4
Duck, roasted, meat without skin	3 oz	170	10
Turkey, roasted:			
Dark meat without skin	3 oz	160	6
Light meat without skin	3 oz	135	3
Egg, hard cooked	1 large	80	6
Seafood			
Flounder, baked:			
With butter or margarine	3 oz	120	6
Without butter or margarine	3 oz	85	1
Oysters, raw	3 oz	55	2
Shrimp, French fried	3 oz	200	10
Shrimp, boiled or steamed	3 oz	100	1
Tuna, packed in oil, drained	3 oz	165	7
Tuna, packed in water, drained	3 oz	135	1
Grain Products*			
Bread, white	1 slice	65	1
Biscuit, 2½ inches across	one	135	5
Muffin, plain, 2½ inches across	one	120	4
Pancake, 4 inches across	one	60	2
Other Foods			
Avocado	½	160	15
Butter, margarine	1 tbsp	100	12
Cake, white layer, chocolate frosting	1 piece	265	11
Cookies, chocolate chip	4	185	11
Donut, yeast type, glazed	one	235	13
Mayonnaise	1 tbsp	100	11
Oils	1 tbsp	120	14
Peanut butter	1 tbsp	95	8
Peanuts	½ cup	420	35
Salad dressing:			
Regular	1 tbsp	65	6
Low calorie	1 tbsp	20	1

*Most breads and cereals, dry beans and peas, and other vegetables and fruits (except avocados) contain only a trace of fat. However, spreads, fat, cream sauces, toppings, and dressings often added to these foods do contain fat.

*Source: Human Nutrition Information Service, U.S. Department of Agriculture. For fat and calorie values for other foods, see *Nutritive Value of Foods*, HG-72, for sale from Superintendent of Documents, U.S. Government Printing Office, Washington, DC 20402.

Figure 73-1 (continued)
Guide To Reducing Dietary Fat

This guide shows the amount of fat in diets with different proportions of calories from fat. For example, a 2,000 calorie diet calculated to have 30 percent of calories from fat has a total of 67 grams of fat, or 600 calories from fat. Food labels can help you find how many grams of fat are contained in packaged foods.

For a 1,500 calorie diet:

Percent of Calories Desired From Fat	Total Calories From Fat Should Not Exceed	Total Grams of Fat Should Not Exceed
40 percent	600 calories	67 grams
35 percent	525 calories	58 grams
30 percent	450 calories	50 grams
25 percent	375 calories	42 grams
20 percent	300 calories	33 grams

For a 2,000 calorie diet:

Percent of Calories Desired From Fat	Total Calories From Fat Should Not Exceed	Total Grams of Fat Should Not Exceed
40 percent	800 calories	80 grams
35 percent	700 calories	78 grams
30 percent	600 calories	67 grams
25 percent	500 calories	56 grams
20 percent	400 calories	44 grams

For a 2,500 calorie diet:

Percent of Calories Desired From Fat	Total Calories From Fat Should Not Exceed	Total Grams of Fat Should Not Exceed
40 percent	1,000 calories	111 grams
35 percent	875 calories	97 grams
30 percent	750 calories	83 grams
25 percent	625 calories	69 grams
20 percent	500 calories	55 grams

of 20–30 g/day. A diet that contains whole wheat products, generous daily servings of fresh fruits and vegetable and dried beans and peas is recommended. Figure 73-2 lists the dietary fiber content of many common foods; Figure 73-3 illustrates how easy it is to include 30 grams of dietary fiber in a day's menu. The dietary fiber content of commonly eaten foods has recently been published by the NCI (68).

It is clear that increasing the proportion of fiber-containing foods while decreasing the amount of fats and oils would be the best preventive dietary strategy. Wise food choices among the wide range of generally available foods will preclude the unnecessary expense of supplementing a diet with purified fiber products such as unprocessed bran and fiber supplements.

Vitamin A/Beta-Carotene

A great deal of research has accumulated supporting a preventive role for vitamin A in human cancer. Epidemiological research has demonstrated an inverse relationship between the consumption of foods rich in beta-carotene, a precursor of vitamin A which is found in plants, and several kinds of cancer (69). Beta-carotene is transformed into vitamin A in the body by enzymatic action. Preformed vitamin A, also known as retinol, exists only in animal products such as liver, butter and milk.

The epidemiological evidence linking vitamin A with lower cancer risk is strongest where vegetables containing beta-carotene have been consumed. Case-control studies have associated a lower risk for lung cancer with a high consumption of beta-carotene foods (70–73). Similar significant associations have demonstrated a lower risk for cancer of the bladder (74), colon-rectum (75), larynx (76), esophagus (77), stomach (78), and prostate (55).

In addition, laboratory experiments with mice and rats also support the concept that vitamin A is protective against cancer (79–85).

It would make good sense to apply these promising research findings by increasing the consumption of foods that are considered good sources of vitamin A/beta-carotene. The dark leafy green and the yellow-orange vegetables (such as broccoli, spinach, collard greens, brussel sprouts, carrots, sweet potatoes, pumpkin and winter squash), and carotene-rich yellow-orange fruits (such as cantaloupe, apricots, or peaches) would be the preferred food choices. According to NCI and ACS cancer prevention recommendations, several servings of these fruits and vegetables should be eaten daily.

The use of vitamin A supplements is not encouraged because high dosages taken over a long period of time can be toxic. The combination of vitamin A in foods and the vitamin supplement could unknowingly result in high doses. Also, all the epidemiological research associates vitamin A/beta-carotene-rich *foods* and not supplements with a reduced cancer risk. Not enough is known to assume that only the vitamin A is producing a benefit for humans. This is currently being investigated further with a large-scale randomized trial employing the beta-carotene supplementation of male physician subjects (86). In any event, increasing consumption of fruits and vegetables will also add beneficial fiber, other vitamins, and minerals.

Vitamin C

There is very limited epidemiological evidence concerning vitamin C and cancer prevention. A few studies have shown that an increased consumption of fruits and vegetables containing vita-

Figure 73-2 Fiber Content of Foods.

Fiber Content of Fruit

Fruit	fruit dietary fiber (gms)
blackberries (½ cup)	5
prunes (4)	4
apple w/skin (1 avg)	4
raisins (¼ cup)	3
rhubarb (½ cup cooked)	3
strawberries (1 cup)	3
raspberries (½ cup)	3
pear w/skin (1 avg.)	3
orange (1 med)	3
blueberries (½ cup)	2
dates (3)	2
apricots (3 med. fresh)	2
banana (2 avg)	2
peach w/skin (1 avg)	2

Fiber Content of Crackers

Cracker	dietary fiber (gms)
Ry-Krisp Ralston (2 triple crackers)	3
Fiber Rich Bran (1)	3
Wasa Fiber Plus (1)	3
Finn crisp (2)	2
Fiber crisp bread (2)	2

Fiber Content of Cereals

Cereal (1 oz. serving)	dietary fiber (gms)
All bran w/Extra fiber (Kellogg)	13
Fiber One (General Mills)	12
All bran (Kellogg)	9
100% bran (Nabisco)	9
Bran Buds (Kellogg)	8
wheat germ	3
Bran chex (Ralston)	5
Ralston High Fiber Hot Cereal	5
Corn bran (Quaker)	5
Weetabix (weetabix)	4
Bran flakes (any brand)	4
Shredded wheat and bran (Nabisco)	4
Fruit and fibre (Post)	4
Cracklin Oat bran (Kellogg)	4
Wheatena (Uhlmann)	4
Raisin Bran (Kellogg & Post)	4
bran, unprocessed (3 Tbsp)	4
Oatmeal (Quaker)	2

High-Fiber Low-Calorie Snacks

snack food	Calories	Fiber
apple w/skin (1 med)	81	4
prunes (4)	80	4
fresh strawberries (1 cup)	45	3
raspberries (½ cup)	35	3
pear w/skin (1 avg)	61	3
apricots (3 med)	51	2
apricots, dried (6 halves)	50	2
banana (1 med)	105	2
peach w/skin (1 avg)	37	2
pineapple (1 cup)	78	2
figs (3)	68	2
Wasa Fiber Plus crackers (1)	36	3
popcorn (3 cups unbuttered)	75	2
whole wheat toast (1 sl.)	61	2

High-Fiber Low-Calorie Snacks

snack food	Calories	Fiber
Rye Krisp (2 triple crackers)	50	2
broccoli (1 stalk)	24	3
carrot (1 med.)	34	2
celery (3 stalks)	21	2

Fiber Content of Vegetables—Greens and Beans

Vegetable (½ c. cooked)	dietary fiber (gms)
peas	4
potato w/skin (1 med)	3
sweet potato (1 med)	3
corn (cnd)	3
spinach	2
broccoli	2
Brussels sprouts	2
turnip	2
zucchini	2
carrots	2

Fiber Content of Legumes

Legumes (½ c. cooked)	dietary fiber (gms)
baked beans (w/tomato sauce)	9
kidney beans	7
lima and pinto beans	5
split peas	5
lentils	4

Fiber Content of Breads and Pasta

Item	dietary fiber (gms)
whole wheat spaghetti (1 c. cooked)	4
bran muffin (1 med.)	3
whole wheat english muffin (1)	3
buckwheat pancakes (2)	3
whole wheat pancakes (2)	3
whole wheat bread (2 slices)	3
whole wheat muffin (1)	2
whole wheat dinner roll (1)	2
whole wheat blueberry muffin (1)	2
brown rice (½ cup cooked)	1

High-Fiber Desserts

baked apple stuffed with chopped prunes and dates	6
blackberry pie (½ of 9" pie)	6
stewed fruit compote (prunes, apricots, peaches) ½ cup	4
fresh blackberries (½ cup)	5
whole-wheat banana-nut bread (1 slice)	3
stewed rhubarb (½ cup)	3
fresh strawberries (1 cup)	3

High-Fiber Desserts	
strawberry/rhubarb pie (½ of 9″ pie)	3
pineapple (¼ whole)	3
fresh raspberries (½ cup)	3
brown rice pudding w/raisins ½ cup	2
3 whole wheat oatmeal cookies w/raisins	2
fruit kebab (3 pieces each: pineapple, strawberry, melon)	2
fresh blueberries (½ cup)	2

Source: 1. Lanz, E. and Butrum, R., "A Critical Review of Food Fiber Analysis and Data" J. Amer. Dietet. Assoc. 86:732–743, 1986. 2. Leveille, Zabik, and Morgan, Nutrients in Foods, The Nutrition Guild, Massachusetts, 1983. 3. USDA Nutrient Data Research Group 4. Product label information

Note: Published figures for dietary fiber vary slightly from one source to another; methods for analyzing dietary fiber have not been standardized.

min C is associated with a lower risk for cancer of the esophagus and stomach (87–90). One case-control study suggests a possible protective effect of vitamin C for laryngeal cancer (91), and another suggests the same protective effect against the early development of cervical cancer (76).

Experimentation with laboratory animals using ascorbic acid (vitamin C) has not been very convincing. However, there are studies that suggest an inhibitory effect for high dosages of ascorbic acid on chemically-induced cancer in rats, although in some cases the number of animals used in the experiments was small (92–94).

It has been well demonstrated that ascorbic acid does inhibit the formation of carcinogenic nitrosamines (95, 96). This is currently the most convincing evidence of a role for vitamin C in a diet to reduce cancer risk. Nitrates and nitrites, naturally present in vegetables but added as preservatives in processed meats and other food products, will react with amines and amides to form nitrosamines. This reaction naturally occurs in the mouth and stomach; it also occurs when preserved meats are cooked. Ascorbic acid inhibits this reaction and for this reason is added to cured meat products such as bacon in the form of sodium erythrobate or sodium ascorbate. Mice fed nitrite and ascorbic acid were found to have fewer tumors than those without the ascorbic acid in their diet (95, 97).

Both the NCI and ACS recommend increasing intake of fruits and vegetables rich in vitamin

Figure 73-3 A 30-Gram Fiber Day

Breakfast	
bran flakes (1/2 cup)	4.0
orange juice (1/2 cup)	0.5
Lunch	
whole wheat bread (2 slices)	4.0
large pear with skin (1)	5.0
carrot sticks (1 medium carrot)	2.0
Snack	
rye krisp crackers (2)	3.0
Dinner	
whole wheat roll (1)	2.0
broccoli (1/2 cup)	2.0
baked potato with skin (1 medium)	3.0
apple with skin (1 medium)	4.0
Total Fiber:	29.5 grams

C. Vitamin C-rich foods include oranges, grapefruit, tangerines, lemons, limes, and strawberries. Many of the green leafy vegetables are rich in vitamin C (as well as beta-carotene). There is no evidence to justify taking vitamin C supplements.

Cruciferous Vegetables

Cruciferous vegetables are vegetables of the cabbage family (Brassicaceae), and include brussels sprouts, cabbage, broccoli, cauliflower, kale, kohlrabi, rutabagas and turnips. Colon cancer studies and some laboratory animal research have provided support for their role in a cancer prevention diet. Case-control studies have shown a lower risk for colon cancer among persons consuming cruciferous vegetables, particularly brussels sprouts and cabbage, compared to persons who never eat these vegetables (98, 99). It should also be noted that some of these cruciferous vegetables are good sources of both beta-carotene and fiber.

In laboratory experiments, rodents on diets that included these cruciferous vegetables have less forestomach cancer after being exposed to a known chemical carcinogen (100). One explanation, demonstrated in laboratory animals, is that natural chemical substances in these vegetables stimulate defensive enzyme systems which allow the body to either neutralize and/or excrete some carcinogens (101). Both the ACS and the NCI recommend that several servings of cruciferous vegetables per week be part of a cancer risk reduction diet.

Cooking Methods and Benzopyrene

Since the early 1960s it has been reported that polycyclic aromatic hydrocarbons are formed on the surface of foods that are grilled or charcoal-broiled.

Most of these compounds are mutagenic, having caused inheritable genetic damage in bacteria. Some of these same mutagens are also carcinogens. One of these carcinogens is benzopyrene, which, in a purified form, is used in laboratory experiments to induce cancer in animals. Investigators have measured the amount of benzopyrene that is formed on the burned or charred surface of foods (101–104) or is permeated throughout foods that have been cured by a smoking process (105). Most of the initial work looked at charcoal-broiled or grilled meat and fish; however, benzopyrene has been found in many other cooked protein foods (106).

There have been no epidemiological studies attempting to investigate an association between smoked-cured foods, or the burned portions of cooked foods, and cancer in humans. Despite this fact, the strength of the laboratory data has encouraged ACS and NCI to recommend moderation in the consumption of smoked and charcoal broiled foods. Cooking methods which minimize the formation of benzopyrene and other mutagens on foods include grilling or frying at lower temperatures (below 300 degrees F) and, when charcoal broiling, wrapping foods in foil to reduce contact with smoke and flame. Using low-fat cuts of meat would also help. Other alternative cooking methods for limiting benzopyrene intake are: baking, steaming, stewing, roasting, or microwaving cooking without a char-producing browning plate.

Alcohol

The consumption of alcohol was first associated with cancer as early as 1910. A number of studies since then have implicated alcoholic beverages as increasing the risk for cancer of the mouth, throat, esophagus, lung, stomach, colon and rectum (107–113). It has been estimated by one study that men who average 3.5 cans of beer a day have three times the risk for rectal cancer of nondrinkers, while whiskey or wine consumption at 50 ounces or more per month would double the risk for lung cancer (114).

Several case-control and cohort studies have been published which associate moderate alcohol consumption with a 40-60% increase in the risk for breast cancer among women (115–119). The case-control studies have shown an increased risk for women consuming more than three drinks per day, but more recent cohort studies suggest that as little as three or more drinks *per week* might increase the risk by 30-60%. Although more research is needed to clarify this issue, it would certainly be a prudent recommendation for women to keep their alcohol intake to a minimum, perhaps an average of less than one drink per day. One drink is defined as a 1-oz. shot of liquor, a 5-oz. glass of wine, or a 12-oz. glass of beer.

The strong relationship between alcohol consumption and cigarette smoking, increasing risk for cancers of the mouth, throat and esophagus is much clearer (109, 120). A person consuming more than 1.5 ounces of alcohol per day and smoking 2 packs of cigarettes daily, has 15.5 times the risk for oral cancer of the person who is a non-drinker and non-smoker (121).

It has also been suggested that this synergism between alcohol and tobacco may increase the risk for respiratory tract cancers (122). These studies should spell caution for heavy consumers of alcohol, particularly those who also smoke. Additionally, the usually impaired nutritional status of heavy drinkers may exacerbate cancer risk. Although the current published recommendations for moderate alcohol consumption are two or fewer drinks per day, it would be wise to revise that to less than one per day.

Obesity

Recently the relationship between obesity and cancer has received attention, due to the fact that laboratory studies have consistently shown that less cancer develops when rats and mice are raised on severe low-calorie diets (123). The epidemiological data are limited, and present several factors that make studies of obesity and cancer risk difficult to interpret. One of these factors is sorting out the effects of specific nutrients, such as dietary fat, as part of the overall caloric intake of obese people. Other factors relate to genetic, metabolic, and/or hormonal differences between the obese and the non-obese.

A person is considered obese if he or she exceeds ideal body weight by 20% or more. Figure 73-4 shows the Metropolitan Life Table standards for ideal body weight for men and women over the age of 25. This table was used in a very large epidemiological study of 750,000 people, conducted by the American Cancer Society. This study concluded that obesity at levels 40% or more above ideal body weight was associated with a 33% increased mortality for men, and a 55% increased mortality for women, from such cancers as uterine, gallbladder, kidney, stomach, colon, prostate and breast (124). The association of obesity with an increased risk for breast cancer is thought to be stronger for postmenopausal women that for premenopausal women (125, 126).

The ACS currently recommends the avoidance of obesity to reduce the risk of cancer. For the person who is already obese, this is a difficult recommendation to follow. However, for the general

Figure 73-4 1983 Metropolitan Height & Weight Table*

Weights are for ages 25-59 based on lowest mortality. Weights include indoor clothing weight 3 lbs. for women and 5 lbs. for men. Heights include shoes with 1″ heels.

Height	Small Frame	Medium Frame	Large Frame
Men			
5′ 2″	128-134	131-141	138-150
5′ 3″	130-136	133-143	140-153
5′ 4″	132-138	135-145	142-156
5′ 4″	134-140	137-148	144-160
5′ 5″	136-142	139-151	146-164
5′ 6″	138-145	142-154	149-168
5′ 7″	140-148	145-157	152-172
5′ 8″	142-151	148-160	155-176
5′ 9″	144-154	151-163	158-180
5′ 10″	146-157	154-166	161-184
5′ 11″	149-160	157-170	164-188
6′	152-164	160-174	168-192
6′ 1″	155-168	164-178	172-197
6′ 2″	158-172	167-182	176-202
6′ 3″	162-176	171-187	181-207
6′ 4″			
Women			
4′ 10″	102-111	109-121	118-131
4′ 11″	103-113	111-123	120-134
5′	104-115	113-126	122-137
5′ 1″	106-118	115-129	125-140
5′ 2″	108-121	118-132	128-143
5′ 3″	111-124	121-135	131-147
5′ 4″	114-127	124-138	134-151
5′ 5″	117-130	127-141	137-155
5′ 6″	120-133	130-144	140-159
5′ 7″	123-136	133-147	143-163
5′ 8″	126-139	136-150	146-167
5′ 9″	129-142	139-153	149-170
5′ 10″	132-145	142-156	152-173
5′ 11″	135-148	145-159	155-176
6′	138-151	148-162	158-179

*Courtesy of Metropolitan Life Insurance Company

population, it is extremely wise to maintain an ideal body weight *throughout life*—not only to reduce any possible excess risk for cancer, but also to reduce the risk of heart disease.

Conclusions

Data from a large body of epidemiological and laboratory research conducted over the past four decades support the hypothesis that some dietary patterns can increase risk of cancer, and other dietary patterns can decrease risk. In addition, what people eat during their lifetime strongly influences the probability of developing certain types of cancer. The potential to prevent as many as one-third of all cancers by modifying dietary intake is under the control of the individual.

NCI's cancer prevention awareness campaign theme, "Every day people can do something to protect themselves from cancer," highlights the importance of taking responsibility for one's health. To increase public awareness regarding the relationship between diet and cancer, to motivate and support personal responsibility, and to provide individuals with skills to change eating behavior has become a public health imperative.

In terms of national policy, both NCI and ACS have moved beyond the debate over the specific dietary guidelines into the area of implementation. Diet has become an important dimension of a national cancer prevention strategy. Both NCI and ACS are actively involved in developing specific strategies to positively influence eating behavior. Such strategies, to successfully influence eating behavior, must target the individual, the community and the food industry. Much needs to be accomplished if NCI's cancer prevention objectives for the year 2000 are to be realized.

References

1. National Cancer Institute. *Cancer Control Objectives for the Year 2000.* 1986

2. American Cancer Society, *1984 Cancer Facts and Figures.* American Cancer Society, National Headquarters, New York, 1984.

3. E. Wynder and G. Gori, Contribution of the environment to cancer incidence: An epidemiologic exercise. *J. Natl. Cancer Inst.* 58, 825–832 (1977).

4. C. DiSogra and L. Groll, *Nutrition and Cancer Prevention: A Guide to Food Choices.* Northern California Cancer Program, Palo Alto, Calif., 1981.

5. American Cancer Society, *Nutrition and Cancer: Cause and Prevention. An American Cancer Society Special Report.* American Cancer Society National Headquarters, New York, 1984.

6. Greenwald, P., and E. Lanza. "Role of Dietary Fiber in the Prevention of Cancer." in *Important Advances in Oncology 1986.* J. B. Lippincott, Philadelphia, 1986.

7. G. H. Beaton, J. Milner, V. McGuire, T. E. Feather, and J. A. Little, Source of variance in 24-hour dietary recall data: Implications for nutrition study design and interpretation. Carbohydrate sources, vitamins, and minerals. *Am. J. Clin. Nutr.* 37, 986–995 (1983).

8. J. H. Hankin, A. M. Y Nomura, J. Lee, T. Hirohata, and L. N. Kolonel, Reproducibility of a diet history questionnaire in a case-control study of breast cancer. *Am. J. Clin. Nutr.* 37, 981–985 (1983).

9. G. Block, A review of validations of dietary assessment methods. *Am. J. Epidemiol.* 115, 492–505 (1982).

10. G. H. Beaton, J. Milner, P. Corey et al., Sources of variation in 24-hour dietary recall data: Implications for nutrition study design and interpretation. *Am. J. Clin. Nutr.* 32, 2546–59 (1979).

11. P. A. Stefanik and M. C. Truison, Determining the frequency intakes of foods in large group studies. *Am. J. Clin. Nutr.* 11, 335–43 (1962).

12. B. S. Burke, The dietary history as a tool in research. *J. Am. Diet. Assoc.* 23, 1041–6 (1947).

13. Tannenbaum A, 1942. The genesis and growth of tumors. III. Effects of a high-fat diet. *Cancers Res* 2:468–475.

14. Silverstone H and Tannenbaum A, 1950. The effect of the proportion of dietary fat on the rate of formation of mammary carcinoma in mice. *Cancer Res* 10:448–453.

15. Carroll KK and Khor HT, 1970. Effects of dietary fat and dose level of 7,12-dimethylbenz(a)anthracene on mammary tumor incidence in rats. *Cancer Res* 30:2260–2264.

16. Carroll KK and Khor HT, 1971. Effects of level and type of dietary fat on incidence of mammary tumors induced in female Sprague-Dawley rats by 7,12-dimethyl-benz(a)anthracene. *J Natl Canc Inst* 62: 1009–1012.

17. Hopkins GJ and Carroll KK, 1979. Relationship between amount and type of dietary fat in promotion of mammary carcinogenesis induced by 7,12-dimethyl-benz(a)anthracene. *J. Natl Canc Inst* 62:1009–1012.

18. IP C, 1980. Ability of dietary fat to overcome the resistances of mature female rats to 7,12-dimethyl-benz(a)anthracene induced mammary tumorigenesis. *Cancer Res* 40:2785–2789.

19. Silverman, J. Shellabarger CJ, Holtzman S, Stone JP and Weisburger JH, 1980. Effect of dietary fat on X-ray induced mammary cancer in Sprague-Dawley rats. *J Natl Canc Inst* 64:631–634.

20. Lea AJ and Birm MB, 1966. Dietary factors associated with death rates from certain neoplasms in man. *Lancet* 2:332–333.

21. Draser BS and Irving D, 1973. Environmental factors and cancer of the colon and breast. *BR J Cancer* 27:167–172.

22. Armstrong B and Doll R, 1975. Environmental factors and cancer incidence and mortality in different countries, with special reference to dietary practices. *Intl J Cancer* 15:617–631.

23. Carroll KK and Khor HT, 1975. Dietary fat in relation to tumorigenesis. *Prog Biochem Pharmocol* 10:308–353.

24. Gray GE, Pike MC, and Henderson BE, 1979. Breast-cancer incidence and mortality rates in different countries in relation to known risk factors and dietary practices. *BR J Cancer* 39: 1–7.

25. Hirayama T, 1978. Epidemiology of breast cancer with special reference to the role of diet. *Prev Med* 7:173–195.

26. Hems G, 1980. Associations between breast cancer mortality rates, childbearing and diet in the United Kingdom. *Br J Cancer* 43:429–437.

27. Haenszel W, 1961. Cancer mortality among the foreign-born in the United States. *J Natl Cancer Inst* 26:37–132.

28. Haenszel W and Kurihara M, 1968. Studies of Japanese migrants. I. Mortality from cancer and other diseases among Japanese in the United States. *J Natl Cancer Inst* 40:43–68.

29. Buell P, 1973. Changing incidence of breast cancer in Japanese American women. *J Natl Cancer Inst* 51:1479–1483.

30. Dunn J, 1977. Breast cancer among American Japanese in the San Francisco Bay area. *Natl Cancer Inst Monogr* 47:157–160.

31. Kolonel LN, Hankin JH, Nomura AM and Chu SY, 1981. Dietary fat intake and cancer incidence among five ethnic groups in Hawaii. *Cancer Res* 41:3727–3728.

32. Phillips RL, 1975. Role of life-style and dietary habits in risk of cancer among Seventh Day Adventists. *Cancer Res* 35:3513–3522.

33. Miller AB, 1978. An overview of hormone-associated cancers. *Cancer Res* 38:3985–3990.

34. Nomura A, Henderson BE, and Lee J, 1978. Breast cancer and diet among the Japanese in Hawaii. *Am J Clin Nutr* 31:2020–2025.

35. Kolonel LN, Hankin JH, Lee J, Chu SY, Nomura AMY,

and Hinds MW, 1981. Nutrient intake in relation to cancer incidence in Hawaii. *Br J Cancer* 44:332–339.

36. Lubin JH, Burns PE, Blot WJ, Ziegler RG, Lees AW and Fraumeni JF Jr, 1981. Dietary factors and breast cancer risk. *Int J Cancer* 28:685–689.

37. Kolonel LN, Nomura AMY, Hinds MW, Hitohata T, Hankin JH and Lee J, 1983. Role of diet and cancer incidence in Hawaii. *Cancer Res* 43(Suppl); 2397–2402.

38. Willett, W. C., M. J. Stampger, G. A. Colditz, et al., Dietary fat and the risk of beast cancer. *New Engl. J. Med.* 316:22–28 (1987).

39. B. Armstrong and R. Coll, Environmental factors and cancer incidence and mortality in different countries, with special reference to dietary practices. *Inst. J. Cancer* 15, 617–631 (1975).

40. M. Jain, G. M. Cook, F. G. Davis, M. G. Grace, G. R. How, and A. B. Miller, A case-control study of diet and colorectal cancer. *Int. J. Cancer* 26, 757–768 (1980).

41. L. G. Dales, G. D. Friedman, H. K. Ury, S. Grossman, and S. R. Williams, A case-control study of relationships of diet and other traits to colorectal cancer in American blacks. *Am. J. Epidemiology* 109, 132–144 (1978).

42. B. S. Reddy, A. R. Hedges, K. Laakso, and E. L. Wynder, Metabolic epidemiology of large bowel cancer: Fecal bulk and constituents of high-risk North American and low-risk Finnish population. *Cancer* 42, 2832–2838 (1978).

43. B. S. Reddy, L. A. Cohen, G. D. McCoy, P. Hill, J. H. Weisburger, and E.L. Wynder, Nutrition and its relationship to cancer. *Adv. Cancer Res.* 32, 237–345 (1980).

44. G. V. Vahouny, M. M. Cassidy, F. Lightfoot, L. Grau, and D. Kritchevsky, Ultrastructural modifications of intestinal and colonic mucosa induced by free or bound bile acids. *Cancer Res.* 41, 3764–3765 (1981).

45. T. Narisawa, N. E. Magadia, J. H. Weisburger, and E. L. Wynder, Promoting effect of bile acids on colon carcinogenesis after intractal instillation of N-methyl-N-nitro-N-nitrosoguanidine in rats. *J. Natl. Cancer Inst.* 533, 1093–1097 (1974).

46. C. Chomchai, N. Bhadrachari, and N. D. Nigro, The effect of bile on the induction of experimental intestinal tumors in rats. *Dis. Colon Rectum* 17, 310–312 (1974).

47. R. C. N. Williamson, F. L. R. Bauer, J. S. Ross, J. B. Watkins, and R. A. Malt, Enhanced colonic carcinogenesis with azoxymethane in rats after panceractico biliary diversion at mid small bowel. *Gastroenterology* 76, 1388–1392 (1979).

48. L. N. Kolonel, J. H. Hankin, J. Lee, S. Y. Chu, A. M. Y. Nomura, and M.W. Hinds, Nutrient intakes in relation to cancer incidence in Hawaii. *Br. J. Cancer* 44, 332–339 (1981).

49. C. H. Lingeman, Etiology of cancer of the human ovary: A review. *J Natl. Cancer Inst.* 53, 1603–1618 (1974).

50. T. Hirayama, Changing patterns of cancer in Japan with special reference to the decrease in stomach cancer mortality. In H. H. Hiatt, J. D. Watson, and J. A. Winsten, eds., *Origins of Human Cancer, Book A: Incidence of Cancer in Humans*. Cold Spring Harbor Laboratory, Cold Spring Harbor, N.Y., 1977, pp. 55–75.

51. A. J. Lea, Neoplasms and environmental factors. *Annals of the Royal College of Surgery, Engl.* 41, 432–438 (1967).

52. B. S. Drasar and D. Irving, Environmental factors and cancer of the colon and breast. *Br. J. Cancer* 27, 167–172 (1973).

53. K. K. Carroll and H. T. Khor, Dietary fat in relation to tumorigenesis. *Prog. Biochem. Pharmacol.* 10, 308–353 (1975).

54. I. D. Rotkin, Studies in the epidemiology of prostate cancer: Expanded sampling. *Cancer Treatment Rep.* 61, 173–180 (1977).

55. L. M. Schuman, J. S. Mandell, A. Radke, U. Seal, and F. Halberg, Some selected features of the epidemiology of prostatic cancer: Minneapolis-St. Paul, Minnesota case-control study, 1976–1979. In K. Magnus, ed., *Trends in Cancer Incidence: Causes and Practical Implications.* Hemisphere Publishing, Washington, D.C., 1982, pp. 345–354.

56. C. E. Woteki, M. G. Kovar, and H. Riddick, Sources of differences in estimates of fat intake in national surveys. Paper presented at the 68th Annual Meeting of the Federation of American Societies for Experimental Biology, St. Louis, Missouri, April 3, 1984.

57. U.S. Congress, Senate, Select Committee on Nutrition and Human Needs. *Dietary Goals for the United States,* 2nd ed., U.S. Government Printing Office, Washington, D.C., December 1977.

58. J. W. Anderson and W. J. Chen, Plant fiber, carbohydrate and lipid metabolism. *American Journal of Clinical Nutrition* 32:346–63, 1979.

59. D. P. Burkitt and H. C. Trowell. *Refined Carbohydrate Foods and Disease. Some Implications of Dietary Fiber.* Academic Press, New York, 1975.

60. K. Liu, J. Stamler, D. Moss, D. Garside, V. Persky, and I. Soltero, Dietary cholesterol, fat, fibre and colon-cancer mortality. *Lancet* 2, 782–785 (1979).

61. O. Manousos, N. E. Day, D. Trichopoulos, F. Gerovassilis, A. Tzonou, and A. Polychronopoulou, diet and colorectal cancer: a case-control study in Greece. *Int. J. Cancer* 32, 105 (1983).

62. B. Modan, V. Barell, F. Lubin, M. Modan, R. A. Greenberg, and S. Grahm, Low-fiber intake as an etiologic factor in cancer of the colon. *J. Natl. Cancer Inst.* 55, 15–18 (1975).

63. L. G. Dales, G. D. Friedman, H. K. Ury, S. Grossman, and S. R. Williams, A case-control study of relationships of diet and other traits to colorectal cancer in American blacks, *Am. J. Epidemiol.* 109, 132–144 (1978).

64. I. Martinez, R. Torres, Z. Frias, J. R. Colon, and M. Fernandez, Factors associated with adenocarcinomas of the large bowel in Puerto Rico. In J. M. Birch, ed., *Advances in Medical Oncology, Research and Education. Volume 3: Epidemiology.* Pergamon Press, New York, 1979.

65. D. M. Fleiszer, D. Murray, G. K. Richards, and R. Z.

Brown, Effects of diet on chemically induced bowel cancer. *Can. J. Surg.* 23, 67–73 (1980).

66. H. J. Freeman, G. A. Spiller, and Y. S. Kim, A double-blind study on the effects of differing purified cellulose and pectin fiber diets on 1,2-dimethydrazine-induced rat colonic neoplasia. 1980. *Cancer Res.* 40, 2661–2665 (1980).

67. S. Bingham, D. R. R. Williams, T. J. Cole, and W. P. T. James, Dietary fibre and regional large-bowel cancer mortality in Britain. *Br. J. Cancer* 40, 456–463 (1979).

68. E. Lanza and R. Burtum, A critical review of food fiber analysis and data. *Journal of the American Dietetic Association.* 86:732–743 (1986).

69. T. Kummet, T. E. Moon, and F. F. Meyskens, Vitamin A: Evidence for its preventive role in human cancer. *Nutrition and Cancer* 5:96–106 (1983).

70. G. Kvale, E. Bjelke, and J. J. Gart, Dietary habits and lung cancer risk. *Int. J. Cancer* 31, 397–405 (1983).

71. E. Bjelke, Dietary vitamin A and human lung cancer. *Int. J. Cancer* 15, 561–565 (1975).

72. C. Mettlin, S. Graham, and M. Swanson, Vitamin A and lung cancer. *J. Natl. Cancer Inst.* 62, 1435–1438 (1979).

73. R. B. Shekelle, S. Liu, W. J. Raynor, Jr., M. Lepper, C. Maliza, and A. H. Rossof, Dietary vitamin A and risk of cancer in the Western Electric Study. *Lancet* 2, 1185–1189 (1981).

74. C. Mettlin and S. Graham, Dietary risk factors in human bladder cancer. *Am. J. Epidemiology* 110, 255–263 (1979).

75. E. Bjelke, Dietary factors and the epidemiology of cancer of the stomach and large bowel. *Aktuel. Ernaehrungsmed. Klin. Prax. Suppl.* 2, 10–17 (1978).

76. S. Graham, C. Mettlin, J. Marshall, R. Priore, and D. Shedd, Dietary factors in the epidemiology of cancer of the larynx. *Am. J. Epidemiology* 113, 675–680 (1981).

77. C. Mettlin, S. Graham, J. Marshall, and M. Swanson, Diet and cancer of the esophagus. *Nutr. Cancer* 2, 143–147 (1981).

78. T. Hirayama, Changing patterns of cancer in Japan with special reference to the decrease in stomach cancer mortality. In H. H. Hiatt, J. D. Watson, and J. A. Winsten, eds., *Origins of Human Cancer, Book A: Incidence of Cancer in Humans.* Cold Spring Harbor Laboratory, Cold Spring Harbor, N.Y., 1977, pp. 55–75.

79. P. Nettescheim and M. L. Williams, The influence of vitamin A on the susceptibility of the rat lung to 3-methylcholanthrene. *Int. J. Cancer* 17, 351–357 (1976).

80. S. M. Cohen, J. F. Wittenberg, and G. T. Bryan, Effect of avitaminosis A and hypervitaminosis A on urinary bladder carcinogenicity of N-[4-(5-nitro-2-fury)-2-thiazoly]formamide. *Cancer Res.* 36, 2334–2339 (1976).

81. T. Narisawa, B. S. Reddy, C.-Q. Wong, and J. H. Weisberger, Effect of vitamin A deficiency on rat colon carcinogenesis by N-methyl-N-nitro-N-nitrosoguanidine. *Cancer Res.* 36, 1379–1383 (1976).

82. R. J. Shamberger, Inhibitory effect of vitamin A on carcinogenesis. *J. Natl. Cancer Inst.* 47, 667–673 (1971).

83. A. E. Rogers, B. J. Herndon, and P. M. Newburn, Induction by dimethylhydrazine of intestinal carcinoma in normal rats and rats fed high or low levels of vitamin A. *Cancer Res.* 33, 1003–1009 (1973).

84. M. B. Sporn and D. L. Newton, Chemoprevention of cancer with retinoids. *Fed. Proc.* 38, 2528–2534 (1979).

85. M. B. Sporn and D. L. Newton, Recent advances in the use of retinoids for cancer prevention. In J. H. Burchenal and F. P. Oettgen, eds., *Cancer. Achievements, Challenges and Prospects for the 1980s,* Vol. 1, Grune and Stratton, New York, 1981, pp. 541–548.

86. C. H. Hennekens, Physicians Health Study Research Group. Strategies for a primary prevention trial of cancer and cardiovascular disease among U.S. physicians (Abstract). *Am. J. Epidemiol.* 118, 453–4 (1983).

87. W. Haenzel and P. Correa, Developments in the epidemiology of stomach cancer over the past decade. *Cancer Res.* 35, 3542–3459 (1975).

88. C. Mettlin, S. Graham, R. Priore, J. Marshall, and M. Swanson, Diet and cancer of the esophagus. *Nutr. Cancer* 2, 143–147 (1981).

89. L. N. Kolonel, A. M. Y. Nomura, T. Hirohata, J. H. Hankin, and M. W. Hinds, Association of diet and place of birth with stomach cancer incidence in Hawaii Japanese and Caucasians. *Ame. J. Clin. Nutr.* 34, 2478–2485 (1981).

90. P. J. Cook-Mozaffari, F. Azordegan, N. E. Day, A. Ressicand, C. Sabai, and B. Aramesh, Oesophageal cancer studies in the Caspian littoral of Iran: Results of a case-control study. *Br. J. Cancer* 39, 293–309 (1979).

91. S. Graham, C. Mettlin, J. Marshall, R. Priore, T. Rzepka, and D. Shedd, Dietary factors in the epidemiology of cancer of the larynx. *Am. J. Epidemiol.* 113, 675–680 (1981).

92. T. Logue and D. Frommer, The influence of oral vitamin C supplements on experimental colorectal tumor induction (Abstract). *Austr. N. Z. J. Med.* 10, 588 (1980).

93. B. S. Reddy and N. Hirota, Effect of dietary ascorbic acid on 1,2-dimethylhydrazine-induced colon cancer in rats. *Fed. Proc.* 38, 714 (1979) Abstract 2565.

94. G. Kallistratos and E. Fasske, Inhibition of benzo(a)pyrene carcinogenesis in rats with vitamin C. *J. Cancer Res. Clin. Oncol.* 97, 91–96 (1980).

95. S. S. Mirvish, Inhibition of the formation of carcinogenic N-nitroso compounds by ascorbic acid and other compounds. In J. H. Burchenal and H. F. Oettgen, eds., *Cancer: Achievements, Challenges, and Prospects for the 1980s,* Vol. 1, Grune and Stratton, New York, 1981, pp. 557–587.

96. National Academy of Sciences. *The Health Effects of Nitrate, Nitrite and N-Nitrosos Compounds.* National Academy Press, 1981.

97. S. Ivankovic, R. Preussman, D. Schmahl, and J. W. Zeller, Prevention by ascorbic acid on *in vivo* formation of

N-nitroso compounds. In P. Bogovski and E. A. Walker, eds., *N-Nitroso Compounds in the Environment.* IARC Scientific Publication No. 9., Intl. Agency for Res. on Cancer, Lyon, France, 1975, pp. 101–102.

98. S. Graham, H. Dayal, M. Swanson, A. Mittelman, and G. Wilkinson, Diet in the epidemiology of cancer of the colon and rectum. *J. Natl. Cancer Inst.* 51, 709–714 (1978).

99. W. Haenszel, F. B. Locke, and M. Segi, A case-control study of large bowel cancer in Japan. *J. Natl. Cancer Inst.* 64, 17–22 (1980).

100. L. W. Wattenberg and W. D. Loub, Inhibition of polycyclic aromatic hydrocarbon-induced neoplasia by naturally occurring indoles. *Cancer Research* 38, 1410–1413 (1978).

101. L. W. Wattenberg, Enzymatic Reactions and Carcinogenesis. *Environment and Cancer,* a collection of papers presented at the 24th annual symposium on fundamental research, M.D. Anderson Hospital and Tumor Institute, University of Texas, Houston (1971).

102. W. Lijinsky and A. E. Ross, Production of carcinogenic polynuclear hydrocarbons in the cooking of food. *Food Cosmet. Toxicol.* 5, 343–347 (1967).

103. C. Lintas, M. C. De Matthaeis, and F. Merli, Determination of benzo(a)pyrene in smoked, cooked and toasted food products. *Food Cosmet. Toxicol.* 17, 325–328 (1979).

104. T. Sugimura and S. Sato, Mutagens-carcinogens in food. *Cancer Res.* (suppl.) 43, 2415s (1983).

105. J. W. Howard and T. Fazio, Analytical methodology and reported findings of polycyclic aromatic hydrocarbons in foods. *J. Assoc. Off. Anal. Chem.* 63, 1077–1104 (1980).

106. L. F. Bjeldanes, M. M. Morris, J. S. Felton, S. Healy, D. Stuermer, P. Berry, H. Timourian, and F.T. Hatch, Mutagens from the cooking of food. II. Survey by Ames/*Salmonella* test of mutagen formation in the major protein-rich foods of the American diet. *Food Chem. Toxic.* 20, 357 (1982).

107. F. Hakulinen, L. Lehtimaki, M. Lehtonen, and L. Teppo, Cancer morbidity among two male cohorts with increased alcohol consumption in Finland. *J. Natl. Cancer Inst.* 52, 1711–1714 (1974).

108. I. D. J. Bross and J. Coombs, Early onset of oral cancer among women who drink and smoke. *Oncology* 33, 136–139 (1976).

109. J. D. Burch, G. R. Howe, A. B. Miller, and R. Semenciw, Tobacco, alcohol, asbestos, and nickel in the etiology of cancer of the larynx: a case-control study. *J. Natl. Cancer Inst.* 67, 1219–1224 (1981).

110. D. Schottenfeld, Alcohol as a cofactor in the etiology of cancer. *Cancer* 43, 1962–1966 (1979).

111. M. Keller, D. M. Promisel, D. Spiegler, L. Light, and M. N. Davies, eds., alcohol and cancer. In *Second Special Report to the U.S. Congress on Alcohol and Health.* Public Health Service, DHEW, Rockville, Md., 1977, pp. 53–67.

112. J. Hoey, C. Montvernay, and R. Lambert, Wine and tobacco: Risk factors for gastric cancer in France. *Am. J. Epidemiol.* 113, 668–674 (1981).

113. J. E. Enstrom, Colorectal cancer and beer drinking. *Br. J. Cancer* 35, 674–683 (1977).

114. E. S. Pollack, A. M. Y. Nomura, L. K. Heilbrun, G. N. Stemmermann, and S. B. Green, Prospective study of alcohol consumption and cancer, *N. Engl. J. Med.* 310, 617–21 (1984).

115. Le M. G., C. Hill, A Kramar, R. Flamant, Alcohol beverage consumption and breast cancer in a French case-control study. *Am. J. Epidemiol.* 120:350–7 (1984).

116. C. La Vecchia, A. Decarli, S. Franceschi, S. Pampallona, G. Tognoni, Alcohol consumption and the risk of breast cancer in women. *JNCI* 75:61–65 (1985).

117. R. A. Hiatt, R. D. Bawol, Alcoholic beverage consumption and breast cancer incidence. *Am. J. Epidemiol.* 120:676–83 (1984).

118. A. Schatzkin, D. Y. Jones, R. N. Hoover, et al., Alcohol consumption and breast cancer in the Epidemiologic Follow-up Study of the First National Health and Nutrition Examination Survey. *N. Engl. J. Med.* 316:1169–73 (1987).

119. W. C. Willett, M. J. Stampfer, G. A. Colditz, B. A. Rosner, C. H. Hennekens, F. E. Speizer, Moderate alcohol consumption and the risk of breast cancer. *N. Engl. J. Med.* 316:1174–80 (1987).

120. L. M. Pottern, L. E. Morris, W. J. Blot, R. G. Ziegler, and J. F. Fraumeni, Jr., Esophageal cancer among Black men in Washington, D.C. I. Alcohol, tobacco, and other risk factors. *J. Natl. Cancer Inst.* 67, 777–783 (1981).

121. Roghman, K., and A. Keller, The effect of joint exposure to alcohol and tobacco on risk of cancer of the mouth and pharynx. *J. Chronic Dis.* 25:711–716 (1972).

122. G. D. McCoy, C. B. Chen, S. S. Hecht, and E. C. McCoy, enhanced metabolism and mutagenesis of nitrosopyrolidine in liver fractions isolated from chronic ethanol-consuming hamsters. *Cancer Res.* 39, 793–796 (1979).

123. The American Society for Clinical Nutrition, Calories and energy expenditure in carcinogenesis. *Am. J. Clinical Nutr., Supplement,* 45:149–372 (1987).

124. E. A. Lew and L. Garfield, Variations in mortality by weight among 750,000 men and women. *J. Chronic Dis.* 32, 563–576 (1979).

125. F. de Waard and E. A. Baanders-van Halewijn, A prospective study in general practice on breast-cancer risk in postmenopausal women. *Int. J. Cancer* 14, 153–160 (1974).

126. F. deWaard, Breast cancer incidence and nutritional status with particular reference to body weight and height. *Cancer Res.* 35, 3351–6 (1975).

127. Committee on Diet, Nutrition and Cancer; National Research Council, *Diet, Nutrition and Cancer.* National Academy Press, Washington, D.C. (1982).

128. National Cancer Institute, *Diet, Nutrition and Cancer Prevention: A Guide to Food Choices.* National Institutes of Health, 1984.

74

Understanding Smoking

Craig Wilson, M.D.

A lone man's companion, a bachelor's friend, a hungry man's food, a sad man's cordial, a wakeful man's sleep, and a chilly man's fire . . .— *Charles Kingsley,* Westward Ho, 1875

WHY SMOKERS SMOKE

Smokers *start* to smoke, usually during adolescence, because of peer and social pressures. But they *continue* to smoke because they are addicted to nicotine. Smokers develop a set of complex behaviors centered around smoking. The same process probably occurs with dippers and chewers.

The incredible thing is that we persist after our first puff. Nearly everyone first experiences nausea, headache, and weakness. This group of symptoms, known as *tobacco cropper's syndrome,* will lessen and then vanish with a few additional cigarettes (exposures)—the condition known as tolerance.

Tolerance to nicotine develops after relatively few exposures, as does dependency. In contrast, chemical dependencies, such as alcohol, may take years of exposure and enormous consumption before chemical dependency sets in.

Nicotine is a highly addictive substance. The hallmarks of chemical dependency, in addition to tolerance, are habituation (always needing the drug) and withdrawal (symptoms occurring on stopping the drug)—both of which are experienced with smoking.

In addition to its purely chemical effects, smoking, early on, becomes tightly woven into lifestyle and deeply ingrained into daily habits, social interactions, and coping.

WOULD MOST SMOKERS RATHER FIGHT THAN QUIT?

An occasional smoker is one who smokes one or two cigarettes a week. They account for less than 7% of smokers. The vast majority of smokers smoke at least one cigarette an hour on a regular daily schedule. Some smokers will wake from sleep to smoke. Frequent use is necessary for the maintenance of normal nervous system function.

The high proportion of continuous daily tobacco users differs significantly from either alcohol or heroin addiction—where the majority are not daily users. Many smokers have never gone more than eight hours without a cigarette.

Most smokers have tried at least once to quit. Few smokers enjoy every cigarette. Smokers are people with a chemical dependency. A number of studies have shown that 80% of smokers want to quit. Most smokers would rather quit than fight.

THREE TYPES OF SMOKERS

There are about as many types of smokers as there are people smoking. However, smokers fall into three general groups: the biochemical smoker, the psychological smoker, and the habitual smoker. All smokers are a combination of all three, but usually one mode predominates.

Being able to identify one's central reason for smoking is an important step to quitting and in choosing the best way to quit. If you are a smoker, or know a smoker you are concerned about, read the following three descriptions to identify the predominant mode in your case.

The Biochemical (Nicotine Dependent) Smoker

Being taken when they goe to bed, it makes one sleepe soundly, and yet being taken when a men is sleepie and drowsy, it will as they say, awake his brain, and quicken his understanding.— *James I, 1604*

All regular smokers are nicotine-dependent, but in some this is the central feature of their smoking behavior. A primarily nicotine-dependent smoker may wake up at night to smoke, and will in any event light up as soon as he or she awakens, and smoke throughout the day, having a cigarette every ten to twenty minutes.

Understanding nicotine is central to understanding smoking behavior. Nicotine resembles the neuro-transmitter acetylcholine (ACh) and affects the central nervous system. It acts as both a stimulant and as a depressant. The effects are unconsciously regulated by the smoker, by the frequency of cigarettes, the frequency of puffs on each cigarette, and the depth of inhalation.

Each smoker has a blood nicotine level that he or she is maintaining. "Favorite" levels—as stimulant or as depressant—vary from smoker to smoker, and may account for why some people smoke, for instance, one pack or two packs per day. Smokers of low-tar and low-nicotine cigarettes have been found to smoke more, deeper, and faster to maintain their desired nicotine blood levels.

Avoiding nicotine withdrawal is a major drive to keep smoking. Nicotine withdrawal symptoms include: irritability, sleep disturbance, difficulty concentrating, preoccupation with smoking (inability to think about anything else besides cigarettes), restlessness, headache, and gastrointestinal disturbances. Some or all of these symptoms are experienced from within 10 minutes to 72 hours of the last cigarette.

The Psychological Smoker

Habit, the instrument of nature, is a great leveler; the familiarity which it induces, taking off the edge of both of our pleasures and of our sufferings.—*Paley, 1819*

Psychological smokers smoke to combat boredom, reduce tension, and legitimize relaxation. They will smoke when they are alone, in moments of conflict or uncertainty, and to relax.

Smoking cigarettes, pipes, and cigars, and chewing tobacco are one way of relieving conflict, uncertainty, frustration, and anger. However, it is a maladaptive coping mechanism because it gives only short-term benefit, and in the long-term it is detrimental.

No one knows more about the behavior of smokers than the tobacco industry. Their highly sophisticated, 2-billion-dollar annual advertising campaign teaches us to choose the right brand (theirs), extract the cigarette from the packet, dismember the matches, light up, put out the flame, get rid of the match, shift the ash tray, flick ash flecks from clothes, and blow smoke thoughtfully into the air (or dramatically out of the nostrils). Over the years, all have become stylized behaviors in ads, books, and movies.

The Habitual Smoker

> 20 puffs/cigarette
> × 20 cigarettes/pack
> × 1.5 packs/day
> × 365 days/year
> = 219,000 puffs/year

Smoking cigarettes thousands of times each year becomes a conditioned, habitual activity. The body becomes trained to automatically respond to external or internal cues.

This pattern of activity becomes associated with external environmental cues such as finishing a meal, drinking coffee or alcohol, talking on the telephone, handling or fiddling with things, and, perhaps most importantly, being around other people lighting up. The habitual smoker will reach for the pack and light up when, for example, after a meal he hears the click of a lighter in a crowded restaurant. Even a year after giving up cigarettes, such a cue in a restaurant will start ex-smokers unconsciously going through their pockets looking for a cigarette, and realizing they still have the urge to smoke. This extraordinary habit is acquired through repetition and the unique pharmacology of nicotine.

THE BARRIERS TO QUITTING

Another reason smokers continue to smoke is fear of quitting. This may include: (1) an overwhelming fear of failure if they try to quit; (2) an exaggerated fear of the consequences of quitting—such as losing control over other areas of their lives (telling the boss to "go to hell," screaming at the kids, etc.); and (3) an avoidance of tobacco withdrawal pain, and the loss of an "old friend"—the cigarette.

Sigmund Freud, himself a victim of tobaccomania (20 cigars/day) underwent 33 operations for throat (laryngeal) cancer, and had heart disease. On attempting to quit, he said: "denouncing the sweet habit of smoking has resulted in a great diminution of my intellectual interests." He considered smoking to be of "erotogenic significance of the labial region." He was unable to overcome his addiction, and died of cancer of the throat at age 83.

PRACTICING SMOKING PREVENTION

This section will present essential smoking prevention and cessation skills. There are three levels of prevention in relation to smoking: primary prevention is never smoking; secondary prevention is quitting before symptoms develop; and tertiary prevention is quitting after symptoms develop.

Primary Prevention

The nation's health strategy must be dramatically recast to emphasize the prevention of disease.—*J. A. Califano, Jr., 1979*

Educational, informational, fiscal, and regulatory measures are key strategies in a national smoking prevention program.

Psychological and social factors, the chief two being parents that smoke and peer pressure, strongly influence whether a teenager becomes a smoker or not.

About 15% of teenagers are regular smokers. Young women between the ages of 18 and 22 are the only group whose tobacco use is increasing; teenage boys, on the other hand, are not increasing but have not reduced their smoking over the last 20 years, and smokeless tobacco and clove cigarettes are increasingly popular. Small wonder that tobacco advertisers have targeted young people, especially young women, as an "up–start market."

Standard educational programs obviously are not enough to influence behavior: ninety percent of third graders know smoking is harmful. However, innovative programs involving social and psychological approaches, peer counseling, and decision-making training have been devised and should become a health education priority in the schools.

Can health professionals, family, and friends also influence the decision not to smoke? Yes!

Remember that decision-making regarding smoking begins at an early age. Most smokers who quit agree that it would have been far easier never to have taken up smoking in the first place.

Secondary Prevention: Asymptomatic Smokers

> Refrain to-night,
> And that shall lend a kind of easiness
> To the next abstinence: the next
> more easy;
> For use almost can change the
> Stamp of Nature.
> Shakespeare, *Hamlet*

Why do 53 million Americans still smoke—about 30% of adult males and 24% of adult females? Eighty percent of smokers say they would quit if their physician urged them to, but only 20% of smokers report being told by their physician to quit. This matches studies of physicians—only 20% urge their smoking patients to quit.

Physicians, nurses, and all health professionals have a major responsibility in educating and motivating their smoking patients to quit, but most smokers simply quit on their own—without a physician's help.

More than 37 million smokers have quit since 1964, when the first Surgeon General's report on "Smoking and Health" was published. How did they do it? Seventy-nine percent did it on their own, 9% did it with the help of their physician, 10% did it with the help of family or friends, and only 2% did it with organized groups or special smoking cessation techniques (e.g., aversion therapy, hypnosis, acupuncture, and smoking cessation classes).

Even though most quitters haven't needed an organized quit smoking program, many have been devised—tending to be about equally successful: 25% who complete the program will not be smoking one year later.

Quit smoking programs vary: in cost—from being free to costing hundreds of dollars; in means—from printed literature to group meetings; in duration—from hours to months; in leadership—from self-help to professional guidance; in approach—from scientific methods to empirical practices; and in devices—from rubber bands to nicotine gum. Most

methods are based on the following steps (actually the same process most ex-smokers go through who quit on their own):

Seven Common Steps

1. Identify the problem—make the diagnosis ("I am a smoker").

2. Understand the smoking habit—(e.g., "I am a nicotine-dependent smoker," or "I am a psychological smoker," and so forth).

3. Choose to quit—(i.e., "I want to quit").

4. Choose a quit date—(e.g., the start of a vacation, your birthday, a Saturday, "now").

5. Learn techniques for quitting, staying quit, and avoiding recidivism (slipping back).

6. Acknowledgement and rewards—(e.g., "I am proud of myself for quitting").

7. Never smoke again—(taking "one day at a time").

Many smokers—like alcoholics—find it important to help others quit.

CASE HISTORIES

• A 32-year-old two-pack-per-day telephone operator quit because his roommate had AIDS and the smoke was affecting his breathing.

• A 68-year-old retired automobile salesman quit because his children gave him a quit smoking clinic tuition on his birthday.

• A 48-year-old accountant quit because his physician asked him to.

• A 38-year-old nurse quit because a close friend urged her to.

• A 50-year-old advertising and newspaper executive quit because she burned a hole in her clothes and didn't like the bondage.

• A 68-year-old single parent with Alzheimer's disease quit (and doesn't miss it) because her son stopped buying her cigarettes.

- A 50-year-old terminal cancer patient (with a non-smoking related tumor) said the most important accomplishment in her life was to quit smoking—during the last six months of her life.

Tertiary Prevention

Tertiary prevention—efforts to quit by people who have symptoms—can be very effective. Studies have shown that up to 60% of smokers who survive their first heart attack will quit for at least one year or more if aggressively told to quit.

Smoking cessation counseling should begin at the hospital bedside by family, friends, and physician—it can be life-saving.

A hard core smoker needn't come to the hospital to become motivated to quit. Many smokers become symptomatic after years of smoking. This may be why male smokers over the age of 55 (most with a greater than 40-year history of continuous smoking) are the fastest growing group of ex-smokers in this country, today. They have developed a chronic cough, shortness of breath, poor exercise tolerance, and other symptoms, and become motivated to quit.

Death and disease rates are higher for smokers and risks are reduced with cessation, at whatever age. Some risks (such as heart attack) are reduced substantially within a short period of time, others over a number of years (lung cancer risk is that of a person who never smoked after about ten years). Benefits accrue from the moment a smoker quits.

SUMMARY

Smoking prevention should be practiced by everyone concerned about smoking—whether for yourself, family, friend, or patient.

Although quitting smoking may prevent recurrent heart attacks and cancer, the best prevention is primary prevention—never smoking.

Most smokers eventually quit on their own. Some smokers need special programs to quit and others can only quit after serious illness. If you smoke, stop—now! If you don't smoke, don't ever start.

RESOURCES AND REFERENCES

Smoking Cessation Resources

Societies and Associations. (local and state offices are listed in the phone book):

AMERICAN CANCER SOCIETY
3340 Peachtree Road, NE
Atlanta, GA 30026
(404) 320-3333

AMERICAN HEART ASSOCIATION
7320 Greenville Avenue
Dallas, TX 75231
(214) 750-5300

AMERICAN LUNG ASSOCIATION
1740 Broadway
New York, NY 10019
(212) 245-8000

OFFICE ON SMOKING AND HEALTH
U.S. Department of Health and Human Services
5600 Fishers Lane
Park Building, Room 110
Rockville, MD 20857
(301) 443-5287

OFFICE OF CANCER COMMUNICATIONS
National Cancer Institute
National Institutes of Health
Bethesda, MD 20205
(800) 638-6694

Also—Proprietary/Volunteer Programs.

Seventh Day Adventist Church
American Cancer Society
University research clinics
Schick Centers for Control of Smoking/Weight
Smoke Enders
Smoke Watchers
Smokers Anonymous

Practitioners: some physicians, acupuncturists, public health nurses, psychologists, hypnotists, etc.

SELECT BIBLIOGRAPHY

The Classics

U.S. Department of Health and Human Services. *Smoking and Health: Report of the Advisory Committee to the Surgeon General of the Public Health Service.* U.S. Department of Health, Education, and Welfare, Public Health Service: January; 387 pp., 1964.

U.S. Department of Health and Human Services. *The Health Consequences of Smoking: Cancer—a report of the Surgeon General.* U.S. Department of Health and Human Services, Public Health Service, Office on Smoking and Health, 1982.

U.S. Department of Health and Human Services. *The Health Consequences of Smoking: Cardiovascular Disease—a report of the Surgeon General.* U.S. Department of Health and Human Services, Public Health Service, Office on Smoking and Health: November; 384 pp., 1983.

Doll R, Peto R. *The Causes of Cancer.* Oxford University Press, Oxford, 1981.

Reviews

CDC—MMWR. Smoking and Cancer. *MMWR:* 31; No 7, 1982.

Fielding J E. Smoking: Health Effects and Control. Part I. *NEJM:* 313; 491–498, 1985.

Fielding J E. Smoking: Health Effects and Control. Part II. NEJM: 313; 555–561, 1985.

Koop C E, Luoto J. The Health Consequences of Smoking: Cancer, Overview of a Report of the Surgeon General. *Public Health Reports:* 97; 318–324, 1982.

Steinfeld J L. Smoking and Lung Cancer: A Milestone in Awareness. *JAMA:* 253; 2995–2997, 1985.

Wynder E L, Hoffmann D. Tobacco and Health: A Societal Challenge. *NEJM:* 300; 894–903, 1979.

Pathophysiology

Albanes D, Jones D Y, Micozzi M S, Mattson M E. Associations between Smoking and Body Weight in the US Population: Analysis of NHANES II. *AJPH:* 77; 439–444, 1987.

Auerbach O, Hammond E C, Garfinkel L. Changes in bronchial epithelium in relation to cigarette smoking, 1955–1960 vs 1970–1977. *NEJM:* 300; 381–386, 1979.

Baird D D, Wilcox A J. Cigarette Smoking Associated with Delayed Conception. *JAMA:* 253; 2979–2983, 1985.

Benowitz N L, Hall S M, Herning R I, Jacob P, Jones R T, Osman A. Smokers of Low-yield Cigarettes do not Consume Less Nicotine. *NEJM:* 309; 139–142, 1983.

Benowitz N L, Jacob P, Kozlowski L T, Yu L. Influence of Smoking Fewer Cigarettes on Exposure to Tar, Nicotine, and Carbon Monoxide. *NEJM:* 315; 1310–1313, 1986.

Churg A. Lung Cancer Cell Type and Asbestos Exposure. JAMA: 253; 2984–2985, 1985. Doll D C, Greenberg B R. Cerebral Thrombosis in Smokers' Polycythemia. *Ann Int Med:* 102; 786–787, 1985.

Hofstetter A, Schutz Y, Jequier E, Wahren J. Increased 24-Hour Energy Expenditure in Cigarette Smokers. *NEJM:* 314; 79–82, 1986.

Macdonald K J S, Green C M, Kenicer K J A. Blood cotinine, carboxyhemoglobin, and thiocyanate concentrations and cigarette consumption. *British Medical J:* 293; 1280, 1986.

Maron D J, Fortmann SP. Nicotine Yield and Measures of Cigarette Smoke Exposure in a Large Population: Are Lower-Yield Cigarettes Safer? *AJPH:* 77, 546–549, 1987.

Michnovicz J J, Hershcopf R J, Naganuma H, Bradlow H L, Fishman J. Increased 2-Hydroxylation of Estradiol as a Possible Mechanism for the Anti-Estrogenic Effect of Cigarette Smoking. *NEJM:* 315; 1305–1309, 1986.

Pojer R, Whitfield J B, Poulos V, Eckhard I F, Richmond R, Hensley W J. Carboxyhemoglobin, Cotinine, and Thiocyanate Assay Compared for Distinguishing Smokers from Non-Smokers. *Clinical Chemistry:* 30; 1377–1380, 1984.

Rogers R L, Meyer J S, Jud B W, Mortel K F. Abstention from Cigarette Smoking Improves Cerebral Perfusion among Elderly Chronic Smokers. *JAMA:* 253; 2970–2974, 1985.

Rosenberg L, Daufman D W, Helmrich S P, Miller D R, Stolley P D, Shapiro S. Myocardial Infarction and Cigarette Smoking in Women Younger Than 50 Years of Age. *JAMA:* 253; 2965–2969, 1985.

Wynder E L, Gramam E A. Tobacco Smoking as a Possible Etiological Factor in Bronchiogenic Carcinoma: A Study of Six Hundred and Eighty Four Cases. *JAMA:* 143; 329–336, 1950.

Psychology

Ashton H, Stepney R. *Smoking Psychology and Pharmacology.* Travistock Publications: London, 1982.

Epstein L H, McCoy J F. Issues in Smoking Control. *Addictive Behav:* 1; 65–72, 1975.

Grabowski J, Bell CS (eds). Measurement in the Analysis and Treatment of Smoking Behavior. *NIDA* Research Monograph 48: Department of Health and Human Services; Alcohol, Drug Abuse, and Mental Health Administration, 1983.

Hansen W B, Malotte K. Perceived Personal Immunity: The Development of Beliefs about Susceptibility to the Consequences of Smoking. *Prev Med:* 15; 363–372, 1986.

Krasbegi N A. Cigarette Smoking as a Dependence Process. *NIDA* Research Monograph 23: Department of Health, Education and Welfare; Alcohol, Drug Abuse, and Mental Health Administration, 1979.

Tamerin J S. The Psychodynamics of Quitting Smoking in a Group. *Amer J Psychiat:* 129; 589–595, 1972.

Select Hazards

Blum A. The Possible Role of Tobacco Cigarette Smoking in Hyponatremia of Long-Term Psychiatric Patients. *JAMA:* 252; 2864–2865, 1984.

CDC—MMWR. Lung Cancer among Women. *JAMA:* 2521; 2806–2811, 1984.

Hagen R. Smoking May be Hazard to Male Sexual Response. *Brain Mind Bulletin:* 7; 1, 1982.

Vandenbroucke J P, Mauritz B J, de Bruin A, Verheesen J H H, van der Heide-Wessel C, van der Heide R M. Weight, Smoking, and Mortality. *JAMA:* 252; 2859–2860, 1984.

Policy

American Cancer Society. Model Policy for Smoking in the Workplace, 1985.

California Nonsmokers' Rights Foundation. A Smokefree Workplace—an Employers' Guide to Nonsmoking Policies. California Nonsmokers' Rights Foundation, 1985.

Federal Trade Commission. The Staff Report on the Cigarette Advertising Investigation. May, 1981.

Marwick C. Changing Climate Seen in Efforts to Tell Public about Smoking, Health. *JAMA:* 252; 2797–2799, 1984.

Marwick C. Effects of 'Passive Smoking' Lead Nonsmokers to Step Up Campaign. *JAMA:* 253; 2937–2944, 1985.

Milio N. Health Policy and the Emerging Tobacco Reality. *Soc Sci Med:* 21; 603–613, 1985.

Warner K E. Health Implications of a Tobacco-Free Society. *JAMA:* October 16, 1987; Vol. 1258, No. 15.

Advertising

Davis R M. Current Trends in Cigarette Advertising and Marketing. *NEJM:* 316, 1987.

Doyle N C. Smoking among Women—An Equal-Opportunity Tragedy. *Am Lung Association Bulletin:* July/August; 10–13, 1980.

Warner K E. Special Report: Cigarette Advertising and Media Coverage of Smoking and Health. *NEJM:* 312; 384–388, 1985.

Cessation

Cummings S R. Kicking the Habit: Benefits and Methods of Quitting Cigarette Smoking. *West J Med:* 137; 443–447, 1982.

Jarvis M J, Russell M. Smoking Withdrawal in Patients with Smoking Related Diseases. *British Med J:* 286; 976, 1983.

Pollin W. Editorial: The Role of the Addictive Process as a Key Step in Causation of All Tobacco-Related Diseases. *JAMA:* 252; 2874, 1984.

Pollin W, Ravenholt R T. Tobacco Addiction and Tobacco Mortality. *JAMA:* 252; 2849–2854, 1984.

Russell M A H. Cigarette Dependence: I—Nature and Classification. *British Med J:* 2; 330–331, 1971.

Physicians' Role and Methods

American Cancer Society. The Impact of Providing Physicians with Quit-Smoking Materials for Smoking Patients. *CA—A Cancer Journal for Clinicians:* 31; 75–78, 1981.

Anda R F, Remington P L, Sienko D G, Davis R M. Are Physicians Advising Smokers to Quit? The Patient's Perspective. *JAMA:* 257; 1916–1919, 1987.

Cummings K M, Giovino G, Sciandra R, Koenigsberg M, Emont S L. Physician Advice to Quit Smoking: Who Gets It and Who Doesn't. *Am J Prev Med:* 3; 69–75, 1987.

Frederickson D T. Helping Smokers Quit: The Physician's Role. *CA—Cancer Journal for Clinicians:* 26; 237–241, 1976.

Goldstein B, Fischer P M, Richards J W, Goldstein A, Shank J C. Smoking Counseling Practices of Recently Trained Family Physicians. *J Fam Pract:* 24; 195–197, 1987.

Green D E, Horn D. Physicians' Attitude toward Their Involvement in Smoking Problems of Patients. Presented at the National Forum on Office Management of Smoking Problems: Chicago, Illinois, 1968.

Green D E, Horn D. Physicians' Attitudes toward Their Involvement in Smoking Problems of Patients. *Diseases of the Chest:* 54; 12–13, 1969.

Hill D. The Family Physician's Influence on Patients' Smoking Habits. *Aust Fam Physician:* 9; 678–679, 1983.

Hjalmarson A I M. Effect of Nicotine Chewing Gum in Smoking Cessation: A Randomized, Placebo-Controlled, Double-Blind Study. *JAMA:* 252; 2835–2838, 1984.

Hughes J R, Miller S A. Nicotine Gum to Help Stop Smoking. *JAMA:* 252; 2855–2858, 1984.

Li V C, Coates T J, Ewart C K, Kim Y J. The Effectiveness of Smoking Cessation Advice Given during Routine Medical Care: Physicians Can Make a Difference. *Am J Prev Med:* 3; 81–86, 1987.

Mason J O, Lindsay G B. A Positive Approach to Smoking Prevention and Cessation. *West J Med:* 139; 721–722, 1983.

Mausner J S, Mausner B, Rial W Y. The Influence of a Physician on the Smoking of His Patients. *AJPH:* 58; 46–53, 1968.

Pederson L L. Compliance with Physician Advice to Quit Smoking: A Review of the Literature. *Prev Med:* 11; 71–84, 1982.

Renneker M, McWaters D. Cancer Prevention and Detection Practices in a County Hospital Family Practice Residency Program. Report to Special Awards: American Cancer Society, 1983.

Rimer B K, Strecher V J, Keintz M K, Engstrom P F. A Survey of Physicians' Views and Practices on Patient Education for Smoking Cessation. *Preventive Medicine:* 15; 92–98, 1986.

Russell M A H. Cigarette Dependence: II—Doctor's Role in Management. *British Med J:* 2; 393–395, 1971.

Russell M A H, Wilson C, Taylor C, Baker C D. Effect of General Practitioners' Advice against Smoking. *British Medical J:* 2; 231–235, 1979.

Burt A, Thornley P, Illingworth D, White P, Shaw T R D, Turner R. Stopping Smoking after Myocardial Infarction. *Lancet:* February 23; 304–306, 1974.

Campbell J L, Valente C M, Levine D, Antlita A M. Using Four Simple Steps, Physicians Do Influence Smoking Behavior. *MMJ:* 34; 50–55, 1985.

Christen A G, Cooper K H. Strategic Withdrawal from Cigarette Smoking. *CA—A Cancer Journal for Clinicians:* 29; 96–107, 1979.

Danaher B G, Ellis B H, Farquhar J W. How to Help Smokers Who Want to Quit. *Patient Care:* 14; 86–121, 1980.

Fredrickson D T. How to Help Your Patient Stop Smoking—Guidelines for the Office Physician. *Diseases of the Chest:* 54; 28–34, 1968.

Horn D. An Approach to Office Management of the Cigarette Smoker. *Dis Chest:* 54; 35–41, 1968.

Richmond R L. Smokescreen: How to Help Your Patients Stop Smoking. *Patient Management:* September; 91–101, 1986.

Richmond R L, Austin A, Webster I W. Three-Year Evaluation of a Programme by General Practitioners to Help Patients to Stop Smoking. *British Med J:* 292; 803–806, 1986.

Richmond R L, Webster I W. A Smoking Cessation Programme for Use in General Practice. *Med J Aust:* 142; 190–194, 1985.

The Hard Core Smoker

Adams E. An Approach to Patients Who Can't Stop Smoking. *Prev Med:* 2, 313–317, 1972.

Kozlowski L T. Less Hazardous Smoking and the Pursuit of Satisfaction. *AJPH:* 77; 539–541, 1987.

Environmental Tobacco Smoke

Committee on Passive Smoking National Research Council. Environmental Tobacco Smoke: Measuring Exposures and Assessing Health Effects. Washington, D.C., National Academy Press, 1986.

Elsner R H. Smokers Are Killing Us. *Calif Physician:* March; 6–7, 1987.

Humble C G, Samet J M, Pathak D R. Marriage to a Smoker and Lung Cancer Risk. *AJPH:* 77; 598–602, 1987.

Tager I B. "Passive Smoking" and Respiratory Health in Children—Sophistry or Cause for Concern? *Am Rev Respir Dis:* 134; 958–961, 1986.

Epidemiology

American Cancer Society. *Dangers of Smoking—Benefits of Quitting and Relative Risks of Reduced Exposure.* Revised ed., 1980.

American Cancer Society. *Facts and Figures on Smoking: 1976–1986,* 1986.

Bohgard F S, Ostrow L B, Sacks S T, McGuire A, Trunkey DD. Fatal Hospital-Acquired Burns. *JAMA:* 252; 2813, 1984.

Friedman G D, Sidney S, Polen M R. Smoking Habits among Multiphasic Examinees, 1979 to 1984. *West J Med:* 145; 651–656, 1986.

Greenberg M A, Wiggins C L, Kutvirt D M, Samet J M. Cigarette Use among Hispanic and Non-Hispanic White School Children, Albuquerque, New Mexico. *AJPH:* 77; 621–622, 1987.

Khoury M J U, Weinstein A, Panny S, Holtzman N A, Lindsay P K, Farrel K, Eisenberg M. Maternal Cigarette

Smoking and Oral Clefts: A Population-Based Study. *AJPH:* 77; 623–625, 1987.

Mattson M E, Pollack E S, Cullen J W. What Are the Odds That Smoking Will Kill You? *AJPH:* 77; 425–431, 1987.

Myers A H, Rosner B, Abbey H, Willet W, Stampfer M J, Bain C, Lipnick R, Hennekens C, Speizer F. Smoking Behavior among Participants in the Nurses' Health Study. *AJPH:* 77; 628–630, 1987.

Office on Smoking and Health—Technical Information Center. Directory: On-Going Research in Smoking and Health. U.S. Department of Health and Human Services: Public Health Service; World Health Organization Collaborating Centre, 1982.

Pincherle G, Wright H B. Smoking Habits of Business Executives: Doctor Variation in Reducing Cigarette Consumption. *The Practitioner:* 205; 209–212, 1970.

Remington P L, Forman M R, Gentry E M, Marks J S, Hogelin G C, Trowbridge F L. Current Smoking Trends in the United States. *JAMA:* 253; 2975–2978, 1985.

Ricer R E. Smokeless Tobacco Use: A Dangerous Nicotine Habit. *Postgrad Med:* 81; 89–94, 1987.

Schuman L M. Progress and Responsibilities of Educators in Smoking Control. *Medical and Pediatric Oncology:* 11; 375–382, 1983.

Soffer A, Auerbach O, Banyai A L, Chadwick D, et al. Discussion of Physicians' Attitude toward Smoking. *Diseases of the Chest:* 54; 14–17, 1968.

Wechsler H, et al. The Physician's Role in Health Promotion—a Survey of Primary Care Practitioners. *NEJM:* 308; 97–100, 1983.

Wells K B, Lewis C E, Leake B, Ware J E. Do Physicians Preach What They Practice? *JAMA:* 252; 2846–2848, 1984.

Wood J C. Stopping Smoking: What the Experts Say. *Healthline:* December; 4–6, 1983.

Stop Smoking Groups

Berecz J M. Superiority of a Low-Contrast Smoking Cessation Method. *Addictive Behaviors:* 9; 273–278, 1984.

Davis A L, Faust R, Ordentlich M. Self-Help Smoking Cessation and Maintenance Programs: A Comparative Study with 12-Month Follow-Up by the American Lung Association. *Am J Public Health:* 74; 1212–1217, 1984.

Hunt W A, Bespalec D A. An Evaluation of Current Methods of Modifying Smoking Behavior.

Kanzler M, Jaffe J H, Zeidenberg P. Long- and Short-Term Effectiveness of a Large-Scale Proprietary Smoking Cessation Program—A 4-Year Follow-Up of Smokenders Participants. *J of Clin Psychol:* 32; 661–669, 1976.

Orlandi M A. Smoking Clinics: Do They Work? *JAMA:* 253; 3017, 1985.

Orleans C S, Shipley R H. Worksite Smoking Cessation Initiatives: Review and Recommendations. *Addictive Behav:* 7; 1–16, 1982.

Stachnik T, Stoffelmayr B. Worksite Smoking Cessation Programs: A Potential for National Impact. *AJPH:* 73; 1395–1396, 1983.

Windsor R A, Cutter G, Morris J, Reese Y, Manzella B, Bartlett E E, Samuelson C, Spanos D. The Effectiveness of Smoking Cessation Methods for Smokers in Public Health Maternity Clinics: A Randomized Trial. *AJPH:* 75; 1389–1392, 1985.

75

Sputum Cytology: A Method to Assess Respiratory Health

Kent W. Sorensen

SMOKING AND DISEASE

"Cigarette smoking is the major single cause of cancer mortality in the United States . . ."

That is the startling conclusion of the U.S. Surgeon General's Report, "The Health Consequences of Smoking." According to this report, smoking would contribute to 30 percent of the estimated 472,000 cancer deaths in the United States in 1986. In addition, the report states that tobacco is primarily responsible for cancers of the lung, larynx, mouth, and esophagus, and also plays a significant role in emphysema, coronary disease and strokes.

The report points out that people fear dying of cancer more than any other disease—and for good reason. One out of every three Americans now living is expected to develop cancer during their lifetime, and it continues to be the second leading cause of death in the United States. While the mortality rates of most chronic diseases in this country have been declining during the last twenty years, only cancer and chronic obstructive pulmonary disease (COPD) continue to claim more lives each year. When the cancer mortality figures are broken down by body site, lung cancer is shown to be the only kind of cancer that is steadily increasing in both men and women. Over 130,000 people in the U.S. die of lung cancer each year. Cigarette smoking represents the major cause for both lung cancer and COPD.

While the percentage of cigarette smokers in the U.S. has declined, the actual number of people who smoke remains the same as 20 years ago. About thirty percent of adults now smoke compared to forty-two percent in 1965. However, there are still 52 million smokers in the country, representing a substantial group at high risk for developing serious lung disease. There is no single action an individual can take to reduce the risk of COPD and lung cancer more effectively than to quit smoking cigarettes. Moreover, smokers are at significantly higher risk to develop several other diseases, including coronary heart disease, strokes and complications from diabetes.

However, the process of quitting smoking is far from easy for many people. Smoking is now considered to be a health behavior which is multifaceted and complex. For example, while the psychological resources of the individual smoker figures into the equation, so does that person's biologic response to smoke inhalation. Thus, it is no longer reasonable, in light of recent scientific evidence, to treat the smoking patient as if the smoking habit were strictly a behavioral problem or strictly a biological problem. It is a bio-behavioral problem that requires a bio-behavioral approach to resolution.

Unfortunately, for most smokers who attempt to quit, the maintenance of their abstinence from cigarettes is extremely difficult to achieve. While there may be many reasons for this, the fact is that smokers have no way of linking their smoking behavior with a biologic outcome that is personally relevant to them. Since the pre-clinical stage of respiratory disease associated with cigarette smoking may exist for years without causing any noticeable symptoms, the cigarette smoker, feeling just fine, sees little reason to make a serious attempt to quit. The return to health after smoking has stopped remains only a vague idea in the minds of most people. The risk ratios and promises of improved health have no personal meaning to ex-smokers who are struggling with urges to return to their former habit.

Figure 75-1 Age Adjusted Death Rates, USA

Causes	1968	1978	Change
Heart disease	386	301	− 22%
Cancer	162	170	+ 5%
Cerebral vascular disease	111	71	− 36%
Accidents	59	46	− 22%
Influenza, pneumonia	38	24	− 37%
Chronic obstructive pulmonary disease	17	22	+ 29%
Diabetes	20	14	− 30%

Figure 75-2 Estimated New Cases and Deaths for Major Sites of Cancer—1988*

Site	No. of Cases	Deaths
Lung	152,000	139,000
Colon-rectum	147,000	61,500
Breast (female)	135,900	42,300
Prostate	99,000	28,000
Urinary	68,900	20,000
Uterus	46,900**	10,000
Oral	30,200	9,050
Leukemia	26,900	18,100
Pancreas	27,000	24,500
Skin	27,300***	7,800
Ovary	19,000	12,000

*Figures rounded to nearest 1,000.
**If carcinoma in situ is included, cases total over 100,000.
***Estimated new cases of non-melanoma over 400,000.
Incidence estimates are based on rates from N.C.I. Seer Program, 1977–1981.

SPUTUM CYTOLOGY TECHNOLOGY

Recent technologic advances in *sputum cytology* now make it possible to link cigarette smoking with its biologic effect on the respiratory tract. Smokers have the opportunity for the first time to establish a personally meaningful connection between their smoking habit and respiratory health.

For the purpose of definition, sputum cytology is the microscopic study of lung cells that are naturally shed from the surface lining of the air passages into the mucus that coats the respiratory tract. A sample is obtained by coughing up phlegm (sputum) and spitting it into a collection container. The specimen is submitted to a cytology laboratory for analysis. The cells are separated from the mucus and expressed onto glass slides, stained, and microscopically examined by cytotechnologists and/or pathologists.

Until now, sputum cytology has been used almost exclusively to detect or diagnose lung cancer. Due to problems associated with specimen collection, test accuracy and lack of conclusive lung cancer survival data, sputum cytology is not widely accepted by the medical community as an early test to detect lung cancer. Nor is it recommended for routine screening by the American Cancer Society.

But, instead of using sputum cytology as a diagnostic test to detect lung cancer, it can be used to assess the general health of the lungs. As such, it then can become a powerful motivational tool to stop smoking. As a result of recent technological advances, eight respiratory components seen in sputum cytology smears have proven to be reliable indicators of bronchial irritation in relation to cigarette smoke exposure. As the exposure increases, the overall number or concentration of these components likewise increases. In the event a person stops smoking, the level of these components will begin to return to normal values as the lungs repair themselves.

The respiratory components are as follows:

1. **Macrophages (Total)**—Macrophage means "big eater." They are giant "white blood cells" that are an important part of your body's

Figure 75-3 The Development of Lung Cancer *Source:* LungCheck, A division of CytoSciences, Inc., Sunnyvale, California. Used with permission

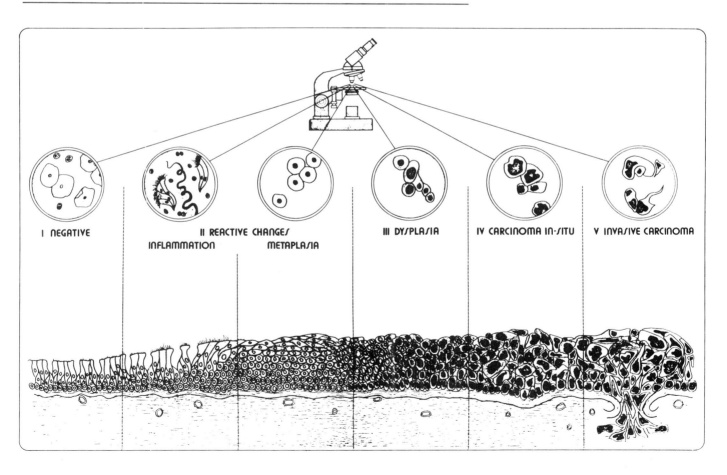

I NEGATIVE II REACTIVE CHANGES INFLAMMATION METAPLASIA III DYSPLASIA IV CARCINOMA IN-SITU V INVASIVE CARCINOMA

immune system. They are capable of identifying foreign substances that have invaded the body and can literally eat them by pulling the matter into their cytoplasm (the jellylike fluid within the cell membrane). Total pulmonary macrophages (both non-pigmented and pigmented) are quantitated. They increase in number in response to the irritating effect of cigarette smoke inhalation.

2. **Macrophages (Pigmented)**—Macrophages ingest carbon pigment and other particulate material found in cigarette smoke. The density of pigment contained in macrophages is assessed, which reflects the dose response to cigarette smoke inhalation.

3. **Neutrophils**—The toxic effect of cigarette smoke stimulates the production of an increased number of small white blood cells called neutrophils. They release elastase, an enzyme that dissolves the biologic "glue" that holds our cells together. When elastase is secreted in the lungs, healthy lung tissue becomes damaged, leading to emphysema.

4. **Mucus**—In response to the effect of cigarette smoke, the cells (lining the airways) that produce mucus begin to multiply. As a result, an overproduction of mucus begins to clog the airways.

5. **Curschmann Spirals**—The overproduction of mucus will eventually accumulate in the small air passages leading to the airsacs. As the mucus stagnates, "rubbery" casts of coiled mucus are formed and are usually dislodged during the process of producing a coughed sputum specimen. They are identified in approximately 90% of sputum samples among cigarette smokers.

6. **Columnar Cells**—As the toxins from cigarette smoke irritate the lungs, the usual rigidly anchored columnar cells (normal cells that line the airways) begin to lose their ability to adhere to the surface. The presence of these columnar cells in sputa reveal chronic lung irritation.

7. **Metaplastic Cells**—When the toxic effect of cigarette smoke continues to irritate the lining of the lungs over a period of time, columnar cells begin to transform themselves into layered "scale-like" metaplastic cells. Such changes may eventually regress to relatively normal epithelium following smoking cessation.

8. **Dysplastic Cells**—Dysplastic cells are potentially premalignant, arising from abnormal changes within metaplastic cells due to prolonged carcinogenic irritation in the lungs. These cells may likewise reverse to healthier tissue after smoking cessation.

Further research has discovered a means to quantify the values of each component, ranging in values from "0" to a maximum of "10." This technologic development is significant, representing the first time that a routine cytology test has been able to be reported in quantifiable and reproducible values. The ability to quantify test results also permits the pathologist to express the values in graphic form, making the report easier to interpret. Moreover, computer systems can automatically retrieve previous test results and display them graphically beside the present values, creating a trend analysis of the test results over time.

Thus, sputum cytology becomes a bio-behavioral tool that links smoking exposure to the current state of health of the lungs, an effective approach to the management of smoking.

References

1. Frost JK, Gupta PK, Erozan YS, Carter D, Hollander DH, Levin ML, and Ball WC: Pulmonary cytologic alterations in toxic environmental inhalation. *Human Pathology* 4:521–536, 1973.

2. Koop, CE: *Chronic Obstructive Lung Disease: A Report of the Surgeon General.* U.S. Department of Health and Human Service. Rockville, MD, 1984.

3. Saccamano G, Saunders RP, Klein MG, Archer VE, and Brennan L: Cytology of the lung in reference to irritant, individual sensitivity and healing. *Acta Cytol* 14:377, 1970.

4. Schumann GB and Colon VF: Sputum cytology. *American Family Physician* 19:81–84, 1979.

5. Madison R, Afifi AA, and Mittman C: Respiratory impairment in coke oven workers: Relationship to work exposure and bronchial inflammation detected by sputum cytology. *J Chron Dis* 37:167–176, 1984.

6. Schmitz B, Pfitzer P: Cellular bodies in sputum. *Acta Cytol* 28:118–125, 1984.

7. Fullmer CD, Short JG, Allen A, and Walker K: Sputum of chronic cigarette smokers: Microscopic observations and incidence of bronchial spirals, fibrils and casts. *Rocky Mountain Med J* 66:42, 1969.

Permission to publish the material in this chapter was given by: LungCheck, A division of CytoSciences, Inc., 1601 Saratoga-Sunnyvale Road, Cupertino, CA 95014.

76

Avoiding
Unnecessary X-Rays

Priscilla W. Laws

Excerpted with permission from Priscilla W. Laws and The Public Citizen Health Research Group. The X-ray Information Book.

Does your doctor know the number of rads you'll be exposed to when he orders an X-ray for you? Does the radiation risk warrant the diagnostic gain? We have reprinted here a chart contained in the guide listing radiation doses for the more commonly ordered X-ray examinations. Referring to an average dose for a chest (radiographic) X-ray examination, the average skin dose is listed as 45 millirads. This is equivalent to .045 rads. Also, it should be mentioned that when discussing radiation exposure, it's usually in terms of the average skin dose. As an indication of how few rads can result in the onset of cancer, bear in mind that thyroid cancers are now appearing in people who were irradiated as children in the 1950s for enlarged thymus glands. They were exposed to from 50 to 500 rads.—*M.R.*

HOW TO MINIMIZE YOUR EXPOSURE TO X-RAYS

Checklist of Questions to Ask

1. Questions everybody should ask medical and dental personnel:

- What benefit should I expect from the proposed x-ray examination?

- Are there clinical indications that an x-ray examination is needed or is this a routine examination?

- Would you like to know about my previous x-ray examinations and would it be possible to use the results of any of them?

- Is this x-ray facility inspected by any licensing agencies?

2. Questions everyone should ask: *Medical Personnel Only:*

- Why is fluoroscopy necessary in my case?

- Is this facility supervised by a full-time radiologist?

- Are you able to adjust the size of the x-ray beam to that of the smallest appropriate film size?

Dental Personnel Only:

- Would it be feasible for me to have one panographic x-ray rather than a series of individual films (for whole mouth x-rays)?

- Do you use a long open-ended lead cylinder?

3. Questions for young adults and children who are potential parents to ask medical and dental personnel:

- Will my reproductive organs be in the main beam, and if so, can you provide me with a lead shield for them?

4. Questions for women who are or may be pregnant to ask medical and dental personnel:

- Do you know that I may be pregnant?

- Can this x-ray examination wait until later in my pregnancy or just after my next menstrual period?

- Will my uterus be in the main beam, and if so, can you provide me with lead shielding for it?

Figure 76-1 Medical and Dental X-Rays—A Consumer's Guide to Avoiding Unnecessary Radiation Exposure (Average Doses for Typical Diagnostic X-Ray Examinations in Millirads)

	Average Skin Dose per Film (a)	Average Integral Bone Marrow Dose per Exam (b)	Average No. of Films per Exam (a)	Estimated Whole Body Equivalent Dose per Exam (c)	Average Gonadal Dose per Exam (d) M	F	Estimated Annual Excess Deaths per Million Exam (e)
Upper GI	519	650	Fluoroscopic**	400–800	30	150	30–100
Lower GI	629	650*	Fluoroscopic	300–700	400	500	25–80
Cholecystography	771	560	3	200–600	10	200	20–70
Intravenous Pyelogram (IVP)	481	400	3	100–500	300	200	15–50
Thoracic Spine	1265	210	3	100–500	30	30	15–45
Lumbar Spine (LS)	1965	280	3	100–500	200	200	15–45
Abdomen or KUB	771	125	3	100–200	150	50	5–25
Mammography***	1500	—	3*	100–200	—	—	5–20
Lumbo-Pelvic	487	135	3	100–200	300	150	5–20
Hip or Upper Femur	1036	100*	3	50–150	300	100	5–20
Cervical Spine	158	50	4	25–75	<10	<10	2–8
Skull	304	35	4	25–75	<10	<10	2–7
Shoulder	213	58	2	25–75	<10	<10	2–6
Chest (photofluoroscopic)	504	80	1	20–60	<10	<10	2–6
Dental (whole mouth)	1100	32	1	10–30	<10	<10	2–6
Chest (radiographic)	45	12	2	5–10	<10	<10	<1
Dental (bite wing)	1100	5	3*	<5	<2	<2	<1
Extremities	100–127	<10	2	<5	<2	<2	<1

(a) Population Dose from X-Rays U.S. 1964 (DHEW/PHS, Washington, D.C., 1969), p. 132.
(b) Ionizing Radiation: Levels and Effects, Vol. 1—UNSCEAR Report (United Nations, New York, 1972), pp. 162, 164.
(c) Laws, P., Estimates of Somatic Risks for Common X-Ray Diagnoses. To be published.
(d) Protection of the Patient in X-Ray Diagnosis. ICRP publication 16 (Pergamon Press, New York, 1970), p. 8.
(e) National Academy of Sciences, National Research Council. The Effects on Population of Exposure to Low Levels of Ionizing Radiation [BEIR Report]. (NAS/NRC, Washington, D.C., 1972), p. 91.

The figures in the last column represent the estimated average number of excess cancer and leukemia deaths under the linear hypothesis in the 30 year period after each million examinations conducted with the given whole body equivalent dose. The ranges are based on figures presented in the BEIR Report. See reference (c) for technical details.

*Estimate by author.
**A fluoroscopic examination is done with continuous radiographic visualization, like taking a movie or watching television. The amount of exposure will necessarily be greater.
***Mammography controversy: Recent attention has been drawn to the possible excessive radiation exposure associated with routine mammograms. The result of this controversy has been a lowering of the radiation dose to perform this procedure. Most mammograms now only utilize 0.5 rads (⅓ of the dose listed in this chart).

Source: The chart "Average Doses for Typical X-ray Examinations in Millirads" from THE X-RAY INFORMATION BOOK by Priscilla W. Laws and The Public Citizen Health Research Group. Copyright 1974, 1983 by Priscilla W. Laws and the Health Research Group. Reprinted by permission of Farrar, Straus and Giroux, Inc.

For Your Information

CT brain scans are reported as using from 0.6 to 3.5 rads. Also, cardiac catheterizations will average about 10 rads but up to 66 rads with fluoroscopy.

Obstetrical X-rays for evaluation of pelvic size may result in a dose to the fetus of from 1 to 4 rads.

77

Environmental Cancer Issues Into the 1990s

Of the issues covered in the following pages, those relating to the first five—water pollution, air pollution, asbestos, radon, and passive smoking—concern documented sources of cancer we encounter daily as we go about our lives; the last two—toxicological testing and genetic screening—concern the means of determining the effects of exposure. They all remain unresolved.

California is the focus of much of this chapter, but the issues obviously apply to the entire United States. For the remainder of the 1980s, and into the 1990s, these are environmental cancer issues you'll read about in the journals and hear about on the evening news.—*M.R.*

WATER POLLUTION

An abundance of cheap water, and a multitude of pesticides and fertilizers, have transformed the arid Central Valley of California into the leading agricultural region of the U.S., generating $14 billion annually. Each year, 85% of the water used in the state and hundreds of different pesticides are employed to grow crops. Historically, little or no toxicological testing of the pesticides has been done prior to sale and application. When water used in irrigation migrates through the soil into the acquifers (underground water), pesticides are carried along. Residents of the Central Valley obtain drinking water from wells which tap this water, and thus thousands of people have been, and are, consuming pesticides on a daily basis. The state Department of Food and Agriculture lists 63 currently used pesticides which are known to cause cancer, birth defects, or other toxic effects in lab animals. Other chemicals, like DBCP, have been banned from application, but may still be found in underground water supplies.

Banned in 1979 because of its ability to cause cancer and birth defects in lab animals, and sterility in human males, DBCP is one of 57 agricultural chemicals which have been found in well water. It has been detected in 80% of the contaminated wells in California, including 1,696 wells in Fresno County alone. In two towns in the Central Valley, Fowler and McFarland, the state has found an unusually high incidence of cancer. Similar clusters have not been found in other California communities.

Urban water also contains chemicals known to cause cancer, although typically at much lower levels than those found in the Central Valley. One example is chloroform, present in tap water throughout the U.S. A National Cancer Institute study concluded that chloroform concentrations are sufficient to cause up to 1.6 cases of cancer per million population per year. Others have disputed this finding, saying that inherent cellular mechanisms detoxify the trace amounts of the chemicals found in tap water.

Most experts accept the statement that water pollution presents a problem in some areas of the U.S., but the extent of the problem has not been identified. A comprehensive study of drinking water quality has not been completed, although many states and municipalities have developed such data. Nor have comprehensive national standards been implemented on safe drinking water. This may be, in part, due to the bureaucracy involved.

In California, municipal water districts implement the guidelines established by the State Department of Health Services, Water Quality Control Board, Regional Water Control Board, the EPA, and the districts themselves. None of these agencies has assumed a dominant role.

But things are changing . . .

• With the passage of the Federal Safe Drinking Water Act more than 10 years ago, Maximum Contaminant Levels (MCLs) were established for 16 chemicals. Later amendments included radionuclides and a group of chemicals termed "trihalomethanes," including chloroform. However, to date, hundreds of chemicals with recognized toxic properties are unregulated nationally. This is about to change. Recommended maximum contaminant levels for a large number of chemicals, including DBCP, were proposed in 1985 and are scheduled to become enforceable limits in two phases, some in June, 1987, the remainder in June, 1988. For the 23 chemicals the Federal Government officially recognizes as carcinogenic, these will be allowed in water at levels no greater than those detectable by analytic techniques available in most labs. Since the limits of detection are continually being lowered as analytic instrumentation improves, the allowable limits will be periodically revised downward.

• An EPA survey, begun in 1987, will check the water in 720 private and 750 municipal wells in 49 states. The results will be used to set acceptable contamination limits, and to enforce the Safe Drinking Water Act.

• The Clean Water Act was renewed in 1987 (over presidential veto). One of its provisions requires states to adopt uniform water quality standards.

• In California, Proposition 65 passed overwhelmingly. It requires the cessation of industrial discharge of chemicals with established carcinogenic or reproductive system effects, unless it can be shown that such discharge does not pose a "significant risk." Although its implementation is currently on schedule, the list of chemicals to be regulated remains a political football.

• Nationally, the EPA requires industries to cease discharge of toxics by March 31, 1989.

AIR POLLUTION

Very little is known about air pollution as a causal agent for cancer. In an attempt to develop an idea of the scope of the problem, the Environmental Protection Agency, in 1983, initiated an air toxics study designed to estimate the cancer risk associated with exposure to selected outdoor air pollutants. Using only existing data, and focusing on only 15 pollutants or pollutant groups, the study concluded that up to 1500 cases of cancer nationally per year are due to air pollution. For residents of urban areas, it was estimated that the risk of developing cancer due to simultaneous exposure to the pollutants is between 1:1000 and 1:10,000. If the numbers are accurate, it appears the risk is low. But are they accurate?

The study had significant limitations:

• It assessed the risk posed by a relative few, though major, pollutants.

• The synergistic or antagonistic health effects of simultaneous exposure to a complex mixture of chemicals remain largely unknown; hence any estimate of risk for such circumstances is essentially guesswork.

• Only routine emissions were addressed, not accidental releases.

• Most of the data used was based on exposure to average, healthy adults. Other age groups, or individual hypersensitivities, were not considered.

One of the authors of the study, when commenting on the assumptions used as the basis for the study, stated that the sum of the assumptions is "a degree of uncertainty that we cannot even begin to quantify. The numerical estimates presented should be viewed as rough indications of the potential cancer risk posed by a few pollutants."

Currently, through the Clean Air Act, the EPA establishes National Ambient Air Quality Standards. In California, the Air Resources Board (ARB) is responsible for implementing Federal air quality regulations, and establishing additional air quality standards to be implemented within the state. Actual *emission* standards are set by 41 local or regional Air Pollution Control Districts. Each district must meet the ARB standards, but, since geography, climate, and industry vary considerably from one area of California to another, the districts are allowed considerable latitude in determining local emission standards which will provide acceptable ambient air quality. Because some districts are much more aggressive than others in fulfilling their mandate, the result can be considerable regional differences in emission standards, and air quality. The ARB presently considers only five materials as toxic— benzene, ethylene dibromide, ethylene dichloride, hexavalent chromium, and asbestos—though many other chemicals of established toxicity, some with carcinogenic potential, are regulated at the local level.

In summary, although it is thought that air pollution does not significantly contribute to cancer incidence, insufficient data exist to either prove or disprove this supposition. Only after considerably more is known about the identity and levels of airborne pollutants, and their toxicology, both individually and in mixture, will it be possible to reach authoritative conclusions on the actual risk presented. Until that time, regulation of air pollution nationally is likely to remain minimal and inconsistent, reflecting local or regional concern rather than national policy.

ASBESTOS

Rarely a week goes by when the hazards of asbestos aren't brought to our attention. In the past decade, we've read of rare forms of cancer occurring in great numbers of workers who, 20 years or more before, were employed by the mining, tire, construction, or ship-fitting industries. And we've read of large corporations forced into bankruptcy under the weight of billion dollar lawsuits. More recently, the media have focused on the risk presented by the buildings in which we work, attend school, and reside. As a consequence you have to wonder, "How much of all this is real, and how much just media hype? Is everyone routinely exposed to asbestos, and, if so, what are the real risks involved?" I'm glad you asked.

Air sampling conducted in rural and urban areas throughout California indicates asbestos is ubiquitous. Although an estimate is not available on natural emissions, the geology of California includes large deposits of minerals in which asbestos is a significant component. Additionally, approximately one million pounds of asbestos per year are emitted into the air by California industry. Consequently, asbestos, and other mineral fibers, originating from both natural and man-made sources, are present in the air we breathe every day.

It has been estimated that, in California, there are typically 8–80 asbestos fibers per cubic meter of air in outdoor areas with *low* asbestos levels. In areas with high levels, 50–500 fibers per cubic meter is the norm. If we use a figure of 100 fibers per cubic meter as an average exposure level, a 70 kg male outside for 3 hours (not exercising) will inhale approximately 100 asbestos fibers.

These counts are for fibers of sufficient size to be seen by traditional methods of analysis, called phase contrast microscopy (PCM) or polarized light microscopy (PLM), and which have historically been associated with the development of the primary asbestos-related cancers: lung cancer and mesothelioma. Using a new method, transmission electron microscopy (TEM), which allows the counting of much smaller fibers, fiber counts in the California survey were found to be 100 to 1000 times greater than the figures quoted above.

If these numbers sound high, consider that the current OSHA-allowed occupational exposure limit, to which, it is believed, nearly all workers may be routinely exposed without significant risk to health, is on the order of one-half million fibers per 8-hour workshift. And these are fibers counted by PCM, not TEM. (For the rest of this section, for consistency's sake, all numbers will be PCM counts, with TEM fiber counts divided by 1000 to generate a PCM-equivalent.)

What about indoor air? It has been established that at least half the buildings in the U.S. are constructed with asbestos-containing materials. In 1981, the National Research Council conducted a nationwide survey to determine asbestos concentrations in public and private schools and Federal buildings. The median results were:

Area Sampled	Fibers/m^3
Schoolrooms without asbestos	540
Schoolrooms with asbestos surfaces	2,080
Schoolrooms with damaged asbestos surfaces	4,050
Buildings with asbestos surfaces[a]	260
Buildings with friable[b] asbestos	640

[a]These surfaces were said to be cementitious; that is, the surface was dense and intact, with the asbestos well contained.
[b]Asbestos material is said to be friable when it can be crushed between your fingers.

The last source of potential exposure is drinking water. In California, because of the abundance of asbestos-containing serpentine rock in watersheds, it is common to find thousands of asbestos fibers per liter of water, and concentrations hundreds of times higher are not uncommon. The good news is that there is no evidence to link ingestion of asbestos fibers with adverse health effects.

In summary, the following are estimates of annual asbestos fiber intakes (counts are in thousands of fibers):

So, it's obvious that we all are routinely exposed to asbestos. What risks are posed? The following are the estimated lifetime risks of lung cancer and mesothelioma due to continuous exposure to 100 fibers/m^3 and 2000 fibers/m^3 (values in parens) of asbestos, expressed as cases per million population. Two thousand fibers was chosen to represent a level to which only 10% of the population is exposed, while 100 fibers may be considered the median level of exposure.

Exposure Group	Lung Cancer	Mesothelioma
Male Smokers	11 (110)	24 (120)
Female Smokers	5 (50)	32 (160)
Male Nonsmokers	2 (15)	32 (160)
Female Nonsmokers	1 (6)	38 (190)

Clearly, a risk is posed, but it is relatively low, and likely to decrease with time as asbestos use is almost entirely phased-out, and asbestos either encapsulated or removed from all public buildings, further reducing the risk. Asbestos-containing materials will continue to be a part of our environment for the rest of our lives but, as long as it is intact and not disturbed, it poses no real hazard. However, routine exposure to friable asbestos leads to increased risk. You can reduce the risk by checking for the presence of friable asbestos in your personal environment, but don't disturb any suspect material. For guidance, call your county health department, or telephone the U.S. Consumer Product Safety Commission and request a copy of "Asbestos in the Home." Their toll-free number is (800) 638-2772.

If you'd like more information on this topic, much of the above data was taken from a draft report (#0171D/0158W) released February 10, 1986 by the California Air Resources Board. You can obtain a

Exposure Route	Child	House Person	Officer Worker
Inhalation			
Ambient Air	20–100	6–30	6–30
Indoor-Schools with asbestos	50–4,000	0	0
Indoor-Office buildings with asbestos	0	10–200	60–1,500
Indoor-Homes with asbestos	1–200	1–300	1–200
Total	**70–4,300**	**20–500**	**70–1,700**
Ingestion			
Tap water	400–90,000,000	500–140,000,000	500–140,000,000

copy by contacting the California Department of Health Services.

RADON

In 1984, officials at a nuclear plant in Pennsylvania were alarmed by an employee's high radiation-badge reading. Unable to find a source of the exposure at work, investigators eventually tested the worker's home. There they found radiation levels far in excess of the guidelines for acceptable exposure. The source: radon and its daughters.

Radon is a gas found in soil across the U.S. which originates from the natural degradation of uranium and radium. It is odorless, tasteless, and invisible, and is said by the EPA to be responsible for 5,000 to 20,000 lung cancer deaths each year.

Radon gas emanates from the soil into the foundation of homes, where it becomes concentrated. Once present, it continues a decay process whereby four, short-lived isotopes (daughters) of other elements are generated. Each decay generates a high-energy alpha particle which, when an unsuspecting inhabitant inhales, bombards the sensitive cells which are found in the lungs at the air-tissue interface, potentially causing lung cancer.

The EPA estimates that 8 million homes nationwide exceed its upper limit for acceptable radon concentration of 4 picocuries per liter of air (1 pico-curie = 3.7 disintegrations per second, each generating an alpha particle). Whether the 4 picocurie guideline is sufficiently protective is the subject of debate. The Environmental Defense Fund estimates that longterm exposure to 4 picocuries presents a "1-in-65" chance of developing lung cancer.

Currently (1987), no epidemiological data exist on the consequences of residential exposure. Results of a recently initiated epidemiological study are expected in 1991. Additionally, the EPA has begun a study to determine radon levels in residences across the country, with results due in 1990.

A recent U.S. General Accounting Office report stated that there is no Federally coordinated effort to manage radon exposure. The EPA has an "action plan" which includes assessment of the problem, developing mitigating procedures, encouraging state programs, and disseminating information, but does not address regulation of exposure.

With the Federal Government assuming only an advisory role, several states have moved to fill the need. In Pennsylvania, New Jersey, and New York, state agencies test homes for radon and provide financial aid to homeowners who choose to reduce concentrations through remedial construction. Several other states are in the process of developing programs.

Two (free) sources of additional information are:

The General Accounting Office report (GAO/RCED-86-170) entitled "Air Pollution, Hazards of Indoor Radon Could Pose a National Health Problem," available from the U.S. General Accounting Office, P.O. Box 6015, Gaithersburg, MD 20877.

"A Citizen's Guide to Radon: What It Is and What to Do about It," and "Radon Reduction Methods: A Homeowner's Guide," are pamphlets available from EPA, Washington, DC 20460.

PASSIVE SMOKING

In the last five years, more than a dozen studies have demonstrated a clear association between the presence of environmental tobacco smoke and an increased incidence of lung cancer in non-smokers. In response:

• In his annual report for 1986, noting that several thousand lung cancer deaths annually may be attributable to passive smoking, U.S. Surgeon General C. Everett Koop called for smoke-free workplaces.

• All but nine states, many municipalities, and approximately 35% of businesses have established some type of smoking prohibition.

• There is legislative momentum to further restrict cigarette advertising.

TOXICOLOGICAL TESTING

There is a clear and pressing need for revolutionary methods of assessing carcinogenic potential. Current methods are slow, expensive, and, ultimately, unreliable, offering limited predictive power on human response to exposure. Epidemiological data remains the only means of accurately evaluating carcinogenicity, but testing on human subjects is unacceptable, not only because of ethical considerations, but because of the long latent period for many carcinogens—20 years is a long time to await results.

Traditionally, laboratory-based animal testing, usually with rodents, has been regarded as the authoritative means of establishing carcinogenic potential in man. However, a recent National Cancer Institute study concluded that the results of testing with animals bred for their susceptibility to cancer cannot be reliably extrapolated to humans. One of the problems with such testing is that, to be timely, it requires administration of high doses in a short duration, with subsequent statistical analysis relied upon to estimate the effects of low doses.

What is needed is a technique which rapidly assesses the effects of exposure, even to low concentrations. As it turns out, such techniques are on the brink of practical application. Often termed "DNA-adduct" tests, they utilize rodents and an array of high-tech analytical instrumentation and techniques, to pick one damaged DNA molecule out of up to 10 million healthy molecules. Based on the assumption that carcinogenic potential is directly associated with the potential to damage DNA, these tests are not only rapid and accurate, they allow researchers to probe into the precise mechanisms by which cancer is initiated, while the results of traditional testing methods—tumors—can only be seen long afterward.

DNA-adduct testing is based on another assumption: that a chemical's ability to damage DNA in a rodent can be directly related to its ability to damage DNA in humans. It is likely that this is true only up to a point, that the effects on DNA are very similar, if not identical, but what happens to the chemical before and after it reaches the DNA can differ greatly, reflecting differences in molecular biology. Mechanisms for deactivating potential carcinogens before they cause damage, and for repairing damage once done, are known to vary considerably from species to species. Only after this problem is surmounted will DNA-adduct testing fulfill its potential to become the predominant method for assessing carcinogenic potential.

GENETIC SCREENING

Within the next decade, present techniques will be refined and new ones developed to allow medical personnel to assess both the current status and the potential of an individual's genetic material. Using DNA-adduct techniques, genetic screening could be used to search for chromosomal damage resulting from exposure to a specific carcinogen, or to predict an individual's susceptibility to hazards he or she may encounter in the workplace. Including genetic screening as part of pre-employment physicals could prevent placement of hypersusceptible individuals in potentially harmful environments. But, before such screening becomes commonplace, two ethical/legal issues will have to be resolved:

1. Is it possible to provide equal opportunity in the workplace when employing a screening process which systematically excludes selected individuals? Differences in susceptibility to chemical damage are likely to reflect ethnic or racial background. To base suitability of employment on such grounds would conflict with the Civil Rights Act. Currently, New Jersey specifically forbids discrimination based on atypical genetic traits.

2. Genetic screening tests may be the ultimate invasion of privacy, revealing medical history, drug use, and predisposition to cancer, heart disease, and other illness. Should an employer be entitled to such knowledge?

In the long run, because the systematic reduction of environment-related disease is of great benefit to both employees and employers, and because technology usually triumphs over tradition, it's likely that current laws will be revised, and restrictive regulations promulgated, to allow limited genetic screening to become common practice.

78

Cancer in the Economically Disadvantaged

American Cancer Society

*Reprinted with the permission of Harold Freeman, M.D.
and The American Cancer Society.*

This chapter consists of material from reports issued in 1986 by the American Cancer Society National Subcommittee on Cancer in the Economically Disadvantaged. The chief finding of the committee's reports: the poor get more cancer and die from it more often. Some of the reasons for this unfortunate truth are explored below.—*M.R.*

In 1971, the President of the United States authorized a national cancer program, hailed by many as the "war on cancer." The following year the historic Howard University study "The Alarming Increase in Cancer Mortality in the United States Black Population" was issued. . . .

In 1979, Dr. Harold P. Freeman discussed the diagnosis and treatment of cancer at Harlem Hospital in New York City, at the American Cancer Society's Science Writers' Seminar.[4] He noted that "half of the 165 consecutive patients with breast cancer seen at Harlem Hospital, were incurable on admission. All of the Harlem patients were black and poor. The five year cure was 20 percent compared to 65 percent in white American women."

"Not able to pay for a private physician in a medical system stressing fee for service," he said, "the poor patient with potential cancer is frequently seen first in an emergency room and referred to a clinic. Long waiting periods and complex registration procedures are common. The emergency room is geared toward treating apparently sick people. A minimally symptomatic patient is likely to be discouraged when faced by a process of diagnosis which may be perceived as being more disturbing than a painless lump. The result is often late diagnosis at an incurable state of disease," Dr. Freeman said.

"By the interplay of all these factors and others, poor people with early cancer are essentially triaged off, later reappearing with advanced stages of disease resulting in death. This triaging off of the disadvantaged is given substance by an establishment which directs its major medical resources to those who can pay the price; a society which apparently views the challenge of fundamentally dealing with the problems of diagnosing and treating cancer in the poor as too enormous. This 'malignant neglect' constitutes a silent death sentence for many thousands of Americans each year."

Subsequently, Dr. Freeman compiled data on studies which had demonstrated the relationship between low socio-economic status and death from cancer. These were presented in part at the Science Writers Seminar of 1981.[5]

He noted among other things that:

1. The California Tumor Registry in 1963 showed that survival rates of cancer patients admitted to city hospitals between 1942 and 1956 were significantly less favorable than those of patients admitted to private hospitals. Their poor prognosis was due to the advanced stage of disease at the time of diagnosis.

2. A study on the influence of socio-economic factors on cancer survival noted a smaller percentage of localized tumors among the indigent. Treatment delays were more frequent among the poor, leading to advanced stage of disease.

3. A 1977 study at the University of Iowa Hospital during 1940–69 on the relation of economic status to survival for 39 different kinds of cancer showed indigent patients had poorer survival than non-indigents. Nearly all patients were white Americans. Both groups of patients were treated in a uniform way by the same clinical team, virtually eliminating the possibility that quality of care in the two groups affected the outcome. The survival of the indigent patients was at least 10 percentage points lower than the non-indigent patients.

He further pointed out that NCI estimates at that time, put the five year cancer survival rate of all Americans at 41 percent, contrasted to a survival rate in black Americans of 30 percent. Incidence of cancer had increased 8 percent in black Americans and decreased 3 percent in white Americans, while during the same time period cancer mortality among black Americans increased 26 percent versus only 5 percent for white Americans.

These searching questions were then posed by Dr. Freeman:

- Are available resources distributed to the American population in such a way that the best survival results are obtained?

- Is there a reasonable balance between allocating resources for cancer research with allocations for education, diagnosis and treatment of people who are candidates for having cancer now?

- Given the fact the poor have a considerably higher incidence and mortality from cancer, is the American establishment willing to fundamentally address this problem?

In the intervening years more and more data pointed to the fundamental conclusion reached by Dr. Freeman, that economic status is the major determinant of the poor survival of black Americans with cancer compared to white Americans and is probably a major factor in cancer survival for American people as a whole. . . .

WHO ARE THE ECONOMICALLY DISADVANTAGED?

... The United States with a population of 238.8 million, has nearly 34 million persons who are below the poverty level—as defined by the poverty index originated by the Social Security Administration in 1964 and revised by Federal Interagency Committees in 1969 and 1980. The poverty thresholds are updated every year to reflect changes in the Consumer Price Index.

These impoverished persons include 23 million white Americans, 9.5 [million] black Americans, and 1.2 million other than blacks or whites. Two-thirds of the poor are white and nearly one-third of the poor are black. Of these, 3,330,000 are elderly persons 65 years and older. Their average annual family incomes range from $6,762 for two to $14,207 for six, according to Bureau of Census figures as of 1984.[15]

Most of the nation's people below the poverty level still live in the South (12,792,000), followed by the Midwest (8,303,000), the West (6,074,000), and the Northeast (6,531,000), according to Bureau of Census figures. This also includes more than a million migrant agricultural workers in all areas of the country, who have a whole range of health, educational, and psychosocial disabilities because of their rootless existence.

In the case of indigenous peoples (American Indians) the nation's smallest minority, cancer incidence and mortality rates are generally lower than for other Americans—because of lower life spans. Of all who die before the age of 70, 54 percent die before the age of 45, according to the Health and Human Services Task Force Report on Black and Minority Health. Their survival rates, however, are much lower than those of white Americans according to SEER Report data. Overall five year relative survival for males was 26 percent compared to 40 percent for white Americans, and 39 percent for females compared to 55 percent for white females. These differences, particularly for mortality, between indigenous peoples and white Americans is believed to be due more to cultural factors and environment than to genetic factors, according to a study of disease among American Indians.

This brief but basic profile of the nation's poor as seen in Bureau of Census findings and other sources reinforce the suggestion that the main features of poverty that impact on overall health and hence on the problem of early detection, treatment, and survival of cancer are:

- Lack of jobs
- Lack of adequate education, overcrowded schools, and underskilled teachers
- Inadequate housing and overcrowding of urban area dwellings
- Lack of medical care
- Chronic malnutrition
- Lack of childcare facilities
- Inadequate recreational space and facilities
- Fatalism born of powerlessness—thinking in terms of the present with little concern for the future. The reality of their situation places a higher priority on sheer survival. Thus, living from day to day precludes concern about future health problems. In the case of cancer, this often makes early detection highly improbable.

All these factors, and the apparent recurrent cycle of poverty are key components in the problem of cancer control. . . .

References

1. Henschke UK, Leffall LD, Mason C, Reinhold AW, Schneider RL, White JE (1973). *Alarming Increase of Cancer Mortality in the U.S. Black Population (1950–1967)*. Cancer, 31: No. 4; 763–768.

2. Dorn, HF. *Illness from Cancer in the United States*. Public Health Report, 59: 33–48, 65–67, 95–115, 1944.

Dorn, HF, Cutler, SJ. *Morbidity from Cancer in the United States: Parts I and II*. U.S. Department of Health Education and Welfare, Public Health Monograph No. 56; U.S. Government Printing Office, 1959.

Cutler, SJ, Young Jr. JL, eds. *Third National Cancer Survey: Incidence Data*. National Cancer Institute Monograph, 41, 1975.

3. Horm JW, Asire AJ, Young Jr JL, Pollack ES, eds. *Cancer Incidence and Mortality in the United States, 1973–1981*, SEER Program, National Institute of Health Publication, No. 85-1837, U.S. Department of Health and Human Services, 1984.

4. Freeman, HP. *Affirmative Action in the Diagnosis and Treatment of Cancer in Blacks, 1979*. American Cancer Society's Twenty-First Science Writers' Seminar, 1979.

5. Freeman HP. *Cancer Mortality: A Socio-Economic Phenomenon, 1981*. American Cancer Society's Twenty-Third Science Writers' Seminar, 1981.

6. Adams, LW. *Black Conference: Vital New ACS Initiative*. ACS Update, From: Executive Vice President, National, To: All Boards of Directors, Vol. 2, No. 1, 1979. American Cancer Society National Office.

7. Caldwell Ph.D. JJ. *Black Americans' Attitudes Toward Cancer and Cancer Tests*. Conducted for: American Cancer Society, Evaxx, Inc. 1981.

8. *A Study of Hispanics' Attitudes Concerning Cancer and Cancer Prevention*. Prepared for: American Cancer Society by Clark, Martire, and Bartolomeo, Inc. 1985.

8A. Howard J (1982). In-reach; *An Approach to the Secondary Prevention of Cancer;* in Behavior, Health Risks, and Social Disadvantage, Parron, DL, Solomon F, Jenkins CD, eds. Washington, D.C., National Academy Press.

9. Berg J. "Cancer in Colorado: A New High, Incidence Data," 1979–81.

10. Pollack ES. *Prognosis among Cancer Patients in Relation to Socio-economic Level of Census Tract of Residence.* Proceedings, Data Use Conference on Small Area Statistics. U.S. Department of Health and Human Services, 1984.

8

Understanding AIDS

79

A History of the AIDS Epidemic

Scott Eberle, M.D. and Mark Renneker, M.D.

AIDS, or the Acquired Immune Deficiency Syndrome, has a unique place among cancers. Aside from being a new epidemic and front-page news story, AIDS is a prime example of a viral infection leading to the development of a cancer. A common manifestation of AIDS is a cancer called Kaposi's sarcoma. An understanding of AIDS will clarify the role of viruses in cancer formation; and, most importantly, will clarify how to prevent the spread of this disease. The best defense against AIDS is information.

WHAT IS AIDS?

The easiest way to define AIDS is to break it down word by word:

ACQUIRED: It is not genetic or inherited or the result of a birth defect, but develops because of other factors (in this case, a viral infection).

IMMUNE: It attacks the immune system, the part of the human body that fights disease.

DEFICIENCY: It creates a weakness in this system by killing a certain cell, the helper T_4-cell; which plays a key role in marshalling the fight against invading organisms and cancerous cells.

SYNDROME: It causes characteristic symptoms that, together, are indicative of an underlying disorder. These symptoms are often the result of "opportunistic" cancers and infections that take advantage of the weakened immune system.

EARLY REPORTS AND THEORIES

In the summer of 1981, 26 cases of Kaposi's sarcoma and 5 cases of Pneumocystis carinii pneumonia in previously healthy gay men were reported to the Centers for Disease Control (CDC) in Atlanta.[1,2,*] Kaposi's sarcoma (KS) was a previously uncommon cancer that had been seen mostly in older men, or patients receiving drug therapy that suppressed their immune system (e.g. kidney transplant patients). Pneumocystis carinii pneumonia (PCP) also was previously uncommon. Caused by a one-cell organism, it was seen mostly in patients with a malfunctioning immune system. The new cases of KS and PCP had occurred in these patients apparently as a result of damage to their immune system. A new disease that attacked the immune system was postulated and given the name Acquired Immune Deficiency Syndrome, or AIDS. Its cause was unknown.

What at first appeared to be a scientific curiosity took on ominous proportions as the CDC began to receive reports of cases at an alarming rate. Every six months the number of new cases doubled and a review of prior records identified cases from as early as 1977.[3,4] Most were in New York or California, but eventually reports began arriving from all over the United States and throughout the world.

Initially, all the people developing AIDS were gay men. This focused attention on a variety of stereotypes about this group, including sexual promiscuity, heavy drug use, and an "immoral" lifestyle. Because a cancer, Kaposi's sarcoma, was one of its manifestations, AIDS was dubbed "the gay cancer." The subsequent appearance of a new risk group, intravenous (i.v.) drug users (people who inject drugs into their veins), modified the gay connection; and, the more frequent occurrence of the deadly Pneumocystis carinii pneumonia led to the cancer label being dropped.

As the number of cases mounted, all evidence pointed to AIDS being caused by an infectious agent (i.e., bacteria, parasite or virus). Factors supporting this infectious theory included: (1) the sudden appearance of cases in geographically limited areas, suggesting that it was contagious; (2) the common infectious symptoms of fever, weight loss and enlarged lymph glands; and (3) information suggesting that the disease was physically transmitted (either sexually or intravenously).[5]

The likelihood that the infectious agent causing AIDS was a virus was supported by other information: (1) viruses are known to suppress the immune system; (2) viruses are known to cause certain cancers; and (3) the greater size of bacteria (10–100 times larger than viruses) and parasites

*Reference numbers in chapters 79–86, refer to the bibliography list at the end of Part 8. See page 422.

(10,000–1,000,000 larger) would have allowed their immediate identification.

RISK GROUPS FURTHER DEFINED

In 1982, reports began to appear of AIDS developing in patients with severe hemophilia, apparently related to their need for frequent transfusions of Factor VIII or Factor IX concentrates (clotting components of blood that hemophiliacs lack).[5,6] In 1983, reports followed of hospitalized patients contracting AIDS as a result of receiving blood transfusions.[7,8] Also appearing in 1983 were reports of infants developing AIDS, presumably as a result of transmission of an infectious agent from the mother prior to, or at the time of birth.[9,10] Along with i.v. drug users, the recognition of these three new risk groups further supported the theory of an infectious agent, and indicated that it was blood-borne.

Initially, transmission of AIDS via sexual contact was confirmed only among gay men. But by 1984, evidence of heterosexual transmission (both male-to-female and female-to-male) began to mount. This evidence included cases of women developing AIDS with their only apparent risk factor being sexual contact with men who either had or were at risk for AIDS.[11] By 1985, several cases had been reported of men developing AIDS who had no known risk factors other then promiscuity and frequent contact with prostitutes (a group at increased risk for AIDS because of multiple sexual partners and a high incidence of intravenous drug use).[12]

In Haiti and central Africa, studies demonstrated that heterosexual transmission played a major role in spreading the virus.[13–15] These studies revealed that the risk increased as a person's number of sexual contacts increased, with female prostitutes being a major source of infection. Women accounted for nearly half of all people with AIDS in these countries.

Another potential risk factor suggested by the Haitian and African studies was poor hygiene in medical practice. For example, it is common in Haiti to receive injections when "not feeling well," and these are frequently administered by non-medical personnel using re-used needles. This has not been a problem in the United States, where better medical hygiene is practiced.

Summarizing the information gained from risk group identification, the development of AIDS requires: (1) direct contact of an infected bodily fluid (e.g. semen) with another person's blood (e.g. genital or rectal tissue traumatized by sex); (2) direct transfusion of infected blood or blood products; or (3) birth by an infected mother. In addition, transmission of the infectious agent can occur before the initial carrier has infectious symptoms.

IDENTIFICATION OF THE CAUSE

Confirmation of the infectious agent theory came in 1984, when two groups (one led by Dr. Robert Gallo of the National Cancer Institute and one led by Dr. Luc Montagnier of the Pasteur Institute in Paris) discovered an RNA retro-virus which appeared to be the cause of AIDS[16,17] Gallo's group called it HTLV-III, short for human T-lymphotropic viruses, the third type (there are also HTLV-I and HTLV-II). Montagnier's group referred to it as LAV, or lymphadenopathy-associated virus. Later work confirmed that HTLV-III and LAV were essentially the same virus, with a less than 5% variation in genetic composition. A compromise name, the Human Immunodeficiency Virus or HIV was eventually agreed upon.

With the later discovery of a different, though related, virus causing immunodeficiency, the original virus is presently called HIV-1, and its relative, HIV-2. For the sake of simplicity, HIV-1 and HIV-2 are referred to as HIV.

The mutation rate of the HIV virus appears to be rapid—about 1% per year. That means that their genetic code is continually changing, making the development of screening tests and vaccines a difficult task. HIV-1 and HIV-2 differ by as much as 35% of their genetic sequence. As for HIV-1 itself, some scientists say that no two AIDS patients carry identical HIV-1 in their blood.

THE NUMBERS—WHERE ARE WE HEADED?

Infection with HIV results in a variety of responses, ranging from no symptoms to a full case of AIDS. Only the rigidly defined full case of AIDS is considered reportable by the Centers for Disease Control or the World Health Organization (see Chapter 81— Clinical Spectrum). Other related conditions are not tabulated, though early estimates have suggested that they are about ten times more common than AIDS. Reportable statistics continue to underestimate the number of people afflicted with an HIV illness.

Although transmission via sex, blood contamination, or contact between mother and baby explain the pattern of HIV infection worldwide, there are significant geographic differences in the relative importance of each mode. The World Health Organization has identified three patterns of infection:

> Pattern I occurs in North America, Europe, parts of South America, Australia, and New Zealand; it is characterized by high incidence of infection among gay men and i.v. drug users and to a lesser extent among heterosexuals.
>
> Pattern II occurs in central, eastern and southern Africa and Haiti; it is characterized by a high incidence of infection among heterosexuals, with an equal number of men and women infected.
>
> Pattern III is seen in parts of South America, the Middle East and Asia; it is charac-

Figure 79-1 HTLV-III
Panel a: A new HTLV-III forming on the surface of a cell. Panel b: The virus after separation. Panel c: The virus viewed from a different angle. *Source:* "Frequent Detection and Isolation of Cytopathic Retroviruses (HTLV-III) from Patients with AIDS and at Risk for AIDS," Gallo, R.C., et. al., Vol. 224, pp. 500–503, May 4, 1984. Copyright 1984 by the AAAS. Used with permission.

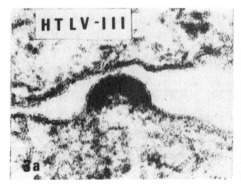
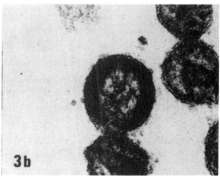
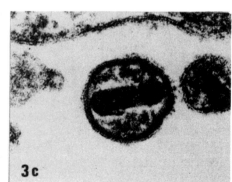

Risk Group Breakdown in the U.S. 1981-88[21]	
ADULTS	**CHILDREN UNDER 13**
61% Gay or bisexual men	78% Child with a parent who had AIDS or was in a high risk group.
20% Intravenous drug users	
7% Gay IV drug users	11% Transfusion recipients
1% Hemophiliacs	4% Hemophiliacs
5% Heterosexual Contacts (partners of someone either with AIDS or at risk for AIDS)	6% None of these categories (risk factor information of parents incomplete)
2% Transfusion recipients	
3% None of these categories	

Age, Race and Sex Breakdown for the United States[21]					
AGE (in years)		**RACE**		**SEX**	
<13	2%	White	59%	Male	91%
13–19	<1%	Black	27%	Female	9%
20–29	21%	Hispanic	13%		
30–39	47%	Other/ Unknown	1%		
40–49	21%				
>49	9%				

terized by a paucity of cases, most of which are attributed to foreign travel or imported blood.[18,19]

The Americas (41 countries, 87% of cases)

By 1988, the number of AIDS cases in the United States had topped 100,000. Of these, over half had died. By 1992, the number of cases is expected to exceed 300,000. Brazil has the second largest caseload in the Americas, having passed the 2000 mark by 1987. Canada, Haiti and Mexico all neared the 1000 mark by the end of 1987.[18,19]

Europe (27 countries, 12% of cases)

Europe's caseload passed 5000 by early 1987 and was approaching 10,000 by early 1988. France, West Germany, United Kingdom and Italy had all passed the 1000 mark by early 1988. The highest rates of infection have been seen in Switzerland (34.9 cases per million people in 1987), France (29.7 cases per million), and Denmark (29.4 cases per million).[18,19]

Africa (37 countries, 10% of cases)

AIDS is underreported in Africa because of poor medical care, patients often not fitting case definitions, and censorship by countries to avoid discrimination. Reporting has improved with time, with Uganda and Tanzania reporting over 1000 by early 1988. HIV infection has reached endemic proportion in many urban populations, with close to 10% of the population being infected. Existing evidence points to a long-standing, widespread problem in this region that may be impossible to control.[18,19,20]

Oceania (4 countries, 1% of cases) and Asia (18 countries, 1% of cases)

Australia's numbers were approaching 1000 by early 1988. New Zealand and Japan, both with less than 100, were next in number.[18,19]

A Global Perspective (107 countries total)

Over 80,000 cases were reported worldwide by early 1988. Experts have suggested the actual number is probably about twice that figure. 5–10 million people are thought to be infected worldwide, with the United States and Africa accounting for the most cases. 1.2 million people are expected to develop AIDS by 1990.[18,19]

ANTIBODY STUDIES

How Large is the Epidemic?

A knowledge of who is infected with HIV is essential for understanding how the virus is transmitted and for planning prevention measures. Large-scale investigations to determine the extent of the epidemic were possible only after the development of a quick, inexpensive test for viral antibodies. Antibodies are substances produced by the body's white cells (part of the immune system) to neutralize foreign particles or organisms trying to invade the body. They persist for years to defend the body from possible subsequent attacks; and they are a good marker of whether someone has been previously infected. The person who tests positive for HIV antibodies may still carry the virus, though they won't necessarily get AIDS.

% OF EACH GROUP WHO ARE ANTIBODY POSITIVE (AS OF 1984, UNLESS OTHERWISE SPECIFIED[35,39,84-96]

United States and Europe	
U.S. General Population	0.5–1.5%
People with AIDS	90–100%
People with an AIDS-Related Condition (ARC)	85–95%
Gay Men (high risk areas, e.g. N.Y., S.F., L.A.)	50–70%
Gay Men (other urban areas, U.S. & Europe)	10–50%
I.V. Drug Users (New York City)	50–60%
I.V. Drug Users (other urban areas, U.S. & Europe)	1–40%
Hemophiliacs (having received non-heat treated Factor VIII concentrate in the U.S.)	70–90%
Heterosexual Partners of People with AIDS (U.S.)	0–60%
Prostitutes (U.S. and Europe)	0–45%
Infants of Mothers who Previously Had an Infant with AIDS (U.S.)	65%
Blood Donors with No Known Risk Factors (U.S. & Europe)	0.01–0.04%

Haiti	
General Population	0–10%
Heterosexual Sex Partners of Men & Women with AIDS	>60%

Central and Eastern Africa	
Urban Populations	6–9%
Rural Populations	0–1%
Prostitutes—1984/85	50-88%
Male Customers of Prostitutes—1984/85	8–28%
Children in Rural Uganda—1973	67%

Venezuela	
General Population—1984/85	0%
Amazonian Tribes—1968/69 & 1984/85	3–13%

The Public Health Service estimated the size of each major risk group. Combining this with seroprevalence studies for each group, they estimated $1–1\frac{1}{2}$ million were infected by 1987. They assumed that the number of men who were exclusively homosexual through their adult life was 2.5 million, the number of i.v. drug users was 900,000, and the number of hemophiliacs was 15,000. These large numbers of high risk people explains how the virus has spread to the estimated $1–1\frac{1}{2}$ million Americans.[108]

Many studies have been done using antibody tests to estimate the extent of HIV infection in specific groups. A review of these studies provides interesting and important information regarding the AIDS epidemic.

A number of observations follow regarding the antibody positive groups:

People with AIDS (90–100%) or an AIDS-Related Condition (85–95%): When contrasted with the 1% antibody positive rate for the general population, these numbers provide excellent proof of the role played by HIV in the development of AIDS.

Gay Men (50–70% in high risk areas, 10–50% elsewhere): Studies of cities with small gay populations (e.g., London and Montreal) have demonstrated a smaller percentage of antibody-positive men, but the level of infection in these cities as of 1984 was the same as it was in New York City or San Francisco back in the early 1980s.[35,108] In other words, the same high degree of spread in all gay male communities can be expected unless prevention practices improve considerably.

The high percentage of antibody positive gay men has necessitated a broadening of the definition of this risk group to include any man that has had sex with another man since 1977, including those who have had only a single homosexual experience.[41]

I.V. Drug Users (50%–60% in New York City, 1–40% in other urban areas): These numbers reflect the time lag affecting cities with a smaller i.v. drug using population. It is reasonable to expect that, unless preventive practices are developed by the i.v. drug using community, the high rate of antibody positive users found in New York City will eventually be matched by other cities, as well.

Hemophiliacs (70–90% for those who have received non-heat treated Factor VIII): By 1983, exposure to HIV was nearly universal among severe hemophiliacs receiving frequent transfusions of Factor VIII concentrate, a product that is pooled from as many as 10,000 donors.[25,97,108] Other products used for bleeding disorders (e.g., Factor IX concentrates and cryoprecipitate) have also been implicated, but to a lesser extent. As of 1985, Factor VIII and Factor IX concentrates are heat treated, a process that kills the virus.[97]

Heterosexual Partners of People with HIV Infection (0–60%): The variable rate of infection presumably reflects the different sexual practices among the studied partners; practices which vary depending on the time and location of a given study. These statistics also confirm the importance of male-to-female and female-to-male sexual transmission.

Prostitutes (0–45%): These numbers reflect either male-to-female transmission or i.v. drug use by prostitutes. Female-to-male transmission is supported by the observation that over a third of men with AIDS and without apparent risk factors have a history of sexual contact with prostitutes.[93,108]

Infants Born to Mothers who Previously had a Child with AIDS (65%): This probably overestimates the risk of HIV transmission from an asymptomatic, antibody-positive mother to a child that she bears.[98] Other evidence suggests that the risk of transmission is greater with vaginal delivery than with Caesarian section.[99] These studies, however, involved very few participants.

Blood Donors (0.01–0.04%): As of January 1985, the antibody test has been used by blood banks to screen all blood. All antibody positive blood is thrown away. Because the test is not 100% accurate, theoretically some infected blood could still go undetected, but the chances of this are small. People receiving blood transfusions after January 1985 are no longer considered a risk group. Several other blood products (e.g., albumin, plasma protein fraction, immune globulin products, and the Hepatitis B vaccine) are also safe, because their preparation involves steps that kill the HIV virus.[108]

Haiti (0-10% in the general population, >60% in heterosexual sex partners of AIDS patients): Early on, being Haitian was an unexplained risk factor for AIDS. Further study determined that the high incidence of AIDS in this country was due to known routes of infection. As with Africa, heterosexual transmission plays a major role in Caribbean countries.

Central and East Africa (6–9% in urban populations, 0–17% in rural populations, 50–88% in prostitutes, and 8–28% in customers of prostitutes): The increased role of heterosexual transmission in Africa has been attributed to several factors.[18,100] The urban migration of the male work force has led to increased contacts with prostitutes. One study of young men in urban areas of Rwanda found that 42% had sexual contact with a prostitute at least once a year.[88]

Another possible factor in Central Africa is the common practice of female circumcision. Referred to as 'infibulation', this operation removes vulval tissue, leaving only a small passage for urine and menstrual blood. Vaginal intercourse often becomes very traumatic and anal intercourse is a common recourse.[101] Both options increase the risk of HIV transmission because of blood and semen contact.

HIV transmission is very dependent on the sexual mores of a country. Further understanding of African and Caribbean cultures will help explain their different pattern of spread.

Children in Rural Uganda (67%): The discovery of HIV antibodies in blood samples, collected in Uganda in 1973, lends support to the theory that the virus originated in Africa.[90] Though inconclusive, other evidence includes: the existence of a related viral infection in African Green Monkeys, named the Simian T-lymphotropic virus (STLV-III); the subsequent discovery of related viruses biochemically midway between HIV and STLV-III that may also cause an AIDS-like illness in humans; evidence of viral infection in Zaire as early as 1959; and the appearance of AIDS in Africa up to ten years prior to other parts of the world.[84,102]

It has been postulated that one ancestor of HIV which infected only monkeys, mutated gradually to several new forms eventually including HIV which could infect humans. Human infection with HIV perhaps began as a childhood epidemic in rural Central Africa, with most people developing immunity by adulthood.[91] Inadequate health care and the difficulty of distinguishing AIDS from other childhood infections would explain the failure to document this initial epidemic. A subsequent influx of this biologically adapted population into urban areas offered new, unprotected hosts for the virus. Heterosexual transmission, particularly via prostitutes, then became a vehicle for further spread. As of 1986, an estimated 10% of sexually mature adults in Uganda were infected.[103]

Venezuela (3–13% in Amazonian Tribes, 0% in urban populations): Studies of blood drawn from Amazonians as far back as 1968 have tested positive for the HIV antibody. Whether this represents a false-positive result (possibly caused by malarial infection) or evidence of HIV infection predating spread to the United States remains to be determined.

80

Cancer and AIDS

Scott Eberle, M.D. and Mark Renneker, M.D.

Much has been learned about AIDS. Not only has this knowledge answered many questions about the disease, but it has also contributed to our understanding of the role of viruses in cancer formation.

OPPORTUNISTIC CANCERS

When applied to a cancer, the term "opportunistic" implies that the cancer developed because of the host's lack of normal defenses. About 25% of AIDS patients have Kaposi's sarcoma and 4% have a non-Hodgkin's lymphoma, which suggests that these cancers opportunistically develop in an immunodeficient patient.[23] This is not unique to AIDS: up to a 100-fold increase in cancer has been observed in other immunodeficiency disorders.[24]

Kidney transplant patients require treatment with drugs that suppress the immune system so that they will not reject the donated kidney. These patients have about a 60-fold increase in the incidence of non-Hodgkin's lymphoma, and a similar increase in the incidence of KS.[24] The cancers develop quickly, taking as little as six months. The incidence and severity of both the lymphomas and KS are in proportion to the duration and dose of immunosuppressive therapy, with dose reduction or discontinuation often leading to regression of the cancer.[23] It is possible that the re-establishment of a normal immune response in an AIDS patient with a cancer could have a similar regressive effect.

CANCER IN PEOPLE WITH AIDS

Kaposi's sarcoma is a cancer involving the lining of the blood vessels, and occurs most often in the skin, lymph nodes, gastrointestinal tract, and other internal organs. Its most apparent signs are pink or purple blotches on the skin or in the mouth, nose or rectum. First described by Moritz Kaposi in 1872, it was a rare cancer seen only in older men of Mediterranean or Jewish extraction, or in African males. This type of KS is called "classical Kaposi's sarcoma."

"AIDS-related Kaposi's sarcoma" differs from the classical form. AIDS-related KS shows no preference for age or race, but has been more common in gay men, though even in this group the frequency has been dropping.[25] Also, AIDS-related KS more commonly involves the gut and other internal organs. Though clinically apparent in only a fourth of AIDS patients, one study reported that the autopsies of 154 people who had died of AIDS revealed unsuspected KS lesions lining the gut in over 90% of cases.[26] (This implies that if the AIDS patients had lived long enough, the cancer would have eventually become apparent.)

Non-Hodgkin's lymphoma is a cancer of the lymph glands that occurs more often in the general population (15,000 cases per year in the U.S.). It typically occurs in people over 40, and starts with painless, enlarged lymph glands. The lymphomas seen in AIDS patients tend to be more aggressive than in the general population, and appear more commonly in the brain. They develop quickly, taking at most a few years.[23]

Research has tried to determine how and why cancers develop in AIDS patients. Because of the opportunistic nature of these cancers, the main research thrust has been directed towards understanding the immune system.

THE IMMUNE SYSTEM

White blood cells are the main component of the immune system. They are found mainly in the blood, the lymph glands, and the spleen. They move to areas that become injured, infected or inflamed. Their functions include protecting against invading organisms and eliminating cells that are potentially cancerous.

There are two basic types of white blood cells, the T-cell and the B-cell. They differ in appearance (e.g. membrane surface markers), and in function. In general, T-cells fight certain viruses and cancers, and are responsible for organ transplant rejection; and B-cells fight certain viruses and bacteria.

T-cells have two subpopulations, identified by the T_4 and T_8 surface markers. They work together in attacking an invader, with the central role played by the T_4-cells (also called helper T_4-cells). Helper T_4-cells orchestrate the entire immune response by recognizing the intruder and activating the T_8-cells and the B-cells. The T_8-cells serve two functions. They are the cytotoxic (or cell-killing) members of the T-cell response; and they also act as suppressers, signaling when the immune response should stop.

The B-cells produce antibodies and release them into the blood. They attach to and hopefully neutralize the intruder.

Depending on the type of invader, either the T-cells or B-cells may be most effective in fighting it off. In any case, the helper T_4-cells trigger the response. If the battle is won, memory cells and antibodies remain that are able to recognize a subsequent attack by the same intruder.

THE IMMUNE SYSTEM IN AIDS

HIV is difficult to overcome because it attacks the immune system itself. The virus focuses its attack on the helper T_4-cell, though it also infects other white cells and, surprisingly, brain cells. HIV uses receptors on the T-cell's surface as docking ports to gain entry into the cell. Once inside, the virus may remain dormant for months to years. If activated,

Figure 80-1. The Immune Response to a Common Cold Virus

Illustration by Ken Miller

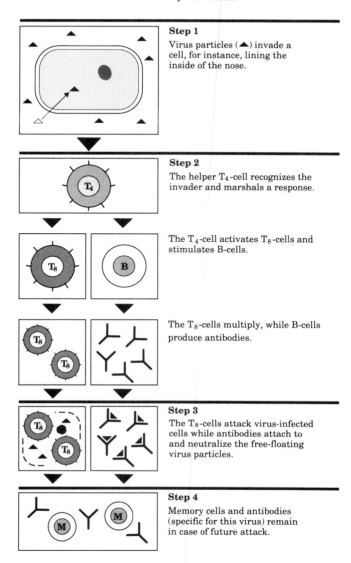

Step 1

Virus particles (▲) invade a cell, for instance, lining the inside of the nose.

Step 2

The helper T_4-cell recognizes the invader and marshals a response.

The T_4-cell activates T_8-cells and stimulates B-cells.

The T_8-cells multiply, while B-cells produce antibodies.

Step 3

The T_8-cells attack virus-infected cells while antibodies attach to and neutralize the free-floating virus particles.

Step 4

Memory cells and antibodies (specific for this virus) remain in case of future attack.

the virus slows the growth of the infected cell, causing it to lose its capacity to recognize invading organisms and to activate other white cells.[27] Eventually, the virus converts the T-cell into a factory that produces more HIV and kills the cell.[28] The body is unable to replace large quantities of lost T-cells, because they normally function for a long time—up to 25 years.

The weakened immune system is left susceptible to invasion by organisms which are normally fought off by T-cells. Being dependent on helper T_4-cells for direction, B-cell function is also impaired. Opportunistic infections result that wouldn't occur in a person with a healthy immune system.

It appears that not everyone infected with HIV develops symptoms. It remains unclear why the immune system can effectively fight the virus in some people, and not in others. Once HIV infection of T-cells is established, viral replication and cell death is triggered by the activation of the T-cell by other invaders.[28] For example, if other viruses, bacteria, blood transfusion products, or semen gain access to the blood stream, the infected T-cells recognize them as foreign and are activated, thereby triggering first viral replication and then their own death. This suggests that frequent infections (e.g. sexually transmitted diseases) or frequent blood transfusions could act as co-factors in the development of AIDS. Lifestyle habits known to lower a body's defenses (e.g. alcohol, cigarettes, recreational drugs, poor diet, high stress levels, lack of sleep, and lack of exercise) are also possible co-factors.

HIV AND OTHER RETROVIRUSES

The discovery of HIV as the cause of AIDS was facilitated by the earlier identification of HTLV-I and HTLV-II. Human T-lymphotropic viruses are members of a special group of RNA viruses called retroviruses. In most biological systems, genetic information is stored as DNA (deoxyribonucleic acid), transcribed into RNA (ribonucleic acid), and then translated into the proteins needed for life. Retroviruses get their name because they reverse this process. They store the information as RNA which, after invading a cell, is transcribed into DNA for incorporation into the host cell's DNA. As with other viral infections, this causes the cell to stop its normal function and, instead, to use its machinery to reproduce the virus.

Early theories postulated that the cause of AIDS might be a retrovirus, because they were known to cause immune suppression and cancer. HTLV-I and HTLV-II both invade T-white cells, but unlike HIV, they attack T-cells indiscriminately rather than focusing on the helper T_4-cell. They also differ in their effect after attack. Rather than killing the T-cell, HTLV-I and HTLV-II cause increased, uncontrollable growth of the T-cell, which results in a leukemia or lymphoma. Despite having an excess of T-cells, these patients are still immunodeficient because the T-cells produced are improperly made and ineffective. HTLV-I is a significant cause of cancer in parts of Japan, the Caribbean, and Africa, while HTLV-II is rare.[29]

Another retrovirus, the feline leukemia virus, or FeLV, has attracted much research and public attention. A leading cause of death among household cats, it is spread by close contact between the animals and results in a leukemia or lymphoma similar to those caused by HTLV-I and HTLV-II. An effective vaccine against FeLV has been introduced, representing the first success in fighting a mammalian retrovirus.

HIV AND CANCER

Instead of causing uncontrollable growth, HIV slows down or kills T-cells. As a result, it causes cancers in a different manner than HTLV-I, HTLV-II, or FeLV. It is still unclear what causes Kaposi's sarcoma. Infected T-cells may secrete a "tumor factor" that causes proliferation of the cells lining the blood vessels. Alternatively, the virus may infect these cells directly, causing the disordered growth.[26] Neither theory, however, explains why an increased incidence of KS is seen in people who are immunosup-

Figure 80-2. Two Different Possible Responses to HIV Infection.

Illustration by Ken Miller

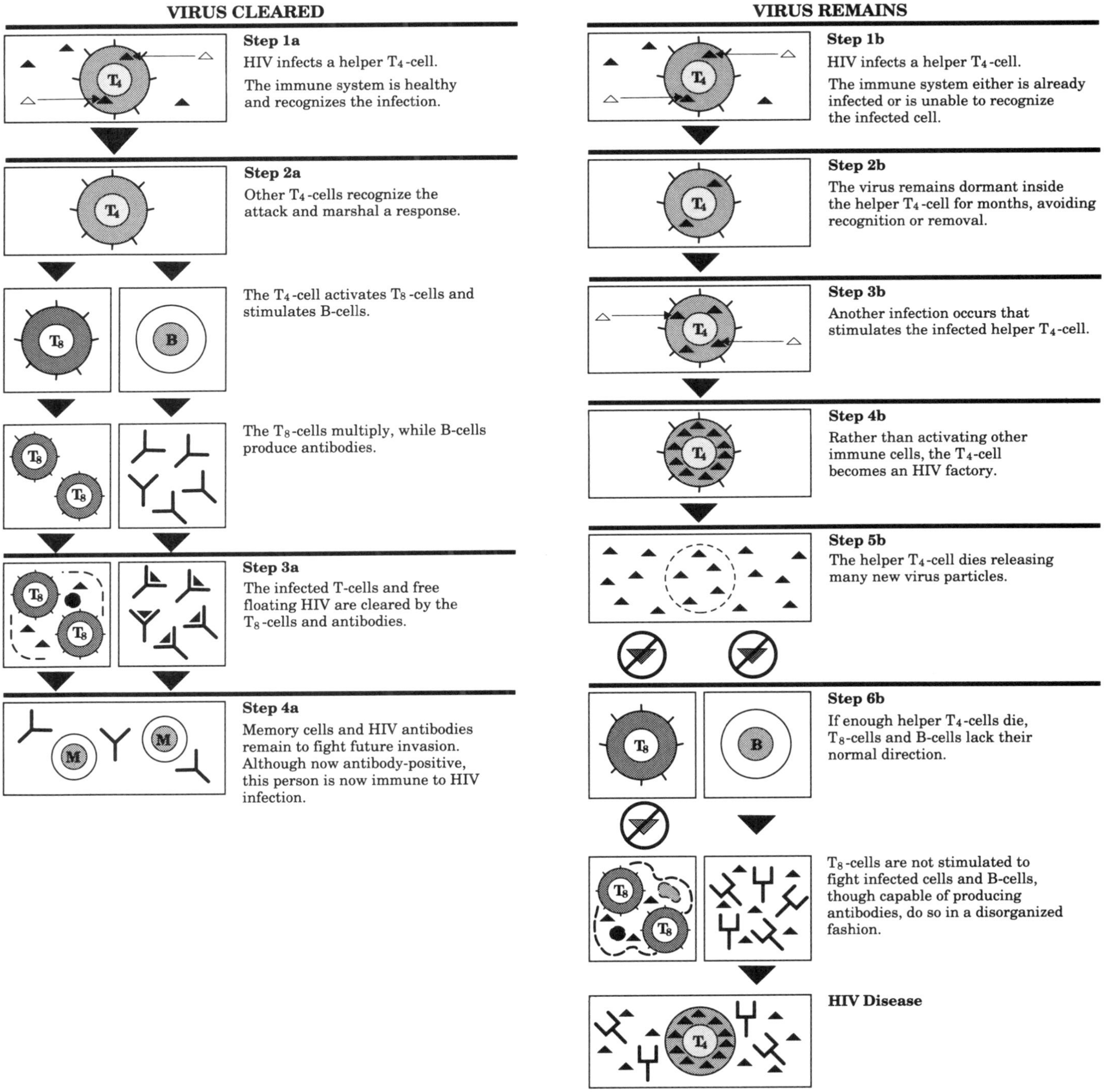

VIRUS CLEARED

Step 1a
HIV infects a helper T$_4$-cell.
The immune system is healthy and recognizes the infection.

Step 2a
Other T$_4$-cells recognize the attack and marshal a response.

The T$_4$-cell activates T$_8$-cells and stimulates B-cells.

The T$_8$-cells multiply, while B-cells produce antibodies.

Step 3a
The infected T-cells and free floating HIV are cleared by the T$_8$-cells and antibodies.

Step 4a
Memory cells and HIV antibodies remain to fight future invasion. Although now antibody-positive, this person is now immune to HIV infection.

VIRUS REMAINS

Step 1b
HIV infects a helper T$_4$-cell.
The immune system either is already infected or is unable to recognize the infected cell.

Step 2b
The virus remains dormant inside the helper T$_4$-cell for months, avoiding recognition or removal.

Step 3b
Another infection occurs that stimulates the infected helper T$_4$-cell.

Step 4b
Rather than activating other immune cells, the T$_4$-cell becomes an HIV factory.

Step 5b
The helper T$_4$-cell dies releasing many new virus particles.

Step 6b
If enough helper T$_4$-cells die, T$_8$-cells and B-cells lack their normal direction.

T$_8$-cells are not stimulated to fight infected cells and B-cells, though capable of producing antibodies, do so in a disorganized fashion.

HIV Disease

pressed for reasons other than HIV infection. One explanation is that KS and other cancers develop in the immunosuppressed person because of a failure of an "immune surveillance system" that seeks out potentially cancerous cells. New information about the immune system has demonstrated that this theory is too simplistic, though it may be the foundation of a more elaborate understanding. Dermatology research investigating the role of the skin in immune function may provide additional understanding. It has been suggested that KS of the skin results from the disruption of a normally close relationship between the skin and T-cells.

Also requiring explanation is the higher incidence of KS in gay men with AIDS, as compared to other groups with AIDS. One theory suggests that a second virus or infectious agent more common to the gay community contributes to formation of the cancer.[25,30] Cytomegalovirus (CMV) has been suspected because of its high prevalence in African children who develop classic KS and in the gay male community. Also suspected is Hepatitis B, as well as non-viral causes such as unlabelled nitrite inhalants (commonly called "poppers").[30,31] A recent decline in the incidence of KS in gay men is probably due to either improved safe sex habits, a reduction in other sexually-transmitted diseases, or a reduction in the use of nitrite inhalants.

Non-Hodgkin's B-cell lymphomas in the immunosuppressed patient appear to be caused by a simultaneous infection with the Epstein-Barr virus (EBV). In a healthy person with an intact immune system, infection of B-cells by EBV can last for months, but healthy T-cells keep the infection in check by suppressing just the infected B cells. A simultaneous HIV infection of helper T_4-cells destroys their ability to suppress the infected B-cells. Uncontrollable growth of the infected B-cells leads to the formation of a B-cell lymphoma.[32]

Many questions regarding AIDS and virally-induced cancers still remain. However, given the remarkable amount learned in a matter of years and the extensive research now being pursued, many of these questions will soon be answered.

81

The Clinical Spectrum of HIV Disease

Scott Eberle, M.D. and Mark Renneker, M.D.

A common misconception regarding infection with HIV is that it always leads to a full case of AIDS. In fact, there is a wide spectrum of responses to an HIV infection. After a mononucleosis-like illness early on, people may develop either no further symptoms, the Persistent Generalized Lymphadenopathy syndrome (PGL), an AIDS-related condition or complex (ARC), or the full syndrome of AIDS. These different categories are artificial as they are all similar manifestations of one disease: infection with HIV. Their main use is to establish a prognosis, but even this is of limited value, as many people with AIDS have outlived others who died of an AIDS-related condition.

The Centers for Disease Control created a system that classifies the clinical spectrum of HIV disease. It highlights the multifaceted nature of the AIDS epidemic, rather than focusing solely on the most severe manifestation, the full AIDS syndrome.

CDC CLASSIFICATION OF HIV INFECTION[33]

Group I: Acute infection (a mono-like illness)

Group II: Asymptomatic infection

Group III: PGL syndrome (i.e., swollen glands)

Group IV: Other Disease

  Subgroup A: Constitutional Disease (e.g. fever, diarrhea)

  Subgroup B: Neurological Disease (e.g. depression, seizures)

  Subgroup C: Secondary Infections (caused by the weakened immune system)

    Subcategory C1: Life threatening infections sufficient to give a diagnosis of AIDS

    Subcategory C2: Other serious, but not life threatening infections

  Subgroup D: Cancers sufficient for a diagnosis of AIDS

  Subgroup E: Miscellaneous conditions not included above

INITIAL HIV INFECTION

Within a few weeks of being infected with the virus, almost everyone develops a mononucleosis-like illness that may include fever, rash, enlarged spleen, and enlarged lymph glands.[34] Antibodies to HIV would by then be present (usually within six months of infection). Earlier on, it was thought that 5–20% of infected individuals would develop AIDS and another 20–30% would develop ARC.[35,36] However, now it remains unclear how many HIV-infected people will escape AIDS or ARC; some scientists predict

no one will, but this would be unprecedented in comparison to all other infectious diseases.

The different responses to an HIV infection represent the varied outcomes in the battle between the virus and the immune system. If the immune system wins the fight, the virus is cleared and the person remains healthy. However, if the virus is successful in destroying enough helper T_4-cells, then the immune system is crippled, allowing a variety of other diseases to opportunistically attack the unprotected body.

The incubation period (from infection to disease) is estimated to be as long as 8 to 11 years, and for some, may be up to 30 years.

An infected person can feel completely healthy, but have diminished T_4-cell levels, elevated T_8 levels (T_4/T_8 ratio reversal), and elevated blood proteins like P24 and Beta-2 microglobulin.

ASYMPTOMATIC PEOPLE AND THE PGL SYNDROME (GROUPS II, III)

The diagnosis of PGL is given to people who develop enlarged lymph glands in two areas besides the groin, lasting for greater than three months. By itself, PGL does not increase the chance of getting AIDS. For both those infected and without symptoms, or those infected who have just PGL, up to 20% go on to get the full AIDS syndrome.[35,36] One study demonstrated that an infected person's chance of remaining healthy are increased if they have: (1) a high level of antibodies when tested for exposure, (2) normal levels of helper T_4-cells and suppressor T_8-cells, (3) no evidence of infection with cytomegalovirus, and (4) no history of sexual contact with someone who has developed AIDS.[37]

AIDS-RELATED CONDITIONS (GROUP IV, SUBGROUPS A,B,C2, AND E)

Because it has been defined in many ways, AIDS-related condition (or ARC) is a hazy term. It describes people who develop mild to moderate immunodefi-

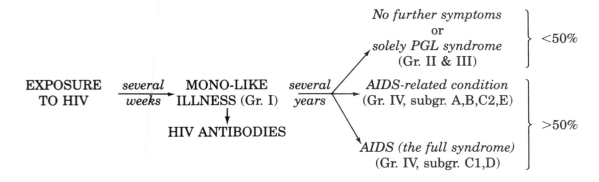

ciency symptoms without developing the infections or cancers necessary for a CDC diagnosis of AIDS. Accurate figures for the number of people with ARC are not available. This is because the definition of ARC is unclear, and reportable cases have been limited to full AIDS. It was estimated in mid-1986 that over 200,000 people had ARC. Close to 50% of people with ARC develop AIDS, while many others die before officially being classified as having AIDS.[38]

The new CDC classification system divides AIDS-related conditions into several subgroups within Group IV: A,B,C2, and E. Subgroup A includes constitutional symptoms (specifically fever, involuntary weight loss, or diarrhea) that last for at least one month and can not be explained by another disease process. It suggests a milder form of immunodeficiency.

Subgroup B includes the neurological manifestations caused by the direct infection of brain cells by the virus. By multiplying in brain cells, the virus creates a reservoir for the infection, while also killing brain tissue and creating a low-grade confusional state.[39] This is particularly devastating in the patient's final months, when it frequently leads to depression, fatigue, confusion, hallucinations, seizures, and coma.[39,40]

Subgroup C includes infections that indicate a more severe malfunction of the immune system. C1 includes infections defined as full AIDS. C2 includes other conditions that usually are not life threatening, but which increase the risk of later developing AIDS. These include tuberculosis, hairy leukoplakia (a viral lesion on the tongue), oral candidiasis (thrush), extensive herpes zoster (shingles), and bacterial infections caused by salmonella or nocardia.

Subgroup E is a miscellaneous category for conditions not mentioned elsewhere.

AIDS (GROUP IV, SUBGROUPS C1, D AND THE SEVERE FORMS OF SUBGROUPS A, B)

Initially, diagnosis of AIDS required that a person have one or more life threatening opportunistic diseases. These included either one of the infections included in subgroup C1 or a cancer included in subgroup D. It is the rigidity of this definition that necessitates the other categories to complete the spectrum of HIV disease. However, the CDC eventually expanded the criteria for a diagnosis of AIDS to include HIV wasting syndrome (the severest form of subgroup A symptoms) and HIV dementia (the severest form of subgroup B symptoms).[110] The criteria will undoubtedly continue to be modified.

Opportunistic cancers have been discussed. Of the opportunistic infections, PCP is the most common and begins with dry persistent cough, shortness of breath, fever, and chills. Other organisms causing opportunistic infections include candida, cytomegalovirus, and cryptococcus. Each organism typically infects only certain parts of the body, with the most common sites being the lungs, the brain, the blood, and the gastrointestinal tract.

The breakdown by illnesses, as of December 1986, reveals the predominance of Kaposi's sarcoma (KS) and Pneumocystis carinii pneumonia (PCP):[18]

% of AIDS patients diagnosed . . .	
. . . with PCP (w/ or w/o other cancers or infections)	64%
. . . with KS alone	15%
. . . with one of the other opport. cancers or infections	21%

The initial onset of AIDS follows one of four patterns:

(1) fever for weeks followed by an opportunistic infection;

(2 abrupt onset of an opportunistic infection;

(3) presentation with an opportunistic cancer; or,

(4) progression from ARC to a cancer or infection.[41]

The typical clinical course of AIDS is one of gradual deterioration, punctuated by bouts with life threatening infections, though intervening periods of well-being with a capacity to work are common. The average life-expectancy from time of diagnosis is eighteen months. In California, 41% of people with AIDS have died during the first year after diagnosis and 49% have died during the second year, leaving only 10% alive after two years.[42] AIDS patients with Kaposi's sarcoma and no opportunistic infections have the best prognosis—some are alive five or more years after diagnosis.[30] Current therapies, however, have yet to cure a single patient.

FUTURE MANIFESTATIONS OF HIV DISEASE

All evidence points to HIV infection as being long-term, so the potential remains for unknown, future manifestations.[36] An increased incidence of cancers (particularly lymphomas) and neurological disorders has been predicted.[33,41] Because of the epidemic's short duration, it remains unclear how many of those infected will eventually develop ARC or AIDS. The possibility remains that all those infected will develop symptoms.

AIDS IN CHILDREN

Older children contracting AIDS from blood or blood products follow a disease pattern similar to adults. But the majority of children with AIDS (at least 75%) were infected either in the womb, during birth, or while breast-feeding.

The development of AIDS in infants differs from adults because they do not have a fully developed immune system. The newborn baby is protected from disease by antibodies received from the mother while in the womb. During the baby's first few years, the immune system gradually matures while the mother's antibodies fade, leaving the child vulnerable to infection. If exposed to HIV, they are more likely than adults to develop AIDS.

Because of the small number of children with AIDS, there is less information about the course of illness. The average age at onset appears to be six months with a range from six weeks to 23 months. Most commonly the infant fails to thrive initially or develops recurrent bacterial infections and/or oral thrush. Much more common in children than in adults is a chronic lung disease called lymphocytic interstitial pneumonitis (or LIP). Conversely, cancers are less common in children.[18,43]

% of children with AIDS diagnosed	
with PCP	58%
with cytomegalovirus	19%
with candida esophagitis	15%
with cryptosporidiosis	6%
with KS	4%
with LIP	specific data unavailable

82

Treatments for HIV Infection

Scott Eberle, M.D. and Mark Renneker, M.D.

Many approaches have been tried in the treatment of AIDS, but none has met with great success. Initially, treatments concentrated on the worst manifestations of the disease—the full AIDS syndrome. Experience has shown that at this late stage, the virus has so weakened the immune system, that a cure is unlikely. Until adequate therapy is developed, the primary focus of medical treatment for people with AIDS remains supportive. This means providing emotional and spiritual support, as well as relief from symptoms. San Francisco's extensive support network of volunteers and health professionals is a model for providing compassionate, home-based care, that actually costs less money by reducing hospital visits.

Increasing attention is being directed towards the treatment of people with ARC or an asymptomatic HIV infection. Clinicians and researchers are recognizing the importance of helping the immune system early on in its fight against the virus. The bulk of treatment is still directed towards people with AIDS, but this imbalance is shifting gradually.

TRADITIONAL TREATMENT FOR HIV INFECTION

Aggressive attempts to treat AIDS continue. Traditional medicine has taken five basic approaches.[27,44]

(1) *Treatment of infections and cancers:* This isn't really a treatment of AIDS itself, but rather a treatment of the diseases that develop after the virus weakens the immune system. Kaposi's sarcoma is treated with different therapies. Small lesions often are left alone, though they can be treated with injections of diluted Vinblastine, radiation therapy, or rarely, surgical excision. More extensive disease is treated with systemic chemotherapy (e.g. alternate courses of Vinblastine and Vincristine) with or without radiation therapy. Spontaneous regression of KS lesions has been reported in a few patients, but the long-term significance of this is unknown.[45]

Opportunistic infections are treated with antibiotics, anti-fungal drugs, and anti-viral drugs—either during an acute infection or prophylactically, in between bouts. Treating the possibility of infection indefinitely (e.g., using aerosolized pentamidine or an oral antibiotic to prevent pneumocystis) has been shown to have life-prolonging effects. Even so, therapy often becomes increasingly difficult if the patient's immune function worsens. The first infection is often responsive to treatment, after which the patient typically does well for many months. As destruction of the immune system proceeds, subsequent opportunistic infections are increasingly difficult to treat and are usually the cause of death.

(2) *Wholescale immune replacement:* This involves replacing or bolstering the weakened immune system with bone marrow or thymus tissue from healthy donors. The bone marrow and the thymus gland are sites for the development and storage of white blood cells. The results have shown only a transient improvement in immune function, with no significant change in the patient's clinical course. This apparently occurs because the virus is able to attack new immune components.[44]

(3) *Enhancement of the immune system:* Many biological agents and drugs with immune enhancing potential have been tried. The "biological agents" are naturally occurring chemicals functioning as messengers for the immune system, and include gamma-interferon, interleukin-2, muramyl tripeptide, thymosin, and gamma globulin. The drugs are man-made products with immune stimulating effects, and include inosine pranobex (Isoprinosine), sodium diethyldithiocarbamate (Imuthiol or DTC), naltrexone, Ampligen, azimexon, cimetidine, indomethacin, transfer factor, and others. With the exception of gamma globulin administered to infants with AIDS, no agent has proven effective.[44] A genetically engineered form of CD4, the docking protein that HIV uses to gain entrance into white blood cells, is being tried as a kind of immune "decoy" therapy.

(4) *Suppression of the immune system:* Paradoxical as it sounds, immune suppression has been tried in the treatment of AIDS. The rationale is that HIV infection of T-cells, and their subsequent transformation into viral factories, is enhanced by the activation of these cells. Therapy that suppresses mature T-cells in the blood stream, without affecting the formation of new ones in the bone marrow, would allow the immune system to rejuvenate itself with uninfected cells.[47] Cyclosporin A, a drug which suppresses T-cell function, was tried initially in France with promising, though inconclusive results.[48] Antibodies directed against helper T_4-cells have also been recommended because this form of suppression would be more easily reversed.[49] Immune suppression therapy, however, compounds the patient's vulnerability to infection and in the long run may actually speed up the progression of AIDS. Large-scale studies are needed.

(5) *Anti-viral therapy:* This has involved the use of a variety of drugs that in lab studies have been shown to inhibit the growth of HIV. Many are directed at an enzyme, reverse transcriptase, which is essential for the reproduction of the virus. The anti-viral drugs include heteropolyanion-23 (HPA-23), azidothymidine (AZT), alpha-interferon, ribavirin, suramin, trisodium phosphonoformate (PFA or Foscarnet), dideoxycytidine, dextran sulfate, d-penicillamine, castanospermine, acyclovir, and ansamycin. HPA-23 received the publicity initially, beginning with stories of actor Rock Hudson traveling to Paris to receive treatment with the drug. But the best results so far, have been obtained with AZT, one of the inhibitors of reverse transcriptase.

A study in early 1986 of both AIDS patients who had a recent bout of PCP, and severe ARC patients, gave half of them AZT and the other half a placebo. After seven months, 17 deaths had occurred in total, 16 of which had received only the placebo. Later studies have shown that success is limited often by side-effects or by failure to receive the drug before severe immune destruction has occurred.[49] Though still considered experimental, the drug has since been made available to patients with HIV infection. Though targeted mainly for people with evidence of immune suppression, infected individuals without symptoms are being tested in experimental trials. Also being studied is the possible synergistic effect of AZT and several other drugs, including Acyclovir and Ampligen.

Widespread screening of chemicals for activity against HIV has identified other potentially beneficial anti-viral drugs, many of which are being readied for controlled testing in HIV-infected patients.[41,44,50]

ALTERNATIVE TREATMENTS FOR HIV INFECTION

Frustration with the failure of the medical establishment to provide a cure for AIDS has led many people to seek treatment elsewhere. Alternative therapies directed towards HIV infection have multiplied rapidly, raising concern within the medical community about the potential for abuse in this unregulated field. By offering hope in the form of a self-directed, personal therapy, these approaches expose the weaknesses of technological medicine.

Alternative therapies for AIDS are numerous, but generally fall into five categories:

(1) *Mind Work:* Recognizing the powerful effect of a positive outlook on the function of the immune system, these techniques attempt to foster spiritual and emotional well-being as a basis for fighting HIV infection. Carl and Stephanie Simonton introduced the concept of teaching cancer patients to visualize the destruction of cancer cells by their immune system. Other people have adapted this system of visualization for the treatment of HIV infection. In a similar fashion, meditation and other spiritual exercises have been utilized by patients in an effort to enhance immune function and to provide peace of mind in the face of a potentially terminal illness.

(2) *Body Work:* A variety of methods, rooted in massage techniques, have been directed toward ARC and AIDS patients. Whether thought of as a stress-reduction tool or as a more developed therapy based on mind-body interconnections, these techniques have offered much of the personal contact lacking in other approaches.

(3) *Nutritional Therapy:* Vitamin and mineral supplementation, modified macrobiotic diets, algae, and yeast-control diets have been suggested as treatment for HIV infection. Though not a complete answer, they partially address the need for lifestyle changes needed to maximize immune function.

(4) *Alternative Drugs:* Receiving much attention are DNCB, AL-721, and Antabuse. DNCB is an inexpensive, powerful chemical used as a photographic solvent, as well as for the treatment of skin warts. First used as a treatment for KS in 1985, DNCB was later found to stimulate helper T_4-cells when painted on healthy skin. Though potentially toxic, it is offered free in "guerrilla clinics," created solely to provide such drugs to HIV-infected people.

AL-721 is a combination of two substances found in egg lecithin, combined with a lipid carrier in the ratio of 7:2:1. In theory, this "active lipid" is incorporated into the membranes of cells and inhibits the attachment of virus particles. AL-721 has not shown the same toxicity problems as DNCB.

Antabuse is a drug prescribed for alcohol cessation treatment. It induces severe nausea and vomiting when ingested with alcohol. Once in the bloodstream, it breaks down into DTC (Imuthiol). DTC is one of the more promising immune inhancers being tested. Because of its immediate availability from willing physicians, Antabuse has been used as a DTC "work-alike" despite the lack of controlled studies.

Other experimental drugs are being obtained from countries that sell them over-the-counter. These include Isoprinosine and Ribavirin, available in Mexico and other underdeveloped countries; and Dextran sulfate, available in Japan.

(5) *Alternative Medical Systems:* Practitioners of both Homeopathy and Chinese medicine are directing their attention to the treatment of HIV infection. Homeopathy is a medical system developed in Europe during the 19th century. It attempts to stimulate the body's normal response to an illness by exposing it to very small doses of a substance that in large doses would create the same symptoms as the treated illness. Directing their treatments at earlier stages of HIV infection, homeopathists claim to have success in increasing the immune function of their patients. Practitioners of Chinese medicine employ acupuncture and a variety of herbs, such as Siberian ginseng. They are used to relieve symptoms (e.g., acupuncture for the pain of peripheral nerve problems), to provide relaxation, and to treat infections.

An exciting cross-over from an alternative to traditional medical system, is the Chinese herb, trichosanthin. Derived from Chinese cucumbers, it appears to selectively kill HIV-infected macrophages. An American biopharmaceutical company has further refined it as an injectable compound called, GLQ 223 (Compound "Q"), and it is being clinically tested.

Numerous anecdotal accounts exist supporting the effectiveness of all the alternative therapies. None, however, has been tested in a controlled study. Ironically, much of their potential value is dependent on their not being tested—their "placebo effect" might be destroyed. Moreover, the benefit of a personal, patient-centered, hopeful therapy may not be measurable by scientific methods, particularly because the very act of studying a method may undermine its subtle healing potential.

There is a role for scientific study of alternative therapies. Potentially toxic treatments, such as DNCB, would benefit from study, both to clarify the value of the treatment as well as the means for its safe administration. Also, given recent information suggesting a strong connection between the mind and immune function, studies evaluating the impact of emotional and spiritual well-being on the progression of HIV infection could be vital.

Otherwise, the value of alternate therapies stand independent of scientific testing. They point the way to a new mode of health care delivery in which the patient takes the lead. With professional advice available from doctors, other traditional health care workers, and alternative healers, the patients take control of their own care, and therefore, of their own lives.

83

Research and AIDS

Scott Eberle, M.D. and Mark Renneker, M.D.

In the face of a deadly epidemic like AIDS, the hopes of many people turn to "science of medicine" to stop the threat. In a very short time, the scientific community has learned a great deal, but unfortunately, science has its limitations. The frustrations and fears of the public are often expressed as anger that more isn't known.

There are constraints dictated by money. Much has been said and written about the failure of our government to respond quickly and fully to this crisis. Whether or not these criticisms are justified, recent trends indicate that funding of research is no longer our major stumbling block. We are now faced with an eternal reality of scientific research—it takes time.

As an example, consider the steps necessary to develop a vaccine: (1) different methods are tried to create a vaccine that will induce protective antibodies in mice; (2) these antibodies are isolated and their ability to inhibit HIV replication in the lab is tested; (3) studies in primates are then done to see how the lab results extend to a human-like organism; (4) small trials with humans are instituted to check for side-effects and effectiveness of the vaccine; (5) larger trials are arranged to confirm its value; and (6) only then, if the studies have proven its value, is the vaccine approved for general use.

Any one of these stages can take months to years. Making them particularly difficult is the apparent genetic variability of the virus. While the basic structure of HIV remains unchanged, the genetic code of its proteins can vary by up to 30%. A vaccine directed against a variable portion of the virus would confer protection against only some of the HIV viruses. Hopes of developing an effective vaccine hinge on creating antibodies that recognize proteins common to all HIV viruses and which are effective in fighting off the virus.[27,53] This process is time-consuming, no matter how fast people work or how much research money is spent. Although human testing of potential vaccines has been initiated, an effective vaccine is probably years away.

In the future, we may be hearing about the discovery of a vaccine or a cure of AIDS. Dr. Robert Gallo, one of the discoverers of HIV, said, "I feel we will get a vaccine and I feel we will get chemical control of the virus." Our best defense, though, remains prevention. As he concludes, "the focus still needs to be on education, so this virus gets to as few people as possible."[21]

84

The Prevention of AIDS

Scott Eberle, M.D. and Mark Renneker, M.D.

Certain specific activities result in the transmission of the HIV. Prevention of infection is possible by avoiding these activities. To better understand how to protect yourself, you must clearly understand how the virus is passed from person-to-person.

HOW IS THE VIRUS TRANSMITTED?

HIV is similar to the Hepatitis B virus, as they are both blood-borne diseases that can be transmitted sexually or intravenously. HIV, however, is present in much smaller concentrations (one-millionth the amount of Hepatitis B), and is very difficult to transmit to another person.[54] Also, HIV is a fragile organism compared to Hepatitis B and is easily killed by bleach, alcohol, or heat.[23,55]

Hepatitis B mainly infects liver cells and HIV mainly infects white blood cells, but both are found in many different bodily fluids. For HIV, these included blood, semen, vaginal secretions, saliva, tears, breast milk, spinal fluid, urine, and feces, with blood and semen being the most infective. Aside from blood and semen, the HIV concentration in other bodily fluids is barely measurable. One study identified HIV in only one of 83 saliva samples taken from antibody-positive people, and even then it was at a minute concentration.[56] It has been suggested that transmission via saliva, tears, or urine would require that at least a quart of infected fluid be introduced directly into the bloodstream.[57]

Fortunately, transmission does not occur simply by an infectious fluid coming in contact with a healthy person's skin or mucous membranes (the linings of the mouth, nose, eyelids, vagina, urethra of the penis, and rectum). The HIV virus has difficulty penetrating these barriers if they are intact, apparently because it is unable to infect the cells lining the skin and mucous membranes. However, the virus does appear capable of entering the body by way of the mucous membranes if they are inflamed or injured.[58] An open sore (for instance, a herpes genital sore) or cut on the skin could also allow the virus to enter. In either case, the transmission of the virus to another person requires that the infected fluid gain access to white cells within their body. How might this happen?

(1) Sexual activity involving the exchange of bodily fluids, especially when associated with genital sores, minor trauma, or irritation of mucous membranes (e.g. sexual intercourse without a condom).

(2) Breaking the skin with an instrument that has previously been contaminated by infected fluids (e.g., reusing needles).

(3) Receiving infected blood or blood products.

(4) Mixing of maternal and fetal blood prior to or during birth.

CAN THE VIRUS BE SPREAD THROUGH CASUAL CONTACT?

Happily, the answer to this important question is NO![59] Evidence comes from several different types of studies, described below.

Excluding sexual partners, none of the family members of over 12,000 AIDS patients has developed AIDS.[60] In addition, six studies have looked for HIV antibodies in the family members and household contacts of people with AIDS. Except for people who had sexual contact with the infected person, or infants born to infected mothers, no one was antibody positive.[61,62]

Only a single case of HIV transmission has been reported involving the care of an AIDS patient in which a needlestick or cut was not implicated. It occurred in a mother who was assisting in the care of her two-year-old son who had received AIDS from a transfusion. She was exposed extensively to blood and other bodily secretion over a seven-month period. She never wore gloves and frequently did not wash her hands after exposure—routine recommendations for those handling infectious fluids. She developed antibodies to HIV during this exposure and at the time of the report was clinically well.[63] There may be additional cases in the future, but they will be extremely uncommon.

Even with direct exposure to infected blood, the risk of transmission is small. By 1986, studies had revealed only five cases of hospital workers being HIV antibody positive because of an accidental needlestick or cut that occurred while handling blood from a patient with AIDS. Each year a few new cases are identified. Available information suggests a less than 1% chance of becoming infected with HIV after an exposure by needlestick, and no risk through routine, daily care.[54,64,106]

Finally, the very low 0.2% rate of HIV infection in San Francisco's low-risk population, despite considerable intermingling with the gay community (including food preparation and sharing, social kissing and hugging, and patient care) is evidence that casual contact is not a significant mode of transmission.[65]

GUIDELINES FOR EVERYONE

Level 1—Self Care

The first level in the prevention of all diseases is to maximize your own health. The healthier you are, the stronger your immune system will be if it encounters the HIV virus. There is evidence that an already damaged immune system is necessary to allow the development of AIDS.

Anything that will maximize your well-being and strengthen your immune system is beneficial. This includes:

(1) Eating well;

(2) Avoiding cigarettes;

(3) Limiting alcohol & drug use;

(4) Exercising regularly;

(5) Managing stress properly;

(6) Keeping involved with friends & interests;

(7) Getting plenty of rest;

(8) Observing spiritual practices central to your life;

(9) Maintaining a positive attitude about your life and health.

Level 2—Preventing Transmission

The second level in AIDS prevention is to avoid exposure to the virus. Given the specific ways that the HIV virus is passed from person to person, it is possible to take specific steps to avoid exposure to it. Every one can and should take these steps— even if they have already been infected in the past (there is evidence that repeated exposures to the virus can increase a person's risk of developing AIDS).

(1) *Know which sexual practices are "safe."*

The following list is not meant to be comprehensive. In general, avoid practices that involve exchange of bodily fluids (especially semen) or that may cause bleeding.

> **Safe Sex Practices:** Massage, Hugging, Social Kissing (dry), Mutual or Self Masturbation.
> **Probably Safe:** French Kissing (wet), Vaginal or Anal Intercourse *with* Condoms, Oral Sex (stopping before climax or using a condom)
> **Unsafe:** Vaginal or Anal Intercourse *without* Condoms, Semen or Urine in the mouth, Sharing Sex Toys or Needles, Blood Contact, Rimming (oral-anal contact), Fisting (insertion of the hand into the anus).

(2) *Use condoms and the spermicide, nonoxynol-9.*

Though not 100% guaranteed to prevent the transmission of the virus, condoms can greatly reduce the risk. Know how to properly use condoms: (1) do not expose them to excess sun or heat before use; (2) use them only once; (3) when putting them on, remove all air bubbles and leave a half inch reservoir at the end to collect semen; and (4) use only water-based lubricants; oil-based ones can make condoms more susceptible to breakage.

The spermicide, nonoxynol-9, kills the HIV virus and can be used as a back-up in case the condom breaks.[66] It comes in foams, creams and jellies as well as in some lubricants (e.g. Forplay) and some pre-lubricated condoms (e.g., Ramses Extra and Trojan Plus). Heterosexual couples can receive maximum protection using a diaphragm coated with a nonoxynol-9 jelly along with a non-oxynol-9 lubricated condom. [Some people are allergic to nonoxynol-9. First test the spermicide on your wrist—if you have a skin reaction, don't use it.]

Other methods of birth control, including the intra-uterine device (IUD) and birth control pill do not prevent the transmission of the HIV virus.

(3) *Limit the number of sexual partners in your life.*

This does not mean to limit the amount of sex, just the number of different partners. The idea is not to stop being sexually active, as intimacy is important for mental and physical well-being.

(4) *Choose healthy partners.*

Be aware of the present and past sexual practices and i.v. drug use of those you are involved with. If you follow safe guidelines and they do not, you may be exposed. Talking honestly with a new or anonymous partner may be difficult, making such encounters potentially risky. Sex with prostitutes, given their large number of partners, may also be risky.

(5) *Be aware of the risks of recreational drugs.*

Using a shared needle to shoot heroin, speed, or cocaine is extremely dangerous. Aside from the risk of viral transmission, these drugs (along with alcohol, nitrite inhalants and marijuana) have been found to weaken the immune system. Drugs and alcohol also cloud judgment about safe sex practices.

Level 3—Community Cooperation

As with any public health crisis, cooperation at the community level can be very important.

(1) *Be aware that casual contact will not cause AIDS.*

At work, school or other public settings, there is no risk of transmission to the co-workers, clients, customers, or classmates of HIV infected people. The only exception is the person with AIDS or a related condition who can not control their bodily fluids (e.g., uncontrollable bleeding, vomiting or diarrhea); but typically someone in this condition is unable to go to work or school anyway.

The Centers for Disease Control recommend that in the typical office or school setting there should be no restricting the use of telephones, office equipment, toilets, showers, eating facilities, coffee pots, and water fountains. If an accident (such as bleeding) does occur, it can safely be cleaned up with alcohol or diluted bleach. Food service workers should observe standard hygiene, avoid skin cuts, and dispose of food potentially contaminated with blood—further restrictions are unnecessary. For work settings in which needles or other skin-penetrating instruments are used (e.g., tattooing, ear piercing, acupuncture, etc.), specific guidelines exist to insure that equipment remains sterile.[67]

(2) *Reach out, don't shy away, if someone you know has AIDS or a related condition.*

One of the great victories of the AIDS epidemic has been the way so many people (patients, friends, family members, healthcare workers, and volunteers) have rallied together. For most every one involved, it has been a chance for positive growth. By helping those with AIDS to cope with the physical and psychological problems brought on by the disease, the lives of many people have been enriched, both by the opportunity to give, as well as the chance to learn firsthand about the process of death and dying. Casual contact does not cause AIDS, but fearful avoidance of those afflicted with AIDS will cause pain and suffering.

(3) *If you are a member of a risk group, refrain from donating blood, plasma, semen, or body organs.*

Risk groups include gay men, i.v. drug users, hemophiliacs, sexual partners of people with AIDS or at risk for AIDS, prostitutes, recipients of blood transfusions before January 1985, people from the Caribbean or Central and East Africa, and anyone who tests positive for HIV antibodies. Along with

screening for antibodies, the voluntary exclusion of these risk groups should greatly reduce the risk of viral transmission by transfusion.

(4) *If you are not at increased risk for AIDS, donate blood to our blood banks.*

It is crucial to a community's well-being that blood be available in case of emergency. Unfortunately, some people have stopped donating blood because they are afraid it might give them AIDS. The supply at some blood banks is dangerously low as a result. There is absolutely no risk of developing AIDS when you give blood. All blood bank equipment is sterile; the needles are new and only used once.

(5) *Support AIDS educational programs in our schools.*

The Surgeon General's 1986 Report on AIDS designated adolescents and pre-adolescents as the group most in need of AIDS education.[68] School-aged children are the group most likely to be exposed to HIV in the coming decade. Health officials have estimated that one-in-seven teenagers currently has a sexually transmitted disease.[69] Because they are just beginning to establish sexual practices that will be continued for years, educating them about safe sex, the use of condoms, and the risks of intravenous drug use is crucial.[70–71]

GUIDELINES FOR PEOPLE AT INCREASED RISK

The preceding guidelines are appropriate for all people. People at increased risk for AIDS should be particularly careful in following them. In addition, there are specific prevention issues to consider:

High Risk Groups

People with an HIV Infection: If a person tests positive for HIV antibodies or has AIDS-related symptoms, infectivity must be assumed and appropriate steps taken (see side-bar on antibody test): (1) Maximizing immune function by lifestyle changes is crucial. A case was reported of a man who initially tested positive for the virus, but then apparently cleared the virus, after giving up cigarettes and alcohol and improving his sleep habits. (2) Safe sex and i.v. drug use guidelines should be followed, both to protect others and to protect the infected person's immune system from further attack. (3) Previous, current, and prospective sexual partners should be informed, so that appropriate precautions can be taken. (4) Guidelines for the protection of caretakers and household contacts should be followed (see below). (5) Childbearing should be postponed. (6) A physician sensitive to the unique issues of AIDS should be consulted for regular medical care.[72]

Gay or Bisexual Men: Given the high rate of HIV infection among gay men, it is crucial that these guidelines be heeded. In particular, certain sexual practices common in the gay community (especially receptive anal intercourse without a condom) involve the greatest risk of transmission and should be avoided. A unique consideration for the gay man is that much of his personal identity is tied to his sexual orientation. Whether it is guilt regarding previous or current sexual activity, or anger at common misconceptions such as "AIDS is a gay plague," the emotional stakes are very high for the gay man practicing AIDS prevention.

Intravenous Drug Users: Unlike such efforts with the gay community, outreach efforts to intravenous drug users have been disappointingly minimal. Guidelines for risk reduction, including those listed above, don't fully address the intravenous drug user's unique circumstances. Suggestions for reducing AIDS transmission in this group have ranged from "effective drug treatment programs, enforcement of drug laws, [and] widespread education of school children," to making sterile syringes available (while keeping the drugs illegal).[35,73] Whatever measures are taken, the priority must be an energetic educational outreach program. Antibody-positive intravenous drug users have been found mostly in American and European cities, and this is where the outreach should be concentrated. The message is simple:

1. Sharing of needles leads to HIV infection and frequently to AIDS.

2. All efforts should be directed at not sharing needles, whether that means: (a) quitting intravenous drug use; or (b) maintaining a sterile kit that is never loaned out.

3. If drug use is continued, take appropriate precautions: (a) do not share equipment; and (b) after each use, wash the needle with a 1:10 dilution of bleach or full strength rubbing alcohol and let it soak in either solution for 10 minutes.

4. Follow safe sex guidelines, particularly when involved with other intravenous drug users.

Hemophiliacs: With the advent of heat-treated Factor VIII and Factor IX concentrates and the screening of donated blood, the risk of further HIV exposure by transfusion has been greatly reduced. Given the existing high rate of infection, "safe sex" precautions are extremely important for hemophiliacs to minimize the degree of spread to others.

Infants of Mothers with an HIV Infection: The risk of transmission from the HIV-infected pregnant mother to her infant could be as high as 65%. Anyone considering having children should minimize exposure to the virus. If they are a member of an intermediate or high-risk group, antibody testing is advised to check for infection. For those considering the use of a sperm donor or a surrogate mother, their health should be verified. If a prospective parent is antibody-positive, s/he should delay having children until more is known abut the transmission and treatment of AIDS. The Centers for Disease Control has considered recommending the inclusion of the antibody test in pre-marital screening.

Intermediate Risk Groups

Heterosexuals with a Potential Sexual Exposure to the Virus: This group includes sexual partners of people who have AIDS or are at increased risk for AIDS, prostitutes and their clients, people with a large number of sexual contacts, and rape victims. The two key issues for this group are determining if previous exposure has occurred, and preventing future exposure. The AIDS antibody test will answer the question of whether an exposure has occurred, and also clarify what guidelines are appropriate in the future (i.e., whether more than the general guidelines is warranted).

People Requiring Blood Transfusions: Since January 1985, the risk of receiving infected blood is quite small. Some people choose to have friends or family members donate blood for their use. Studies, however, found no significant difference in the rate of HIV antibody positive results when comparing designated donors (friends and family) with donors from the general population. Donations made for specific people reduce the blood bank's general supply, while complicating storage and record-keeping. Therefore, it is best to rely on the blood bank's regular supply and to encourage donations to replenish the bank. If the need for blood can be anticipated and health permits, the safest option is to donate one's own blood, up to six weeks before an operation.

People who received a blood transfusion between 1977 and January 1985 are at increased risk for AIDS, although this risk is small. The CDC has estimated that about 12,000 people were exposed to the virus by transfusion in this eight year period.[107] Having the HIV antibody test should be considered to confirm or deny this possibility.

Caretakers or Household Contacts of People with AIDS (including family and friends): As stressed earlier, casual contact is not a significant concern, but special measures should be taken to avoid exposure to bodily secretions. Health professionals and personal contacts should be informed of the potential for transmission, so that the measures can be followed. The Centers for Disease Control recommend:

(1)   Sharp items (needles in particular) should be considered potentially infective, handled with extreme care, and disposed of in puncture-resistant containers. Needles should not be recapped.

(2)   Gloves should be worn when exposed to bodily fluids (including blood or soiled linens). If someone is exposed, they should wash thoroughly with soap. Gowns, masks, and eye-coverings are needed when performing procedures that might cause splattering of blood or other fluids (e.g., dental and medical procedures).

(3)   Masks are only needed if the patient has tuberculosis, or if a worker or household contact has a respiratory infection that they might transmit to the patient. In either case, both people should wear a mask.

(4)   Spills of blood or other bodily fluids should be cleaned up with a 1 to 10 dilution of household bleach while wearing gloves.

(5)   Soiled or potentially contaminated items should be flushed down the toilet or double-bagged with sturdy plastic bags.

(6)   Other laundry should be washed at high temperatures, using bleach whenever possible.

(7)   Razors, toothbrushes, and other items easily contaminated with blood should not be shared.[67,106]

The HIV Antibody Test

Though available, isolation and culture of HIV is unsuitable for large-scale screening at this time. Testing for evidence of the virus in blood by other techniques is improving and will probably replace some of the current uses for antibody testing. Several accurate, inexpensive tests for detecting antibodies against the virus are being used to identify those infected. Tests are also becoming available to test for the actual presence of the virus.

The most commonly used antibody tests are the ELISA (enzyme-linked immunosorbent assay) and the Western blot. ELISA is useful as a screening test because it is economical (less than $10 per test) and it seldom misses an antibody-positive sample. However, it sometimes will incorrectly identify a sample as positive (i.e., it overcalls rather than undercalls). If a blood sample is tested by ELISA as negative, no further tests are done. If a sample tests positive, it will be tested a second time by the "gold standard' of tests, the Western blot. Any test that is read as positive usually has been tested at least twice, once by each of these two methods.

Other methods, both for detecting the virus and antibodies, are being developed. Future screening procedures may change, if they prove to be more accurate or economical.

What the Test Tells You

The HIV antibody test is not a test for AIDS. If positive, it will not tell you that you have AIDS or that you will get AIDS. If negative, it doesn't mean you are definitely free of infection or that you won't later be infected.

If you test **POSITIVE,** it means

(1)   Your blood sample has been tested more than once and the tests indicate you have antibodies to HIV; **and**

(2)   You have in the past been infected and your body's immune system produced antibodies to the virus to fight it off; **and**

(3)   You are probably contagious. Studies have shown that the majority of people with antibodies still have the virus present (perhaps as high as 60%).

If you test **NEGATIVE,** it means one of three things:

(1)   You have not been in contact with the HIV virus; **or**

(2)   You came into contact with the virus, but were not infected: **or**

(3)   You have been infected by the virus but have not yet produced antibodies. Usually it takes 2 – 8 weeks after infection to produce antibodies, but occasionally up to 6 months. For some, antibodies are never produced despite infection.[104]

Large-Scale Screening

In large studies, the antibody test has been useful in determining the extent of the HIV epidemic. Large-scale screening of the general population is not so clearly beneficial.

The Centers for Disease Control has recommended that HIV antibody testing not be used as a screening device in work or school settings. Regardless of test results, there is no risk of transmission in these settings, and needless discrimination could result.

In addition, mass screening of the public has been strongly discouraged by most experts. Aside from questions of personal civil rights violations, quarantining or monitoring the activity of HIV-infected people would be unfeasible for both economic and logistical reasons. In addition, mandatory testing is likely to alienate those at risk for infection and limit chances for positively influencing their prevention practices.

The question of routine pre-marital screening is less clear. Although it would help prevent spread to newborns, routine testing would be expensive and would only identify a small number of infected mothers. Testing people with increased risk (e.g., people attending drug rehabilitation centers or sexually transmitted disease clinics, prostitutes, or partners of people who are at risk for AIDS) is a logical— but also complex option.

Individual Testing:

What about individuals who want to know if they have been infected with the virus, should they get the test? The test may clarify issues regarding prevention practices. For some, anxiety may be relieved (even by a positive result), while others may experience increased anxiety or depression. Given the sensitive, complicated issues involved, such a decision should be carefully thought out. Consulting trusted friends and health professionals will help. Here are some points to consider.

High Risk Groups: These include gay or bisexual men, i.v. drug users, hemophiliacs, infants born to infected mothers. The key issue for these people is to minimize further exposure or spread of the virus, regardless of whether they are antibody positive or negative. Consequently, all recommendations for prevention will be identical, regardless of test results. The test should be taken if it will enhance prevention measures or allay anxieties.

Intermediate Risk Groups: These include spouses or lovers of a person with AIDS or at high risk for AIDS, heterosexuals with multiple sexual contacts (including prostitutes and their clients), people from Central and East Africa or the Caribbean, caretakers or household contacts who are directly exposed to bodily secretions of an HIV-infected person, and people who received a blood transfusion between 1978 and January 1985. Because these people have had a limited or uncertain past exposure, their prevention guidelines would be altered by the test result. If no further exposure is anticipated, a negative test would change a person's perception of their risk level from intermediate to low. If positive, however, they become high-risk and an increase in prevention efforts is advised. The test is most suitable for this group.

Low Risk Groups: Here, the issue is clouded by the frequency of "false-positive" results. Even after multiple testing, an antibody-free blood sample still has a small chance of being read as positive (a "false-positive"). In the testing of low-risk populations, very few people are "true-positives" (i.e., their blood is correctly read as positive), and they roughly equal the number of "false-positives". Therefore, of the 0.25% of low-risk people who test positive, about half are incorrectly identified.[105] Because of the inconclusive results when testing low risk people, many are subject to needless anxiety. Other than for screening blood donations, the test is of questionable value for this group.

If You Want to be Tested

If antibody results become public, people might encounter insurance, housing, or employment discrimination. California and other states have established alternative test sites (i.e., alternatives to blood banks) that maintain anonymity and assure protection. Elsewhere, sites exist that offer test confidentiality (e.g., in New York). Though confidential, results are recorded, however, and future laws may require their disclosure. Contact your local department of public health to find out if there is an anonymous or confidential site near you.

Another concern with the antibody test is the problem of incorrect results (false positives and false negatives). These errors can be minimized by repeat testing. A second test after six months is advised if a possible exposure to the virus occurred shortly before the first test. Antibody formation can take up to several months and could be missed by the first test.

85

The Psychosocial Aspects of AIDS

Scott Eberle, M.D. and Mark Renneker, M.D.

THE RESPONSE BY A PERSON WITH AIDS

Easily lost in the scientific story of AIDS are the personal accounts of individual people, often quite young, who develop the disease, struggle with its physical and emotional hardships, and die. I am reminded of my first encounter with one such person.

As a first-year medical student in 1982, I worked in the office of a physician who had a large number of gay male patients. While there, I came to know first-hand about AIDS from one particular patient, David.

David was returning to see the doctor after he had been referred to a specialist to evaluate a nickel-sized, purple lesion inside his mouth. He almost certainly knew the diagnosis in advance, but would not believe it until he heard it from his personal family physician. When told he had "K.S.," he accepted it stoically at first, but it wasn't long before he and the physician were arm-in-arm, both in tears. With time, the sobs were replaced by quiet ruminations of, "so now what?" The question of support from friends or family was discussed and finally a temporary resolution was reached. Arrangements were made for his return visit and also for follow-up in an AIDS clinic. I was struck by the physician's willingness to embrace David as a human being and not simply to categorize him as a diagnosis. Sadly though, the effect wasn't positive enough. David hung himself that very evening in Golden Gate Park (in San Francisco).

David's story is an exception, of course. Most people do not commit suicide when told they have a terminal illness. But it illustrates a reality—AIDS is a disease that affects individual people.

A diagnosis of AIDS carries an impact potentially larger than the simple declaration that life will end. A group of psychiatrists working with AIDS patients at San Francisco General Hospital found that these patients were dealing with many of the same issues facing any one coping with the death and dying process. However, they found three psychological themes specific to this group of predominantly gay male patients: (1) uncertainty; (2) isolation; and (3) illness as retribution.[74]

(1)   *Uncertainty* regarding the cause, treatment and prognosis of their illness is a major concern of many. Given the epidemic's brief history, the lack of information about AIDS is inevitable. Extensive publicity compounds this uncertainty by constantly reminding the person with AIDS that scientific advances are being made at a pace that seems agonizingly slow.

(2)   *Isolation* issues grow out of a sense of not being 'socially acceptable' because of their illness.

This isolation often is reinforced by visits from gowned and gloved hospital personnel, as well as avoidance by family and friends. For the "queer," "junkie," or "whore" who has already been labeled an outcast, this isolation may hurt even more.

(3)   The notion that the illness is *retribution* for past sexual exploits develops in some guilt-ridden patients. Not having fully come to terms with their homosexuality, they may see their sexual orientation as an answer to the question: "Why me?" People struggling with this issue were found to be in the greatest discomfort and needed the most support.

It is quite possible that David's despair resulted from these same issues, particularly the last two: that his disease had made him "socially unacceptable" and therefore very isolated; and that his diagnosis revealed a societally-taught label that being a homosexual was inherently "bad."

THE RESPONSE TO AIDS BY OTHERS

The fear which caused David's despair is no longer restricted to a few high risk groups. With the growing realization that AIDS can be spread by both heterosexual and homosexual contact, this fear is now widespread. What is the source of this fear? Probably and quite simply, it is a fear of death. As Elizabeth Kübler-Ross wrote in her book, *On Death and Dying:*

> ". . . death is never possible in regard to ourselves. It is inconceivable for our unconscious to imagine an actual ending of our own life here on earth, and if this life of ours has to end, the ending is always attributed to a malicious intervention from the outside by someone else. In simple terms, in our unconscious mind we can only be killed; it is inconceivable to die of a natural cause or of old age. Therefore death in itself is associated with a bad act, a frightening happening, something that in itself calls for retribution and punishment".[75]

Our society teaches us little about how to die or how to live with an acceptance that we will die. To cope with this, we focus our unconscious fears on something outside of ourselves. Susan Sontag in her 1979 book, *Illness as Metaphor,* described how, in the 20th Century, cancer has replaced tuberculosis as the repository of many of these unconscious fears.[76] Since she wrote her book, AIDS has taken on much of this role and is now the disease most commonly equated with death. The result is that AIDS (or death) is conveniently dismissed as something that doesn't happen to the average, up-standing citizen. It happens to "bad people" (queers, junkies or whores) or innocent victims (hemophiliacs, transfusion-recipients and, worst of all, infants). A poll in May of 1987 found that AIDS had surpassed cancer as the disease most feared by Americans. The same poll revealed a major contradiction: While 53% said everyone or almost everyone was at risk for AIDS, only 16% thought that they were at risk themselves.

THE RESPONSE TO AIDS BY THE GOVERNMENT AND SOCIETY

As chronicled by Randy Shilts' book, *And the Band Played On: Politics, People, & the AIDS Epidemic*, the Federal Government has contributed to the attempted dismissal of this epidemic. From the outset, only people with opportunistic diseases were officially given the diagnosis of 'AIDS'. Other people, with "lesser" manifestations of immune deficiency, were not considered reportable. As a result, people with ARC have been denied access to government support and the enormity of the epidemic has been greatly underestimated.

A common practice has been to downplay AIDS "because it only effects a small number of people." In 1985, there were over 8,000 reported cases of AIDS—close to the number of cases that year of testicular cancer, cancer of the cervix, and Hodgkin's disease. Add to this the ARC and lesser AIDS cases and the total number would approach 100,000—equal in incidence to lung, colorectal or breast cancer, the major causes of cancer in the United States. With the ever increasing numbers, it can no longer be said that AIDS afflicts only a small number of people.

The days of ignoring AIDS, for whatever reason, are behind us. Even so, there is still some question about the Government's commitment to AIDS education. Dr. Lewis Kuller, an epidemiologist, estimated that $100 million was needed for education in 1986 compared to a "foolish" $7 million allocated by the Federal Government.[77] By 1988, Congress was considering bills with funding in the $100 million range though with considerable resistance from conservative forces. In mid-1988, after months and months of numerous delays, the Federal Government issued a booklet to all households in America titled, "Understanding AIDS."*

With a legacy of fear and dismissal threatening our future approach to AIDS, we should take our cue from those whose lives are being shortened by the disease. Anthony Ferrara, a person who has since died of AIDS, summed up the situation powerfully:

> "To those of you not afflicted goes the task of ensuring that our care is not forgotten by the politicians and civic leaders responsible for allocating funds to carry on the research that feeds our hopes. To you is assigned the work of keeping our plight in the public eye so that those who would ignore the problem in the hope that it will go away, or those who would declare it to be a problem afflicting a single segment of society, cannot accomplish what people of good conscience know is patently wrong. . . . We are not bad people and [there] is no reason to regard us with disdain. Those of us physically unable to carry on this message look to you for champions".[78]

*The identical titling of this part of *Understanding Cancer* preceded the Federal Government's use of the title.

86

The Future— Spread or Control

Scott Eberle, M.D. and Mark Renneker, M.D.

Current projections concerning the spread of AIDS are complicated by the long lag time from initial HIV infection to the development of AIDS. The lag time in adults is at least 15 months (it can be shorter in children); and no clear upper limit of the possible delay has been determined.[36,58] Because of the lag time, AIDS would continue to develop in previously infected people, even if HIV transmission were stopped today.

Fortunately, the development of new AIDS cases is slowing. The nationwide doubling rate (the time needed for the total number of cases to double) was initially about six months, but is now about one year.[18] Evidence suggests that the rate of transmission in urban gay communities has decreased markedly. Screening of blood and heat treatment of blood products has minimized these risks. However, i.v. drug users have not been successfully reached with educational campaigns. They remain the main source of heterosexual and perinatal transmission, two modes of transmission that could become more prevalent in the future. This pattern is already being seen in the poor sections of major urban centers.

Many disturbing statistics and trends remain. Along with the projected 1–1½ million people infected in the United States, there are a total of 5–10 million infected worldwide. Future predictions of numbers of people with AIDS include 270,000 in the United States by 1991 (CDC prediction) and 1.2 million worldwide by 1990 (WHO prediction).[18,19] Although the rate of new cases in New York City, San Francisco and Los Angeles is leveling off, other cities and towns are seeing an increasing incidence. World-wide, a similar problem is emerging. Particularly distressing is the continued lack of planning and preparedness by governments around the globe.

SUMMARY

In summary, education and prevention can halt the spread of AIDS. The material presented in this section is part of that effort. It is meant to be referred to as often as necessary. Although specific details will become outdated, the large amount already learned about AIDS insures that the "big picture" will be unchanged.

But, learning about AIDS is not as simple as just reading this account. As Dr. Constance Wofsy, an infectious disease specialist, has said:

> ". . . information about AIDS isn't heard with just one go-round. The first go-round leads to fear and denial. The second go-round leads to acceptance that maybe this is something that I'm going to have to know about . . . The third go-round leads to just a little bit of intellectual curiosity because it really is kind of an interesting topic. The fourth go-round tends to lead to real interest, and the fifth go-round usually puts people in a place where they finally become a little bit more concerned about the other person than themselves."[80]

Which go-round has this been for you?

87

Resources for Information & Support

Scott Eberle, M.D. and Mark Renneker, M.D.

The best weapon in the fight against AIDS is information. If you have questions, want some pamphlets or need some support, here are resources to contact.

TOLL-FREE HOTLINES

- Nationwide Hotline (toll-free from any-where in the continental U.S., collect calls accepted from Hawaii and Alaska at 202-245-6867)

Basic information (any hour, any day): 800-342-AIDS [or in Atlanta: 404-329-1290]

More details (9am-7pm EST, Mon-Fri): 800-447-AIDS [or in Atlanta: 404-329-1295]

- Statewide Hotlines

No. California	800-FOR-AIDS
So. California	800-922-AIDS
Delaware	800-342-4012
New Hampshire	800-852-3345
New York	800-462-1884
Ohio	800-332-2437
Pennsylvania	800-692-7234
Texas	800-392-2040

STATE & LOCAL ORGANIZATIONS— UNITED STATES

S.F. AIDS Foundation, 333 Valencia St., S.F. CA 94103   415-863-AIDS

AIDS Project Los Angeles, 937 North Cole Ave., L.A. CA 90038   213-871-AIDS

Gay Men's Health Crisis, Inc., 354 W. 18th St., N.Y. NY 10011   212-807-6655

AIDS Action Project, 2676 Halstead St., Chicago IL 60614   312-871-5696

AIDS Center, Jackson Memorial Hospital, Miami FL 33136   305-547-6231

KS/AIDS Foundation, 3317 Montrose Blvd., Houston TX 77006   713-529-3211

Other similar organizations can be found in most major cities. Contact the national hotline to find the one nearest you.

OUTSIDE THE UNITED STATES

Australia: National AIDS Coordinating Committee, Commonwealth Dept. of Health, P.O. Box 100, Woden 06 (Canberra)

Victorian AIDS Council, P.O. Box 174 Richmond, Melbourne 3121 03-417-1759

Canada: AIDS Vancouver, P.O. Box 4991 MPO, Vancouver, BC V6B 4A6

AIDS Committee, P.O. Box 55, Station F, Toronto, Ontario M4Y 1R3 416-926-1626

England: Terrance Higgins Trust, BM AIDS, London WC1N 3XX   01-833-2971

Holland: AIDS Policy Coordination, Burgo GVO, Prins Hendricklaan 12, 1075 BB Amsterdam

Puerto Rico: Fundacion AIDS de Puerto Rico, Call Box AIDS, Louisa Street Station, San Juan, Puerto Rico 00914 809-754-9119

West Germany: Deutsch AIDS-Hilfe, Niebuhr-strasse 71, 1000 Berlin 12 030/323-60-27

REFERENCES

These references can be found in chapters 79–86, pages 387-420.

1. CENTERS FOR DISEASE CONTROL. *MMWR.* 1981; 30:250-2.

2. CENTERS FOR DISEASE CONTROL. *MMWR.* 1981; 30:305-8.

3. FAUCI AS, MACHER AM, LONGO DL, et al. *Ann Intern Med.* 1984; 100:92-106.

4. SELIK RM, HAVERKOS HW, CURRAN JW. *Am J Med.* 1984; 76:493-500.

5. EVATT BL, RAMSEY RB, LAWRENCE DN, et al. *Ann Intern Med.* 1984; 100:499-504.

6. CENTERS FOR DISEASE CONTROL. *MMWR.* 1982; 31:365-7.

7. AMMANN AJ, COWAN MW, WARA DW, et al. *Lancet.* 1983; i:956-8

8. CURRAN JW, LAWRENCE DN, JAFFEE HW, et al. *N Engl J Med.* 1984; 310:69-75.

9. RUBENSTEIN A, SICKLICK M, GUPTA A, et al. *JAMA.* 1983; 249:2350-6.

10. OLESKE J, MINNEFOR A, COOPER R, et al. *JAMA.* 1983; 249:2345-9.

11. HARRIS C, SMALL CB, KLEIN RS, et al. *N Engl J Med.* 1983; 308:1181-4.

12. CENTERS FOR DISEASE CONTROL. *MMWR.* 1985; 34:561-3.

13. PAPE JW, LIAUTAUD B, THOMAS F, et al. *Ann Intern Med.* 1985; 103:674-8.

14. VAN DER PERRE P, LEPAGE P, KESTELYN P, et al. *Lancet.* 1984; ii:62-5.

15. PLOT P, TAELMAN H, MINLANGU KB, et al. *Lancet.* 1984; ii:65-9.

16. GALLO RC, SALAHUDDIN SZ, POPOVIC M, et al. *Science.* 1984; 224:500-3.

17. BARRE-SINOUSSI F, CHERMANN JC, MONTAGNIER L, et al. *Science.* 1983; 220:868-70.

18. VON REYN C, MANN JM. *West J. Med,* 1987; 147:694-701

19. MANN JM. Unpublished presentation, The First International Conference on the Global Impact of AIDS. 1988, March 8.

20. GALLO RC. Quoted in *San Francisco Chronicle.* 1986, April 21.

21. CENTERS FOR DISEASE CONTROL. *MMWR.* June 12, 1986. Vol. 38 No. 54

22. BRUNET JB, ANCELLE RA. *Ann Intern Med.* 1985; 103:670-4.

23. AMERICAN CANCER SOCIETY, *Circular Letter to All Units of the California Division, Inc.* 1986: 86-7.

24. KINLEN LJ. Immunologic Factors, from *Cancer Epidemiology and Prevention.* W.B. Saunders Co.; 1982: 494-505.

25. STEIS R, BRODER S. AIDS: A General Overview, from *AIDS: Etiology, Diagnosis, Treatment and Prevention.* J.P. Lippincott Co.; 1985:299-338.

26. MOSKOWITZ LB, HENSLEY GT, GOULD EW, et al. *Hum Path.* 1985; 16:47-56.

27. LAURENCE J. *Sci Amer.* Dec 1985; 85-93.

28. ZAGURY D, BERNARD J, LEONARD R, et al. *Science.* 1986; 231:850-3.

29. SHAW GM, BRODER S, ESSEX M, et al. *Adv Intern Med.* 1984; 1-24.

30. SAFAI B, JOHNSON KG, MYSKOWSKI PL, et al. *Ann Intern Med.* 1985; 103:744-50.

31. LEVINE AM, MEYER PR, BEGANDY MK, et al. *Ann Intern Med.* 1984; 100:7-13.

32. BIRX DL, REDFIELD RR, TOSATO G. *N Engl J Med.* 1986; 314:874-9.

33. CENTERS FOR DISEASE CONTROL. *MMWR.* 1986; 334-9.

34. COOPER D, MACLEAN P, GOLD J, et al. *Lancet.* 1985; i:537-40.

35. CURRAN JW. *Ann Intern Med.* 1985; 103:657-62.

36. JAFFE HW, DARROW WW, ECHENBERG DF, et al. *Ann Intern Med. 1985; 103:210-4.*

37. POLK GF, FOX R, BROOKMEYER R, et al. *N Engl JMed* 1987; 316: 61-66.

38. MURRAY HW, HILLMAN JK, RUBIN BY, et al. *N Engl J Med.* 1985; 313:1504-10.

39. HO DM, ROTA TR, SCHOOLEY RT. *N Engl J Med.* 1985; 313:1493.

40. LEVY RM, BREDESEN DE, ROSENBLUM ML. *J Neurosurg.* 1985; 62:475-95.

41. FOOD AND DRUG ADMINISTRATION. *FDA Drug Bulletin.* 1985; 15:27-32.

42. KIZER KW, RODRIGUEZ J, MCHOLLAND GF, et al. *A Quantitative Analysis of AIDS in California.* State of California Department of Health Services; 1986.

43. RUBINSTEIN A, BERNSTEIN L. *Clin Immun and Immunopath.* 1986; 40:115-21.

44. LANE HC, FAUCI AS. *Ann Intern Med.* 1985; 103: 714-8.

45. REAL FK, KROWN SE. *N Engl J Med.* 1985; 313:1659.

46. MASUR H, KOVACS JA, OGNIBENE F, et al. Infectious Complications of AIDS, from *AIDS: Etiology, Diagnosis, Treatment and Prevention.* J.P. Lippincott Co.; 1985: 161-84.

47. WALGATE R. *Nature.* 1985; 318:3.

48. SINGER A, SHEARER GM. *Nature.* 1986; 320:113.

49. VOLBERDING PA. *Aidsfile.* 1986; 1(4):2-3.

50. HIRSCH MS, KAPLAN JC. *Ann Intern Med.* 1985; 103:750-5.

51. POMIDOU A, ZAGURY D, GALLO RC, et al., *Lancet.* 1985; ii:1423.

52. MARIMAN EC, TELLIER R, WEBER JM. *Nature.* 1985; 318:414.

53. FRANCIS DP, PETRICCIANI JC. *N Engl J Med.* 1985; 313: 1586-90.

54. GEDDES AM. *Br Med J.* 1986; 292:711-2.

55. RESNICK L, VEREN K, SALAHUDDIN SZ, et al. *JAMA.* 1986; 255:1887-91.

56. HO DH, BYINGTON RE, SCHOOLEY RT, et al. *N Engl J Med.* 1985; 313:1606.

57. LEVY J. Interviewed in the video, *An Epidemic of Fear—AIDS in the Workplace* The S.F. AIDS Foundation; 1985.

58. FRANCIS DP, JAFFE HW, FULTZ PN, et al. *Ann Intern Med.* 1985; 103:719-22.

59. SANDE M. *H Engl J Med.* 1986; 314:380-2.

60. CENTERS FOR DISEASE CONTROL. *MMWR.* 1985; 34:517-21.

61. CENTERS FOR DISEASE CONTROL. Cited in *Answers About AIDS.* American Council on Science and Health; 1985.

62. FRIEDLAND GH, SALTZMAN BR, ROGERS MF. *N Engl J Med.* 1986; 314:344-9.

63. CENTERS FOR DISEASE CONTROL. *MMWR.* 1986; 35:76-9.

64. MCCRAY E. *N Engl J Med.* 1986; 314:1127-32.

65. SCIENTIFIC AFFAIRS COMMITTEE, BAY AREA PHYSICIANS FOR HUMAN RIGHTS. *Medical Evaluation of Persons at Risk of Acquired Immunodeficiency Syndrome.* Bay Area Physicians for Human Rights; 1985.

66. HICKS DR, MARTIN LS, GETCHELL JP, et al. *Lancet.* 1985; ii:1422-3.

67. CENTERS FOR DISEASE CONTROL. *MMWR.* 1985; 34:681-95.

68. KOOP CE. Surgeon General's Report on the Acquired Immune Deficiency Syndrome. 1986.

69. GUINAN M. *JAMA.* 1986; 255:1665-7.

70. SCIENTIFIC AFFAIRS COMMITTEE, BAY AREA PHYSICIANS FOR HUMAN RIGHTS. *Guidelines for AIDS Risk Reduction.* S.F. AIDS Foundation Pamphlet; 1984.

71. SAN FRANCISCO AIDS FOUNDATION, KPIX. *AIDS Lifeline.* S.F. AIDS Foundation Pamphlet; 1985.

72. COUNCIL ON SCIENTIFIC AFFAIRS. *JAMA.* 1985; 254:1342-5.

73. ANDREYEV HJ. *Lancet.* 1985; ii:1192-3.

74. DILLEY JW, OCHITILL HN, PERL M, et al. *Am J Psychiatry.* 1985; 142:82-5.

75. KUBLER-ROSS E. *On Death and Dying.* MacMillan Publishing Co.; 1969; p. 2.

76. SONTAG S. *Illness as Metaphor.* Vintage Books; 1979.

77. KULLER LH, cited by PERLMAN D. *San Francisco Chronicle.* 1986; May 21:5.

78. FERRARA AJ. *Amer Psychologist.* 1984; 39:1285-7.

79. PUBLIC HEALTH SERVICE. *Public Health Rep* 1986; 101:341-8, 459-66.

80. WOFSY C. Interviewed in the video, *An Epidemic of Fear—AIDS in the Workplace.* The S.F. AIDS Foundation; 1985.

81. SIVAK SL, WORMSER GP. *N Engl J Med.* 1985; 313:1352.

82. FUCHS D, DIERICH MP, HAUSEN A, et al. *Lancet.* 1985: ii:1130.

83. LANDESMAN SH, GINZBURG HM, WEISS SH. *N Engl J Med.* 1985; 312:521-5.

84. MELBYE M. *Br J Med.* 1986; 292:5-12.

85. CENTERS FOR DISEASE CONTROL. *MMWR.* 1985; 34:5-11.

86. BLATTNER WA, BIGGAR RJ, WEISS SH, et al. *Ann Intern Med.* 1985; 103:665-70.

87. KREISS JK, KOECH D, PLUMMER FA, et al. *N Engl J Med.* 1986; 314:414-8.

88. VAN DE PERRE P, CARAEL M, CLUMECK N, et al. *Lancet.* 1985; ii:524-6.

89. BAYLEY AC, CHEINGSONG-POPOV R, DOWNING RG, et al. *Lancet.* 1985; i:359-61.

90. SAXINGER WC, LEVINE PH, DEAN AG, et al. *Science.* 1985; 227:1036-8.

91. BIGGAR RJ, MELBYE M, KESTENS L, et al. *Br Med J.* 1985; 290:808-10.

92. RODRIGUEZ L, SINANGIL F, DEWHURST S, et al. *Lancet.* 1985; ii:1098-100.

93. CENTERS FOR DISEASE CONTROL. *MMWR.* 1985; 34:561-3.

94. CENTERS FOR DISEASE CONTROL. *MMWR.* 1985; 34:721-6.

95. BARTON SE, BRENKY-FAUDEUX D, TIRELLI U, et al. *Lancet.* 1985; ii:1424.

96. LUZI G, ENSOLI B, TURBESSI G, et al. *Lancet.* 1985; ii:1018.

97. LEVINE PH. *Ann Intern Med.* 1985; 103:723-6.

98. SCOTT GB, FISCHL MA, KLIMAS N, et al. *JAMA.* 1985; 253:363-6.

99. CHIODO F, RICCHI E, COSTIGLIOLA P, et al. *Lancet.* 1986; i:739.

100. BIGGAR RJ. *Lancet.* 1986; i:59-62.

101. LINKE U. *Science.* 1986; 231:203.

102. WALGATE R, PALCA J. *Nature.* 1986; 320:385.

103. AKEHURST CJ, FITZSIMONS DW. *AIDS Newsletter.* London: Bureau of Hygiene & Tropical Diseases. 1986; 8:item 207.

104. SAN FRANCISCO AIDS FOUNDATION. *AIDS Antibody Testing at Alternative Test Sites.* S.F. AIDS Foundation Pamphlet; 1985.

105. PETRICCIANI JC. *Ann Intern Med.* 1985; 103: 726-9.

106. CENTERS FOR DISEASE CONTROL. *MMWR.* 1987, 36 (25): 38-18S.

107. CENTERS FOR DISEASE CONTROL. Quoted by *SF Chronicle,* February 12, 1988.

108. CENTERS FOR DISEASE CONTROL. *MMWR* 36 (5-6): 1-46.

109. SHILTS R. *And the Band Played On: Politics, People & the AIDS Epidemic,* St. Martin's Press, Inc. 1987.

110. CENTERS FOR DISEASE CONTROL. *MMWR* 36 (1S):3S-15S.

Glossary

This "dictionary" will help you with some of the medical and scientific terms most often used by physicians, nurses, researchers, and technicians who deal with cancer on an everyday basis. Principal sources for the following definitions, include: Victor Richard's *Cancer—The Wayward Cell* (1972), the American Cancer Society's "Cancer Word Book" (1977), Michael Shimkin's "Science and Cancer" (1973), and David Prescott's "Cancer—the Misguided Cell" (1973). An excellent and easy-to-use additional reference is Dorland's Pocket Medical Dictionary (updated regularly).

Abdomen. The belly.

Ablation. Removal of a part.

Actinic rays. Rays of light beyond the violet end of the spectrum.

Adenine. One of the four bases of DNA (deoxyribonucleic acid). See also Guanine, Cytosine, and Thymine. One of the four bases of RNA (ribonucleic acid). *See also* Guanine, Cytosine and Uracil.

Adenoma. Cancer originating in glandular tissue.

ADP (Adenosine diphosphate). A product, along with organic phosphates, of the hydrolysis of adenosine triphosphate (ATP).

Adrenalectomy. Removal of the adrenal glands.

Adrenal glands. Two small glands located just above the kidney that produce hormones essential for life.

Aerobic system. An oxygen-dependent respiratory system. Cells in the animal kingdom operate on an aerobic system; they are dependent on oxygen for their life.

Agglutination. Collection into clumps of the cells distributed in a fluid.

AGL (anti-lymphocyte globulin). Powerful immunosuppressive agent made against the lymphocytes or the lymphocyte globulins.

AIDS. Acquired Immune Deficiency Syndrome.

Alkaptonuria. Excretion in urine of alkapton bodies, causing the urine to turn dark.

Alkylating agents. Chemcial carcinogens. Other cancer-producing chemicals are: the Nitroso compounds, the Lactones, the Azo dyes and the Polycyclic hydrocarbons.

Alleles. Dominant or recessive forms of the same genetic trait on the chromosomes.

Allogenic grafting. Transplantation of tissues between genetically nonidentical animals belonging to the same species.

Alpha helix. Name given to the helical configuration of the proteins by Linus Pauling.

Alpha particles. High-energy particles dispensing their energy in a very limited range within the tissues but highly destructive of the tissues they encounter.

Amenorrhea. The absence of menstrual cycles.

Amino acids. Organic compounds, building blocks of proteins; about 20 amino acids are essential for life.

Anaerobic system. The chlorophyll system of plants. Cells in the plant kingdom do not depend upon oxygen for life but absorb carbon dioxide and return oxygen to the atmosphere. Aerobic and anaerobic systems are inter-dependent.

Anaphase. The stage in mitosis following metaphase in which the halves of the divided chromosomes move apart to the poles of the spindle.

Anaplastic. Cancerous; reverted to a more primitive or undifferentiated form.

Anaploid cells. Cells containing an abnormal number of chromosomes. They are cancerous cells. See also Hypoploid, Heteroploid, Tetraploid cells.

Androgens. Male sex hormones.

Anorexia. Lack of appetite for food.

Antibiotic. A substance produced by living organisms such as bacteria, or molds, which can destroy other bacteria. Penicillin is the most familiar example. Some antibiotics have shown effective anticancer activity.

Antibody. Substance manufactured by cells to fight invading antigens.

Antigen. Foreign substance (such as the antigen of a virus) invading a cell and eliciting the formation of antibodies.

Ascorbic acid. Vitamin C.

Atom. Smallest element of matter having distinct chemical properties. Atoms group together into molecules constituting all substances found in nature. An atom is made in the form of a miniature solar system: at its center is the nucleus around which electrons orbit at enormous speeds.

ATP (adenosine triphosphate). A nucleotide compound occurring in all cells which represents an energy source for cellular function.

Atrophy. Wasting away of tissue.

Axilla. A small hollow beneath the arm where it joins the shoulder (also called the armpit).

Axillary lymph nodes. Lymph nodes in the axilla.

Azo dyes. Chemical carcinogens. *See* Alkylating Agents.

"B" cells. Lymphocytes that mediate humoral immunity (B = bursa equivalent). See "T" cells.

Bacteria. Single-celled organisms. Many are infectious.

Bacteriophage. A virus that multiplies in bacteria.

Barium enema. The use of barium sulfate introduced into the intestinal tract by an enema to allow X-ray exam of the lower bowel.

Basal cell carcinoma. The most common type of skin cancer. It forms in the lowermost layer of the skin, grows slowly and seldom spreads. It is easily detected and readily cured when treated promptly.

BCG (Bacillus Calmette-Guerin). A vaccine against tuberculosis, consisting of attenuated living cultures of bovine tubercle bacilli.

Benzopyrene. Purified form of polycyclic aromatic hydrocarbons, from charred or burnt foods.

Benign tumor. An abnormal swelling or growth that is not a cancer and is usually harmless.

Beta-carotene. A precursor of vitamin A which is found in plants. It is transformed to vitamin A in the body by enzymatic action.

Biochemistry. The chemistry of living organisms or living processes.

Biological predeterminism. Concept expressing the fact that each individual organism's response to cancer and other diseases is unique and, to an extent, "predetermined."

Biopsy. The removal of a small portion of tissue from the body for examination under the microscope.

Blood count. An examination of the blood to count the number of white and red blood cells and platelets.

Brachytherapy. Treatment by inserting radioactive isotopes into and around a tumor.

Breast self-examination. Simple procedure to examine breasts thoroughly, recommended once a month for all women to do themselves between regular physician checkups.

Burkitt's lymphoma. A cancer of lymphoid tissues, frequent in South Africa.

Cachexia. Severe generalized weakness/malnutrition, and emaciation.

Cancer. A large group of diseases characterized by uncontrolled growth and spread of abnormal cells.

Carcinogen. An agent (viral, chemical, irradiating) capable of inducing cancer.

Carcinogenesis. Development of cancerous cells.

Carcinoma. A form of cancer which arises in the tissues that cover or line such organs of the body as skin, intestines, uterus, lung, breast, etc.

Carcinoma in situ. A stage in the growth of cancer when it is still confined to the tissue in which it started.

Catalase. An enzyme which specifically hastens the decomposition of hydrogen peroxide which is found in practically all cells.

Catalyst. A substance that does not initiate but facilitates a chemical reaction.

Cell. Unit of living tissue, both in plants and animals.

Cell-free system. A system which reproduces artificially the composition of a cell. All the elements of a cell are present but they are not structured into a cell.

Cell fusion. Coherence of adjacent cells.

Cellular antibodies. Or cell-bound antibodies. Many circulate throughout the organism but are bound to the cell, generally the lymphocyte.

Centromere. Clear region where the arms of a chromosome meet.

Centrosomes (or centrioles). Two small bodies in the cell cytoplasm which travel to either side of the cytoplasm at the time of cell division.

Cervix. Any neck or neck-like structure in the body; in cancer terminology it usually refers to the neck of the uterus.

Chalones. Substances produced in an organ which diminish or inhibit function in the organ.

Chemotherapy. Treatment by drugs.

Chlorophyll. Green pigment of plants.

Choriocarcinoma. A highly malignant tumor developed from the epithelium of the protective and nutritive covering of the growing zygote or fertilized ovum.

Chromatin strands. The readily stainable portion of the cell nucleus forming a network of fibrils of DNA and serving as the carrier of the genes in inheritance.

Chromatography. Chemical analysis of compounds through examination of the rate of migration on an absorbent column.

Chromosomes. Minute structures in the cell nucleus made up of genes; the carriers of heredity.

Chronic cystic mastitis. Breast disease characterized by nodular cysts; the breast is tender and painful.

Classical radical mastectomy. Operation of Halsted for breast cancer. Removal of the breast with its tumor, together with the pectoral muscles and the lymph nodes of the axilla.

Clinical. Pertaining to the study and treatment of disease in human beings by direct observation, as distinguished from laboratory research.

Clone. A strain of cells descended in culture from a single cell.

Co-carcinogen. Environmental agent which acts with another to cause cancer.

Colon. The part of the large intestine that extends from the end of the small intestine to the rectum.

Colonoscopy. Technique for direct visual examination of the entire large bowel by means of a lighted, flexible tube.

Colostomy. A surgical procedure which creates an artificial opening from the colon through the abdominal wall in order to permit elimination of wastes.

Colposcopy. Examination of the vagina and cervix with a magnifying instrument called a colposcope to check pre-stained tissues for abnormality.

Combination therapy. The use of two or more modes of treatment—surgery, irradiation, chemotherapy, immunotherapy—in combination, alternately or together, to achieve optimum results against cancer.

Compton effect. A change in wavelengths of scattered rays and emission of recoil electrons in deep radiation.

Computerized tomography. See CT Scan.

Contact inhibition. A mechanism of growth control in cells, whereby cells cease to grow when they touch each other. Cancer cells have lost the capacity for contact inhibition.

Control genes. Genes that stimulate or inhibit the action of structural genes. (Jacob and Monod.) (*See* Structural genes.)

COPD. Chronic obstructive pulmonary disease (e.g., asthma, bronchitis, emphysema).

Crossing-over. Exchange of genes between homologous chromosomes of a hybrid.

Cryogenic. Pertaining to the production of very low temperatures.

Cruciferous. Vegetables of the cabbage family (Brassicaceae), including brussels sprouts, cabbage, broccoli, cauliflower, kale, kohlrabi, rutabagas and turnips. Cruc- refers to a cross-like component common to these plants.

CT Scan. Computerized tomography—a scanning, diagnostic procedure using x-rays and computer processing.

Cyclic accelerator (or cyclotron). One of the machines producing high-energy radiations.

Cytology. The science which deals with the study of living cells. Cells which have been sloughed off, or scraped off, from such organs of the body as uterus, lungs, bladder or stomach are examined under the microscope for early signs of abnormality. The Pap test used for early detection of cervical cancer is an example of this method; also referred to as exfoliative cytology.

Cytoplasm. Protoplasm of the cell, its living matter. Makes up the bulk of a cell, excluding the nucleus and membrane.

Cytosine. One of the four bases of DNA—see Adenine. One of the four bases of RNA—see Guanine.

Decarboxylic acid. An organic acid having a carboxyl (COOH) group at each end of the organic carbon chain.

Defective virus. A virus which does not destroy the cell and replicate itself but which inserts its genome into the cell it attacks.

Diagnosis. Identifying a disease by its signs, symptoms, course and laboratory findings.

Diethylstilbestrol (DES). Synthetic compound with estrogenic activity. Used in meat industry and "morning after" pill. Linked to adenocarcinoma of the vagina.

Differentiation. The development of form and function in a cell or tissue.

Dimerization. Fusion or joining of two similar purine or pyrimidne bases by cross-linkage of carbon rings.

Diploid cell. A normal cell containing the normal number of chromosomes, in a human being 46 chromosomes.

Diverticulosis. A common condition affecting the intestines whereby there are small outpockets (diverticula) as a result of weak points in the bowel wall. When they become infected, the condition is called diverticulitis.

DNA (deoxyribonucleic acid). The informational macromolecules of the cell nucleus, wound together in the form of a double helix.

Dominant trait. A strong genetic trait.

Double helix. The coil-like configuration of the nucleic acid molecule as demonstrated by Watson and Crick, forming the backbone of DNA.

Dysplasia. Disturbance in the usual orderly organization of cells and tissues, often part of a developmental phase of many neoplasms. The epidermic and mucosal surfaces are frequent sites of this disturbance.

Edema. The presence of large amounts of fluid in the intercellular space of the body.

Effusion. The escape of fluid into a part or tissue.

Electron. The unit of negative electricity which revolves about the nucleus of an atom or which flows in a conductor to produce an electric current.

Electron microscopy. A technique for visualizing material through the microscope that uses beams of electrons instead of light beams, and thereby permits clearer magnification than is possible with the ordinary microscope.

Electron therapy. Direct cancer therapy by electrons.

Embryogenesis. The process of embryo formation.

Endocrine glands. Glands secreting internally into the blood or lymph.

Endogenous. Originating or developing within the organism.

Endometrial. Having to do with the lining of the uterus or body of the womb, used in describing a form of uterine cancer.

Endometrium. The mucous coat or lining of the uterus.

Endoplasmic reticulum. System of connected channels in the cell cytoplasm. It is involved in protein synthesis and also has a role in the action of drugs on cells.

Endoscopy. The use of a scope to examine the body cavity.

Energy metabolism. Cellular processes directly related to the production of energy.

Enterostomal therapist. An allied health professional trained in the care of stomas, or openings in the abdominal wall, constructed to permit the elimination of wastes from the digestive or urinary tract.

Enzymes. Proteins stimulating cell functions or acting as catalysts.

Epidemiologist. A health professional/statistician who detects disease patterns through the evaluation of data on the incidence of the disease.

Epidemiology. The study of incidence, distribution, environmental causes and control of a disease in a population.

Epithelium. The external covering of a tissue or organ.

Epizootiology. The study of diseases and disease factors in animals.

Escape mechanisms (from immunological surveillance). Mechanisms through which the body favors tumor growth.

Esophageal speech. An acquired technique by which laryngectomees (those who have lost their voice boxes) are taught to speak again by swallowing and expelling air through the mouth from the esophagus (gullet).

Estrogen. A hormone secreted by the ovaries which is essential to reproduction; involved in the menstrual cycle; produces female secondary sex characteristics, such as breast development.

Etiocholanolone. A reduced form of testosterone (hormone produced by testes) excreted in the urine.

Etiology. The study of the causes of disease.

Excision. Surgical removal of a diseased part of the body, including cancerous growths.

Excoriation. A break in the skin surface, usually covered with blood or serous crusts.

Exogenous. Originating or developing outside an organism.

Fascia. A thin tissue covering muscles and internal structures of the body.

Femoral. Pertaining to the femur (thigh bone) or to the thigh.

Fiber. The structural component of plant cell walls that is not digested by human gastrointestinal enzymes. Can be soluble or insoluble.

Filial. Pertaining to offspring.

Fractionation. The dividing into fractions.

Gamete. One of two cells, male and female, whose union is necessary to initiate the development of a new individual (in sexual reproduction).

Gamma rays. Electromagnetic radiations of short wavelength emitted by the nucleus of an atom during a nuclear reaction.

Genes. Units of hereditary material grouped into chromosomes and constituted of DNA.

Genetic code. A sequence of purine and pyrimidine bases in DNA which carries the hereditary message for protein synthesis.

Genome. The complete set of hereditary factors contained in the haploid chromosome.

Glycoprotein. Chemical conjugation of carbohydrate and protein, found especially in cell membranes.

Gonadectomy. Excision of an ovary or testis.

Gonads. The gamete-producing glands, the ovaries and testes.

Guaiac test. A chemical test used to detect occult (hidden) blood in the stool. A simple method allows stool specimens to be placed on special guaiac-treated paper slides. These slides are then treated and checked by a doctor or lab technician. The test is well-suited to screening programs for colon-rectal cancer because the specimen can be prepared at home.

Guanine. One of the four bases of DNA; see also Adenine. One of the four bases of RNA; the other three bases of RNA are: Adenine, Cytosine, Uracil.

Haploid cell. A germ cell, in human beings, containing 23 chromosomes. In fertilization, when male and female germ cells unite, the total number of chromosomes is again 46.

Heme. The nonprotein, insoluble iron protoporphyrin constituent of hemoglobin (oxygen-carrying pigment of the blood).

Heteroploid cell. A cell containing more than the normal number of chromosomes.

HIV. Human immunodeficiency virus—the AIDS virus (also called HTLV-3 and LAV).

Hodgkin's disease. A disease of the lymphoid tissues.

Homeostasis. The essential stability of an organism.

Homografts (or allografts). Grafts of tissue between genetically different animals of the same species.

Horizontal Transmission (of tumors). Transmission from individual to individual. *See* Vertical transmission.

Hormones. Substances secreted by the endocrine glands and discharged through the blood and lymph streams. They stimulate the organs (the so-called "target organs") to specific action.

Hormonotherapy. Treatment by the use of hormones; used in controlling cancers in conjunction with other modalities such as chemotherapy.

Huggins' tumor. An experimental breast cancer in inbred rats produced by 7, 12 DMBA (7, 12 dimethylbenz (a) anthracene).

Humoral antibodies. Free circulating antibodies.

Hydroxy acids. Acids containing the hydroxyl (OH) group.

Hydroxy corticoids. Hormones of the adrenal cortex.

Hyperplasia. The abnormal multiplication of cells in a tissue.

Hyperthermia. Abnormally high body temperature, especially that induced for therapeutic reasons.

Hypopysis. See Pituitary gland.

Hysterectomy. A surgical procedure for removal of the uterus; may be combined with removal of ovaries (oophorectomy).

Ileostomy. A surgical procedure which constructs an artificial opening of the small intestine through the abdominal wall for elimination of body wastes.

Immunity. Rejection of an antigen by the organism.

Immunological surveillance. Body mechanisms for the rejection of foreign cells.

Immunological tolerance. A state of body reaction to antigens varying from total tolerance to total immunity.

Immunology. The science of immunity, or the study of the mechanisms whereby the host reacts to foreign substances in its environment to resist disease, poison, or infection.

Immuno-suppression. Suppression of the body's immuno responses. Certain chemicals initiate immuno-suppression.

Immunotherapy. Treatment of disease by stimulating the body's own defense mechanism against the disease.

Industrial hygienist. A health professional trained to recognize and evaluate workplace hazards, and to recommend means to control them.

Initiation (of cancer process). The silent beginning of the cancer process.

Initiator. An agent that initiates the growth of a cancer.

In situ. Confined to a small site of origin (cancer in situ).

Interferon. Special proteins made by cells to fight virus infections.

Interleukin. A chemical produced as part of an immune response.

Internal mammary chain. Chain of lymph nodes within the chest.

Interphase. "Resting" period of cell, when it is not dividing.

In utero. Still in the womb (the uterus).

Invasive. Manner of growth of some cancers in which lesions expand by sending cells singly and in groups through the surrounding tissues, veins, and lymphatic vessels.

In vitro. In the test tube.

In vivo. Within the living body.

Ion. Electrically charged atom.

Ionic bond. Organic molecules commonly contain one or more units of net positive or negative charge in a group known as an ionic group or an ionic bond.

Ionizing radiation. X-ray or gamma ray radiation which produces ion pairs in matter.

Isogenic. Of identical genetic composition.

Isotopes. Variants of a given chemical element. Their constitutions are about identical to that of the original element but their nuclei weigh more or less, therefore their atomic weights are different.

Karyotype. Constant grouping of chromosomes in a normal cell; also arrangement in pairs according to length and shape.

Lactones. Chemical carcinogens. See also Alkylating agents.

Laparotomy. Incision through the abdominal wall.

Laryngectomy. A surgical procedure which removes the larynx or voice box. A laryngectomy is someone who has undergone this surgery.

LASER. *L*ight *a*mplification by *s*timulated *e*mission of *r*adiation, an intensely powerful narrow beam of radiation.

Lesion. Describes any abnormal change in tissue due to disease or injury.

Leucosis (or leukosis). Proliferation of leukocyte-forming tissue—the basis of leukemia.

Leukemia. Cancer of the blood-forming tissues (bone marrow, lymph nodes, spleen); characterized by the over-production of white blood cells.

Leukemogenic. Causing leukemia.

Leukoplakis. Whitish, thickened patch of the epithelium which is sometimes a forerunner of cancer.

Ligation. To bind or tie-off.

Linear accelerator. A machine producing high-energy radiation.

Lipid. An organic fatty substance which is insoluble in water but soluble in alcohol, ether, chloroform, and other fat solvents.

Lymph. A clear fluid which circulates throughout the body, containing white blood cells called lymphocytes, antibodies and nourishing substances.

Lymph gland. Tissue which is made up of lymphocytes and connective tissue and produces lymph and lymphocytes (also called lymph node). These lymph glands, or nodes, normally act as filters of impurities in the body.

Lymphadenopathy. Enlarged large nodes.

Lymphangiography. Radiography of the lymph nodes after the introduction of an opaque iodinated oil into the lymph channels.

Lymphedema. Swelling as a result of obstruction of lymphatic vessels or lymph nodes.

Lymphoblastoma. Tumor of the lymph glands.

Lymphocytes. White blood corpuscles arising in lymph glands and nodes, instrumental in the immunological processes of the body.

Lymphoma. Malignant growths of lymph nodes.

Lymphosarcoma. Cancer of lymphoid tissue.

Lysosomes. Bodies situated in the cell cytoplasm, containing enzymes active in the digestion of foodstuff.

Lysozyme. An enzyme within cells which is capable of destroying the cell or certain of its functions.

Macromolecules. Large molecules that are bio-chemically complex; (i.e., proteins).

Magnetic Resonance Imaging—See MRI.

Male gamete (and female gamete). *See* Gamete.

Malignant tumor. An abnormal tissue growth which tends to destroy the host by direct spread or metastasis.

Mammography. Low-dose X-ray technique for studying the structure of breast tissue in order to locate any abnormality at the earliest possible stage; permits detection of a breast cancer before the lump can be felt.

Mass spectrometry. Analysis of substances by breaking them down into their basic atoms and measuring the weight, or mass, of the atoms by the rate of their migration in a strong electric field.

Mastectomy. Surgical removal of a cancerous breast to prevent spread of the disease. Simple mastectomy refers to removal of the entire breast. Radical mastectomy involves removal of the entire breast, underlying muscle tissue and lymph nodes in the armpit. A mastectomee is someone who has had the breast removed.

Meiosis. Division of sex (or germ) cells.

Melanoma. A pigmented, highly malignant form of cancer of the skin. The tumor may vary in color from nearly black to almost white.

Mesothelioma. A tumor formed from cells that line the inside of the body. Malignant mesothelioma of the lung is an increasingly common—but still rare—cancer associated with asbestos exposure. Almost always fatal.

Messenger RNA. The messenger between nuclear DNA and the ribosomes of the cell cytoplasm, site of protein synthesis.

Metabolism. All the physical and chemical processes in living organisms necessary for maintaining life.

Metaphase. The middle phase of mitosis during which the lengthwise separation of the chromosomes in the equatorial plate occurs.

Metastasis. Secondary tumor centers at a distance from the original tumor, and resulting from the transportation of tumor cells by blood or lymph streams.

Mitochondria. Fine structure in the cell cytoplasm, "power house" of the cell; center of photosynthesis in plants, and of oxidation of foodstuffs in animals.

Mitosis. Cell division.

Molecule. Small mass of matter, made up of atoms.

Mongolism. Mental retardation associated with flat skull, flat nose, short fingers, wide fingerwebs, and a chromosomal abnormality.

Monoclonal antibody. An antibody produced in the laboratory using recombinant DNA technology.

Morbidity. Conditions of being diseased.

MRI. Magnetic resonance imaging, a non-radiation producing form of imaging used for diagnostic purposes.

Mutagenesis. The process of genetic changes within the cell.

Mutant. The result of a mutation.

Mutation. Change in a cell which is permanent and transmissible to offspring.

Myelocytic. Related to myelocytes, or marrow cells.

Myelomatosis. Multiple myeloma.

Necrosis. Death of a tissue.

Neoplasia. The process of new growth; commonly cancer formation.

Neoplasm. Any new abnormal growth of cells or tissues; may be benign or malignant but is customarily used to describe a cancerous tumor.

Neoplastic transformation. The change from normal growth to abnormal growth such as a tumor.

Neurofibromatosis. Familial changes in the nervous system, muscles, bones, and skin, with appearance of soft tumors over the whole body of nerve tissue and fibrous tissue origin.

Nitrates/Nitrites. Chemicals naturally present in vegetables, but added as preservatives in processed meats and other food products.

Nitroso compounds. Compounds containing nitrogen and oxygen in a univalent linkage.

Nosocomal. Hospital-acquired infection.

Nuclear sap. Amorphous protein matrix which bathes all the nuclear structures of the cell.

Nucleic acids. DNA (deoxyribonucleic acid) and RNA (ribonucleic acid); chemical constituents of genes, simplest forms of "life" (capable of reproducing themselves).

Nucleolus. A round granular structure found in the nucleus of the cell, which is involved in ribosomal RNA synthesis.

Nucleotide. Purine or pyrimidine base bound to a 5-carbon sugar and a phosphate group.

Nucleus (of cell). A steroid body within the cell which is circumscribed by a thin nuclear membrane and contains nucleoli, granules of chromatin, and the main core of DNA in the cell.

Obstructive edema. Swelling of the limbs due to choking of the lymphatic channels by cancer cells.

Oncogenesis. The development of a tumor or growth.

Oncogenic. Leading to the development of a tumor or growth.

Oncology. The study of cancer, which has become a specialty branch of modern medicine.

Oophorectmy. Removal of an ovary or the ovaries.

Operator gene. The gene responsible for synthesis of a specific enzyme or protein.

Operon. A genetic unit of functions at the subcellular level under the control of a so-called operator and a repressor.

Ostomy. A surgical procedure that creates a stoma, or artificial opening. A stoma of the intestinal and urinary tracts permits the elimination of wastes through the abdominal wall. A stoma of the respiratory tract permits the passage of air through the neck. An ostomate is someone who has had this form of surgery.

Oxidation. The act of combining with oxygen, generally consisting in either an increase in the positive charges on the atom or the loss of negative charges.

Oxygen effect. Enhancement of radiosensitivity of cells because of the presence of oxygen.

Ozone. A more active form of oxygen resulting from exposure of oxygen to the silent discharge of electricity.

Palliative treatment. Providing relief from symptoms of a disease but not directly curing the disease; alleviating pain.

Palpation. The application of the fingers to the body for the purpose of diagnosis.

Pap test. Developed by the late Dr. George Papanicolaou, to examine, under the microscope, cells found in vaginal secretions. Its major purpose is to detect cancer of the cervix in its earliest stage. (See Cytology)

Parametrium. Soft tissues adjoining the uterus.

Parenteral. Not given orally. (IV)

Pathology. The science which studies the nature, cause and development of disease through examination of tissues and fluids of the body. A pathologist does autopsies and examines urine, blood, tissues removed for biopsies, etc.

PCP. Pneumocystis carinii pneumonia.

Pelvic examination. Examination of the organs of the pelvis, through the vagina and rectum.

Philadelphia chromosome. An abbreviated chromosome, found in certain leukemias, such as chronic granulocytic leukemias.

Photons. "Quanta" of energy delivered by X-rays and other rays of the electromagnetic spectrum (Planck).

Photosynthesis. Metabolism of plants. The sunlight energy is captured by the plants' chlorophyll and transformed into chemical energy.

Phylogeny. The complete developmental history of a race or group of animals.

Pituitary gland (or hypophysis). An endocrine gland situated at the base of the brain; the master gland.

Platelets. A small circular or oval disk present in blood which is necessary for the ability of the blood to clot and/or retract.

Pneumonectomy. A surgical procedure for removal of an entire lung.

Polycyclic hydrocarbons. Chemical carcinogens. See Alkylating agents.

Polymer. Variation of a given chemical compound. In polymerization the molecules of the compound; in consequence, the polymer has a heavier molecular weight than that of the compound.

Polynucleotide. A linear sequence of nucleotides in which the 3 prime position of the sugar of one nucleotide is linked through a phosphate group to the 5 prime position on the sugar of the adjacent nucleotide.

Polyoma virus. A DNA virus inducing a variety of cancers in mammals.

Polyp. An overgrowth of tissue projecting into a cavity of the body, e.g., the lining of the colon, the nasal passage, or the surface of vocal cords.

Polypeptide. A polymer of amino acids linked together by peptide bonds.

Polyposis. The development of multiple polyps in an organ or structure.

Polyvalent vaccine. A vaccine prepared from cultures of more than one strain of virus or bacterium.

Procto. Short for proctosigmoidoscopy, an examination of the first 10 inches of the rectum and colon with a hollow, lighted tube.

Progeny. Offspring; descendants.

Prognosis. The prospect of a disease, its outcome or future.

Progression (of cancer process). The appearance of cancer in clinical form.

Promoter. An agent that sets a cancer to growing after it has been initiated.

Promotion (of cancer process). The intermediate stages of cancer growth wherein the cell is altered by extraneous factors either within the patient or from the environment.

Prophase. Followed by Metaphase, Anaphase, Telophase; the four main phases of cell division.

Prostate. A gland located at the base of the bladder in males.

Prosthesis. An artificial replacement for a missing body part, e.g., breast form, leg, arm, eye.

Proteins. Combinations (polymers) of amino acids, constituting animal tissues.

Proton. The unit of positive electricity equivalent in charge to an electron and equal to the hydrogen ion in mass.

Provirus. A latent stage of virus.

Purine base, pyrimidine base. Organic compounds of carbon, hydrogen, and nitrogen; in cyclic form these are the primary components of DNA.

Quackery. The practice of using untested or unproved methods of treatment for a disease; alleged recoveries cannot be validated or equaled in subsequent tests under controlled situations.

Rad. A measure of the amount of any ionizing radiation which is absorbed by tissues.

Radiation sickness. Illness sometimes caused by radiation therapy; characterized by nausea, lack of appetite, vomiting, and diarrhea.

Radiation therapy. Treatment of cancer with radiant energy of extremely short wave lengths which damages or kills cancer cells. Radioactive elements such as cobalt 60, radium and radon, gallium and Cesium 27 are used to produce gamma rays. Supervoltage machines, such as betatrons and linear accelerators are used as sources of X-rays.

Radioactive isotopes. Isotopes having radioactive properties.

Radiopaque. Not permitting the passage of X-rays or other radiant energy.

RBE. Relative biological effectiveness of a radiation: the effect of a given radiation on a given tissue is dependent upon the energy absorbed and the wavelength used.

Recessive trait. A weak genetic trait.

Regional involvement. When cancer has spread from its original site to nearby areas. (*See* Metastasis)

Regression. The subsidence of a disease, or symptom.

Remission. Complete or partial disappearance of the signs and symptoms of a disease; or the period during which a disease is under control.

Replication. Transcription and translation: biological processes of the cell. Replication is the self-copying process; transcription, the passage of a message from DNA to RNA; translation, the actual carrying out of the message by messenger RNA.

Repressor gene. The gene suppressing the active, or operator, gene.

Retinoblastoma. A malignant tumor of the retina of the eye.

Retinol. The form of vitamin A found in mammals, especially high in the liver and milk.

Ribonucleotide. A compound that consists of a purine or pyrimidine base bonded to a ribose sugar which in turn is connected to a phosphate group.

Ribosome. Substance of the cell cytoplasm, site of protein synthesis.

RNA (Ribonucleic acid). Polymer of ribonucleotides.

Roentgen. Unit of radiation (after the name of the German physicist who discovered X-rays).

Roentgen rays. X-rays.

Rous sarcoma virus. An RNA virus, producing cancer in chickens.

Sarcoma. A form of cancer that arises in the connective tissue and muscles, such as bone and cartilage.

Senescence. The process or condition of growing old.

Sex-linked. Invariably related to male or female sex.

Sigmoidoscopy. Visual inspection of the lower portion of the large bowel (the sigmoid colon).

Sputum test. A study of cells from the lungs contained in material coughed up in the sputum. (also called sputum cytology)

Staging. Determining the extent of growth of a cancer so that results of treatment can be compared and prognosis offered.

Structural genes (Jacob and Monod). Genes which determine the complexity and differentiation of a cell. *See* Control genes.

Substrate. A substance upon which an enzyme acts.

Supraclavicular nodes. Lymph nodes above the clavicle.

Synergism. Joint action of agents whereby their effects together are greater than the sum of their individual actions.

Syngenic grafting. Transplantation of tissues between genetically identical animals.

"T" Cells. Lymphocyte responsible for cell-mediated immunity. (T = thymus dependent).

Telecobalt unit. A machine producing high-energy radiations.

Telophase. The last of the four stages of mitosis.

Template surface. Copying surface of the DNA strands; in replication, when the DNA helix unwinds into two separate strands, each of these strands serves as the template on which the second half is paired off.

Thanatology. Study of death (and dying).

Thermography. A technique for measuring the surface temperature of parts of the body to detect underlying disease; used along with mammography and palpation for discovering breast cancer in its earliest stage.

Thymine. One of the four bases of DNA.

Tissue. A collection of similar cells. There are four basic tissues in the body: (1) epithelial; (2) connective; (3) muscle; (4) nerve.

Tissue culture. Technique of growing plant or animal cells in test tubes outside of the body (in vitro), but using a medium containing a variety of nutrients.

Tolerance. State of acceptance of an antigen by the cell, or an organism to a drug.

Tomograms. Cross-sectional x-rays.

Toxicologist. A scientist who investigates, in a laboratory, the association between exposure to a chemical and its biological effect.

Tracheostomy. A surgical procedure to create a stoma or permanent opening of the trachea or windpipe through the neck. Tracheotomy is the surgery that temporarily provides direct passage of air into the windpipe.

Transcription. The formation of messenger RNA from the template DNA.

Transduction. The transfer of a genetic fragment from one cell to another.

Transfer RNA. The adaptor molecule between messenger RNA (bringing DNA's message to the ribosomes) and the ribosomes themselves. It is a free RNA molecule in the cell cytoplasm, which "searches" for each required amino acid and brings it to each exact spot on messenger RNA for protein synthesis.

Transformation. Conversion of a normal cell into an abnormal cell, usually a cancer cell, under the influence of radiation, chemicals, or viruses.

Translation. The formation of protein coded by the messenger RNA.

Triplet. Assemblage of any three of the four bases of DNA (A, G, T, C) codifying the formation of a particular amino acid.

Tumor. A swelling or enlargement; an abnormal mass, either benign or malignant, which performs no useful body function.

Tumoricidal. Destroying tumor cells.

Ultrasound. An imaging method using sound waves (no radiation).

Univalent vaccine. A vaccine prepared from the culture of one strain of virus or bacterium.

Uracil. One of the four bases of RNA. See also Adenine.

Urostomy. A surgical procedure which creates a stoma or opening in the urinary tract through the abdominal wall to permit the elimination of urine.

Uterus. Organ in the female for receiving the fertilized egg and nourishing the embryo during development prior to birth.

Vertical transmission (of tumors). Transmission from generation to generation, from mother to offspring.

Virology. The branch of biology dealing with the study of viruses.

Virus. Minute living organism composed of an inner nucleic acid core and an outer protein coat. Parasitic, it needs to live in a cell to reproduce itself.

Wilms' tumor. An embryonal tumor of the kidney, affecting young children primarily.

Xeroradiography. A photographic way of recording X-ray images; useful in early detection of breast cancer (from Xerox).

X-ray. Radiant energy of extremely short wave length, used to diagnose and treat cancer.

Yttrium. A rare metal producing isotopes that emit X-rays.

Zenogenic grafting. Transplantation of tissues between animals of different species.

Appendix I

Cancer Statistics

AMERICAN CANCER SOCIETY FACTS AND FIGURES

- Estimated new cases and deaths from major sites of cancer—1988
- Cancer's Seven Warning Signals
- Guidelines for the cancer related checkup
- Cancer incidence and deaths by site and sex—1988 estimates
- Five year cancer survival rates for selected sites
- Cancer death rates by site, United States, 1930–85
- Trends in survival by site of cancer, by race
- Mortality for leading causes of death: United States, 1977
- Estimated new cancer cases and deaths for all sites—1988

NATIONAL CANCER INSTITUTE—Cancer Risks and Rates

- Changes for 19 sites among whites
- Changes for 19 sites among blacks
- International range of cancer incidence
- Earnings lost due to cancer in 1977

American Cancer Society

Estimated New Cases and Deaths from Major Sites of Cancer—1989*

Site	No. of Cases	Deaths
Lung	155,000	142,000
Colon-Rectum	151,000	61,000
Breast (Female)	142,000	43,000
Prostate	103,000	28,500
Urinary	70,200	20,260
Uterus	47,000	10,000
Oral	31,000	8,700
Leukemia	27,000	18,100
Pancreas	27,000	25,000
Skin	27,000	8,200
Ovary	20,000	12,000

*Figures rounded to nearest 1,000.
†Melanoma 6,000; other skin 2,200

Cancer's Seven Warning Signals*

1. Change in bowel or bladder habits
2. A sore that does not heal
3. Unusual bleeding or discharge
4. Thickening or lump in breast or elsewhere
5. Indigestion or difficulty in swallowing
6. Obvious change in wart or mole
7. Nagging cough or hoarseness

If you have a warning signal, see your doctor.

*Ed: The American Cancer Society has long advocated teaching the "Seven Warning Signals" to the public. They've even arranged them as an acronym—CAUTION—in the hope that more people will remember them. However, by the time a person has a cancer that is causing any of these symptoms, it is almost certainly not an *early* cancer. Emphasizing the Seven Warning Signals is not part of a prevention or early detection plan. Cancers need to be found before there are symptoms.

Guidelines for the Cancer Related Checkup

In 1981, after studying at length all available research data on cancer screening, the American Cancer Society released the following guidelines. Significantly, chest x-rays were no longer recommended, Pap smears were no longer automatically recommended yearly, and mammography was recommended with greater frequency.

The guidelines were modified in 1985, 1987, and 1989, and will no doubt require future modifications.

Bear in mind that these guidelines are for the screening of asymptomatic people, and do not account for possible significant factors in a person's medical history.

Test or Procedure	Sex	Age	Frequency
Chest x-ray		—not recommended—	
Sputum cytology		—not recommended—	
Sigmoid-oscopy	M&F	over 50	after 2 neg. exams 1 year apart
Stool hidden blood slide test	M&F	over 50	every year
Digital rectal examination	M&F	over 40	every year
Pap test	F	all women 18 or older; all women who are sexually active	yearly, after 3 negative exams, may be less frequent
Pelvic examination	F	20–40 over 40	every 3 years every year
Endometrial tissue sample (biopsy)	F	at menopause women at high risk[1]	at menopause
Breast self examination	F	over 20	every month
Breast physical examination	F	20–40 over 40	every 3 years every year
Mammography	F	between 35–39 40–49 over 50	baseline every 1–2 years every year
Health counseling and cancer checkup[2]	M&F M&F	over 20 over 40	every 3 years every year

[1] history of infertility, obesity, failure of ovulation, abnormal uterine bleeding, or estrogen therapy.
[2] to include examination for cancers of the thyroid, testicles, prostate, ovaries, lymph nodes, oral region, and skin.

CANCER INCIDENCE AND DEATHS BY SITE AND SEX—1989 ESTIMATES

CANCER INCIDENCE BY SITE AND SEX†

SKIN	3%		3%	SKIN
ORAL	4%		2%	ORAL
LUNG	20%		28%	BREAST
COLON & RECTUM	14%		11%	LUNG
PANCREAS	3%		15%	COLON & RECTUM
PROSTATE	21%		3%	PANCREAS
URINARY	10%		4%	OVARY
LEUKEMIA & LYMPHOMAS	8%		9%	UTERUS
ALL OTHER	17%		4%	URINARY
			7%	LEUKEMIA & LYMPHOMAS
			14%	ALL OTHER

CANCER DEATHS BY SITE AND SEX

SKIN	2%		1%	SKIN
ORAL	2%		1%	ORAL
LUNG	35%		18%	BREAST
COLON & RECTUM	11%		21%	LUNG
PANCREAS	5%		13%	COLON & RECTUM
PROSTATE	11%		5%	PANCREAS
URINARY	5%		5%	OVARY
LEUKEMIA & LYMPHOMAS	9%		4%	UTERUS
ALL OTHER	20%		3%	URINARY
			9%	LEUKEMIA & LYMPHOMAS
			20%	ALL OTHER

†Excluding non-melanoma skin cancer and carcinoma in situ.

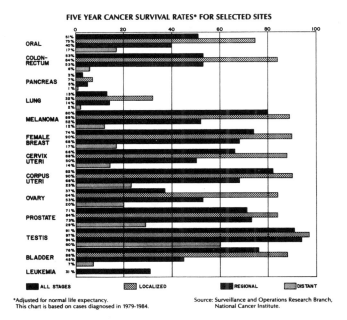

FIVE YEAR CANCER SURVIVAL RATES* FOR SELECTED SITES

■ ALL STAGES   ▨ LOCALIZED   ■ REGIONAL   ▨ DISTANT

*Adjusted for normal life expectancy.
This chart is based on cases diagnosed in 1979-1984.

Source: Surveillance and Operations Research Branch, National Cancer Institute.

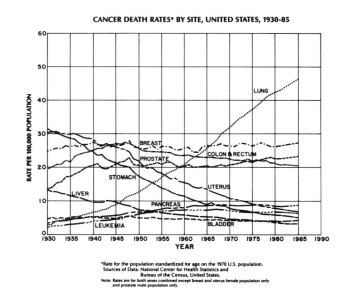

CANCER DEATH RATES* BY SITE, UNITED STATES, 1930-85

*Rate for the population standardized for age on the 1970 U.S. population.
Sources of Data: National Center for Health Statistics and
Bureau of the Census, United States.
Note: Rates are for both sexes combined except breast and uterus female population only
and prostate male population only.

TRENDS IN SURVIVAL BY SITE OF CANCER, BY RACE
Cases Diagnosed in 1960-63, 1970-73, 1974-76, 1977-78, 1979-84

SITE	WHITE					BLACK				
	RELATIVE 5-YEAR SURVIVAL					RELATIVE 5-YEAR SURVIVAL				
	1960-63[1]	1970-73[1]	1974-76[2]	1977-78[2]	1979-84[2]	1960-63[1]	1970-73[1]	1974-76[2]	1977-78[2]	1979-84[2]
All Sites	39%	43%	50%	50%	50%	27%	31%	38%	38%	37%
Oral Cavity & Pharynx	45	43	54	53	54	–	–	35	35	31
Esophagus	4	4	5	6	7	1	4	4	2	5
Stomach	11	13	14	15	16*	8	13	15	16	17
Colon	43	49	50	52	54*	34	37	45	44	49
Rectum	38	45	48	50	52*	27	30	40	40	34
Liver	2	3	4	3	3	–	–	1	1	5
Pancreas	1	2	3	2	3	1	2	2	3	5
Larynx	53	62	66	69	66	–	–	58	59	55
Lung & Bronchus	8	10	12	13	13*	5	7	11	10	11
Melanoma of Skin	60	68	78	81	80*	–	–	62##	–	61#
Breast (females)	63	68	74	75	75*	46	51	62	62	62
Cervix Uteri	58	64	69	69	67	47	61	61	63	59
Corpus Uteri	73	81	89	87	83*	31	44	61	58	52*
Ovary	32	36	36	37	37*	32	32	41	40	36
Prostate Gland	50	63	67	70	73*	35	55	56	64	60*
Testis	63	72	78	86	91*	–	–	77#	–	82#
Urinary Bladder	53	61	73	75	77*	24	36	47	53	57*
Kidney & Renal Pelvis	37	46	51	50	51	38	44	49	54	53
Brain & Nervous System	18	20	22	23	23	19	19	27	24	31
Thyroid Gland	83	86	92	92	93	–	–	88	92	95
Hodgkin's Disease	40	67	71	73	74*	–	–	67#	79#	69
Non-Hodgkin's Lymphoma	31	41	47	48	49*	–	–	47	46	49
Multiple Myeloma	12	19	24	24	24	–	–	28	30	29
Leukemia	14	22	34	37	32	–	–	30	31	27

Source: Surveillance and Operations Research Branch, National Cancer Institute.

[1] Rates are based on End Results Group data from a series of hospital registries and one population-based registry.

[2] Rates are from the SEER Program. They are based on data from population-based registries in Connecticut, New Mexico, Utah, Iowa, Hawaii, Atlanta, Detroit, Seattle-Puget Sound and San Francisco-Oakland. Rates are based on follow-up of patients through 1985.

* The difference in rates between 1974-76 and 1979-84 is statistically significant (p < .05).

The standard error of the survival rate is between 5 and 10 percentage points.

The standard error of the survival rate is greater than 10 percentage points.

– Valid survival rate could not be calculated.

Mortality for Leading Causes of Death: United States, 1985

Rank Cause of Death	Number of Deaths	Death Rate Per 100,000 Population	Percent of Total Deaths
All Causes	**2,086,440**	**739.0**	**100.0**
1 Heart Diseases	771,113	261.4	37.0
2 Cancer	461,563	170.5	22.1
3 Cerebrovascular Diseases	153,050	51.0	7.3
4 Accidents	93,457	36.0	4.5
5 Chronic Obstructive Lung Diseases	71,047	25.0	3.4
6 Pneumonia & Influenza	67,615	22.0	3.2
7 Diabetes Mellitus	36,969	13.1	1.8
8 Suicide	29,453	11.2	1.4
9 Cirrhosis of Liver	26,767	10.6	1.3
10 Arteriosclerosis	23,926	7.6	1.1
11 Nephritis	21,349	7.3	1.0
12 Homicide	19,893	7.5	1.0
13 Diseases of Infancy	19,246	8.8	0.9
14 Septicemia & Pyemia	17,182	6.0	0.8
15 Aortic Aneurysm	15,112	5.3	0.7
Other & Ill-defined	258,698	96.1	12.5

Source: Vital Statistics of the United States, 1985.

ESTIMATED NEW CANCER CASES AND DEATHS BY SEX FOR ALL SITES—1989*

	ESTIMATED NEW CASES			ESTIMATED DEATHS		
	Total	Male	Female	Total	Male	Female
ALL SITES	1,010,000*	505,000*	505,000*	502,000	266,000	236,000
Buccal Cavity & Pharynx (ORAL)	30,600	20,600	10,000	8,650	5,775	2,875
Lip	4,200	3,700	500	100	75	25
Tongue	6,000	3,900	2,100	1,950	1,300	650
Mouth	11,700	7,000	4,700	2,600	1,600	1,000
Pharynx	8,700	6,000	2,700	4,000	2,800	1,200
Digestive Organs	227,800	115,200	112,600	123,000	64,400	58,600
Esophagus	10,100	7,200	2,900	9,400	6,900	2,500
Stomach	20,000	11,900	8,100	13,900	8,200	5,700
Small Intestine	2,700	1,400	1,300	900	500	400
Large Intestine } (COLON-RECTUM)	107,000	50,000	57,000	53,500	26,000	27,500
Rectum	44,000	23,000	21,000	7,800	4,000	3,800
Liver & Biliary Passages	14,500	7,500	7,000	11,400	5,800	5,600
Pancreas	27,000	13,000	14,000	25,000	12,500	12,500
Other & Unspecified Digestive	2,500	1,200	1,300	1,100	500	600
Respiratory System	171,600	114,000	57,600	147,100	96,900	50,200
Larynx	12,300	10,000	2,300	3,700	3,000	700
LUNG	155,000	101,000	54,000	142,000	93,000	49,000
Other & Unspecified Respiratory	4,300	3,000	1,300	1,400	900	500
Bone	2,100	1,200	900	1,300	700	600
Connective Tissue	5,600	3,000	2,600	3,000	1,400	1,600
SKIN	27,000**	14,500**	12,500**	8,200†	5,200	3,000
BREAST	142,900***	900***	142,000***	43,300	300	43,000
Genital Organs	181,800***	109,900	71,900***	52,200	29,100	23,100
Cervix Uteri	13,000***	—	13,000***	6,000	—	6,000
Corpus, Endometrium } (UTERUS)	34,000	—	34,000	4,000	—	4,000
Ovary	20,000	—	20,000	12,000	—	12,000
Other & Unspecified Genital, Female	4,900	—	4,900	1,100	—	1,100
Prostate	103,000	103,000	—	28,500	28,500	—
Testis	5,700	5,700	—	350	350	—
Other & Unspecified Genital, Male	1,200	1,200	—	250	250	—
Urinary Organs	70,200	49,000	21,200	20,200	12,900	7,300
Bladder	47,100	34,500	12,600	10,200	6,900	3,300
Kidney & Other Urinary	23,100	14,500	8,600	10,000	6,000	4,000
Eye	1,900	1,000	900	300	150	150
Brain & Central Nervous System	15,000	8,200	6,800	11,000	6,000	5,000
Endocrine Glands	12,600	3,700	8,900	1,750	775	975
Thyroid	11,300	3,000	8,300	1,025	375	650
Other Endocrine	1,300	700	600	725	400	325
Leukemia	27,300	15,200	12,100	18,100	9,800	8,300
Lymphocytic Leukemia	13,000	7,500	5,500	7,000	3,900	3,100
Granulocytic Leukemia	13,300	7,200	6,100	10,600	5,600	5,000
Monocytic Leukemia	1,000	500	500	500	300	200
Other Blood & Lymph Tissues	51,800	27,000	24,800	27,400	14,100	13,300
Hodgkin's Disease	7,400	4,200	3,200	1,500	900	600
Non-Hodgkin's Lymphomas	32,800	16,800	16,000	17,300	8,900	8,400
Multiple Myeloma	11,600	6,000	5,600	8,600	4,300	4,300
All Other & Unspecified Sites	41,800	21,600	20,200	36,500	18,500	18,000

NOTE: The estimates of new cancer cases are offered as a rough guide and should not be regarded as definitive. Especially note that year-to-year changes may only represent improvements in the basic data. ACS six major sites appear in boldface caps.

*Carcinoma in situ and non-melanoma skin cancers are not included in totals. Carcinoma in situ of the uterine cervix accounts for more than 50,000 new cases annually, and carcinoma in situ of the female breast accounts for about 10,000 new cases annually. Non-melanoma skin cancer accounts for more than 500,000 new cases annually.

**Melanoma only.   ***Invasive cancer only.   †Melanoma 6,000; other skin 2,200

INCIDENCE ESTIMATES ARE BASED ON RATES FROM NCI SEER PROGRAM 1983-85.

National Cancer Institute

CHANGES FOR 19 SITES AMONG WHITES

The overall, 5-year relative survival rate for cancer patients in the United States is now 48 percent or greater. These data show the changes in survival rates for all whites in this country for 19 major cancers. There have been some gains in survival rates for almost all cancers in the 20 years spanned by these data.

The most notable gains have been seen for endometrial, cervical and breast cancers among women, testicular and prostatic cancers among men, and for Hodgkin's disease, melanoma skin cancer, and bladder cancer among both men and women.

Survival for colorectal cancer patients has improved over the 20-year period but is still less than 50 percent. Survival rates for cancers of the lung, stomach, pancreas, and esophagus remain low.

Five-year Relative Survival Rates for Selected Sites for White Cancer Patients.

	1960–63*	1970–73*	1973–79*
Bladder	53	61	71
Brain	18	20	20
Breast (females)	63	68	72
Cervix	58	64	66
Colon	43	49	48
Endometrium (corpus)	73	81	87
Esophagus	4	4	4
Hodgkin's disease	40	67	68
Kidney	37	46	48
Leukemia	14	22	28
Lung	8	10	11
Melanoma of the skin	60	68	76
Non-Hodgkin's lymphoma	31	41	43
Ovary	32	36	34
Pancreas	1	2	2
Prostate	50	63	64
Rectum	38	45	46
Stomach	11	13	13
Testicular cancer	63	72	80

*Data for 1960–63 and 1970–73 are from three hospital registries and one State registry, and appear in Cancer Patient Survival Experience, 1980. Data for 1973–79 are from SEER, and represent 10 percent of the U.S. population. Thus, the earlier data and the SEER data are not strictly comparable, but each set represents the best available data for the time period covered.

CHANGES FOR 19 SITES AMONG BLACKS

Substantial gains in 5-year survival rates can be seen for endometrial, cervical and breast cancers among women and for cancer of the prostate among men.

Some gains in survival are also apparent for bladder cancer, kidney cancer and colorectal cancers in both sexes. The outlook for stomach cancer and for cancers of the lung, pancreas, ovary and esophagus remains poor.

Although white patients survive longer than black patients for more than half of these sites, the survival rates are almost equal for cancers of the stomach, lung and esophagus, and for Hodgkin's disease and non-Hodgkin's lymphoma. Black patients with cancers of the pancreas, ovary, kidney, and brain survive slightly longer than whites.

The differences in survival rates is a subject of concern and is under intense study at the National Cancer Institute.

Five-year Relative Survival Rates for Selected Sites for Black Cancer Patients.

	1960–63*	1970–73*	1973–79*
Bladder	24	36	43
Brain	19	19	21
Breast (females)	46	51	60
Cervix	47	61	61
Colon	34	37	44
Endometrium (corpus)	31	44	54
Esophagus	1	4	3
Hodgkin's disease	**	**	66
Kidney	38	44	49
Leukemia	**	**	24
Lung	5	7	9
Melanoma of the skin	**	**	**
Non-Hodgkin's lymphoma	**	**	43
Ovary	32	32	35
Pancreas	1	2	4
Prostate	35	55	54
Rectum	27	30	35
Stomach	8	13	14
Testicular cancer	**	**	62

*Data for 1960–63 and 1970–73 are from two hospital registries and appear in Cancer Patient Survival Experience, 1980. The later data are from SEER, and represent 10 percent of the U.S. population. Thus, the earlier data and the SEER data are not strictly comparable, but each set represents the best available data for the time period covered.
**Rates could not be calculated because the number of cases was too small.

	Males					
	High			Low		Ratio
Site	Population	Rate		Population	Rate	H/L
Lip	Canada, Newfoundland	22.8		Japan, Osaka	0.1	228.0
Tongue	India, Bombay	10.2		Romania, County Cluj	0.5	20.4
Mouth	France, Bas Rhin, Urban	13.0		Japan, Miyagi	0.5	26.0
Oropharynx	France, Bas Rhin, Urban	13.4		Norway	0.3	44.7
Nasopharynx	Hong Kong	32.9		Japan, Miyagi	0.3	109.7
Hypopharynx	France, Bas Rhin, Rural	11.0		Israel, All Jews	0.2	55.0
Esophagus	Shanghai	24.7		Hungary, Szabolcs, Rural	1.1	22.5
Stomach	Japan, Nagasaki	100.2		U.S., Atlanta, White	5.7	17.6
Colon	U.S., Connecticut	32.3		India, Poona	3.1	10.4
Rectum	Canada, N.W. Territory & Yukon	22.6		Israel, Non-Jews	3.1	7.3
Liver	Hong Kong	34.4		Australia, New South Wales, Rural	0.6	57.3
Gallbladder	U.S., New Mexico, Amerindian	7.7		India, Bombay	0.5	15.4
Pancreas	U.S., Bay Area, Black	18.3		India, Bombay	2.0	9.2
Larynx	Italy, Varese	16.0		U.K., North Scotland	1.8	8.9
Lung & Bronchus	U.S., New Orleans, Black	107.2		U.S., New Mexico, Amerindian	8.1	13.2
Melanoma	Australia, New South Wales, Urban	17.2		Japan, Osaka	0.2	86.0
Prostate	U.S., Alameda, Black	100.2		Shanghai	0.8	125.3
Testis	Switzerland, Vaud, Rural	10.5		Cuba	0.3	35.0
Penis	Jamaica, Kingston	5.7		U.S., Los Angeles, White	0.2	28.5
Bladder	Switzerland, Geneva	30.2		India, Poona	2.4	12.6
Kidney, etc.	U.S., Hawaii, White	11.2		India, Bombay	1.3	8.6
Brain	Australia, South	8.2		Japan, Miyagi	0.9	9.1
Thyroid gland	U.S., Hawaii, Chinese	7.8		India, Poona	0.4	19.5
Lymphosarcoma	Switzerland, Geneva	8.5		Poland, Warsaw, Rural	1.2	7.1
Hodgkin's disease	Switzerland, Vaud, Urban	4.9		Japan, Miyagi	0.5	9.8
Multiple myeloma	U.S., Bay Area, Black	8.4		India, Poona	0.6	14.0
Lymphatic leukemia	Switzerland, Neuchatel	7.9		Japan, Fukuoka, Urban	0.5	15.8
Myeloid leukemia	U.S., Hawaii, Hawaiian	8.7		Romania, County Cluj	0.7	12.4

*Age-standardized to the Standard World Population (Waterhouse et al, 1982).

INTERNATIONAL RANGE OF CANCER INCIDENCE

Although cancer occurs in every country in the world, there are wide geographic variations in incidence. Among men, for example, lip cancer occurs at a rate of 22.8 cases per 100,000 population in Newfoundland and 0.1 cases per 100,000 in Osaka, for a high-low ratio of 228.

The incidence of cancer of the prostate is highest among black men living in Alameda County, California, and lowest among men in Shanghai. The high-low ratio is 125.3. Stomach cancer occurs at a rate of 100.2 cases per 100,000 among Japanese men in Nagasaki and 5.7 cases per 100,000 among U.S. white men in Atlanta, for a high-low ratio of 17.6.

Both the world's highest and lowest incidence rates of lung cancer in men are found in the United States: the highest incidence rate—107.2 cases per 100,000—is found among black men in New Orleans and the lowest—8.1 per 100,000—is found among American Indians living in New Mexico. This

	Females					
	High			Low		Ratio
Site	Population	Rate		Population	Rate	H/L
Lip	Romania, County Cluj	2.3		U.K., Birmingham	0.1	23.0
Tongue	India, Bombay	4.1		Czechoslovakia, W. Slovakia	0.2	20.5
Mouth	India, Bombay	5.8		Yugoslavia, Slovenia	0.2	29.0
Oropharynx	U.S., Hawaii, White	2.7		Japan, Osaka	0.1	27.0
Nasopharynx	Hong Kong	14.4		Trent, U.K.	0.1	144.0
Hypopharynx	India, Bombay	2.2		Canada, British Columbia	0.1	22.0
Esophagus	India, Bombay	10.7		U.S., Utah	0.4	26.8
Stomach	Japan, Nagasaki	51.0		Israel, Non-Jews	2.4	21.3
Colon	U.S., Bay Area, Japanese	27.4		India, Poona	2.8	9.8
Rectum	Switzerland, Neuchatel	13.4		Israel, Non-Jews	1.5	8.9
Liver	Shanghai	9.1		Norway, Rural	0.4	22.8
Gallbladder	U.S., New Mexico, Amerindian	22.2		India, Bombay	0.7	31.7
Pancreas	U.S., New Mexico, Amerindian	10.4		India, Bombay	0.9	11.6
Larynx	India, Bombay	2.6		Norway	0.2	13.0
Lung & Bronchus	New Zealand, Maori	48.8		Spain, Navarra	2.6	18.8
Melanoma	Australia, New South Wales, Rural	19.1		Japan, Osaka	0.2	95.5
Breast	U.S., Hawaii, Hawaiian	87.5		Japan, Osaka, Rural	8.9	9.8
Cervix uteri	Colombia, Cali	52.9		Israel, Non-Jews	2.1	25.2
Corpus uteri	U.S., Alameda, White	38.5		Japan, Fukuoka, Rural	1.0	38.5
Ovary	Israel, Jews born in Europe & America	17.2		Japan, Osaka, Rural	2.1	8.2
Bladder	U.S., New Orleans, White	6.5		Hungary, Szabolcs, Rural	0.5	13.0
Kidney, etc.	Canada, N.W. Territory & Yukon	15.3		India, Poona	0.6	25.5
Brain	Poland, Warsaw City, U.S., Hawaii	6.6		Japan, Miyagi, Rural	0.6	11.0
Thyroid gland	Hawaiian	17.6		Poland, Warsaw, Rural	0.7	25.1
Lymphosarcoma	U.S., Hawaii, Hawaiian	6.3		Poland, Katowice	0.5	12.6
Hodgkin's disease	Switzerland, Vaud, Rural	4.3		Japan, Osaka	0.3	14.3
Multiple myeloma	U.S., Hawaii, Hawaiian	5.9		Poland, Katowice	0.4	14.8
Lymphatic leukemia	U.S., New Mexico, Other White	3.3		Japan, Fukuoka	0.4	8.3
Myeloid leukemia	New Zealand, Maori	5.4		Hungary, Szabolcs	0.8	6.8

*Age-standardized to the Standard World Population (Waterhouse et al, 1982).

latter group has the world's highest incidence rate of gallbladder cancer—7.7 cases per 100,000—compared with 0.5 cases per 100,000 among men in Bombay.

Among women, the greatest worldwide variation in incidence is found for cancer of the nasopharynx. It occurs at a rate of 0.1 cases per 100,000 population in Trent, England, and at a rate 144 times greater, 14.4 cases per 100,000, among women in Hong Kong. The highest incidence rate of breast cancer in the world, 87.5 cases per 100,000, is found among Hawaiian women and the lowest rate, 8.9 cases per 100,000, is found among Japanese women in Osaka. The high-low rate is 9.8.

Cancer of the uterine corpus, or endometrium, occurs at a rate of 38.5 cases per 100,000 among white women in Alameda County, California, and at a rate of 1.0 cases per 100,000 among rural Japanese women in Fukuoka, a 38.5-fold difference.

The world's highest incidence of melanoma is found in New South Wales, Australia. It occurs there at a rate of 19.1 cases per 100,000 among women and 17.2 cases per 100,000 among men. The lowest incidence of this cancer is found among Japanese men and women in Osaka.

By comparing the worldwide incidence of cancer among men and women, it can be seen that cancer is generally less common among women. The table also shows that the United States has the highest incidence rates in the world of a number of cancers: breast and bladder cancers among women, prostate and kidney cancers among men, and cancers of the colon, pancreas, and gallbladder and myeloid leukemias in both sexes. The U.S. incidence rates for stomach cancer among men, lung cancer among American Indian men, and cancer of the esophagus among women are the lowest in the world.

The charts on the preceding two pages are based on data obtained by the International Agency for Research on Cancer (IARC), a part of the World Health Organization. IARC was formed in 1965 to collect and evaluate international data on cancer and to identify potential risk factors through epidemiologic and laboratory studies.

EARNINGS LOST DUE TO CANCER IN 1977

The value of lost earnings due to cancer and benign tumors was estimated to be $26.4 billion in 1977. "Lost earnings" are those lost because of premature death from cancer. They are computed by multiplying the number of cancer deaths at various age levels by adjusted projections of lifetime earnings.

Even though 60 percent of 1977 cancer deaths occurred in persons 65 and older, that age group accounted for only 11 percent of lost earnings. Those aged 45 to 64 accounted for 34 percent of deaths and for 62 percent of lost earnings. Persons under age 45 at time of death were responsible for 6 percent of cancer deaths and for 27 percent of lost earnings.

Lung cancer deaths accounted for the largest single portion of lost earnings: almost $6 billion. Cancers of the digestive organs include colorectal cancer and cancers of the stomach, esophagus, and pancreas.

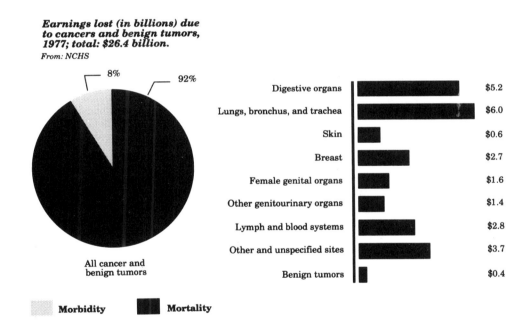

Earnings lost (in billions) due to cancers and benign tumors, 1977; total: $26.4 billion.
From: NCHS

8%   92%

All cancer and benign tumors

Morbidity   Mortality

Digestive organs	$5.2
Lungs, bronchus, and trachea	$6.0
Skin	$0.6
Breast	$2.7
Female genital organs	$1.6
Other genitourinary organs	$1.4
Lymph and blood systems	$2.8
Other and unspecified sites	$3.7
Benign tumors	$0.4

Appendix I

Cancer Statistics

AMERICAN CANCER SOCIETY FACTS AND FIGURES

- Estimated new cases and deaths from major sites of cancer—1989
- Cancer's Seven Warning Signals
- Guidelines for the cancer related checkup
- Cancer incidence and deaths by site and sex—1989 estimates
- Five year cancer survival rates for selected sites
- Cancer death rates by site, United States, 1930–85
- Trends in survival by site of cancer, by race
- Mortality for leading causes of death: United States, 1977
- Estimated new cancer cases and deaths for all sites—1989

NATIONAL CANCER INSTITUTE—*Cancer Risks and Rates*

- Changes for 19 sites among whites
- Changes for 19 sites among blacks
- International range of cancer incidence
- Earnings lost due to cancer in 1977

Table I Drugs Commonly Used for Different Types of Cancer

Cancer Type	Drugs Currently Preferred	Alternative Drugs
DISEASES IN WHICH CHEMOTHERAPY HAS MAJOR ACTIVITY		
Acute lymphocytic leukemia (ALL)	Induction: vincristine + prednisone ± asparaginase ± doxorubicin or daunorubicin	Cyclophosphamide, cytarabine, thioguanine, vindesine*, teniposide*, mitoxantrone*, etoposide, ifosfamide*
	CNS prophylaxis: intrathecal methotrexate ± radiotherapy	CNS prophylaxis: high dose IV methotrexate + intrathecal methotrexate
	Maintenance: combination chemotherapy with methotrexate + mercaptopurine or other combinations Bone marrow transplant for chemotherapy failures	Maintenance: doxorubicin and/or asparaginase in addition to methotrexate and mercaptopurine
Acute myelocytic leukemia (AML)	Daunorubicin + cytarabine ± thioguanine Marrow transplantation with cyclophosphamide and total body irradiation	High dose cytarabine, mitoxantrone*, azacitidine*, etoposide, amsacrine*, teniposide*, ifosfamide*
Breast cancer**	Tamoxifen, progestins Cyclophosphamide + methotrexate + fluorouracil ± prednisone (CMF or CMFP) Cyclophosphamide + doxorubicin ± fluorouracil (AC or CAF)	Vincristine, vinblastine, mitomycin, mitolactol*, mitoxantrone*, teniposide*, estrogens, androgens, progestins, prednisone, aminoglutethimide, etoposide, ifosfamide*
Choriocarcinoma	Methotrexate ± dactinomycin	Vinblastine, chlorambucil, bleomycin, etoposide, cisplatin, methotrexate with leucovorin rescue
Embryonal rhabdomyosarcoma**	Vincristine + dactinomycin + cyclophosphamide (VAC) ± doxorubicin Vincristine + doxorubicin + cyclophosphamide	Methotrexate, thiotepa, cisplatin, dacarbazine
Ewing's sarcoma**	Cyclophosphamide + doxorubicin + vincristine (CAV)	Dactinomycin, etoposide ± ifosfamide*
Hairy cell leukemia	Interferon or deoxycoformycin*	Chlorambucil
Hodgkin's disease	Mechlorethamine + vincristine + procarbazine + prednisone (MOPP) Doxorubicin + bleomycin + vinblastine + dacarbazine (ABVD) + cyclophosphamide MOPP alternated with ABVD Chlorambucil + vinblastine + procarbazine + prednisone (CVPP) ± carmustine Mechlorethamine + vincristine + procarbazine + doxorubicin + bleomycin + vinblastine (MOP/ABV)	Lomustine, carmustine, etoposide, teniposide*, streptozocin, methotrexate, ifosfamide*, mitoguazone* Marrow transplantation with lomustine, cyclophosphamide, etoposide
Lung		
small cell (oat cell)	Cyclophosphamide + doxorubicin + vincristine (CAV) Etoposide + cisplatin ± vincristine Cyclophosphamide + doxorubicin + etoposide (CAE) Methotrexate + doxorubicin + cyclophosphamide + lomustine (MACC)	Cyclophosphamide + doxorubicin + vincristine + etoposide (CAVE) Methotrexate, vincristine, cyclophosphamide, lomustine, procarbazine, mechlorethamine, ifosfamide*, carboplatin*
Non-Hodgkin's lymphoma Burkitt's lymphoma	Cyclophosphamide Cyclophosphamide + vincristine + methotrexate Cyclophosphamide + high dose cytarabine ± methotrexate with leucovorin	Carmustine, methotrexate, ifosfamide*
Diffuse histiocytic lymphoma	Cyclophosphamide + doxorubicin + vincristine + prednisone (CHOP) Bleomycin + doxorubicin + cyclophosphamide + vincristine + prednisone (BACOP) Bleomycin + doxorubicin + cyclophosphamide + vincristine + prednisone + methotrexate with leucovorin rescue (M-BACOP) Prednisone + methotrexate-leucovorin + doxorubicin + cyclophosphamide + etoposide–mechlorethamine + vincristine + procarbazine + prednisone (ProMACE-MOPP) Bleomycin + doxorubicin + cyclophosphamide + vincristine + prednisone + procarbazine (COP-BLAM)	Bleomycin, chlorambucil, lomustine, carmustine, cytarabine, etoposide, teniposide*, amsacrine*, methotrexate, high dose cytarabine, ifosfamide* Bone marrow transplantation with high dose cyclophosphamide and total body irradiation

*Available only for investigational use
**Drugs have major activity only when combined with surgical resection, radiotherapy, or both (adjuvant chemotherapy).

Table I   Drugs Commonly Used for Different Types of Cancer

Cancer Type	Drugs Currently Preferred	Alternative Drugs
DISEASES IN WHICH CHEMOTHERAPY HAS MAJOR ACTIVITY		
	Methotrexate with leucovorin + doxorubicin + cyclophosphamide + vincristine + prednisone + bleomycin (MACOP-B)	
	Cyclophosphamide + vincristine + methotrexate-leucovorin + cytarabine (COMLA)	
Osteogenic sarcoma**	Doxorubicin and/or high-dose methotrexate + leucovorin rescue + cisplatin + bleomycin ± cyclophosphamide + dactinomycin	Melphalan, mitomycin, ifosfamide*
Testicular	Cisplatin + vinblastine + bleomycin (PVB) Bleomycin + etoposide + cisplatin (BEP) Vinblastine + dactinomycin + bleomycin + cyclophosphamide + cisplatin (VAB-6)	Doxorubicin, vincristine, ifosfamide*, carboplatin*, etoposide, cyclophosphamide, methotrexate, plicamycin, dactinomycin, melphalan, chlorambucil
Wilms' tumor**	Dactinomycin + vincristine ± doxorubicin	Doxorubicin, cyclophosphamide, cisplatin, ifosfamide*, etoposide
DISEASES IN WHICH CHEMOTHERAPY HAS MODERATE ACTIVITY		
Adrenocortical carcinoma	Mitotane Cisplatin	Doxorubicin, aminoglutethimide, cyclophosphamide
Bladder	Cisplatin and/or doxorubicin + methotrexate + vinblastine (M-VAC) Instillation of thiotepa or doxorubicin or BCG* or mitomycin	Mitomycin, fluorouracil, vinblastine, methotrexate, instillation of interferon
Brain glioblastoma	Carmustine or lomustine	Semustine*, procarbazine, vincristine, cisplatin, cyclophosphamide, mechlorethamine
medulloblastoma	Vincristine + carmustine ± mechlorethamine ± methotrexate Mechlorethamine + vincristine + procarbazine + prednisone (MOPP) Vincristine + cisplatin	
Cervix	Cisplatin + bleomycin ± methotrexate Bleomycin + mitomycin + vincristine ± cisplatin	Cyclophosphamide, vincristine, methotrexate, mitomycin, fluorouracil, doxorubicin, vinblastine
Chronic lymphocytic leukemia	Chlorambucil + prednisone	Cyclophosphamide, vincristine, deoxycoformycin*
Chronic myelocytic leukemia (CML) Chronic phase	Busulfan Hydroxyurea Bone marrow transplantation with cyclophosphamide and total body irradiation	Mitobronitol*, mercaptopurine, thioguanine, melphalan, interferon
Acute phase	Daunorubicin + cytarabine + vincristine + prednisone ± thioguanine Vincristine + prednisone for lymphoid variant	Amsacrine*, azacitidine*, vincristine, high-dose cytarabine, plicamycin
Endometrial	Megestrol acetate or hydroxyprogesterone caproate or medroxyprogesterone acetate Doxorubicin ± cyclophosphamide ± cisplatin	Fluorouracil, tamoxifen, melphalan
Gastric	Fluorouracil + doxorubicin + mitomycin (FAM) Fluorouracil + doxorubicin + semustine*	Cisplatin, fluorouracil
Head and neck, squamous cell	Bleomycin + cisplatin ± methotrexate Cisplatin + fluorouracil	Vinblastine, cyclophosphamide, mitomycin, doxorubicin
Islet cell carcinoma	Streptozocin + fluorouracil	Cyclophosphamide, doxorubicin, dacarbazine, somatostatin*

*Available only for investigational use
**Drugs have major activity only when combined with surgical resection, radiotherapy, or both (adjuvant chemotherapy).

Table I   Drugs Commonly Used for Different Types of Cancer

Cancer Type	Drugs Currently Preferred	Alternative Drugs
DISEASES IN WHICH CHEMOTHERAPY HAS MAJOR ACTIVITY		
Kaposi's sarcoma (epidemic)	Etoposide or interferon	Cyclophosphamide, vinblastine, vincristine
Mycosis fungoides	Combination chemotherapy as in Hodgkin's disease or non-Hodgkin's lymphoma Mechlorethamine (topical)	Vinblastine, methotrexate, psoralen + ultraviolet light (PUVA), interferon, deoxycoformycin*, etretinate
Myeloma	Melphalan (or cyclophosphamide) + prednisone Melphalan + carmustine + cyclophosphamide + prednisone Dexamethasone + doxorubicin + vincristine	Carmustine, vincristine, lomustine, doxorubicin, interferon
Neuroblastoma	Doxorubicin + cyclophosphamide + cisplatin + teniposide* Doxorubicin + cyclophosphamide Cisplatin + cyclophosphamide	Mechlorethamine, daunorubicin, dacarbazine, vinblastine, prednisone, cisplatin, teniposide*, etoposide
Non-Hodgkin's lymphoma Follicular lymphoma	Cyclophosphamide or chlorambucil ± vincristine and prednisone or etoposide (combinations not demonstrably superior to single agents)	Cytarabine, asparaginase, methotrexate, interferon
Ovary	Melphalan (or cyclophosphamide) ± cisplatin + doxorubicin (CP, CAP) Cyclophosphamide + hexamethylmelamine* + doxorubicin + cisplatin (CHAP)	Hexamethylmelamine*, fluorouracil, chlorambucil, thiotepa, ifosfamide*, megestrol acetate, carboplatin* Intraperitoneal: fluorouracil, methotrexate, melphalan, cisplatin, doxorubicin
Prostate	Diethylstilbestrol, other estrogens, leuprolide or depot-formulation of LHRH analogs Cisplatin ± cyclophosphamide ± doxorubicin ± fluorouracil	Estramustine, megestrol acetate, fluorouracil, cyproterone*, flutamide*, methotrexate, mitoguazone*, streptozocin
Retinoblastoma	Doxorubicin + cyclophosphamide Doxorubicin + cyclophosphamide + cisplatin + teniposide*	
Sarcomas (soft tissue, adult)	Doxorubicin + dacarbazine + cyclophosphamide ± vincristine Doxorubicin + dacarbazine Doxorubicin + dacarbazine + ifosfamide*	Methotrexate, cisplatin
DISEASES IN WHICH CHEMOTHERAPY HAS MINOR ACTIVITY		
Colorectal	Fluorouracil Intra-arterial floxuridine (hepatic metastases)	Methotrexate, fluorouracil + leucovorin, ifosfamide*
Liver	Doxorubicin Fluorouracil ± methotrexate ± semustine*	Fluorouracil, floxuridine, etoposide, intra-arterial floxuridine
Lung non-small cell	Cyclophosphamide + doxorubicin + cisplatin (CAP) Vindesine* + cisplatin ± mitomycin Vinblastine + cisplatin ± mitomycin Fluorouracil + doxorubicin + mitomycin (FAM) Methotrexate + doxorubicin + cyclophosphamide + lomustine (MACC)	Methotrexate, etoposide, lomustine, fluorouracil, ifosfamide*, mitomycin, mitomycin + vinblastine, carboplatin*, procarbazine
Melanoma	Dacarbazine or semustine*	Dactinomycin, carmustine, procarbazine, vinblastine, interferon, ifosfamide*
Pancreatic	Fluorouracil + doxorubicin + mitomycin (FAM) Streptozocin + mitomycin + fluorouracil (SMF)	Mitomycin, doxorubicin, streptozocin, semustine*, ifosfamide*
Renal	Interferon	Vinblastine, lomustine, lymphokine-activated killer (LAK) cells + interleukin-2*, progestins

*Available only for investigational use
**Drugs have major activity only when combined with surgical resection, radiotherapy, or both (adjuvant chemotherapy).

Table II   Some Commercially Available Anticancer Drugs and Hormones (Dose-limiting effects are in **bold** type)

Drug	Acute Toxicity	Delayed Toxicity*
Aminoglutethimide (*Cytadren*–Ciba)	Drowsiness; nausea; dizziness; rash	Hypothyroidism (rare); bone marrow depression; fever; hypotension; masculinization
Asparaginase (*Elspar*– Merck; *Kidrolase*– Rhône-Poulenc)	**Nausea and vomiting; fever,** chills; headache; hypersensitivity, anaphylaxis; abdominal pain; hyperglycemia leading to coma	CNS depression or hyperexcitability; acute hemorrhagic pancreatitis; coagulation defects; thrombosis; renal damage; hepatic damage
Bleomycin (*Blenoxane*– Bristol-Myers)	Nausea and vomiting; fever; anaphylaxis and other allergic reactions	**Pneumonitis and pulmonary fibrosis; rash and hyperpigmentation;** stomatitis; alopecia; Raynaud's phenomenon
Busulfan (*Myleran*– Burroughs Wellcome)	Nausea and vomiting; rare diarrhea	**Bone marrow depression;** pulmonary infiltrates and fibrosis; alopecia; gynecomastia; ovarian failure; azoospermia; leukemia; chromosome aberrations; cataracts; Addisonian syndrome
Carmustine (BCNU; *BiCNU*–Bristol-Myers)	**Nausea and vomiting;** local phlebitis	**Delayed leukopenia and thrombocytopenia** (may be prolonged); pulmonary fibrosis (may be irreversible); delayed renal damage; gynecomastia; reversible liver damage; carcinogenesis
Chlorambucil (*Leukeran* Burroughs Wellcome)	Seizures	**Bone marrow depression;** pulmonary infiltrates and fibrosis; leukemia; hepatic toxicity; sterility
Cisplatin (Cis-Diamminedichloroplatinum; Cis-DDP; *Platinol*–Bristol-Myers)	**Nausea and vomiting;** anaphylactic reactions; fever; hemolytic-uremic syndrome	**Renal damage;** bone marrow depression; ototoxicity; hemolysis; hypomagnesemia; peripheral neuropathy; hypocalcemia; hypokalemia; Raynaud's syndrome; sterility
Cyclophosphamide (*Cytoxan*–Bristol-Myers; *Neosar*–Adria; *Procy-tox*–Horner)	**Nausea and vomiting;** Type I (anaphylactoid) hypersensitivity; facial burning with IV administration	**Bone marrow depression;** alopecia; hemorrhagic cystitis; sterility (may be temporary); pulmonary infiltrates and fibrosis; hyponatremia; leukemia; bladder cancer; inappropriate ADH secretion
Cytarabine HCl (cytosine arabinoside; *Cytosar-U*–Upjohn)	**Nausea and vomiting;** diarrhea; anaphylaxis	**Bone marrow depression;** conjunctivitis; megaloblastosis; oral ulceration; hepatic damage; fever; pulmonary edema and encephalopathy with high doses
Dacarbazine (DTIC; *DTIC-Dome*–Miles; and others)	**Nausea and vomiting;** diarrhea, anaphylaxis; pain on administration	**Bone marrow depression;** alopecia; flulike syndrome; renal impairment; hepatic necrosis; facial flushing, paresthesia; photosensitivity; urticarial rash
Dactinomycin (actinomycin D; *Cosmegen*–Merck)	**Nausea and vomiting;** diarrhea; local reaction and phlebitis; anaphylactoid reaction	**Stomatitis; oral ulceration; bone marrow depression;** alopecia; folliculitis; dermatitis in previously irradiated areas
Daunorubicin (*Cerubidine*–Wyeth)	**Nausea and vomiting;** diarrhea; red urine (not hematuria); severe local tissue damage and necrosis on extravasation; transient EKG changes; anaphylactoid reaction	**Bone marrow depression; cardiotoxicity;** alopecia; stomatitis; anorexia; diarrhea; fever and chills; dermatitis in previously irradiated areas
Doxorubicin (*Adriamycin*–Adria)	**Nausea and vomiting;** red urine (not hematuria); severe local tissue damage and necrosis on extravasation; diarrhea; fever; transient EKG changes; ventricular arrhythmia; anaphylactoid reaction	**Bone marrow depression; cardiotoxicity;** alopecia; stomatitis; anorexia; conjunctivitis; acral pigmentation; dermatitis in previously irradiated areas
Estramustine phosphate sodium (*Emcyt*–Roche)	Nausea and vomiting; diarrhea	Mild gynecomastia; increased frequency of vascular accidents; myelosuppression (uncommon); edema; dyspnea; pulmonary infiltrates and fibrosis; leukemia
Etoposide (VP16-213; *VePesid*–Bristol-Myers	**Nausea and vomiting;** diarrhea; fever; hypotension	**Bone marrow depression;** alopecia; peripheral neuropathy; allergic reactions; hepatic damage with high doses
Floxuridine (*FUDR*–Roche)	**Nausea and vomiting;** diarrhea	**Oral and gastrointestinal ulceration; bone marrow depression;** alopecia; dermatitis; hepatic dysfunction with hepatic infusion
Fluorouracil (5-FU; *Flu-orouracil*–Roche; and others)	**Nausea and vomiting;** diarrhea; hypersensitivity reaction	**Oral and GI ulcers; bone marrow depression;** neurological defects; usually cerebellar; alopecia; hyperpigmentation

*Cutaneous reactions (sometimes severe), hyperpigmentation, and ocular toxicity have been reported with virtually all nonhormonal anticancer drugs.

Table II Some Commercially Available Anticancer Drugs and Hormones *(Dose-limiting effects are in **bold** type)*

Drug	Acute Toxicity	Delayed Toxicity*
Hydroxyurea (*Hydrea*–Squibb)	Nausea and vomiting; allergic reactions to tartrazine dye	**Bone marrow depression;** stomatitis; dysuria; alopecia; rare neurological disturbances
Interferon (*Roferon-A*–Roche; *Intron-A*–Schering)	Fever; chills; myalgias; fatigue; headache; arthralgias; hypotension	Bone marrow depression; anorexia; renal damage; hepatic damage
Leuprolide (LH-releasing hormone analog; *Lupron*–TAP)	Transient increase in bone pain; hot flashes	Impotence; amenorrhea; testicular atrophy
Lomustine (CCNU; *Cee-NU*–Bristol-Myers)	**Nausea and vomiting**	**Delayed (4 to 6 weeks) leukopenia and thrombocytopenia** (may be prolonged); transient elevation of transaminase activity; neurological reactions; pulmonary fibrosis; renal damage
Mechlorethamine (nitrogen mustard; *Mustargen*–Merck)	**Nausea and vomiting;** local reaction and phlebitis	**Bone marrow depression;** alopecia; diarrhea; oral ulcers; leukemia; sterility
Melphalan *Alkeran*–Burroughs Wellcome)	Mild nausea; hypersensitivity reactions	**Bone marrow depression** (especially platelets); pulmonary infiltrates and fibrosis; leukemia; inappropriate ADH secretion
Mercaptopurine (6-MP; *Purinethol*–Burroughs Wellcome)	Nausea and vomiting; diarrhea	**Bone marrow depression; cholestasis and rarely hepatic necrosis; oral and intestinal ulcers;** pancreatitis; allopurinol may increase overall toxicity
Methotrexate (MTX; *Methotrexate*–Lederle; and others)	**Nausea and vomiting;** diarrhea; fever; anaphylaxis	**Oral and gastrointestinal ulceration,** perforation may occur; **bone marrow depression;** hepatic toxicity including cirrhosis and acute hepatic necrosis; renal toxicity; pulmonary infiltrates and fibrosis; osteoporosis; alopecia; depigmentation; menstrual dysfunction; encephalopathy and anaphylactoid reactions with high doses; chemical arachnoiditis and rarely necrotizing encephalitis with intrathecal administration
Mitomycin (*Mutamycin*–Bristol-Myers)	**Nausea and vomiting;** local reaction; fever	**Bone marrow depression** (cumulative); stomatitis; alopecia; acute pulmonary toxicity; pulmonary fibrosis; hepatotoxicity; renal toxicity; hemolytic-uremic syndrome
Mitotane (o,p'-DDD; *Lysodren*–Bristol-Myers)	**Nausea and vomiting;** diarrhea	**CNS depression;** rash; visual disturbances; adrenal insufficiency; brain damage with long-term high dosage; hematuria; hemorrhagic cystitis; albuminuria; hypertension; orthostatic hypotension; cataracts
Plicamycin (*Mithracin*–Miles)	**Nausea and vomiting;** diarrhea; fever	**Hemorrhagic diathesis; bone marrow depression** (thrombocytopenia); coagulation abnormalities; hepatic damage; hypocalcemia and hypokalemia; stomatitis; renal damage
Procarbazine HCl (*Matulane*–Roche; *Natulan*–Roche of Canada)	**Nausea and vomiting;** CNS depression; Antabuse-like effect with alcohol	**Bone marrow depression;** stomatitis; peripheral neuropathy; pneumonitis; leukemia
Streptozocin (streptozotocin; *Zanosar*–Upjohn)	**Nausea and vomiting;** local pain; chills and fever	**Renal damage;** hypoglycemia; hyperglycemia; liver damage; diarrhea; bone marrow depression (uncommon); fever; eosinophilia
Tamoxifen citrate *Nolvadex*–Stuart)	Nause and vomiting; hot flashes; transient increased bone or tumor pain	Vaginal bleeding and discharge; rash; hypercalcemia; thrombocytopenia; peripheral edema; depression; dizziness; headache; decreased visual acuity; corneal changes; retinopathy
Thioguanine (*Thioguanine*–Burroughs Wellcome)	Occasional nausea and vomiting	Bone marrow depression; hepatic damage; stomatitis
Thiotepa (triethylene-thiophosphoramide; *Thiotepa*–Lederle)	**Nausea and vomiting;** local pain	**Bone marrow depression;** menstrual dysfunction; interference with spermatogenesis; leukemia

*Cutaneous reactions (sometimes severe), hyperpigmentation, and ocular toxicity have been reported with virtually all nonhormonal anticancer drugs.

Table II Some Commercially Available Anticancer Drugs and Hormones (*Dose-limiting effects are in **bold** type*)

Drug	Acute Toxicity	Delayed Toxicity*
Vinblastine sulfate (*Velban*–Lilly; and others)	**Nausea and vomiting;** local reaction and phlebitis with extravasation	**Bone marrow depression;** alopecia; stomatitis; loss of deep tendon reflexes; jaw pain; muscle pain; paralytic ileus; inappropriate ADH secretion
Vincristine sulfate (*Oncovin*–Lilly; *Vincasar*–Adria)	Local reaction with extravasation	**Peripheral neuropathy;** alopecia; mild bone marrow depression; constipation; paralytic ileus; inappropriate ADH secretion; hepatic damage; jaw pain

*Cutaneous reactions (sometimes severe), hyperpigmentation, and ocular toxicity have been reported with virtually all nonhormonal anticancer drugs.

Table III Some Investigational Drugs

Drug	Acute Toxicity	Delayed Toxicity
Amasacrine (AMSA; Bristol-Myers, *Amsidyl*–Parke-Davis, Warner-Lambert)	Nausea and vomiting; diarrhea; pain or phlebitis on infusion; anaphylaxis	Bone marrow depression; hepatic injury; convulsions; stomatitis; ventricular fibrillation; alopecia
Azacitidine (*Mylosar*–Upjohn)	Nausea and vomiting; diarrhea; fever; drowsiness	Leukopenia (may be prolonged); thrombocytopenia; hepatic damage; muscle pain and weakness; bone marrow depression; possibly cardiotoxicity
Bisantrene HCl (ADC, ADAH; Lederle)	Nausea and vomiting; hypotension; flu-like illness; fever; phlebitis	Leukopenia; thrombocytopenia
Carboplatin (*Paraplatin*–Bristol-Myers)	Nausea and vomiting	Bone marrow depression; peripheral neuropathy (uncommon)
Deoxycoformycin (DCF; *Pentostatin*)	Nausea and vomiting	Nephrotoxicity; CNS depression; leukopenia; thrombocytopenia
*Flutamide (antigen; *Eulexin*; *Euflex*–Schering; *Anandron*)	Nausea	Gynecomastia; hepatotoxicity
Hexamethylmelamine (HMM)	Nausea and vomiting	Bone marrow depression; visual disturbances (reversible); CNS depression; peripheral neuritis; visual hallucinations; ataxia
Ifosfamide (*Ifex*–Bristol-Myers)	Nausea and vomiting; confusion	Bone marrow depression; hemorrhagic cystitis (prevented by concurrent 2-mercaptoethanol sodium sulphonate [mesna]); alopecia; sterility (may be temporary); nephrotoxicity; inappropriate ADH secretion
Interleukin-2 (*Cetus*–Biogen)	Fluid retention; hypotension; rash; anemia; thrombocytopenia; nausea and vomiting; diarrhea; capillary leak syndrome; nephrotoxicity; myocardial toxicity; hepatotoxicity	Unknown
Mitobronitol (*Myelobromol*–Sinclair, UK)	GI disturbances	Bone marrow depression; alopecia
Mitoguazone (methyl-GAG; methylglyoxal Bisguanylhydrazone; MGBG)	Nausea and vomiting, fatigue	Myopathy, paresthesia, bone marrow depression, ventricular arrhythmias, stomatitis, gastrointestinal ulcerations
Mitolactol	Mild nausea	Bone marrow depression
*Mitoxantrone HCl. (DHAD; *Novantrone*–Lederle)	Blue-green pigment in urine; blue-green sclera; nausea and vomiting	Bone marrow depression; cardiotoxicity; stomatitis; alopecia; white hair
Semustine (methyl-CCNU; Bristol-Myers)	Nausea and vomiting	Delayed leukopenia and thrombocytopenia (may be prolonged); pulmonary fibrosis; leukemia; renal failure
*Teniposide (VM-26; *Vumon*–Bristol-Myers)	Nausea and vomiting; diarrhea; phlebitis; anaphylactoid symptoms	Bone marrow depression; alopecia; peripheral neuropathy
*Vindesine sulfate (*Eldisine*–Lilly)	Local reaction if extravasation; fever; nausea and vomiting; diarrhea	Bone marrow depression; alopecia; peripheral neuropathy; jaw pain

*Commercially available in Canada

PARTIAL LIST OF BRAND NAMES

Adriamycin—doxorubicin
*Adrucil—fluorouracil
Alkeran—melphalan
BiCNU—carmustine
Blenoxane—bleomycin
CeeNU—lomustine
Cerubidine—daunorubicin
Cosmegen—dactinomycin
Cytadren—aminoglutethimide
Cytosar-U—cytarabine
Cytoxan—cyclophosphamide
Depo-Provera—medroxyprogesterone acetate
*DTIC Dome—dacarbazine
Eldisine—vindesine
Elspar—asparaginase
Emcyt—estramustine phosphate sodium
Eulexin—flutamide
*Folex—methotrexate
FUDR—floxuridine
Hydrea—hydroxyurea
Ifex—ifosfamide
Intron-A—interferon
Leukeran—chlorambucil

Lupron—leuprolide
Lysodren—mitotane
Matulane—procarbazine
Megace—megestrol acetate
*Mexate—methotrexate
Mithracin—plicamycin
Mustargen—mechlorethamine
Mutamycin—mitomycin
Myelobromol—mitobronitol
Myleran—busulfan
Mylosar—azacitidine
Neosar—cyclophosphamide
Nolvadex—tramoxifen citrate
Novantrone—mitoxantrone
Oncovin—vincristine sulfate
Paraplatin—carboplatin
Platinol—cisplatin
Purinethol—mercaptopurine
Roferon-A—interferon
*Velban—vinblastine sulfate
Vepesid—etoposide
Vincasar—vincristine
Zanosar—streptozocin

*Also available generically

Appendix III

Helping Organizations

Edward J. Larschan, J.D. Ph.D.
Richard J. Larschan, Ph.D.

Source: The Diagnosis is Cancer, *Bull Publishing Company, 1986.*

These national organizations offer information, practical assistance and emotional support to cancer patients and their families. Services are provided by local chapters which can be found either through your telephone directory or the national offices of each organization. Responses to my phone calls or letters to all of them indicated greatly varied knowledgeability and efficiency, depending on the person I happened to reach. So if the answers you get at first aren't altogether satisfactory, talk with someone else and you'll eventually receive the advice or information you want.

Organizations have been organized under categories: General, Specific, Emotional, Financial, Practical, Experimental/Alternative. (Where more than one service is provided, subsequent listings are by agency name alone.)

GENERAL

General information and educational material

The American Cancer Society, Inc.

National Headquarters
3340 Peachtree Road, NE
Atlanta, GA 30326
Tel. (404) 320-3333

Local offices can supply the free booklet, *Cancer Facts and Figures,* in addition to other literature on specific subjects. All ACS materials and service are provided free of charge. Numerous services are itemized below under various categories.

The Cancer Information Service (CIS)

Office of Cancer Communications
National Cancer Institute
Building 31, Room 10A18
Bethesda, MD 20205
National office Tel: 1-800-638-6694; *but* better to phone your Regional office Tel: 1-800-4-Cancer (1-800-422-6237); *except* Alaska: 1-800-638-6070; Hawaii-Oahu: (808) 524-1234 (other islands call collect);
Oklahoma: 1-800-522-0220
Washington, D.C., MD, and VA suburbs:
(202) 636-5700.

Nationwide toll-free telephone system provides authoritative answers to a broad range of questions concerning cancer: causes; prevention; detection; diagnosis; treatment methods and facilities; rehabilitation; home care; financial help; emotional support. Information provided both by telephone and a series of over 80 free pamphlets (many of them excellent).

The Candlelighters Foundation

1901 Pennsylvania Avenue
Suite 1001
Washington, DC 20006
Tel. (202) 659-5136

Free quarterly *Newsletter:* Up-to-date information on treatment, services, etc. for parents of children with cancer. Free *Youth Newsletter:* Stories and poems mainly for and by youngsters with cancer. Free *Progress Reports:* Summaries of research, rehabilitation, psychological support, etc. *Annotated Bibliography and Resource Guide* ($1.00)—sample topics: Parents' basic cancer library; how to obtain materials; information on specific diseases; survival skills; effects on patients and families; death and bereavement.

National Cancer Institute

See *Cancer Information Service*

National Cancer Foundation, Inc.

Cancer Care
1180 Avenue of the Americas
New York, NY 10036
Tel. (212) 221-3300

Sponsors *Cancer Care,* which promotes social services to cancer patients worldwide (see specific services below); conducts educational programs for professionals; supports research on social, emotional and economic effects of cancer; publishes *Lamp,* research studies, professional papers, bibliographies and other informational materials.

National Library of Medicine (NLM)

Office of Inquiries/MEDLARS Management Section
8600 Rockville Pike, Building 38A, Room 4N-421
Bethesda, MD 20209
Tel. (301) 496-6193

Largest professional research library in U.S., with access by computer terminals in local hospitals, medical schools or by individuals with personal computers through 3 commercial networks: TYMNET, TELENET AND UNINET; access code through MEDLARS. Five databases: CANCERLIT (abstracts of publications on all aspects of cancer worldwide); CANCERPROJ (summaries of ongoing research worldwide); CLINPROT (summaries of clinical trials of new anticancer agents or treatment modalities); CANCER-EXPRESS (fourth-month file of literature citations, updated monthly); PDQ (descriptions of approximately 1,000 ongoing cancer therapy research programs; designed to be understandable by cancer patients). For nearest library, contact NLM in Bethesda, MD. Free bibliographies on various subjects (name and address on gummed label required, no postage).

United Cancer Council, Inc.

410 W. 86th Street, Suite H
Indianapolis, IN 46268
Tel. (317) 879-9900

Publishes a wide variety of brochures. Other services itemized below.

SPECIFIC

Information about specific forms of cancer

Breast Cancer

Reach to Recovery
(contact **American Cancer Society**)

Sponsors visits before and after surgery by recovered mastectomy volunteers; advice on physical, emotional and cosmetic needs; assistance to family as well.

Breast, Vaginal and Cervical Cancer

DES Action National, Inc.
Long Island Jewish-Hillside Medical Center
New Hyde Park, NY 11040
Tel. (516) 775-3450

Informs women who have been exposed to DES (and their daughters and sons) of need for medical monitoring; offers counseling and physician referral service, speakers bureau, and library. Publishes *DES Action Voice,* fact sheets, and large bibliography—available from West Coast Office: 2845 24th Street, San Francisco, CA 94110.

Childhood Cancer

The Candlelighters Foundation (see page 453)

Ronald McDonald Houses

Children's Oncology Services
500 North Michigan Avenue
Chicago, IL 60611
Tel: (312) 836-7100

Provides low-cost lodging ($6 to $15 per day—no charge in cases of economic hardship) for families of children undergoing treatment for cancer at medical centers away from home; a caring, family atmosphere for parents and children, with mutual support and comfort from others in a similar situation; locations supplied by national office or from telephone directory.

Wish Fulfillment Group for Children
(contact **Candlelighters**)

Aims to fulfill wishes of dying children such as by sending toys, arranging for child to act as police chief for a day, sending child and family on vacations, or setting up visits with celebrities important to the child, etc.

Cancer of the Larynx

International Association of Laryngectomees
(contact **American Cancer Society**)

Pre- and post-operative support by recovered laryngectomee volunteers; speech lessons by speech pathologists or lay teachers. Educational materials and programs for patients and families.

Cancer of the Digestive System

United Ostomy Association, Inc.
36 Executive Park, #120
Irvine, CA 92714
Tel. (714) 660-8624

Sponsors hospital and home visits by recovered ostomy patients to assist rehabilitation through moral support and education in ostomy care (though not to answer specific medical questions); lobbies manufacturers for improved equipment and supplies; publishes numerous informative materials, including the *Ostomy Quarterly,* many books and pamphlets.

Rehabilitation Program
(contact **American Cancer Society**)

Sponsors pre- and post-surgical visits, for moral support by selected volunteers working under medical supervision.

Leukemia

Leukemia Society of America
205 Lexington Avenue
New York, NY 10016
Tel. (212) 679-1939

Provides up to $750 for outpatient costs not covered by other sources, including approved drugs, blood transfusions, transportation, x-ray therapy, etc. Applications available at local chapter offices. Also supplies information on medical, psychological and financial help; special summer camps, transportation, etc. for patients and families.

National Leukemia Association
585 Stewart Ave., Suite 536
Garden City, NY 11530
Tel. (516) 222-1944

Provides financial aid to leukemia patients and families, based on need. Contact for qualifications.

EMOTIONAL
Agencies offering emotional support

American Cancer Society

- *CanSurmount*
For those not eligible for *Reach to Recovery,* laryngectomy and ostomy programs, provides carefully selected and trained volunteers—themselves cancer patients—for emotional support at home or in hospital, on short-term basis; visitors matched by age, type of cancer and family situation; direct supervision by professionals.

- *I Can Cope*

An 8-week series of 2-hour classes on human anatomy, cancer development, treatment, physical and emotional side effects, etc.; taught by doctors, nurses, social workers and other professionals.

Cancer Care, Inc.
(contact **National Cancer Foundation, Inc.**)

Offers free individual counseling by professional social workers to determine patient's personal needs, concerns and fears; also, group therapy, to discuss physical and emotional effects of cancer and draw strength from others; counseling in "relatives" groups (spouses, children, parents, siblings); "spouses bereavement" groups to help widows and widowers talk about and accept their loss. Located throughout metropolitan NY, NJ, CT; new Los Angeles office; provides information in response to requests worldwide.

CHUMS (Cancer Hopefuls United for Mutual Support)
3310 Rochambeau Avenue
New York, NY 10467
Tel. (212) 655-7566

Offers nationwide crisis intervention and information service; self-help discussion groups for cancer patients/survivors; educational meetings where prominent cancer specialists speak and answer questions; phone and visit cancer patients to give them emotional support; parties and social gatherings; newsletter with up-to-date information for and about cancer patients/survivors. Overall: aims to strengthen 'psychological weapons': positive outlook, cheerful attitude, optimism, determination to live.

Make Today Count
101½ S. Union Street
Alexander, VA 22314
Tel. (703) 548-9674

Provides emotional self-help to patients and families through monthly peer support meetings with cancer patients, families, health professionals and community members.

We Can Do!
601 Wapello
Altadena, CA 91001
Tel. (818) 797-3919

Addresses psychological aspects of cancer by encouraging peer emotional support and patients taking an active role in their own treatment; emphasizes music, laughter, relaxation, visualization and positive attitudes; offers therapy using stress reduction, guided imagery and biofeedback. Distributes tapes and published pamphlets.

National Self-Help Clearing House
33 West 42nd Street
New York, NY 10036
Tel. (212) 840-1259

Provides name, description and location of local peer-support and education groups of all kinds, including those for cancer patients and their families.

American Psychiatric Association
1400 K Street, NW
Washington, DC 20005
Tel. (202) 682-6000

Can provide the name of a psychiatrist in your area through its membership directory.

American Psychological Association
1200 Seventeenth Street, NW
Washington, DC 20036
Tel. (202) 955-7600

National professional organization of psychologists; has a directory of psychologists practicing in every state and can assist in locating private clinical counselor in your community through its membership directory.

American Society of Clinical Hypnosis
2250 East Devon Avenue, Suite 336
Des Plaines, IL 60018
Tel. (312) 297-3317

Can supply the name of trained clinical hypnotists in your area (psychiatrists, psychologists, social workers) through its membership directory.

National Association of Social Workers
7981 Eastern Avenue
Silver Springs, MD 20910
Tel. (301) 565-0333

Can assist in locating a social worker-counselor in your area through membership directory.

FINANCIAL

Agencies offering financial advice and assistance

Direct Financial Assistance

United Cancer Council, Inc.
410 W. 86th St., Suite H
Indianapolis, IN 46032
Tel. (317) 879-9900

Provides financial assistance to help pay for medications and cancer treatments.

Credit

National Foundation for Consumer Credit, Inc.
8701 Georgia Avenue, Suite 507
Silver Springs, MD 20910
Tel. (301) 589-5600

Privately supported by lending organizations, merchants and individuals; provides free or inexpensive help with money management and credit problems (not a "debt consolidation" service); trained counselor helps devise budgeting plan for expenditures; intervenes with creditors to extend payment time or eliminate interest and service charges; at your request will place your funds in insured trust account, from which payments are made directly to creditors.

Bankruptcy Division of the U.S. Courts
Admis. Office, U.S. Corps.
Washington, DC 20544
Tel. (202) 633-6234

Provides information on location of your nearest district bankruptcy court, filing fees and limited help with preparation of bankruptcy forms; interpretation of Bankruptcy Act is available, but not legal advice for your case.

Legal

American Bar Association
750 North Lakeshore Drive
Chicago, IL 60611
Tel. (312) 988-5000

Publishers *Directory of Lawyer Referral Services* listing attorney referral services in each state; from which you can find names of lawyers in your community who concentrate on particular types of legal problems and services.

Clearinghouse on the Handicapped
External Affairs Staff–USERS
U.S. Department of Education
Switzer Building, Room 3132; Mailstop 2319
330 C Street, SW
Washington, DC 20202
Tel. (202) 732-1245

Federal agency providing information and referral services to individuals and helping organizations dealing with the handicapped generally; contact for related problems.

Disabled in Action National
c/o Disabled in Action of Metropolitan New York
PO Box 30954
New York, NY 10011-0109
Tel. (718) 261-3737

National civil rights organization promoting equal access for the disabled through legislation and education; initiates or joins lawsuits to enforce existing laws protecting rights of the disabled in employment, housing, transportation, etc.

Foundation for Dignity
Cancer Patients' Employment Rights Project
37 S. 20th St., Suite 601
Philadelphia, PA 19103
Tel. (215) 567-2828

Non-profit foundation devoted to eliminating cancer-based discrimination: Offers free legal counseling; serves as clearinghouse and referral service, providing public and professional education; and works with federal and state legislatures toward expanding legal rights of people with a cancer history.

- *Cancer Patients' Employment Rights Project:* Doesn't represent clients in direct litigation, but counsels free of charge on legal options, and refers to appropriate resources for pursuing a potential claim.

Insurance

American Council of Life Insurance and Health Insurance Association of America
1001 Pennsylvania Ave., NW
Washington, DC 20004-2599
Tel. 1-800-423-8000

Represents commercial insurers (not Blue Cross/Blue Shield or Health Maintainance Organizations); provides information on availability of medical/health, disability income and life insurance for cancer patients. For specific information, write to:

National Underwriters Company
420 East 4th Street
Cincinnati, OH 45202
Tel. (513) 721-2140

Ask for book called *Who Writes What in Life and Health Insurance*. Six states (CT, IN, MN, WI, ND, NE) have "risk pools"—forcing insurance companies to provide health insurance to those disqualified from buying individual policies because of pre-existing diseases.

Blue Cross and Blue Shield Associations
233 North Michigan Avenue
Chicago, IL 60601
Tel. (312) 938-6000

Provides information regarding coverage offered in each state, or refers you to local association; resource for information about "open enrollment" periods, eligibility and coverage requirements for pre-existing conditions; resolves disputes about unpaid medical claims.

Group Health Association of America
Membership Department
1129-20th St., NW, Suite 600
Washington, DC 20001
Tel. (202) 778-3200

Provides information about eligibility for group health plan coverage with commercial insurers (not Blue Cross/Blue Shield), including people with pre-existing conditions like cancer.

National Association of Insurance Commissioners
1120 W. 12th St.
Kansas City, MO 64105
Tel. (816) 842-3600

Provides information about Blue Cross/Blue Shield on a state-by-state basis. Note particularly "open enrollment" periods (every year or two) when anyone may apply for coverage without medical examination; starts covering pre-existing cancer after varying periods (3 months is typical).

Office of Health Maintenance Organizations
Parklawn Building, Room 9-11
5600 Fishers Lane
Rockville, MD 20857
Tel. (301) 443-2300

U.S. agency, providing information on Health Maintenance Organizations (HMOs) in each state (HMOs offer comprehensive medical services to members enrolled on pre-paid basis; generally fixed premium covers outpatient visits for diagnosis and treatment, x-rays, emergency-room visits, ambulance service, as well as hospital inpatient care); federally qualified HMOs provide group coverage, but some take individual members—find out waiting period for pre-existing conditions, and what's covered.

Consumer Information Center (U.S. Government)
Pueblo, CO 81009
Tel. toll-free from many areas

Publishes inexpensive *Consumer's Resource Handbook* (100-plus pages and detailed index), listing commercial trade organizations in health and insurance fields; also federal, state, county and city government consumer protection agencies.

PRACTICAL
Agencies offering practical assistance

American Cancer Society

May provide home care services and equipment, including wheel chairs, walkers, beds and bedside tables, etc., recreational and other aids for the care and comfort of patients; transportation for patients and family members to and from doctor's offices; clinics or hospitals for diagnosis, treatment, rehabilitation and hospice-type care—either free through "Road to Recovery" volunteer program, or inexpensively through community agencies referral. Services vary widely from community to community.

Association of Junior Leagues, Inc.
660 First Avenue
New York, NY 10016-3241
Tel. (212) 683-1515

Various local branches offer different services, many in conjunction with *Ronald McDonald Houses* for children, and hospice programs for cancer patients. *New York Junior League* publishes *Access:* 130-page guide to Manhattan for the disabled and elderly, describing wheel chair access to public facilities.

Cancer Care, Inc.
(contact **National Cancer Foundation, Inc.**)

Offers help in finding homemaking and child care services; referrals to health and social service agencies and supplementary contributions for needed home care services.

CAN (Corporate Angels Network)
Westchester County Airport, Building One
White Plains, NY 10604
Tel. (914) 328-1313

Offers free transportation for cancer patients and a family member aboard a corporate airplane already traveling to and from locations of specialized treatment centers far from home—on limited 'space available' basis. Requirements: patients don't require special equipment or services en route, have proper medical authorization, and arrange own ground transportation.

National Hospice Organization
1901 North Fort Myer Drive, Suite 402
Rosslyn, VA 22209
Tel. (703) 243-5900

Provides care emphasizing the management of pain and other symptoms related to terminal illness; professional health care workers (doctors, nurses, social workers, therapists, clergy) and trained volunteers available around the clock daily; offers care to family also, for one year after patient's death.

United Cancer Council, Inc.

Provides free direct services to cancer patients, including transportation for medical care, loan of hospital beds, wheel chairs and other equipment to aid in caring for cancer patients at home.

Continental Association of Funeral & Memorial Societies

20001 S Street, NW, Suite 630
Washington, DC 20009
Tel. (202) 462-8888

Not in undertaking business; for a one-time fee of approximately $25, these non-profit societies provide accurate information about prices and legal requirements for funerals, how to notify newspapers and other organizations, planning memorial services, spiritual and emotional considerations, etc.; offers various informational material, including the book, *Dealing Creatively with Death: A Manual of Death Education and Simple Burial,* by Ernest Morgan, (The Celo Press, 1984); common sense approach to death, emphasizing unemotional choice-making.

EXPERIMENTAL/ALTERNATIVE—SCIENTIFICALLY GROUNDED

Organizations engaged in experimental or alternative treatment

Cancer Research Institute, Inc.

133 East 58th Street
New York, NY 10022
Tel. (212) 688-7515

Devotes all resources to immunological approach to cancer, through grants to cancer researchers worldwide; maintains communications network and information clearinghouse for scientists and patients seeking guidance about diagnosis, treatment, prevention, and rehabilitation; offers information regarding effects of nutrition in maintaining health and fighting cancer; free nutritional guides and immunological information also available.

Institute for the Advancement of Health

16 East 53rd Street
New York, NY 10022
Tel. (212) 832-8282

Provides research support on mind-body interactions, including biofeedback, hypnosis, meditation, imagery, and stress management; publishes *Advances,* containing articles for scientists and patients on mind-body research; *Mind and Immunity: Behavioral Immunology* contains annotated bibliography of 1300 entries on connections between the brain and the immune system; sponsors conferences to inform scientists and the public about latest developments in research and clinical care.

COMPREHENSIVE CANCER CENTERS

The institutions listed have been recognized as Comprehensive Cancer Centers by the National Cancer Institute. These centers have met rigorous criteria imposed by the National Cancer Advisory Board. They receive financial support from the National Cancer Institute, the American Cancer Society and many other sources.

Alabama

University of Alabama in Birmingham Comprehensive Cancer Center
Lurleen Wallace Tumor Institute
1824 6th Avenue South
Birmingham, Alabama 35294
Phone: (205) 934-5077

California

University of Southern California Comprehensive Cancer Center
1441 Eastlake Avenue
Los Angeles, California 90033-0804
Phone: (213) 224-6416

UCLA-Jonsson Comprehensive Cancer Center
Louis Factor Health Sciences Bldg.
10833 LeConte Avenue
Los Angeles, California 90024
Phone: (213) 825-5268

Connecticut

Yale Comprehensive Cancer Center
Yale University School of Medicine
333 Cedar Street
New Haven, Connecticut 06510
Phone: (203) 785-4095

District of Columbia

Georgetown University/Howard University Comprehensive Cancer Center

- *Vincent T. Lombardi Cancer Research Center*
  Georgetown University
  Medical Center
  3800 Reservoir Road, N.W.
  Washington, D.C. 20007
  Phone: (202) 625-7721

- *Howard University Cancer Research Center*
  College of Medicine
  Department of Oncology
  2041 Georgia Avenue, N.W.
  Washington, D.C. 20060
  Phone: (202) 636-7697

Florida
Comprehensive Cancer Center for the State of Florida
University of Miami School of Medicine, Dept. of Oncology
1475 N.W. 12th Avenue
Miami, Florida 33101
Phone: (305) 548-4800

Illinois
Illinois Cancer Council
36 South Wabash Avenue, Suite 700
Chicago, Illinois 60603
Phone: (312) 346-9813

- *Northwestern University Cancer Center*
  303 East Chicago Avenue
  Chicago, Illinois 60611
  Phone: (312) 266-5250

- *University of Chicago Cancer Research Center*
  950 East 59th Street
  Chicago, Illinois 60637
  Phone: (312) 702-6180

- *University of Illinois*
  Department of Surgery,
  Division of Surgical Oncology
  840 South Wood Street
  Chicago, Illinois 60612
  Phone: (312) 996-6666

- *Rush Cancer Center*
  Suite 820
  1725 West Harrison Street
  Chicago, Illinois 60612
  Phone: (312) 942-6028

Maryland
Johns Hopkins Oncology Center
600 North Wolfe Street
Baltimore, Maryland 21205
Phone: (301) 955-8822

Massachusetts
Dana-Farber Cancer Institute
44 Binney Street
Boston, Massachusetts 02115
Phone: (617) 732-3555

Michigan
Michigan Cancer Foundation
Meyer L. Prentis Cancer Center
110 East Warren Avenue
Detroit, Michigan 48201
Phone: (313) 833-0710

Minnesota
Mayo Clinic
200 First Street, S.W.
Rochester, Minnesota 55905
Phone: (507) 284-8964

New York
Columbia University Cancer Research Center
701 West 168th Street, Rm. 1208
New York, New York 10032
Phone: (212) 305-6904

Memorial Sloan-Kettering Cancer Center
1275 York Avenue
New York, New York 10021
Phone: (212) 794-6561

Roswell Park Memorial Institute
666 Elm Street
Buffalo, New York 14263
Phone: (716) 845-5770

North Carolina
Duke Comprehensive Cancer Center
P.O. Box 3814
Duke University Medical Center
Durham, North Carolina 27710
Phone: (919) 684-2282

Ohio
Ohio State University Comprehensive Cancer Center
Suite 302
410 West 12th Avenue
Columbus, Ohio 43210
Phone: (614) 422-5022

Pennsylvania
Fox Chase/University of Pennsylvania Cancer Center

- *The Fox Chase Cancer Center*
  7701 Burholme Avenue
  Philadelphia, Pennsylvania 19111
  Phone: (215) 728-2781

- *University of Pennsylvania Cancer Center*
  3400 Spruce Street
  7th Floor, Silverstein Pavilion
  Philadelphia, Pennsylvania 19104
  Phone: (215) 662-3910

Texas

The University of Texas System Cancer Center
M.D. Anderson Hospital and
Tumor Institute
1515 Holcombe Blvd.
Houston, Texas 77030
Phone: (713) 792-6000

Washington

Fred Hutchinson Cancer Research Center
1124 Columbia Street
Seattle, Washington 98104
Phone: (206) 292-2930 or 292-7545

Wisconsin

Wisconsin Clinical Cancer Center
University of Wisconsin
Department of Human Oncology
600 Highland Avenue
Madison, Wisconsin 53792
Phone: (608) 263-8610

Index

Page numbers in bold type represent key discussions
Page numbers followed by *g* refer to the glossary

Ablation 426g
Acceptance
    and facing death 302
    discussed by Kübler-Ross 303
Accessory organs 57
Acid phosphatase
    serum test for prostate 149
Acne
    radiation for 185
    and thyroid cancer 185
Acquired Immune Deficiency
        Syndrome (AIDS) 426g
    adults, table 390
    age groups and 390
    AL-721 and 405
    alternative treatments 405–06
    and antabuse
    anti-viral therapy for 405
    antibody positive percentages,
        table 391
    and ARC 400–01
    asymptomatic infection 400
    and cancer 91
    cases per country 389
    and casual contact 411–12
    CDC worksite recommendations
        413
    chemotherapy for 404
    children 402
    children, table 390
    clinical course 401
    clinical spectrum, diagrammed 400
    clinical spectrum of HIV disease
        399–402
    community cooperation 412
    and condom use 411
    defined 386
    diagnosis 401
    DNCB 405
    and DTC 405
    education in school 412
    educational program 412

guidelines for everyone 410–11
guidelines for people at risk
    412–13
hairy leukoplakia 401
Haiti 388
hemophiliacs 388
herpes zoster 401
heterosexuals, first cases 388
history of cancer and 12
history of the epidemic 387–93
HIV dementia 401
HIV wasting syndrome 401
how HIV is transmitted 410
immune system and 395–96
IV drug users, first cases 388
in males vs females 390
in schools 412
infections and AIDS 91
infections in specific groups 391
initial infection 400
large-scale screening 410
lymph node self-examination 320
measuring helper T4 cell level
    400
and medical hygiene 388
neurological manifestations 401
nocardia 401
opportunistic cancers 395
oral candidiasis 401
patterns of 401
persistent generalized lym-
    phadenopathy 400
preventing transmission 412
prevention 409–15
prognosis 401
projections of degree of spread
    420
prostitutes, first cases 388
psychiatric manifestations 401
psychosocial aspects 416–18
publics' misconceptions 417–18
race and 390

radiation therapy for 404
research 407–08
resources for information and sup-
    port 421–24
response by government and
    society 418
risk group breakdown, table 390
risk groups defined 388
routes of transmission, sum-
    marized 388
salmonella 401
self care and 410–11
sexual practices and 411
steps to develop vaccine for 408
survival in 401
symptoms of 400
table of CDC classifications 400
traditional treatments 403–05
treatment 403–06
tuberculosis 401
in the world of viruses, illustration
    63
Acrylonitrile 97
    and lung cancer 133
Actinic keratoses 126
    during skin self-examination 319
Acute lymphocytic leukemia (ALL)
        203
    drugs used in treatment 445
    in children 203
Actinic rays 426g
Acute myelocytic leukemia (AML)
    drugs used in treatment 445
Adenine 33, 426g
Adenocarcinoma 22
    of the colon and rectum 136
    defined 21
    and hepatobiliary cancers 180
    of the kidney 166
    of the lung 132
    of the prostate 148
    of salivary glands 169

Adenoids
   radiation for 185
   and thyroid cancer 185
Adenoma 22, 426g
Adenosine diphosphate (ADP) 426g
Adenoviruses 67
Adrenal gland 184, 426g
   described 185
Adrenal gland cancer
   diagnosis 185
   prognosis 185
   symptoms 185
   treatment 185
   types 185
Adrenalectomy 426g
Adrenocortical adenoma 22
Adrenocortical carcinoma 22
   drugs used in treatment 446
Adriamycin 223
Aerobic system 426g
Aflatoxin
   and carcinogenesis 49
   and liver cancer 181
AFP
   see Alpha-feto protein
African sleeping sickness 91
Africans, Central
   and HIV infection 392
Age
   summary table 119–21
Agent Orange
   and non-Hodgkin's lymphoma 193
Agglutination 426g
AGL (anti-lymphocyte globulin)
   426g
Agran, L. 50
Agranulocytes 190
AIDS
   see Acquired Immune Deficiency
      Syndrome
AIDS foundations and resources
421–24
AIDS-related conditions
   see ARC
AIDS treatments
   alternative
   traditional
Air pollution 114–16, 375–76
   and lung cancer 33
Air Quality Standards 376
Air Resources Board (ARB) 376
AL-721
   described 405
   use for HIV therapy 405
Albinos 124
Alcohol 352
   and breast cancer 142
   and cigarette smoking 352
   and esophagus cancer 175
   general recommendation 84
   and laryngeal cancer 173
   list of cancers from 315

and liver cancer 181
and oral cancers 170
and pancreatic cancer 179
and smoking 87
summary table 119–21
and ulcers 88
Alienation 270
Alkaptonuria 426g
Alkyl iysophospholipids (ALP) 230
Alkylating agents 426g
Alleles 426g
Allogenic grafting 426g
Allogeneic immunization 230
Alopecia
   and chemotherapy 229
Alpha-feto protein (AFP) 164
   in liver cancer 181
   and ovarian cancer 158
Alpha helix 426g
Alpha particles 426g
Alternative treatments
   alternative drugs 405
   alternative medical systems 406
   body work 405
   mind work 405
   nutritonal therapy 405
Aluminum
   in prostate cancer 148
Alveolar soft part sarcoma 206
Alzheimer's disease
   and Hodgkin's disease 193
Amazonian Tribes
   and AIDS test 393
   and HIV infection 392
Amblyopia
   and smoking 88
Amenorrhea 426g
Ameobiasis 91
American Cancer Society 27, 453,
   454–55, 457
   check-up guidelines, table 316
   defined 14
   dietary guidelines 83
   guidelines for cancer-related check-
      ups 12, 316
   history of 10, 14
   structure of 14
   volunteering for 14, 317
American College of Obstetrics and
   Gynecology 155
American College of Surgeons 39
American Heart Association
   dietary guidelines 83
American Indians
   and cancer rates 381
   and cervical cancer 151
   and gall bladder cancer 181
   and pancreas cancer 179
American Indians, New Mexico
   gall bladder cancer 442
American Medical Association
   described 248

American Psychiatric Association
   455
American Psychological Association
   455
American Society of Clinical Hyp-
   nosis 455
Ames test 45
Ames, Bruce 45, 231
Amino acids 426g
   defined 27
Aminoglutethimide (Cytraden-Ciba)
   side effects 447
Amitrole 97
Anaerobic system 426g
Anal cancer
   also see Colon and rectal cancer
   prognosis 138
   and sex 138
   symptoms 138
   treatment 138
Anal self-examination 316
   how to 328
   rationale 327–28
Anaphase 4020426g
Anaplastic 426g
Anaploid cells 426g
Androgens 112, 426g
Aneuploidy, defined 19
Anger 268
   and facing death 302
Angiography
   digital subtraction for breast can-
      cer detection 143
Angiosarcoma
   see Liver cancer
Animals
   cancer in 72–76
Anklyosing spondylitis 197
Annulus
   illustrated 129
Anorexia 426g
Anoscopy 341
Ansamycin
   and AIDS 405
Antabuse 405
Antibiotic 426g
Antibodies 426g
   general 58
Antigen 426g
   general 58
Antigrowth factors 230
Anus cancer
   see Anal cancer
Anus, illustrated 339
Anxiety
   and nutrition 273
Apocrine glands 184
Appendix
   see Colon and rectal cancer
Appetite
   and exercise 275
   loss of 272

ARC (AIDS-related conditions)
   also see *Acquired Immune Deficiency Syndrome*
   classifications 400–01
   defined 400–01
   number of cases 400–01
Argentaffinomas
   see *Carcinoid tumors*
Arsenic 97
   and leukemia 197
   and lung cancer 133
   and multiple myeloma 201
   in water 118
Aryl hydrocarbon hydroxylase (AHH)
   and laryngeal cancer 173
Asbestos **97**
   cancers associated with 98
   fiber counts 376
   future issues 376
   in the air 376
   in water 118
   and laryngeal cancer 173
   measured amounts, table 377
   and multiple myeloma 201
   and ovarian cancer 158
   and pollution 117
   regulations 98
   in schools 376
   and smoking 86, 98
   types of fibers 376
   uses of 97
Asbestos workers
   and urinary tract cancers 167
Asbestosis
   see *Lung cancer*
Ascaris 91
Ascending colon
   illustrated 288
Ascorbic acid 426g
Asimov, Isaac 53
Asire, Ardyce J. 95–99, 108–09,
   110–13, 114–16
Asparaginase
   side effects 447
Asthma
   and smoking 88
Astrocytomas 22
   in children 204
   prognosis 183
Astruc, Jean 9
Ataxia telangiectasia
   and Hodgkin's disease 193
Atherosclerosis
   and smoking 87
ATL (adult T-cell leukemia)
   and Evan's postulates 68
Atom 426g
   defined 27
Atomic bombs 27
   also see *Radiation*
   hazards of 106
ATP (adenosine triphosphate) 426g

Atrophy 426g
Attitude 270
   also see *Emotions*
   also see *Stress*
   positive **283**
   physician's 295
Auramine and cancer 97
Autopsy
   of thyroids 184
Axilla 426g
Axilary lymph nodes 426g
Azathioprine 112
Azidothymidine (AZT)
   and AIDS 405
Azimexon 230
   and AIDS 404
Azo dyes 426g

B-cells 426g
B-cell growth factor (BCGF) 230
B-cell response 58
B-lymphocytes
   also see *Lymphocytes*
   and lymphoma 190
Bacillus Calmette Guerin (BCG)
   230, 427g
   immunotherapy and **230–31**
Back pain
   see *Multiple myeloma*
   see *Prostate cancer*
Bacon, Francis 73
Bacteria 426g
   and bronchitis 91
   and cancer 91
   and digestion 91
   mechanisms 91
Bacteriophage 426g
Bailer, J. C. 50
Baldness
   and chemotherapy 229
Baltimore, David 11
Bargaining
   and facing death 137, 302
Barium enema 426g
   for colorectal cancer detection 137
Bartlett, Irene 243
Basal cell carcinoma 426g
   see Skin cancer
Basophils 58, 190
Bayh, Marvella 11
BCG, see *Bacillus Calmette Guerin*
Bed rest
   effects of 274
Behavioral approach to quitting
   smoking 370
Behavioral aspects
   and physicians 241
   rights of patients 241
Bence-Jones protein
   and multiple myeloma 200
Benign
   described 18, 43

Benign prostatic hyperplasia (BPH)
   148
Benign tumor 427g
Beneze 97, **98**
   and cacer 98
   history of 98
   in the air 98, 376
   and leukemia 98
   uses 98
Benzidrine 97
and urinary tract cancer 167
Benzo(a)pyrene 97, 351–**52, 427g**
Benzotrichloride 97
Bergonie, J. 101
Berry, Carol 327
Beryllium 97
   and lung cancer 133
Bestatin 230
Beta-2 400
Beta-Carotene 427g
   see *Vitamin A*
Betel nuts
   and oral cancers 170
Betatrons
   and radiation therapy 214
Bichat, Marie Francoise 9
Bilharzia 91
Biliary tract cancer
   see *Liver cancer*
   see *Gall bladder cancer*
Biochemistry 427g
Biofeedback 264
   and stress 283
   for pain 222
Biological predeterminism 426g
Biological response modifiers 221,
   229–30
   also see *Biolociagl treatments*
   also see *Chemotherapy*
   table 230
Biological treatments 220–32,
   229–30
   and AIDS 404
   flavonoids 232
   history of 221
   interferon 231
   interleukin 231
   monoclonal antibodies 232
   principles 230
   retinoids 232
   table 230
Biology of cancer
   college courses 25–51, 81
   future of 49
   general 25–51
   history ix
   introduction 27
   overview 27
Biopsy 427g
   aspiration biopsy 20, 211
   CNS tumors 183
   cone biopsy of cervix 155

Biopsy *continued*
  excisional biopsy 20, 210
  fine-needle biopsy 211
  incisional biopsy 20, 210
  with laser, of the cervix 155
  methods of 20
  needle biopsy 20
  principles 210–11
  in prostate cancer 149
  techniques for breast 144
  of thyroid gland nodules 185
Birth control
  and HIV prevention 411
Birth control pill
  and blood clots 88
  and cancer **111**
  and ovarian cancer 158
  and smoking 88
Bis (chloromethyl) ether (BCME)
Bishop, Michael 50, 71
Bittner particles 142
Black, Shirley Temple 11
Blacks
  cancer in 381
  and cervical cancer 151
  5-year survival rates and cancer 440
  and multiple myeloma 201
  and stomach cancer 177
Bladder, illustrated 288
Bladder cancer 166–68
  anatomy 166
  chlornaphazine and 113
  diagnosis 167
  drugs used in treatment 446
  early detection 167
  and parasites 90
  physiology 166
  prevention 167
  screening for 167
  and smoking 87
  survival rate, table 440
  symptoms 167
  types 166
Bladder/kidney cancer
  summary table **120**
Bleomycin
  side effects 448
Blood
  illustrated 190
  in the urine 167
  in the stool 328
  types of blood cells 190
Blood and lymphoid tissue cancers
  189–91
Blood count 427g
Blood donors
  and AIDS 412
  and HIV infections 392
Blood products
  and AIDS 410
Blood transfusions
  risk of acquiring AIDS from 413

Body image
  and sexuality 278
Bone cancer **187–88**
  diagnosis 188
  during infant/child exam by
    mother 329
  early detection 188
  epidemiology 188
  prevention 188
  prognosis 188
  and radiation 104
  and radioactive drugs 112–13
  risk factors 188
  symptoms 188
  treatment 188
Bone marrow 189, **190**
  illustrated 190
  in the immune system 57
  suppression by chemotherapy
    228–29
Bone marrow transplantation 230
  for leukemia 198
Bone metastases
  radiation therapy for 218
tumors
  benign or malignant 188
Bowel
  see *Small intestines* or *Colon and
    rectum*
BPH
  see *Benign prostatic hyperplasia*
Brachytherapy 427g
  and radiation therapy 214
Brain cancer 182–83
  drugs used in treatment 446
  survival rate trends, table 440
Brain tumors
  also see *Central nervous system
    tumors*
  diagnosis 193
  early detection 183
  epidemiology 183
  in children
    detection methods 204
    survival 204
    symptoms 204
    treatment 204
  as metastases 182
  prevention 183
  prognosis 183
  radiation therapy for 218
  risk factors 183
  summary table **121**
  survival rate trends, table 440
  symptoms 183
  treatment 183
  treatment with biopsy proof 210
Braun, A. C. 50, 75
Bray, Judith 274
Bray, Stephen vi, 253–54
Breast
  anatomy 140

  and cysts 142
  and fibrocystic conditions 142
  illustrated 140
  lymph nodes, illustrated 144
  physiology 140
Breast cancer 139–46
  and alcohol 142
  BCDDP Study 143
  blacks vs whites 141
  and breast feeding 94, 142
  Breast Cancer Detection
    Demonstration Project 12
  breast self-examination 315
  computed tomography (CT) 143
  control of 139
  detection 330–37
  diagnosis 20, 143
  diaphanography 143, 337
  dietary fat and 345
  drugs used in treatment 445
  ductal 140
  early detection 142
  in the elderly 145
  emotional consequences 145
  epidemiology 141
  and estrogen exposure 142
  and family history 141
  and fat intake 141
  general statistics 4
  Halsted, William S. 10
  and heredity 79
  history of treatment 10
  hyperplasia 142
  and hysterectomy 142
  imaging techniques, other
    methods 330–37
  immunotherapy for 145
  in situ 140, 143
  in the elderly 145
  infection 142
  and lactation 94
  lobular 140
  lymph node controversy 144
  magnetic resonance imaging
    (MRI) 143, 337
  mammography 315, 330–37
  and menstruation 94
  and Nancy Reagan 142
  natural history 140
  nipple aspiration cytology 143
  nipple discharge 143
  pattern of reappearance 144
  and pregnancy 142
  prevention 142
  prostheses 142
  and radiation 141
  radiation therapy for 144, 218
  radical mastectomy 10
  Reach to Recovery 145
  receptor studies 144
  risk factors 141
  reconstructive surgery 145

sizes at diagnosis 142
summary table **119**
survival rate trends, table 440
survival rates 145
symptoms 143
thermography 143, 337
treatment 144
tumor sizes, illustrated 143
types 140
types, percentages 23
ultrasound 143, 336–37
Women's Health Trial 142
Breast Cancer Detection Demonstra-
    tion Project 12, 143
Breast feeding
    and breast cancer 94
Breast self-examination (BSE) 315,
    427g
    guidelines for check-ups 315
    history 11
    how-to **323–24**
    nipple discharge 324–25
    patterns of search, illustrated 324
Breast physical examination
    guidelines for check-ups 315
Breslow, Lester and Devra 12, 14, 16
Brill-Symmer's disease 22
Bronchogenic carcinoma
    see *Lung cancer*
Bronchoscope
    principle 211
Bronchoscopy
    defined 134
Brucella abortus 230
Bullard, David G. 276
Burkitt, Denis 136
Burkitt's lymphoma 63, 69, 192, 427g
    a cluster case 193
    and Epstein-Barr virus (EBV) 69
    drugs used in treatment 445
Burns
    and skin cancer 124
Busulfan
    side effects 448

CA 19–9 179
CA-125 158
Cachexia 427g
    described 21
Cadium 97
    and lung cancer 133
Cairns, John 45, 90
Califano, Joseph A. 11, 360
Calories
    also see *Obesity*
    and cancer risk 82, 345
    fat 84
    recommended amount 347
    table 348
Canadian Task Force
    Pap guidelines 316
Cancer 427g

also see Prevention
and AIDS **394–98**
and aging 80
as a contagious disease 80
in animals 72–76
and asbestos 97–100
from bacteria 90–92
benign or malignant 43
benign or malignant, table 187
biological treatments for **220–32**
breast self-examination **323–26**
cancer registries 238–39
causes, overview 78–80
causes, table 79, 83
check-up guidelines, table 316
chemotherapy for **220–32**
chemotherapy, table 444–51
and chronic irritation 80
classifications of tumors 20
cure rates, historical 3
death, how patients die 21
defined 3, 18, 21
and dentures 80
diagnosis 20, 296, 302
and diet 81, 84
and discrimination 290–91
early man 9
and ecology 74
economic aspects 260–61
economically disadvantaged and
    380–83
in Egyptians 9
environmental issues 374–80
and Epstein-Barr virus 91
essential concepts 3
and evolution 72–76
field of 13–16
general 27
general description 43
and genetics 47
growth rates 3
in Harlem 381
histological types 21
r'#home stool blood testing 329
home stool blood testing 329
homosexuality and 388
and hormones 111
how cancers spread 19
and iatrogenesis 110–13
identification of 19
immune response to 58
immune system and AIDS 395
immunotherapy for **220–32**
impact on society 260–61
infant exam by mother 329
infections and 80
infections of patients, types 22
major site, overview 117–206
malaria and 91
metastasis 18
mode of growth 18
as a model illness 258

natural history of 6
nomenclature 20
number of types 21
oncogenes 67
opportunistic cancers 394–98
overview 2–4
pain 222
from parasites 90–92
percent from diet 82
in plants 73
poem about 25
poor and 3
practicing cancer prevention
    314–17
prevention 5–7, **313**
quackery 243–49
and radiation 100–07
rate of growth 18
rates in families 3
rehabilitation **274–75**
rights of the patient 240–42
self-examinations for **318–29**
self-examinations, general 7
seven warning signs **436**
and sexuality 276–78
small intestine 135–38
small or large tumor, illustrated
    225
smoking and 358–66
from smoking, list 86
social aspects 257–62
spontaneous regression 233–35
staging 20
statistics
statistics, table 4
stress and 80, **279–84**
surgery, overview **209–12**
from surgery 80
and tidepools 74
and tobacco 85–89
and trauma 80
tumor board 236–37
U.S. numbers 4
understanding smoking **358–66**
and venereal wart 70
viruses 67
and weight loss 272
world numbers 4
worldwide, table 441
Cancer Care, Inc. 455
Cancer cells
    compared to normal cells 45
    described 45
Cancer centers
    general description 15
    history of 15
    listing of 458–60
Cancer chemotherapy
    see *Chemotherapy*
Cancer control
    objectives for the year 2000 344
    state service 15

Cancer Control Society 16
Cancer Education and Prevention
    Center vi
Cancer field 13–16
Cancer Information Services (CIS)
    453
Cancer of cartilage 187–88
Cancer of fat 187–88
Cancer of muscles 187–88
Cancer of tendons 187–88
Cancer of the gall bladder
    see Gall bladder cancer
Cancer of the Liver
    see Liver cancer
Cancer of the pituitary gland
    see Pituitary gland cancer
Cancer of the stomach
    see Stomach cancer
Cancer of the thyroid
    see Thyroid cancer
Cancer oncogenes 67
Cancer prevention 4, 313
Cancer registry 238–39
    defined 239
    function 239
    history of 11
Cancer-related organizations 452–60
Cancer research
    with monoclonal antibodies 232
    also see Cancer field
Cancer Research Institute, Inc. 458
CANCER REVIEW 118–21
Cancer specialists
    defined 15
Cancer surgery
    overview 209–12
Cancer treatments
    overview 201
Cancerphobia 2
Cancers
    incurable 212
Cancers in children
    see Childhood cancers
Cancers of bone 187–88
Cancers of lymph systems 189–91
Cancers of soft-tissues 187–88
Cancers of the blood 189–91
Candida 22
    and AIDS 401
Candlelighters Foundation 14, 453
CanSurmount 14
Carbon monoxide 86
    from smoking 87
Carbon tetrachloride 97
Carcinoembryonic antigen (CEA) 158
Carcinogen 427g
Carcinogenesis 427g
    chemical 47
    chemical, drugs 111
    environmental (chemical) 48
    illustrated 44
    vs mutagenesis 47

occupational 95–99
    radiation 46, 100–07
    radiation vs. 102
    viral 46
Carcinogens
    in the air 117
    in water 118
Carcinoid tumors 186
Carcinoma 427g
    defined 21
Carcinoma in situ 427g
    see In situ
Carcinomas
    how they spread 19
Cardiovascular disease
    and tobacco 87
Carmustine
    side effects 448
Carotene, low intake
    list of cancers form 315
Cartilage cancer 187–88
Cases
    summary table 119–21
Catalase 427g
Catalyst 427g
Causes of cancer 79
    Doll and Peto's 12
    general 12
    see specific causes
Causes/risk factors
    summary table 83–84
Cauterization
    for cervical cancer 156
CEA
Cell 427g
    cancer cell 43
    cell cycle 39, 224–25
    contact inhibition 30
    doubling time in breast cancer 331
    effects of radiation 101
    eucaryotic 27, 39
    lung types 369–70
    meiosis 40
    membrane 28
    mitosis 39
    normal or cancer 45
    nucleotides 33
    nucleus described 32
    number in human body 27
    procaryotic 27, 29
    and radiation, table 101
    transport of molecules, types 30
    types 27
Cell cycle 224–25
    described 39
    illustrated 40, 225
    steps 39
Cell-free system 427g
Cell fusion 427g
Cell membrane
    illustration 30
Cell theory 37

Cellular antibodies 427g
Celsus 9
Centers for Disease Control
    classification systems of HIV infec-
        tion 399–400
    worksite recommendations for
        AIDS 412
Central dogma 33
Central nervous system
    cancer, types 22
    described 182
Central nervous system cancers
    in children 203
Central nervous system tumors
    182–83
    and chemicals 183
    and childhood cancers 183
    diagnosis 183
    early detection 183
    and EB virus 183
    epidemiology 183
    heredity 183
    natural treatment 183
    prevention 183
    prognosis 183
    and radiation 183
    risk factors 183
    and sick pets 183
    treatment 183
Centriole 427g
    illustrated 29
Centromere 40, 427g
Centrosomes (or centrioles) 427g
Cerf, Arthur Z. 274
Cervical cancer 63, 150–56
    also see Uterine cervix
    anatomy 151
    and American Indians 151
    and blacks 440
    and circumcision 151
    and condoms 70
    culposcopy 155
    definition 151
    diagnosis 155
    and dietary factors 153
    and douching 152
    dysplasia 151
    early detection 154–55
    epidemiology 153
    genetic factors 153
    and intercourse 94
    and IUD 151
    natural history 153
    and Pap test 151
    and pregnancy 153
    prevention 154–44
    prognosis 156
    and prostitution 151
    and radiation therapy 217
    risk factors 151
    risk factors, table 154
    and sexual practices 151

and smoking 71, 87
symptoms 155
treatment 156
types, percentage 23
and viruses 70
Cervix 427g
illustrated 152, 153
Cervix cancer
drugs used in treatment 446
survival rate trends, table 440
Chaga's disease 91
Chalones 230, 427g
Change
and stress 283
Charcoal broiling 352
Charred food 352
Chemical carcinogenesis 10, 47
also see *Environmental
cancers*
also see *Occupational cancers*
and brain tumors 184
and drugs 111
Chemical workers
and urinary tract cancers 167
Chemoprevention
and oral cancers 170
Chemotherapy 220–32, 427g
adjuvant chemotherapy 221, 226,
227
alkylating agents 223
anti-androgen drugs 149
antimetabolites 223
antitumor antibiotics 223
basic principles 223–26
biological response modifiers 223
Bondonna's studies 228
and bone cancers 188
for brain tumors 183
for breast cancer 145, 228
causing cancer 112
caution when administering
229
cell cycle 224–25
for central nervous system tumors
183
classes of chemotherapeutic
agents 223
combination chemotherapy
225–26, **226–27**
cycle specific drugs 224–25
decision for the patients 229
drugs, table 444–51
and esophagus cancer 175
and estrogen receptors 228
enzymes 223
evaluating response 226
first cis-platinum use 11
first leukemia remission 111
and gall bladder cancer 181
and gastrointestinal disturbances
272
hair loss and 229

high-dose chemotherapy 226
history 11, **221**
history of drug development,
graph 221
for Hodgkin's disease 194
hormones and hormone inhibitors
223
intra-arterial for oral cancer 171
intraperitoneal 228
and laryngeal cancer 173
and leukemia 198
leuprolide 149
list, complete 444–51
and liver cancer 181
log kill hypothesis 223–24
and loss of appetite 272
for lymphomas 194
malaria 231
medical oncologists and 221
MOPP regimen 221
and multiple myeloma 201
and nutrition 272
nutritional therapy 229
and oral cancers 171
and osteogenic sarcoma 206
for ovarian cancer 158
overview 208
overview, diagram 226
palliation 221
and pancreas cancer 179
photochemotherapy 195
plant alkaloids 222
for prostate cancer 149
protocols 226
pump infusions 228
regional chemotherapy 226, **228**
risk-benefit 229
role of the immune system 224
and sarcomas 188
side effects of 228–29, 444–51
site of action, illustration
223
solid tumors vs hematologic
tumors 225
and stomach cancer 177
supportive care 229
tables of drugs **444–51**
tamoxifen 145, 228
and testicular cancer 165
and thyroid cancer 185
toxicity 228
tumor resistance 225
and urinary tract cancers 168
uses for 221
and uterine cancer 156
and vulvar cancer 161
vomiting and 228
Chest x-ray
guidelines for check-ups 315
Chew
see *Tobacco*
Child-bearing

see *Pregnancy*
Childhood cancers **202–06**
also see specific types of cancer
and AIDS 402
brain cancer **203**
central nervous system **203**
epidemiology 203
Ewing's sarcoma 206
germ cell tumor **205**
incidence 203
lymphomas **205**
neuroblastoma **204–05**
osteogenic sarcoma **206**
other types 206
reasons for better survival 203
retinoblastoma **205**
rhabdomyosarcoma **205**
summary table **122**
types, as per age groups 203
Wilms' tumor 204
Children
infant exam by mother 329
Children's Oncology Services 454
Chlamydia
and cervical cancer 151
Chlorambucil
and leukemia 197
side effects 448
Chloramphenicol
and leukemia 197
Chlornaphazine 113
Chloroform
and water pollution 375
Chloromethyl ethers
and lung cancer 133
Chloromethyl methyl ether (CMME)
96
Chlorophyll 427g
Cholangiocarcinoma 22
Cholangioma 22
Chondroma 22
Chondrosarcoma 22
Choriocarcinoma 22, 163, 427g
drugs used in treatment 445
Chromatin
illustrated 29
Chromatin stands 427g
Chromatography 427g
Chromium **97**
and lung cancer 86, 98, 133
and South Africa 98
in water 116
uses 98
Chromosomes 427g
Chronic bronchitis
and smoking 88
Chronic cystic mastitis 427g
Chronic irritation 80
Chronic lymphocytic leukemia
drugs used in treatment 446
Chronic myelocytic leukemia (CML)
drugs used in treatment 446

Chronic obstructive pulmonary disease (COPD) 368, 428g
  and pollution 117
  and smoking 88
CHUMS (Cancer Hopefuls United for Mutual Support) 455
Cigarettes
  see *Tobacco*
Cilia
  illustrated 29
Cimetidine 230
  and AIDS 404
Circumcision
  and cancer of the penis 165
  and cervical cancer 151
Cirrhosis 69
  and liver cancer 181
Cis-platinum 223
  first uses of 11
  side effects 448
Citrovorum factor 226
Clark, William R. vi, 52, 57
Classical radical mastectomy 427g
Clean Air Act 376
Clear cell cancer
  and DES 161
  of the vagina 161
Clear cell carcinoma
  see *Kidney cancer*
Clinical 427g
Clone 427g
Clostridia
CNS
  see *Central nervous system*
Cobalt machines
  see *Radiation therapy*
Cobalt unit
  illustration 215
Co-carcinogen 427g
Coffee
  and pancreas cancer 179
  and ulcers 88
  and urinary tract cancers 167
Coggle, J. 101, 102–104
Cohen, Elie 298
Cohnheim, Julius 10
Colds 6
Cole, Warren H. 233
Colon 427g
Colon and rectal cancer **135–38**
  anatomy 136
  and bile acids 136
  Denis Burkitt 136
  diagnosis 137
  and dietary fat 345
  drugs used in treatment 447
  epidemiology 136
  and fat 136
  and fiber 136, 345
  general statistics 4
  hemorrhoids 137

and heredity 79, 137
immunotherapy for 137–38
and parasites 91
and polyps 136
prognosis 137–38
proximal migration of polyps 136
radiation therapy for 137–38
risk factors 136
and schistosomiasis 91
self-testing for 137
summary table **119**
surgery for 137–38
symptoms 137
treatment 137–38
types, percentages 23
and ulcerative colitis 137
Colon cancer
  and asbestos 98
  survival rate trends, table 440
Colonoscopy 338–342, 427g
  also see *Sigmoidoscopy*
Colony-stimulating factor (CFS) 230
Colostomy 3, 427g
  defined 138, 286
  illustrated 288–89
Colposcope
  principle 211
Colposcopy 155, 427g
Columnar cells
  in the lungs 370
Combination therapy 427g
Committee for Freedom of Choice in Cancer Therapy 16
Communication
  and sexuality 278
  difficulties in 302
  with physicians 210
  with surgeon 210
Community
  cancer prevention plan 317
Comparative neoplasia 72
Comparative oncology
  summary 75
Complement
  described 58
Compound BW A509U
  and AIDS 405
Compton effect 428g
Computer tomography (CT) 428g
  for breast cancer 143
  for breast tumors 337
  and central nervous system tumors 183
  and pituitary gland cancer 183
  and radiation 203
  radiation dose 373
Condoms
  and HIV prevention 411
Condyloma accuminatum
  see *Venereal wart*
Contact inhibition 428g

described 30, 43
and viral transformation 66
Control genes 428g
Cooking methods 351–52
COPD 428g
  See *Chronic obstructive pulmonary disease*
Copper
  and multiple myeloma
Cornybacterium parvum 230, 231
Cough
  morning cough and smoking 88
Craniopharyngioma
  in children 204
  prognosis 183
Credit organizations 456
Crick, Francis 33
Crossing-over 428g
Cruciferous vegetables 315, **351, 428g**
Cryogenic 428g
Cryotherapy
  for cervical cancer 156
Cryptococcus 23
  and AIDS 401
Cryptorchidism
  defined 164
  factor in testicular cancer 164
Cryptosporidiosis
  and AIDS 402
Cure rate
  summary table **120–22**
Curie, Madame 10, 214
Curie, Pierre 10, 214
Curschmann sprials
  in the lungs 370
Cyclamates
  and urinary tract cancer 167
Cyclic accelerator 428g
Cyclophosphamide
  side effects 228, 448
Cyclosoprin A 112
  and AIDS 404
Cyrosurgery
  and skin cancer 129
Cystadenocarcinoma 22
Cystadenoma 22
Cystosarcoma phylloides 22
Cystoscopy
  and bladder cancer 167–68
Cysts, ganglion 188
Cytarabine HCI
  side effects 448
Cytokines 230, 232
Cytological studies
  principles 211
Cytology 428g
  nipple aspiration 143
Cytomegalovirus (CMV) 23, 398
  and AIDS 401
Cytoplasm 428g

described 31
Cytosine 33, 428g
Cytotoxic T-cell clones 230

D & C
  see *Dilation and curettage*
Dacrabazine
  side effects 448
Dactinomycin
  side effects 448
Daunorubicin
  side effects 448
Dawe, Clyde J. 22
DBCP
  and water pollution 375
DDT 97
Death
  and acceptance 299–300
  and anger 299
  and Auschwitz 298
  and technology 296
Death (and dying) 292–300, **301–04**
  living will 309
Decarboxylic acid 428g
Defective virus 428g
Delay 259
Dementia
  from AIDS 401
  and smoking 87
Denial
  and facing death 302
  discussed by Kübler-Ross 303
Dental x-rays 372
Dentists
  and detection of oral cancers 170
Dentures
  and oral cancers 170
Deoxyribonucleic acid (DNA) 428g
  described 32
  diagram 34, 35
  effects of radiation on 101
  pronounced 32
  recombinant DNA 38
  recombinant, treatments involving 231
  repair 38
  replication 37
Depression
  and facing death 302
  and nutrition 273
Dermoid (benign teratoma) 22
DES (diethylstilbestrol) 11
  and cancer 46–47
  daughters 111, 161
  exam for those exposed 161
  history of 111, 161
  iatrogenesis 11
  sons 111, 161
  and vaginal cancer 111, 161
DES Action 454
Detection
  see *Early detection*

DeVita, V. T. 119
deVries, Peter 300
Diagnosis 428g
  discussing with patient 296
  methods of 20
  telling the patient 302
  use of mammography 331
Diaphanography 143
Diaphragm
  illustrated 288
3, 3'-Dichlorobenzidine 97
Dideoxycytidine
  and AIDS 405
Diet
  and alcohol 352
  benzopyrene 351–52
  and Beta-Carotene 349
  and breast cancer 141
  calorie, table 348
  and cancer prevention 343–57
  and cervical cancer 153
  cooking methods 351–52
  cruciferous vegetables 351
  fat and colorectal cancer 136
  fat, table 348
  fiber 347
  fiber and colorectal cancer 136, 345
  fiber content, table 350–51
  and gall bladder cancer 181
  guide to reducing fat 349
  and laryngeal cancer 173
  and lung cancer 133
  and obesity 352
  and pancreas cancer 179
  and placental neoplasia 161–62
  and stomach cancer 177
  summary table **119–21**
  and thyroid cancer 185
  types of research 344
  U. S. Dietary Goals 347
  and urinary tract cancers 167
  and Vitamin A 349
  and Vitamin C **349–51**
  and Women's Health Trial 142
Diet and cancer 81–84, **345–53**
  brief history 12
  dietary fat **345–47**
  overview 81–84, **345–53**
  recommendations, table 84
Diethylstilbesterol 428g
  see *DES*
Differentiation 17, 18, 428g
  as a method of classification 21
Diffuse histiocytic lymphoma
  drugs used in treatment 445
Diffusion 30
Digital rectal examination
  guidelines for check-ups 315
Dilation and curettage 155
Dimethyl sulphate 97
3, 3'-Dimethoxybenzidine (ortho-Dianisidine) 97

Dimethylcarbamoyl chloride 97
Dinosaurs 9
1,4-Dioxane 97
Diploid cell 428g
Direct black 38 (technical grade) 97
Direct blue 6 (technical grade) 97
Direct brown 95 (technical grade) 97
Discrimination
  Cancer Patients' Employment Rights Project 456
  job discrimination 290–91
DiSogra, Charles A. 81, 343
DiSogra, Lorelei K. 81, 343
Diverticulitis 342
Diverticulosis 342, 428g
DNA
  see *Deoxyribonucleic acid*
DNA probes 379
DNA synthesis 38
  illustrated 38
DNA-adduct tests 379
DNCB
  and skin cancer 129
  described 405
  use for HIV therapy 405
Doctor-patient models 259
Doll, Sir Richard 12, 79, 82, 93–94
Dominant trait 428g
Doolittle, Mark J. 279
Dosimetrists
  and radiation therapy 216
Double helix 428g
Doubling times
  in breast cancer 331
  in colon cancer 7
  in natural history 6
Douching
  in cervical cancer 152
Down's syndrome
  and leukemia 197
Doxorubicin 223
  side effects 448
Drasin, Harry 271
Dronabinol 229
Drugs
  abused drugs and AIDS 411
  and spontaneous regression 234
Drugs and cancer **110–13**
  androgens 112
  anticancer drugs causing cancer 112
  DES 111
  immunosuppressive drugs 112
  radioactive drugs 112
DTC (Imuthiol) 405
Duodenum 135
Dust
  and cancer 99
Dyes
  and urinary tract cancer 167
Dysentary 91

Dysgerminoma
   of the ovary 159
Dyspareunia
   defined 155
Dysplasia 19, 428g
   of the cervix 151
Dysplastic cells
   in the lungs 370
Dysplastic nevi syndrome 127

Early detection **313–83**
   brain and central nervous system
      cancer 183
   breast cancer 142
   cervical cancer 154–55
   colon and rectal cancer 137
   endometrial cancer 155
   esophagus cancer 175
   gall bladder cancer 181
   laryngeal cancer 173
   liver cancer 181
   leukemias 197–98
   lung cancer 133
   lymphomas 193–94
   mouth and throat cancer 170
   multiple myeloma 201
   ovarian cancer 158
   pancreas cancer 179
   prostate cancer 148
   sarcomas 188
   skin cancer 126
   stomach cancer 177
   testicular cancer 164
   thyroid cancer 185
   urinary tract cancers 167
Eberhart, Richard 25
Eberle, Scott 385–420
EBV
   see *Epstein-Barr virus*
Ecology 74
Economic aspects of cancer 260–61
   earnings lost due to cancer, table
      443
Economically disadvantaged 380–83
   also see *Poor people*
Edema 428g
   defined 18
Education
   professional 17
   public 7
Effusion 428g
Egyptians and cancer 9
Electrodissecation
   and skin cancer 129
Electron 428g
Electron microscopy 428g
Electron therapy 428g
ELISA
   and HIV antibody test 414
Embryogenesis 428g
Embryonal carcinomas 163
Embryonal rest theory 10

Embryonal rhabdomyosarcoma
   drugs used in treatment 445
Emotional care
   for leukemia 198
Emotional response
   to AIDS 417
Emotions 79
   also see *Stress*
   and breast cancer 145
   LeShan's studies 282
   positive role 282
   support for AIDS patients 412
   and will to live **266–70**
Emphysema
   and smoking 88
Endocrine gland 184, 428g
Endocrine gland cancers 184–86
   also see by glands' name
   defined 184
   types 184
Endocrine tumors
   pancreas 185–86
Endocrinologist
   defined 184
Endogenous 428g
Endometrial 428g
Endometrial biopsy 155
   guidelines for check-ups 315
   secondary prevention 316
Endometrial cancer **150–56**
   also see *Uterine cancer*
   also see *Uterine corpus*
   anatomy 151
   biopsy for 155
   definition 151
   diagnosis 155
   drugs used in treatment 446
   early detection 155
   endometrial biopsy 155
   epidemiology 154
   and estrogens 154
   and fibroid tumors 154
   genetic factors 154
   high-risk groups 155
   and hormones 111
   and obesity 154
   physiology 151
   and pregnancy 154
   prevention 155
   prognosis 156
   risk factors 154
   and smoking 154
   staging 155
   symptoms 155
   treatment 156
   types, percentages 23
   radiation therapy for 218
   in whites 154
Endometrium 428g
Endometrium cancer
   survival rate trends, table 440
Endoplasmic reticulum 428g

   illustrated 29
   small 31
   smooth 31
Endoscopy 428g
   of the stomach 177
Endotoxin 230
Energy metabolism 428g
Enterstomal therapist 428g
Environment
   as cause of cancer 79
   and lung cancer 86
   and smoking 89
Environmental cancer 9
   also see *Occupational cancer*
   air pollution 375–76
   asbestos 376
   California cases
   future issues 374–80
   genetic screening 379
   passive smoking 378
   percentage of cancers 27
   radon 378
   second-hand smoke 378
   toxicological testing 378–79
   and water pollution 375
Environmental carcinogenesis
   general 45
   illustrated 48
   ozone 45
Environmental Protection Agency
   375
Enzymes 429g
   see *Protein*
Eosinophils 58, 190
Ependymoma
   prognosis 183
   in children 203
Epichlorohydrin 97
Epidemiologist 429g
Epidemiology 429g
   and diet research 344
   summary table **119–21**
   world-wide, table 441
Epidermal carcinoma 22
Epidermal papilloma 22
Epididymis
   illustrated 327
Epididymitis 164, 327
Epithelium 429g
Epizootiology 73, 429g
Epstein, S. 50
Epstein-Barr virus (EBV) 398
   and brain tumors 183
   early detection 183
   and malaria 69
   and mononucleosis 69
   prevention 183
Erections
   after prostate surgery 149
Erthyrocytes, illustrated 190
Erythroblast 190
Erythroleukemia 22

Erythroplasia 322
  and oral cancers 170
Escape mechanisms 429g
Escherichia (E.) coli bacteria 28
Esophageal cancer belt 175
Esophageal speech 173, 429g
Esophagitis
  and AIDS 402
Esophagus
  illustrated 288
Esophagus cancer **174–75**
  anatomy 174
  and asbestos 98
  diagnosis 175
  early detection 175
  and EB virus 175
  epidemiology 174
  and genetics 175
  physiology 174
  primary prevention 175
  prognosis 175
  risk factors 175
  and smoking 87
  summary table **120**
  survival rate trends, table 440
  symptoms 175
  treatment 175
Estramustine phosphate sodium
  side effects 448
Estrogen 429g
  also see *DES (diethylistlbesterol)*
  and the breast 140
  and breast cancer 142
  and cancer **111**
  and kidney cancer 167
  and liver cancer 181
Estrogen receptors
  and breast cancer 143
  and chemotherapy 228
Ethylene dibromide 97
  in the air 376
Ethylene dichloride
  in the air 376
Ethylene oxide 97
Ethylene thiourea 97
Etiocholanolone 429g
Etiology 429g
Etoposide
  side effects 448
Eucaryotic cell 28
  illustrated 29
Evan's postulates 67
Everson, Tilden 234
Evolution 75
  and oncogenes 66–67
Evolution and cancer 72–76
Ewing's sarcoma
  also see *Bone cancer*
  described 206
  drugs used in treatment 445
  prognosis 206
  radiation therapy for 218

symptoms 206
treatment 206
Excision 429g
Excoriation 429g
Exercise
  after surgery 264
  and breast cancer 141
  and recovery form cancer 264
  for the cancer patient 274–75
Exocrine gland, pancreas 177
Exogenous 429g
Experimental/alternative
  organizations 458
Extravasation
  defined 228
Eyes
  damage from pituitary gland
    cancer 185

Facia 429g
Facial nerve
  in parotid gland surgery 171
Fallopian tube 160
  illustrated 152, 153
Fallopian tube cancers **161**
Familial cancers 79
Fantastic Voyage 53
Farber, Sidney 11
  and chemotherapy history 221
Farmers
  and multiple myeloma 201
Fat
  and breast cancer 345
  cancers of 187–88
  guide to reducing fat 349
  and other cancers 347
  percent of calories 84
  recommended amount 347
  table 348
  unsaturated vs saturated 345
Fatigue
  see *Human B-cell lymphotrophic*
    virus (HBLV)
Fatty tumors
  see *Lipomas* or *Fibromas*
Fear 259, **267**
  and nutrition 273
Federal Safe Drinking Water Act 375
Feldman, Frances L. 291
Feline leukemia virus (FeLV) 397
Femoral 429g
Ferrara, Anthony 418
Ferfuson, Tom 327
Fiber 429g
  and Denis Burkitt 136–37
  and colon and rectal cancer 136,
    345
  content in foods, table 350–51
  function 347
  health benefits from 347
  planning a high-fiber diet 350–51
  recommendation 137

types of 347
Fiberoptics
  in use with sigmoidoscopy 339
Fibrodenoma
Fibroid tumor
  of the endometrium (uterus) 154
Fibroma 22, 188
Fibrosarcoma 22, 206
Filial 429g
Financial aspects 443
Flagellum
  illustrated 29
Flavonoids 232
Flexible sigmoidoscope
  illustration 340
Flexible sigmoidoscopy 338–42
  and polyps 340
  preparation for 340–41
  procedure 341
  rationale 339
  risks of 341
  after sigmoidoscopy 342
Floxuridine
  side effects 448
Fluid Mosaic Model 30
Flukes 91
Fluorocarbons
  and ozone 109
5-Fluorouracil (5-FU) 223, 228
  side effects 448
Follicular carcinoma
  of the thyroid 184
Food and Drug Administration
  described 248
Formaldehyde (gas) 97
Fowler, California
  cases and water pollution 375
Fractionation 429g
Freeman, Dr. Harold P. 381
Freese, Arthur S. 284
Freud, Sigmund
  and smoking 360
Furniture manufacture
  and cancer 97, **98**

Galen 9
  and melancholy 281
Gall bladder
  anatomy 180
  physiology 180
Gall bladder cancer 180–81
  and American Indians 181
  diagnosis 181
  early detection 181
  epidemiology 181
  prevention 181
  prognosis 181
  risk factors 181
  symptoms 181
  treatment 181
Gall bladder disease
  and multiple myeloma 201

Gallo, Robert 12, 389
  and vaccines 11, 408
Gallstones
  and gall bladder cancer 181
Gamete 40, 429g
Gamma globulin
  and AIDS 404
Ganna rays 429g
Ganglion cysts 188
Ganglioneuroma 22
Gardner's Syndrome 137
Garrett, Laurie 26
Gastric cancer
  drugs used in treatment 446
Gastric carcinoma 22
Gastric polyp 22
Gay men
  and HIV infection 391
Genes 429g
  defined 33
  see Deoxyribonucleic acid
Genetic code 429g
  central dogma 33
  history of discovery 33
Genetic engineering
  see Biological treatment
Genetic screening 379
Genetics
  also see Heredity
  and breast cancer 141
  as cause of cancer 79
  and esophagus cancer 175
  and Hodgkin's disease 193
  and laryngeal cancer 173
  and leukemia 197
  and leukemia in children 203
  and retinoblastoma 205
  and stomach cancer 177
Genetics/heredity
  summary table 119–21
Genome 429g
Geology
  and asbestos 376
Germ cell tumors
  described 205
  in children 205
  treatment 205
Gerson and Hoxsey therapy 16
Gestational choriocarcinoma 221
Gestational neoplasia
  see Placental neoplasia
Giardiasis 91
Ginseng 406
GLQ 223, 406
Glioblastoma multiforme 22
Glioma
  in children 182
Glucan 230
Glycoprotein 429g
Goiter
  and thyroid cancer 185
Golgi apparatus 32

Golgi complex
  illustrated 29
Golgi, Camillo 32
Gonad 429g
Gonadectomy 429g
Gonorrhea
  and cervical cancer 151
Gori, Gio 82
Grant, Ronald N. 243
Granulocytes 190
  illustrated, 190
Granuloma
  defined 21
Granulosa cell tumor 22
Graphite 86
Greene, Bob, story 205
Guaiac test 429g
  see Stool test for hidden blood
Guanine 33, 429g
Gynecological cancers 160–62
  also see chapters on Uterine can-
    cer, Ovary cancer and Vaginal/
    Vulvar and less common cancers
  and parasites 91

Hairdressers
  and urinary tract cancers 167
Hairy cell leukemia
  durgs used in treatment 445
  and interferon 231
Hairy leukoplakia
  in AIDS 401
Haitians
  and HIV infection 392
Halsted radical mastectomy
  see Surgery, breast cancer
Halsted, William S. 10
Haploid cell 429g
Hawaiians
  and pancreas cancer 179
HBLV
  see Human B-cell lymphotrophic
    virus
HCG
  see Human chorionic gonadotropin
Head and neck cancers
  drugs used in treatment 446
  also see Oral cancers from smoking
  also see specific site
Headache
  and CNS tumor symptoms 184
Health care workers
  and HIV/AIDS transmissions 410
Health Insurance Plan (HIP) of
    Greater New York 143
Heart disease
  and smoking 87
Helper cells (T4) 190, 395
Hemangioblastoma 182
Hemangiopericytoma 206
Hematogenous spread (by blood) 19
Hematology

described 189
Heme 429g
Hemoccult
  see Stool test for hidden blood
Hemophiliacs
  and HIV infection 392
Hemorrhage
  from 22
Hemorrhoids 328, 341
  also see Colon and rectal cancer
Hepandna viruses 63, 64
Hepatic tumors
  see Liver cancer
Hepatitis B virus (HBV) 63
Hepatitis B
  and liver cancer 69, 181
Hepatobiliary cancer
  see Liver cancer, Gall bladder
    cancer
Herbicides
Herbst, Arthur 11
Heredity
  also see Genetics
  as cause of cancer 70
  and Hodgkin's disease 193
  and multiple endocrine neoplasms
    (M.E.N.) 186
  and pancreas cancer 179
  and sarcomas 188
  summary table 119–21
Herpes 63
Herpes genitalis
  and cervical cancer 151
Herpes simplex 23
Herpes simplex virus (HSV) 70
Herpes virus 67
  and laryngeal cancer 173
Herpes zoster 23
  in AIDS 401
Heteroploid cell 429g
Heteropolyanion-23 (HPA-23)
  and AIDS 405
Hexavalent chromium
  in the air 115
High-fat diet
  list of cancers from 315
Hippocrates 9
  chemotherapy, history 221
Histiocytes
  and lymphoma 191
Histiocytosis X syndromes 206
Histology
  defined 20
History of cancer 8–12
HIV
  see Human Immunodeficiency
    Virus
HIV antibody test 414–15
  guidelines per risk group 415
  if you want to be tested 415
HIV treatments
  alternative 405–06

traditional 404–05
HIV virus
  and brain tumors 183
HIV wasting syndrome 401
Hodgkin, Thomas 192
Hodgkin's disease 22, 192–95 , 429g
  also see *Lymphomas*
  biopsing for 194
  and chemotherapy 227
  classification for treatment 194
  compared to other lymphomas 191
  described 191
  diagnosis 194
  drugs used in treatment 445
  early detection 193–94
  epidemiology 193
  history 11
  Kaplan, Henry 11
  lymph node self-examination 194
  possible infectious causes 193
  prevention 193–94
  prognosis 195
  radiation treatment for 194, 217
  and Reed-Sternberg cells 192
  risk factors 193
  staging 194
  and Sternberg-Reed cells 192
  summary table **121**
  survival rate trends, table 440
  symptoms 194
  treatment 194
  types 192
Holleb, Arthur I. 16, 233
Holmes, Thomas 280
Homeopathy 406
Homosexuality
  and AIDS 388
  HIV infections in gays 391
Homeostasis 429g
Homografts 429g
Horizontal transmission 429g
Hormonal treatments
  and chemotherapy 228
Hormone therapy
  for prostate cancer 149
  and uterine cancer 156
Hormones 429g
  and breast cancer treatment 144
  and cancer 111
  and endometrial cancer 154
  and vaginal cancer 161
Hormonotherapy 429g
Hospice 305–07
  discussed by Kübler-Ross 304
  National Hospice Organization
    306, 457
Hospitals
  first cancer hospital 10
  Memorial hospital 10
Housman, A. E. 293
Hoxsey therapy 13
HPV, see Human papilloma virus

HTLV 11
  HTLV-1, also see Leukemia 12, 68
  HTLV-2, see *Human immuno-*
    deficiency virus
  HTLV-3, see *Human immuno-*
    deficiency virus
HTLV-I
  in Africa 396
  in Caribbean 396
  in Japan 396
Huggins' tumor 429g
Human B-cell lymphotrophic virus
  (HBLV) 91
Human chorionic gonadotropin 162,
  164
Human immunodeficiency virus
  (HIV) 429g
  also see *Acquired Immunodefi-*
    ciency Syndrome (AIDS)
  and AIDS-related conditions
    (ARC) 400–01
  alternative treatments 405–06
  anti-viral therapy for 405
  antibody positive percentages,
    table 391
  asymptomatic infection 400
  and cancer 397
  and casual contact 410
  CDC worksite recommendations
    412
  chemotherapy for 404
  in children 401
  clinical course 401
  clinical spectrum, diagrammed 400
  clinical spectrum of disease
    399–402
  community cooperation 412
  compared to hepatitis B 410
  and condom use 411
  diagnosis of 401
  education in schools 412
  educational programs 412
  future manifestations 401
  guidelines, general 410
  guidelines for blood tranfusions
    413
  guidelines for caretakers or
    household contacts 413
  guidelines for gay or bisexual men
    413
  guidelines for hemophiliacs 413
  guidelines for heterosexuals 413
  guidelines for infants of mothers
    with an HIV infection 413
  guidelines for intravenous drug
    users 413
  guidelines for people at risk
    412–13
  guidelines for people with an HIV
    infection 413
  hairy leukoplakia 401
  herpes zoster 401

  how named 389
  how virus can be killed 410
  and the immune system 395–96
  infections in specific groups 391
  initial infection 400
  large-scale screening 414–15
  measuring helper T4 cell level 400
  neurological manifestations 401
  nocardia 401
  oral candidiasis 401
  patterns of 401
  and persistant generalized lymph-
    adenopathy 400
  preventing transmission 411
  prognosis 401
  projections of degree of spread 420
  psychiatric manifestations 401
  radiation therapy for 404
  responses to infection, illustrated
    397
  retroviruses 396
  salmonella 401
  in schools 412
  and self care 410–11
  and sexual practices 411
  size of the epidemic 390–91
  steps to develop vaccine for 408
  survival in 401
  symptoms of 400
  traditional treatments 403–5
  transmission to health care
    workers 410
  tuberculosis 401
Human papilloma virus (HPV)
  and cancer of the penis 165
  and cervical cancer 152
Human T-lymphocyte leukemia
  virus (HTLV-I)
  and AIDS 68
  discovery of 68
  Gallo and 68
Human T-lymphotropic virus
  see *Human immunodeficiency*
    virus (HIV)
  see *Human T-lymphocyte leukemia*
    virus (HTLV)
Humoral antibodies 429g
Humoral theory 9
Hybridoma
  and monoclonal antibodies 232
Hydatiform mole 22
Hydrazine 97
Hydroxy acids 429g
Hydroxyurea
  side effects 448
Hyperlipidemia
  and smoking 87
Hypernephroma
  see *Kidney cancer*
Hyperplasia 429g
Hyperthermia 212, 429g
  described 216

Hyperthermia *continued*
   and kidney cancer 168
   and urinary tract cancers 168
Hypnosis
   for pain 222
Hypopysis 429g
Hysterectomy 430g
   for cervical cancer 156
   types 156

I Can Cope 14, 455
Iatrogenesis
   and cancer 110–13
   described 10
   and urinary tract cancers 167
Ichikawa, Korchi 10
Ikiru 252
Ileostomy 430g
   defined 286
   illustrated 288–89
Ileum 135
   illustrated 288
Immonuosuppression
   and brain tumors 183
Immune RNAs 230
Immune surveillance 60, 398
Immune system
   also see *Immunology*
   accessory organs 57
   in AIDS **395–96**
   and aging 80
   antibodies
   antigen 58
   bone marrow 57
   bone marrow transplantation and
     AIDS 404
   cells of 58
   and chemotherapy, diagrammed
     226
   in chemotherapy 224
   complement 58
   effects of drugs on 112
   enhancement for AIDS therapy 404
   illustrated 59
   immune surveillance 60
   immunoglobulin, illustrated 60
   in kidney transplant 60
   killer cell 58
   leukocytes 58
   lymph nodes 57
   lymphocytes 58
   macrophages 58
   memory cells 58
   molecules 58
   natural killer cells (NK) 60
   and nutrition 272
   organization 58
   organs 57
   and parasites 91
   principles of biological
     treatment 30
   response 58

response to a common cold virus,
   illustrated 396
response to cancer 58
   and smoking 88
   and sperm 152
   spleen 57
   and spontaneous regression 235
   suppression of, as a treatment for
     AIDS 404
   T-4 cells and AIDS 395
   T8 cells and AIDS 395
   thymus gland 57
   transplant patients 112
Immune therapy 16
Immunity 430g
Immunoabsorbents 230
Immunoassay
   CA 19–9 179
   and central nervous system
     tumors 183
Immunoglobulin
   illustrated 60
Immunological surveillance 430g
Immunological tolerance 430g
Immunology 430g
   and cancer cells, general 45
   general 52–60
   introduction 57–60
   lymphatic system, illustrated 54
   self vs non-self 57
Immuno-suppression 430g
   and brain tumors 184
Immunotherapy 220–32, **229–30,**
   430g
   and bone cancers 188
   for breast cancer 145
   for cervical cancer 156
   flavonoids 232
   intra-operataive and CNS tumors
     183
   for leukemia 198
   for lung cancer 134
   for lymphomas 194–95
   for melanoma 130
   and multiple myeloma 201
   non-specific 230
   for ovarian cancer 158
   overview 208
   and pancreas cancer 179
   retinoids 232
   and sarcomas 188
   specific 231
   table 230
   and urinary tract cancers 168
   use of DNCB for skin cancer 129
   and uterine cancer 156
In situ 19, 430g
   breast cancer 143
   cervical cancer, treatment 156
   of the cervix 151
   defined 4
   statistics 4

In situ cancer
   in breasts 140
In utero 430g
In vitro tests 344, 430g
In vivo 430g
Incidence
   summary table **119–21**
Inclusion granules
   illustrated 29
Indomethacin
   and AIDS 404
Industrial hygienist 430g
Infant exam by mother 316, **328**
Infection 80
   is cancer infectious? 91
   as a cause of cancer 90–92
   summary table **119–21**
Initiation 430g
Initiator 430g
   defined 3
Inosine pranobes
   and AIDS 404
Insecticides
   and brain tumors 183
Institute for the Advancement of
   Health 458
Insurance companies 456
Intercourse
   painful 155
Interferon 12, 223, **231,** 232, 430g
   and AIDS 404, 405
   described 231
   side effects 448
   types 230, 231
   use 231
Interleukin 231, 232
Interleukin-2 12, 223
   and AIDS 404
Interleukin-3 (IL-3) 230
Internal mammary chain 430g
International Agency for Research
   on Cancer (IARC) 96, 442
International Association of Cancer
   Victims 16
International Association of Laryn-
   gectomees 454
International cancer incidence
   441–442
   table 441
International Union Against Cancer
   16
Interpersonal considerations **257–62**
Interphase 39, 430g
Interstines
   see *Small intestines* or *Colon and
     rectum*
Intracranial pressure
   increased death from 22
Intrauterine device (IUD)
   and cervical cancer 151
Intravenous drug use
   and AIDS 388

Intravenous drug users
    and HIV infection 391
Intravenous pyelogram (IVP)
    described 167
    and urinary tract
        cancers 167
Invasive 430g
Ion 430g
Ionic bond 430g
Ionizing radiation 430g
    list of cancers from 315
Irritation Theory 10
Ischemia
    defined 18
Islet cell carcinoma
    drugs used in treatment 446
Isogenic 430g
Isolation
    and AIDS 417
Isoprinosine
    and AIDS 404
Isoprophyl alcohol manufacture
    and cancer 97
Isotopes 430g

Japanese
    and stomach cancer 177
Jaundice
    and pancreas cancer 179
Jaw cancer **169–71**
Jejunum 135
John Birch Society 16

Kala-azar 91
Kaplan, Henry 11
Kaposi's sarcoma **395**
    AIDS related 12, 395
    autopsy studies 395
    classical 395
    compared to other sarcomas 188
    described 188
    drugs used in treatment 446
    first reports of in AIDS 12, 388
    history of 395
    and interferon 231
    radiation therapy for 404
    treatment for 404
    types 395
Kaposi, Moritz 395
Karyotype 430g
Kennaway, Ernest L. 10
Ketoconazole
    for prostate cancer 149
Kidney
    illustrated 288
Kidney cancer
    anatomy 166
    and asbestos 98
    diagnosis 167
    early detection 167
    and kidney stones 167
    and obesity 167

physiology 166
prevention 167
screening for 167
and smoking 87
survival rate trends, table 440
symptoms 167
types 166
Killer cell
    see *Immune system*
Kingsley, Charles 359
Koch's postulates 378
Kornberg, A. 50
Krant, Melvin J. 240
Krestin 230
Kübler-Ross, Elisabeth 301, 417
Kurosawa, Akira 252

L-asparaginase 223
Lactate dehydrogenase (LDH)
    and kidney cancer 167
Lactation
    defined 94
Lactones 430g
Laetrile 16
LaLanne, Jack 275
Laparoscopy
    for ovarian cancer 158
Laparotomy 430g
    for ovarian cancer 158
    for staging lymphomas 194
Large bowel
    see *Colon and rectum*
Large intestine
    see *Colon and rectum*
Larschan, Edward J. 306, 308
Larschan, Richard J. 306, 308
Laryngeal cancer **172–73**
    diagnosis 173
    early detection 173
    epidemiology 173
    and genetics 173
    glottic 173
    prevention 173
    prognosis 173
    risk factors 173
    supraglottic 173
    symptoms 173
    treatment 173
Laryngectomy 430g
Larynx
    anatomy 172
    and smoking 173
    summary table **120**
Larynx cancer
    also see *Laryngeal cancer*
    and asbestos 98
    and smoking 87
Laser 430g
    biopsy 155
    for brain tumors 183
    for CNS tumors 183
Laser surgery

and vulvar cancer 161
Laser therapy
    for cervical cancer 156
    and laryngeal cancer 173
Lawrence Livermore National
        Laboratory
    and melanoma 125
Laws, Priscilla W. 371
Lead
    and brain tumors 183
    and lung cancer 133
    and multiple myeloma 201
LeBlanc 10
Ledran, Henri 9
Legal aspects
    rights of the cancer patient 240–42
Legal organizations 456
Legionnaire's disease 91
Lehninger, A. L. 50
Leib, Steven 255
Leiomyoma 22
Leiomyosarcoma 22, 206
Leishmaniasis 91
Lentinan 230
LeShan, Lawrence
    emotional life history studies 282
Lesion 430g
Leucosis 430g
Leukemia 22, 63, **190, 196–99**, 430g
    acute lymphocytic leukemia (ALL)
        197
    acute lymphocytic leukemia
        (ANLL) 199
    acute myelogenous leukemia
        (AML) 197
    acute myelomonocytic leukemia
        (AMML) 197
    acute vs chronic 190
    adult T-cell 67
    and AIDS 67
    aminopterin 11
    and atomic bombs 103
    and benzene 98
    blastic vs cystic 197
    blood counts 67
    and bone marrow biopsy 198
    and bone marrow transplantation
        198
    and chemotherapy 198
    from chemotherapy 112
    in children 203
    in children, story 204
    chronic lymphocytic leukemia
        (CLL) 197
    chronic myelogenous leukemia
        (CML) 197
    compared to lymphoma 189
    described **190**, 197
    diagnosis 198
    early detection 197
    emotional therapy for 198
    epidemiology 197

Leukemia *continued*
  family cluster 197
  Farber, Sidney 11
  and fluorscopy 197
  hairy cell and interferon 231
  heredity 197
  Hiroshima and Nagasaki studies 197
  history 11
  human T-cell leukemia virus, (HTLV-1) 12
  immunotherapy for 198
  and Philadelphia chromosome 197
  pre-leukemia 198
  prevention 197
  prognosis 199
  radiation and 103, 197
  and radiation therapy 198
  radiation therapy for 218
  risk factors 197
  and spontaneous regression 199
  summary table **121**
  survival rate trends, table 440
  symptoms 198
  table **191**
  treatment 198
  types 197
  types of chemotherapy 198
  types of leukemia and radiation 103
Leukemia Society of America 454
Leukemogenic 430g
Leukocytes 58, 190
Leukocytes
  also see *White blood cell*
Leukopenia
  and chemotherapy 229
Leukopheresis
  for leukemia 198
Leukoplakia 322
  cytological methods 170
  detection techniques 170
  and laryngeal cancer 173
  natural history, in the mouth 170
  and oral cancers 170
  of the penis 165
  treatment 170
Leukoplakis 430g
Leuprolide
  for prostate cancer 149
  side effects 448
Levamisole 230, 231
Levy, Barry S. 96
Ligation 430g
Linear accelerator 430g
  illustration 215
  see *Radiation treatment*
Lip cancer **169–71**
  and smoking 86
  and sun exposure 170
Lipid 430g
Lipoma 22, 188

Liposarcoma 22
Liposome-encapsulated biologicals 230
Lissauer, Heinrich
  chemotherapy, history 221
Listeria 22
Liver
  anatomy 180
  physiology 180
Liver cancer 63, 180–81
  diagnosis 181
  drugs used in treatment 447
  early detection 181
  epidemiology 181
  and hepatitis B virus 69
  and parasites 90
  prevention 181
  primary hepatocellular carcinoma 69
  prognosis 181
  risk factors 181
  symptoms 181
  treatment 181
Liver flukes (clonorchis) 91
Liver transplantation
Liver/biliary cancer
  summary table **120**
Living Will 308–11
  example of 310
  right to die laws 309
  Society for the Right to Die 311
Loa loa 91
Log kill hypothesis 223–24
Lomustine
  side effects 449
Low-fiber diet
  list of cancers from 315
Lumpectomy
  see *Mastectomy, partial*
Lung cancer **132–34**
  and asbestos 97, 133
  and chest x-rays 133
  and chromium 98
  defined 132
  detection 133
  development, illustrated 369
  diagnosis 134
  and diet 133
  drugs used in treatment 445, 447
  epidemiology 133
  filtered vs non-filtered 133
  from smoking 86
  and furniture dust 99
  general statistics 4
  genetics 133
  history of 133
  lost earnings related to 443
  mesothelioma 97, 133
  oat-cell and work exposure 96
  oat-cell (small cell anaplastic) 132
  and pollution 117
  prevention 133

  prognosis 133
  and radiation 104
  radiation therapy for 218
  risk factor 133
  scarring of lung 133
  second-hand smoke 133
  and sputum cytology 133
  summary table **119**
  survival rate trends, table 440
  symptoms 134
  treatment 134
  types and percentages 23
  types of 132
Lung cells
  types 369–70
Lung, small cell (oat-cell)
  used in treatment 445
Lye burn
  of the esophagus 175
Lymph 430g
Lymph gland 430g
Lymph node
  and breast cancer 143
  of the breast and armpit, illustrated 321
  described 320
  in immune system 57
  of the groin, illustrated 321
  of the neck, illustrated 320
  removal in breast cancer 144
  scalene, in lung cancer 134
  self-examination 193, **320–21**
  swelling and AIDS 399
Lymphadenopathy 430g
  in AIDS 399
  in HIV infection 399
Lymphadenopathy-associated virus 389
Lymphangiography 430g
  defined 158
  for ovarian cancer 158
Lymphatic spread 19
Lymphatic system
  illustrated 54
Lymphedema 430g
Lymphoblast 190
Lymphoblastoma 430g
Lymphocyte activation factor 230
Lymphocytes 190, 430g
  and lymphoma 190
  defined 58
  illustrated 190
  T or B 58, 190
  T, general 58
Lymphocytic interstitial pneumonitis (LIP)
  in AIDS 402
Lymphocytic leukemia 22
Lymphoid system, illustrated 190
Lymphokines 230
Lymphoma **190–91, 192–95,** 430g
  also see *Hodgkin's disease*

and AIDS 398
and B-lymphocytes 190
biopsing for 194
in children 205
classification for treatment 194
a cluster case 193
compared to leukemias 189
described 190
diagnosis 194
discovered during infant/child
    exam 329
and drugs 193
early detection 193–94
epidemiology 193
and heredity 193
and HIV 193
and immune suppression 193
and infections 193
lymph node self-examination 194
mycosis fungoides 195
naming described 21
non-Hodgkin's
and occupation 193
and parasites 91
prevention 193–94
prognosis 195
radiation therapy for 218
risk factors 193
Sezary's syndrome 195
of the small bowel 135
staging 194
symptoms 194
and T-lymphocytes 190
table **191**
treatment 194
Lymphomatoid granulomatosis 191
Lymphosarcoma 22, 430g
Lymphotoxin 230
Lysosome 430g
    illustrated 29, 31
Lysozyme 430g

Machinists
    and urinary tract cancers 167
Macromolecules 431g
Macrophage 58, 230
    and smoking 88
    illustrated 190
    and lymphoma 191
    in the lungs 230
Macrophage activation factor (MAF)
    230
Macrophage cytoxic factor (MCF) 230
Macrophage chemotactic factor 230
Macrophage growth factor (MGF) 230
Magenta 97
Magnesium
    and esophagus cancer 175
Magnetic resonance imaging (MRI)
    431g
    for breast cancer 143

and central nervous system
    tumors 183
and cost 203
data from MRI
and pituitary gland cancer 185
and retinoblastoma 205
Make Today Count 455
Malabsorption 272
Malaria 69, 91, 393
Male cancers 148
Male genetalia cancers
    see specific site of cancer
Maleic anhydride-divinyl ether
    (MVE-2) 230
Malignant
    described 18, 43
Malignant melanoma 22
    also see *Melanoma*
Malignant myeloma
    vs bone cancer 188
Malignant teratoma 22
Malignant tumor 431g
Mammography **330–37,** 431g
    BCDDP study 143
    calcifications 331
    cost 335
    dedicated equipment, described
        335
    false-positives and false-negatives
        335–36
    getting a mammogram 333
    guidelines 143, 336
    guidelines for check-ups 315
    HIP study 143
    history of 12
    history of development **331**
    illustration of abnormal breast 332
    illustration of normal breast 333
    and in situ cancer 143
    machine, illustrated 143, 334
    and Nancy Reagan 143
    other imaging techniques 336–37
    and radiation 143
    radiation dose 373
    radiation risks 335
    secondary prevention 316
    table of recommendations 337
    what it shows 331–21
    why don't women get more mam-
        mograms? 334
    xeromammography 333
Manuel, Francine 274
Margolin, Frederick 331
Marijuana
    and cancer 88
    and chemotherapy 229
    oral use 229
Marsee, Sean 87
Mass spectrometry 431g
Massachusetts General Hospital 11
Massage therapy 274

Mastectomy 431g
    also see *Breast cancer*
    Halsted and 10, 144
    history 10
    modified 144
    partial (segmented) 145
    radical mastectomy, defined 10
    simple 144
    types 144
    types, illustrated **145**
Maturation factors 230
Maximum Contaminant Levels
    (MCLs) 375
McFarland, California
    cases and water pollution 372
McGinn, Kerry Anne 285, 330
McWaters, David S. 220
Measles 23
Meat
    see *Diet*
    table 348
Mechlorethamine 227
    side effects 449
Mediastinoscopy
    defined 134
Medical oncologists
    defined 221
Medical practice
    list of cancers from 315
Medications and urinary tract
    cancers 167
Meditation 264
    and stress 283
    for pain 222
Medullary carcinoma
    of the thyroid 184
Medulloblastoma
    in children 182, 203
    drugs used in treatment 446
    prognosis 203
    radiation therapy for 218
Megakaryoblast 190
Meiosis 40, 431g
    and gametes 40
    illustrated 42
Melanoma **123,** 431g
    ABCD rule 126
    appearance 126, 130
    appearance comparison tables 129
        –30
    in Australians 125, 442
    biopsing 129
    and congenital moles 127
    diagnosis 129
    drugs used in treatment 447
    and dysplastic nevi 127
    epidemiology 125
    genetics 125
    and hormones 125
    immunotherapy for 130
    monoclonal antibodies 130
    name described 21

Melanoma *continued*
non-skin sites 123
and occupational exposure 125
prognosis 130
risk factors 125
and seborrheic keratosis 127
spontaneous regression 130
summary table **119**
survival rate trends, table 440
symptoms 129
treatment 130
Melphalan
and leukemia 197
side effects 449
Membrane
described 28
phospholipids in 28
transport of molecules through 31
Memorial Hospital 10
Memory cells 58
Meningeal sarcoma 22
Meningioma 22, 182
Menopause
as a factor in breast cancer
and hormone replacement 111
Menstruation
and breast cancer 94
and the breast 140
Mercaptopurine
side effects 449
Mesothelioma 133, 431g
and asbestos 98
and smoking 98
Messenger RNA 431g
Metabolism 431g
Metal workers
and urinary tract cancers 167
Metaphase 39, 40, 431g
Metaplastic cells
in the lungs 370
Metastasis 18, 431g
defined 18
Methotrexate 223, 226, 228
and chemotherapy history 221
side effects 449
Methoxpsoralens 113
Microfiliments
described 30
illustrated 30
Microtubules
described 30
illustrated 30
Microvilli
illustrated 29
Microwave cooking 352
Migration inhibitory factor (MIF) 230
Mind
and recovery 264
Mind-body
and stress 281
Misonidazole 168
Mitochondria 431g

described 31
illustrated 29
Mitomycin
side effects 449
Mitoses
identifying cancer 19
Mitosis 39, 431g
defined 18
illustrated 41
steps 39
Mitotane
side effects 449
Mitotic figures 18
Mixed bacterial vaccines 230
MOHS' technique 212
MOHS' surgery diagrammed 130
Molecule 431g
defined 27, 129
Moles
found during skin self-examination 319–20
Mongolism 431g
Monoclonal antibodies 431g
for breast tumors 337
CA-125 158
history and 12
history of development 232
how they are made 232
and lung cancer testing 133
for ovarian cancer detection 158
in melanoma treatment 130–31
for research 232
Monocytes
illustrated 190
and lymphoma 191
Mononucleosis 63, 69
and Hodgkin's disease 193
mono-like illness and AIDS 401
Montagnier, Dr. Luc 389
MOPP regimen 194, 227
Morbidity 431g
Mormons
and pancreas cancer 179
Morning after pill 161
Mortuis vivos docent 293
Mouth self-examination 315
how to **322–23**
Mouth and throat cancer
also see *Oral cancers*
summary table **120**
Mouth cancer **169–71**
MRI
see *Magnetic Resonance Imaging*
Mucositis
and radiation treatment 171
Mullen, Barbara Dorr 285
Muller, Johannes 9
Multidisciplinary approaches
and childhood cancers 203
and surgery 211
team approach 264
treatment 208

treatment team 212
Multiple endocrine neoplasms
(M.E.N.) 186
Multiple myeloma 22, 200–01
and back pain 201
compared to lymphoma and
leukemia 191
described 191
diagnosis 201
early detection 201
epidemiology 201
and mink ranchers 201
and occupation 201
prevention 201
prognosis 201
and radiation 201
risk factors 201
summary table **121**
symptoms 201
treatment 201
whites vs blacks 201
Multiple sclerosis
and Hodgkin's disease 193
Mumps 63
and testicular cancer 164
Muramyl tripeptide
and AIDS 404
Muramyldipeptide (MDP) 230
Muscles
cancers of 187–88
Mustard gas
and chemotherapy, history 221
and laryngeal cancer 173
and lung cancer 133
Mutagenesis 431g
Mutagens
and carcinogeneses 47
described 38
Mutant 431g
Mutation 431g
frameshift mutation 39
thymine dimer 39
Mycosis fungoides 191
and interferon 231
drugs used in treatment 446
Myeloblast 190
Myelocytic 431g
Myelogenous leukemia 22
Myeloma
drugs used in treatment 447
Myelomatosis 431g

N, N-Bis (2-chloroethyl)-2 naph-
thylamine (Chlornaphazine)
table 197
N-137 230
Nasal cancers
and furniture dust 99
Nasopharynx cancer 169–71
symptoms **171**
Nathan, Laura E. 257
National Academy of Sciences

diet and cancer report 82
National Ambient Air Quality Standards 376
National Association of Social Workers 455
National Cancer Act 11, 49
National Cancer Foundation, Inc. 453
National Cancer Institute
    defined 14
    described 248
    history and 11, 14
National Hospice Organization 457
National Institute for Occupational Safety and Health 98
National Leukemia Association 454
National Library of Medicine (NLM) 453
National Self-Help Clearing House 455
Natural history of cancer 6
Necrosis 431g
    defined 18
Neoplasia 431g
    described 43
    discussion 73
Neoplasm 41g
    defined 18
    described 43
Newplastic transformation 431g
Nephroblastoma
    see *Wilms' tumor*
Neurilemoma 182
Neuroblastoma 22, **204–05**
    described 204
    drugs used in treatment 447
    prognosis 205
    and spontaneous regression 205
    symptoms 205
    treatment 205
Neurofibromatosis 431g
    CNS cancer in children 203
Neurofibrosarcoma 206
Neutron generators
    and radiation therapy 214
Neutrophils 58, 190
    in the lung 370
Nevi
    defined 127
New York Cancer Hospital 10
Nickel 97
    and laryngeal cancer 173
    and lung cancer 86, 133
    in water 118
Nickel refining
    and cancer 97
Nicolson, Garth 30, 51
Nicotine 86, 359
    chemistry of 359
    physiology of 359
Nicotinic acid
    and esophagus cancer 175

Nipple
    deviation 143
    discharge 143
    retraction 143
Nitrates 431g
    in water 118
Nitrite inhalants
    and AIDS 398
Nitrogen mustard 223, 227
Nitrosamines 87
    and stomach cancer 177
    in smokeless tobacco 87
Nitroso compounds 431g
NK (natural killer) cell 60, 230, 232
    see *Immune system, natural killer cells*
Nocardia 23
    in AIDS 401
Nocardia rubra cell wall skeleton (CWS) 230
Non-Hodgkin's lymphoma
    compared to other lymphomas 191
    described 191
    drugs used in treatment 447
    summary table **121**
Non-melanoma skin cancer
    see *Skin cancer*
    summary table **119**
Nonoxynol-9 411
Nosocomal infections 431g
    defined 23
Nuclear sap 431g
Nucleic acids 431g
Nucleoli 32
Nucleolus 431g
    illustrated 29
Nucleotide 431g
Nucleus 431g
    described 32
    illustrated 29
Nuns
    and cervical cancer 94
Nurse oncologists 212
Nutrition
    and AIDS 411
    and AIDS therapy 405
    cancer patient and 271–73
    causes of problems 272
    and chemotherapy 229
    and menstruation 94
    and recovery from cancer 264
    after surgery 212

Oat cell cancer
    see *Lung cancer*
Obesity 167, **352**
    and endometrial cancer 154
    list of cancers from 315
Obstruction
    of vital organ, death from 22
Obstructive edema 431g
Occupation

and asbestos 117
    and bladder cancer 167
    and Hodgkin's disease 193
    list of cancers from 315
    and lung cancer 75
    and lymphoma 193
    and multiple myeloma 201
    and pollution 114–16
    and smoking 89
    summary table **119–21**
    and urinary tract cancer 167
    workers 10
Occupational cancer 95–99
    and airborne dust 99
    and asbestos 97–98
    in chimney sweeps 9
    history of 9
    list of chemicals associated with cancer 97
    Pott, Sir Percivall 9
    scrotal cancer 8
Occupational therapists 264
Odell, Rollin 213
Oils 97
OK-432 156
Oligodendroglioma 22
    prognosis 183
Oncogene theory 66
Oncogenes 66, 75
    described 46
    proto-oncogenes 67
    and transformation 67
    and viruses 67
Oncogenesis 431g
Oncogenic 431g
Oncogenic viruses
    and feline leukemia 67
Oncologist
    gynecological oncologist 15
    medical 16
    pediatric 16
    radiation 16
    surgical 15
    urological 15
Oncology 431g
    comparative 73
    compared to hematology 189
    defined 15, 18
Oncovin 227
Operator gene 431g
Operon 432g
Opportunistic cancers
    in AIDS 395
    Kaposi's sarcoma 395
    non-Hodgkin's lymphoma 395
    in transplant recipients 395
Oral cancers
    diagnosis 170–71
    early detection 170
    epidemiology 170
    erythroplasia 170
    leukoplakia 170

Oral cancers *continued*
  prevention 170
  prognosis 171
  radiation therapy for 171, 217
  risk factors 170
  symptoms 170–71
  treatment 171
Oral candidiasis
  in AIDS
Oral cavity cancer
  and smoking 87
Oral cavity
  mouth self-examination, how to
    323
  torus palatinus 323
  uvula 323
Oral hygienists
  and detection of oral cancers 170
Oral methoxalen 195
Oral self-examination
  for oral cancers 170
  see *Mouth self-examination*
Orchitis 327
Organ failure
  death from 22
Organ transplant
  and brain tumors 183
Organelles
  defined 28
Organizations
  cancer-related 452–60
  experimental/alternative 458–60
Ortho-toluidine 97
Osler, Sir William 282
Osteogenic sarcoma 22, **206**
  also see *Bone cancer*
  described 206
  drugs used in treatment 446
  locations 206
  prognosis 206
  symptoms 206
  treatment 206
Osteoma 22
Osteomyelitis
  multiple myeloma 201
Osteoporosis
  and smoking 88
Ostomate
  defined 286
Ostomy 285–89, 432g
  abdominal ostomy 286
  defined 286
  and digestion 286
  illustrated 288–89
Ovarian cancer 157–59
  AFP for 158
  blood tests for 158
  CA-125 for 158
  CEA for 158
  diagnosis 158
  drugs used in treatment 447
  early detection 158

epidemiology 158
intraperitoneal
  prevention 158
  prognosis 158
  reproductive factors 158
  risk factors 158
  summary table **119**
  survival rate trends, table
  symptoms 158
  treatment 158
  types 157
Ovaries
  anatomy 157
  illustrated 152, 153
  physiology 157
  removal for breast cancer 145
Ovary cancer
  see *Ovarian cancer*
Oxidation 432g
Oxidative phosphorylation 31
Oxygen effect 432g
Ozone 45, 432g

P-24 400
PABA (para-aminobenzoic acid)
  and sunscreens 126
Page, Harriet S. 95–99, 108–09, 110
  –13, 114–16
Paget
  and emotions 281
Paget's disease
  and bone cancer 188
  of the breast 140
Pain
  addiction myth 222
  from cancer 222
  causes 222
  prevention of 222
  treatment of 222
Painters
  and urinary tract cancers 167
Palliation
  history of 221
Palliative treatment 432g
Palpation 432g
Pan
  and oral cancers 170
Pancreas 184
  anatomy 178
  described 178
  endocrine tumors 178, 185–86
  insulin and 178
  physiology 178
Pancreas cancer **178–79**
  in American Indians 179
  diagnosis 179
  drugs used in treatment 447
  early detection 179
  epidemiology 179
  in Hawaiians 179
  prevention 179
  prognosis 179

risk factors 179
  and smoking 87
  summary table **120**
  survival rate trends, table 440
  symptoms 179
  treatment 179
Pap test 12, 20, 432g
  categories (classes) 20
  for endometrial cancer 155
  guidelines for check-ups 315
  in high-risk women 154
  history 11
  methods of taking a Pap 20
  politics 155
  rationale for recommendations 154
  recommendations 154
  squamocolumnar junction, defined
    151
  technique 20, 151
Papanicolaou, George 11
Papillary
  defined 21
Papillary adenocarcinoma
  of the thyroid 184
Papovarviruses 67
Parametrium 432g
Parasites 167
  and bladder cancer 167
  and cancer 90–92
  list of cancers from 315
  and liver cancer 91
  major types 91
Parasitic theory of cancer 10
Parathyoid 184
Parenteral 432g
Parotid gland
  cancer in 171
  importance of the facial nerve 171
Partnerships 267
Pathology 432g
  benign vs malignant 17
  benign vs malignant, table 23
  defined 17
  differentiation 18
Pathology of cancer 17–23
  identifying a cancer cell 19
Patient
  and alienation 270
  anger 268
  attitude 270
  fear 267
  feelings 253–54
  and hope 270
  and loneliness 270
  needs for physician 256
  rights 240–42
  self-esteem 269
  social services 265
  support teams 265
  total patient care **263**
PCP 432g
Pelletier, Kenneth 284

Pelvic examination 432g
  for detection of ovarian cancer 158
  for endometrial cancer 157
  guidelines for check-ups 315
  technique of 158
Penis cancer 165
  detection 165
  epidemiology 165
  prognosis 165
  risk factors 165
  symptoms 165
  treatment 165
Pesticides
  and brain tumors 183
  and water pollution 375
Peto, Richard 12, 79, 82, 93–94
Petroleum workers
  and urinary tract cancers 167
Peutz-Jeughers Syndrome 137
Peyer's patches 57
Peyrilhe, Bernard 9
Pharyngeal cancer **169–71**
Pharynx cancer
  and smoking 87
Phase contrast microscopy (PCM)
  376
Phenacetin 113, 167
Phenoxyacetic acid herbicides 97
Phenylbutazone
  and leukemia 197
Pheochromocytoma 22
  also see *Adrenal gland cancer*
Philadelphia chromosome 432g
Phospholipids 30
Photochemotherapy 195
Photoflurography
  for stomach cancer 177
Photons 432g
Photosynthesis 432g
Phycomycetes 23
Phylogeny 432g
Physical rehabilitation 264
Physical therapists 264
Physician
  attitude 295
  needs of patients 256
Physician-patient relationship
  293–94
  honesty in 299
Physicians' checkup
  what should be included 316
Picibanil (OK432) 230
Pigmented nevus 22
Pill
  see *Birth control pill*
Pineal tumors 182
Pinocytic vesicle
  illustrated 29
Pitot, Henry C. 12
Pituitary adenoma 182
  prognosis 183
Pituitary gland 432g

described 185
Pituitary gland cancer
  diagnosis 185
  locations 185
  prognosis 185
  symptoms 185
  treatment 185
Placebo effect 282–83
Placenta 162
Placental neoplasia 161
  diagnosis 161
  epidemiology 161
  HCG in 161
  prognosis 161
  treatment 161
  types 161
Plasma cell
  illustrated 190
  and multiple myeloma 200
Plasmapheresis 230
Platelets 432g
  illustrated 190
Plato 279
Pleomorphism
  defined 19
Plicamycin
  side effects 449
Pneumocystis 23
Pneumonia 63
Pneymocystis carinii 91
Pneumocystis carnii pneumonia
  (PCP)
  described 388
  first reports of in AIDS 388
Pneumonectomy 432g
Polarized light microscopy (PLM) 376
Polio 63
  and Hodgkin's disease 193
Politics
  and AIDS 418
  and genetic screening 379
  legislation for clean water 375
  and Pap recommendations 155
Pollution **114–16**
  air 375–76
  and asbestos 117
  and benzo(a)pyrene or B(a)P 117
  cigarette smoke 117
  radon 117
  water 375
Poly A:U 230
Poly IC-LC 230
Polychlorinated biphenyls (PCBs)
  97, 118
Polycyclic aromatic hydrocarbons 10,
  96
  and lung cancer 133
  and skin cancer 124
Polycyclic hydrocarbons 432g
Polycythemia vera 22
Polymers 432g
  described 28

Polymorphic reticulosis 191
Polynucleotide 432g
Polyoma virus 432g
Polyp 136, 432g
  also see *Colon and rectal cancer*
  adenomatous 136
  size vs cancer 136
  villous adenoma 136
Polyp (intestinal)
  described 340
  incidence 340
  and President Reagan 340
  removal of 340
  and sigmoidoscopy 340
Polypeptide 432g
Polyposis 432g
Polyvalent vaccine 432g
Poor people
  and cancer 380–83
  oral cancer in 170
  and stomach cancer 177
Poppers
  and AIDS 398
Positron emission tomography (PET)
  184
Pott, Percivall 9
  and chimney sweeps 96
  and prevention 96
Poverty
  and cancer 382
Pre-cancer
  see *Dysplasia*
Prednisone 227
Pregnancy
  and the breast 140
  and cancer risk 94
  and cervical cancer 153
  and endometrial cancer 154
  and neoplasia 162
  and ovarian cancer 158
Preservatives
  and stomach cancer 177
Preserved foods
  list of cancers from 315
Prevention
  of AIDS 409–15
  and breast cancer **142**
  cancer prevention study 1 (CPS-I)
    14
  cancer prevention study 2 (CPS-II)
    14
  cervical cancer **154–55**
  community plan 317
  endometrial cancer 155
  esophagus cancer 175
  family plan 317
  and gall bladder cancer 181
  general 5–7
  laryngeal cancer 173
  liver cancer 181
  pancreas cancer 179
  personal plan 317

Prevention *continued*
  primary prevention, defined 6
  secondary prevention, defined 6
  skin cancer 126
  stomach cancer 177
  tertiary prevention, defined 6
  thyroid cancer 185
  upstream thinking 7
Primary prevention 315
  and smoking 360
  list of cancers that can be primarily prevented 315
  list of factors to be avoided 315
  practicing primary cancer prevention 315
  summary table **119–21**
Printers
  and urinary tract cancers 167
Procarbazine 227
Procarbazine HCl
  side effects
Procaryotic 28
  illustrated
Procto 432g
Proctosigmoidoscopy
  see *Sigmoidoscopy*
Progeny 432g
Progesterone
  and the breast 140
Progesterone receptors
  and breast cancer 144
Progestin 111
Prognosis 432g
Progression 432g
Promoter 432g
  defined 3
Promotion 432g
Prophase 432g
Prostaglandin inhibitors 230
Prostate 432g
Prostate antigen
  serum test 148
Prostate cancer **147–49**
  in Alameda, Calif. blacks 441
  and alcoholism 148
  anatomy 148
  autopsy studies 148
  and benign prostatic hyperplasia 148
  biopsy 149
  in blacks 148
  blood tests for 148
  chemotherapy 149
  detection by ultrasound 148
  diagnosis 148–49
  and diet 148
  drugs used in treatment 447
  early detection 148
  epidemiology 148
  and erections 149
  inheritability 148
  MRI in 149

physiology 148
prevention 148
prognosis 149
prostate self-examination 148
prosthesis 149
radiation
radiation therapy for 149, 218
risk factors 148
serum phosphate acid phosphatase 148
serum prostate antigen 148
and sex 148
summary table **119**
surgery for 149
survival rate trends, table 440
symptoms 148–49
treatment 149
types, percentages 23
Prostate self-examination 148, 316
  how to **327**
  rationale 327
Prosthesis 212, 432g
  oral cancers 171
  laryngeal cancer 173
  testicular cancer 165
Prostitutes
  and cervical cancer 151
  and HIV infection 392
Protease-antiprotease 88
Protein 432g
  defined 27
  enzymes 28
  functions of 27
  unwinding protein 37
Protein synthesis
  control of 35
  described 34
  illustrated 36–37
  steps in 34
  transcription 34
  translation 34
Proton 432g
Protozoa 23, 91
Provirus 432g
Psammomatous
  defined 21
Pseudomonas 22
Psychological aspects
  of AIDS 416–18
  an essay 253–54
  patients' needs 256
Public education
  about AIDS 412
  about Pap tests 155
Pulmonary embolus
  death from 22
Purine 33
Purine base 432g
Pyrimidines 33
Pyrmidine base 432g

Quackery 432g
  costs 243
  how cancer patients become involved 245
  investigation of unproven methods 247–48
  list of scientifically unproven methods of cancer treatment 246
  major sources of information 248
  overview 243
  proponents 244
  also see *Unproven methods*

Rabies 63
Rad 433g
  see *Radiation*
Radiation
  avoiding unnecessary x-rays 371–73
  and breast cancer 217
  cosmic radiation 105
  definition 214
  dose for cancer 185
  ionizing 105
  ionizing radiation 101
  law of radiosensitivity 101
  and leukemia 197
  and lung cancer 133
  measurement 214
  and multiple myeloma 201
  non-ionizing radiation 101
  and ovarian cancer 158
  and pancreas cancer 179
  for prostate cancer 218
  radiobiology 215
  risks from mammography 335
  and sarcomas 188
  summary table **119–21**
  table of doses 373
  terrestrial radiation 105
  and thyroid cancer 185
  types of 105
  ultraviolet radiation 101
  and urinary tract cancers 167
Radiation and cancer 100–07
  acute radiation syndrome 105
  and atomic bomb radioactivity 104
  and atomic energy 105
  atomic holocaust 106
  biological effects 102
  bone marrow effects 106
  of the breast 141
  frequency of mutation 105
  genetic effects 105
  Hiroshima and Nagasaki 105
  induction of cancer by radiation 102
  introduction to radiation 101
  long-time delay 102
  physics of radiation 101
  rad, defined 102

radiation hazards in peace and
war 105
radiologists' cancers 104
roentgen, defined 102
solar radiation **108–09**
sources of ionizing radiation 105
summary table 101, 107
threshold dose 102
and thymus gland 102
and thyroid cancer 104
Radiation biology 101
Radiation carcinogenesis
also see *Radiation and cancer*
in man 103
Radiation exposure
and stomach cancer 177
Radiation oncology **213–19**
also see *Radiation therapy*
described 213
history of 214
Radiation sickness 433g
Radiation therapy 432g
also see *Radiation and cancer*
adjuvant treatment 218
and bone cancers 188
brachytherapy 214, 215
for brain tumors 183
for breast cancer 144
for CNS tumors 183
for cervical cancer 156
and cobalt machines 214
cobalt unit, illustration 215
complications 218–19
definition 214
and esophagus cancer 175
future prospects 219
and gall bladder cancer 181
and gastrointestinal disturbances
272
history 10
for Hodgkin's disease 194, 217
and hyperthermia 216
interstitial implants 215
for Kaposi's sarcoma 404
and laryngeal cancer 173
law of radiosensitivity 10
and leukemia 198
linear accelerator 214
linear accelerator, illustration 215
and liver cancer 181
localization 217
and loss of appetite 272
for lymphomas 194
measurement 214
and multiple myeloma 201
and nutrition 272
and oral cancers 171
for oral cancers, side effects 171
and orthovoltage machines 214
and osteogenetic sarcoma 206
for ovarian cancer 158
overview 208

palliation 221
and pancreas cancer 179
for penile cancer 165
and pituitary gland cancer 185
planning treatment 215
for prostate cancer 149
psychosocial aspects 216
rad, defined 214
radiobiology 215
radiotherapy team 216
reontgen, defined 102
Wilhelm von Roentgen and 10
and sarcomas 188
side effects 217, 218–19
for specific cancers 217–18
staging 215
and stomach cancer 177
and supra-voltage machines
214
and testicular cancer 165
and thyroid gland cancer 185
and urinary tract cancers 168
and uterine cancer 156
for vaginal cancer 161
and vulvar cancer 161
Radical masteceomy (classical) 427g
Radioactive isotopes 433g
Radiobiology
also see *Radiation therapy*
in radiation therapy 215
Radiology
mammography 330–337
needle localization 144
Radiopaque 433g
Radon 117, **378**
and lung cancer 133
Rahe, Richard 280
Raymond, Greg 95–99, 374–80
RBE 433g
Reach to Recovery 14, 145, 453
Reagan, Nancy 143
Reagan, Ronald
and colon cancer 12
and polyps 12, 340
and sigmoidoscopy 12, 340
Recessive involvement 433g
Recombinant DNA 38
Recreational therapists 264
Rectal cancer
radiation therapy for 218
survival rate trends, table 440
Rectal self-examination
how to **327**
illustrated 327
rationale 327
Rectum
illustrated 288, 339
Red blood cells 190
Regression 433g
Rehabilitation **263**
Rehabilitation exercises
for the cancer patient 274–75

Relaxation
for pain 222
Remission 433g
Renal cancer
drugs used in treatment 447
see *Kidney cancer*
Renneker, Mark vi
Replication 433g
Repressor gene 433g
Reproductive factors
as causes of cancer
list of cancers from 93–94, 315
Rescue factor 226
Research
and AIDS 407–08
criteria for association 344
diet and cancer research 344
dietary research issues 344–45
rights of the cancer patient 240–42
toxicological testing 378–79
Resources
cancer-related, list **452–60**
Reticulum cell sarcoma 22
Retinoblastoma 205, 433g
described 205
detection of 205
drugs used in treatment 447
discovered during infant/child
exam by mother 328
genetics and 205
prognosis 205
radiation therapy for 218
symptoms 205
treatment 205
Retinoic acid
for leukoplakia treatment 170
Retinol 433g
Retribution
and AIDS 417
Retroid viruses 63
Retroviruses 46, 64
and AIDS 396
discovery of 46
feline leukemia virus 397
general 63
replication 63
reverse transcriptase 46
Reverse transcriptase 11, 46, 64, 65
Rhabdomyoma 22
Rhabdomyosarcoma 22, **205**
described 205
discovery during infant/child exam
by mother 328
prognosis 205
symptoms 205
treatment 205
Rheumatoid arthritis
and multiple myeloma 201
Ribavirin
and AIDS 405
Riboflavin
and esophagus cancer 175

Ribonucleic acid (RNA) 433g
  defined 33
  diagram 35
  messenger 34
  ribosomal 34
  transfer 34
Ribonucleotide 433g
Ribosome 32, 433g
  illustrated 29
Richards, Victor 12, 51
Richmond, J. B. 86
Ringworm
  radiation for 185
  and thyroid cancer 185
RNA polymerase 33
Robbins, Stanley L. 17, 71, 252
Rockefeller, Happy 11
Roentgen rays 433g
Roentgen, Willhem 10, 433g
Ronald McDonald Houses 454
Rosenbaum, Ernest H. 263, 267, 271,
    274, 276
Rosenbaum, Isadora R. 267, 271, 276
Rous, F. Peyton 10, 66
Rous sarcoma virus 433g
Rubber industry
  and cancer 97
Rubin, Philip 118, 226

Saccharine
  and urinary tract cancers 167
Safe Drinking Water Act
Safe sex
  and ovarian cancer 158
Salivary gland cancer 169–71
  symptoms 171
Salmonella 22
  in AIDS
Sarcoma **187–88,** 433g
  defined 187
  diagnosis 188
  drugs used in treatment 447
  early detection 188
  epidemiology 188
  how they spread 19
  prevention 188
  prognosis 188
  risk factors 188
  summary table **121**
  symptoms 188
  treatment 188
  types 188
Scalp fungal infections
  and sarcomas 188
Scars
  and skin cancer 124
Schistosoma haematobium
  and bladder cancer 167
Schistosomiasis 91
Scleroderma
  and multiple myeloma 201
Scrotal cancer 165

  and Sir Percivall Potts 165
Scrotum
  see *Testes*
Seborrheic keratosis 127
  discovery during skin self-
    examination
Secondary prevention 315
  practicing secondary cancer
    prevention 315
  and smoking 360
  summary table **119–21**
Seizures
  and symptoms of CNS tumors 183
Selenium
  in prostate cancer 148
Self-esteem 269
Self-examinations for cancer **318–29**
  list of 315–16
Selye, Hans 284
Semen
  and cervical cancer 152
Seminoma 22, 163
Senescence 433g
Serpentine rock
  and asbestos 376
Serratia 22
Seven warning signs of cancer 436
Seventh Day Adventists
  and pancreas cancer 179
Sex
  summary table **119–21**
Sex-linked 433g
Sexual behavior
  as causes of cancer 93–94
Sexual functions
  after prostate surgery 149
Sexual partners
  and HIV infection 392
Sexual practices
  and AIDS 411
  list of cancers from 315
Sexuality **264**
  and cancer 276–78
  and counseling 160
  and gynecological cancers 160
  stereotypes about gays 388
  and testicular cancer 165
Sexually-transmitted disease (STD)
  and cervical cancer 151
  and gynecological cancers 151
Sezary syndrome 191, 195
Shakespeare 361
Shilts, Randy
Shimkin, Michael B. 12, 51
Shoe manufacture
  and cancer 97
Sigmoid colon
  illustrated 288, 339
Sigmoidoscope
  flexible, illustrated 340
Sigmoidoscopy **137,** 338–42, 433g
  guidelines for check-ups 315

described 339
secondary prevention 316
Simonton approach 283–84
  for HIV therapy 405
  and imaging 284
  and positive attitude 284
  and stress 284
Singer, S. J. 51
Skin cancer 123–31
  and actinic keratoses (AK) 126
  in albinos 124
  appearance 126
  biopsing 129
  and burns 124
  dermatology and KS (in AIDS) 398
  diagnosis 128–29
  and dysplastic nevi 127
  early detection 126
  epidemiology 124
  epithelialomas vs carcinomas 123
  genetic dispositions to 124
  and heredity 79
  and MOHS' surgery 129
  and ozone layer 124
  prevention 126
  prognosis 129
  radiation therapy for 217
  risk factors 124
  and scars 124
  and seborrheic keratosis 127
  and skin types, table 126
  and solar radiation **109**
  solar radiation, table 125
  and sunscreens 126
  symptoms 128–29
  and tanning parlors 124
  treatment 129
  in whites vs blacks 124
Skin self-examination 315
  how to **319–20**
Skin types, table 126
Small intestine 135
Smell
  changes in from cancer 372–73
Smoking 358–66
  and AIDS 411
  and babies 88
  and bad breath 88
  biochemical smoker 359
  case histories of quitters 361–62
  and the community 88
  and disease 368
  and esophagus cancer 87
  and the family 88
  and gum disorders 88
  habitual smoker 360
  in history of cancer 12
  how people quit 361
  and the immune system 412
  and laryngeal cancer 173
  and leukemia 197
  list of cancers from 315

marijuana 88
message to stop 133
and morning cough 88
non-smokers risk 86
numbers of smokers 88
and oral cancers 170
and pancreas cancer 179
passive smoking 88, **378**
preventing smoking 360
psychological smoker 360
reverse smoking used in India 170
steps to quitting 361
and stomach cancer 177
stopping 360
types of smokers 359
and urinary tract cancers 167
why smokers smoke 359
at work 88
Smoking and cancer
first Surgeon General report 11
Smoking cessation
how to **358–66**
resources 362–66
Smokeless tobacco
list of cancers from 315
Snuff
see *Tobacco*
Social aspects **257–62**
job discrimination 291
Social readjustment rating scale 281
Social services 265
Society for the Right to Die 311
Socio-economic status
and cancer rates 381
Sodium diethyldithiocarbamate
(DTC) 230
Sodium diethyldithiocarbamate
(imuthiol)
and AIDS 404
Sodium nitrate
and stomach cancer 177
Sodium nitrite
and brain tumors 183
and stomach cancer 177
Soft-tissue cancer 187–88
Solar radiation **108–09**
aging of skin, table 125
cancer, table 125
and melanoma 109
and ozone 109
and skin cancer 109
tanning, table 125
UVA, UVB 109
Sontag, Susan 417
Soots 97
Sorensen, Kent 367
South Africa
and chromium 98
Spinal cord tumors 183
Spleen
in the immune system 57
Spontaneous regression **233–35**

defined 234
documented case 234
explanations for 234
and leukemia 199
in melanoma 130
and neuroblastoma 205
rate 234
sites, table 235
types of cancers 24
Sputum cytology **367–70**
and lung cancer 133
guidelines for check-ups 317
secondary prevention 315–16
technology 369
Sputum test 433g
Squamocolumnar junction
illustrated 153
Squamous cell
of the esophagus 174
of the vagina 161
see site of cancer (e.g., skin cancer)
Squamous cell carcinoma
of the lung 132
Squamous cell type
layrnx cancer 172
Staging 433g
principle 211
stages explained 20
TNM system explained 20
Starr, Kevin 62
Stem cell
illustrated 190
Steroids 112
Stitt, Carol A. 271
Stoklosa, Jean M. 276
Stoma
illustrated 289
Stomach
illustrated 288
Stomach cancer **176–77**
and asbestos 98
blacks and 177
diagnosis 177
early detection 177
epidemiology 177
history of incidence 176
in history 10
in Japan 177
prevention 177
prognosis 177
risk factors 177
and smoking 87
summary table **120**
survival rate trends, table 440
symptoms 177
treatment 177
types, percentage 23
and water pollution 118
Stool
self-testing for blood 328
Stool hidden blood test **137**
guidelines for check-ups 316–17

Streptococcal preparation (OK-432)
156
Streptozocin
side effects 449
Stress 79
and biofeedback 283
and cancer **279–84**
and change 283
and coping 282
described 280
fight-or-fright response 280
LeShan's studies 282
and meditation 283
and other diseases 279
and the placebo effect 282–83
rating scale 281
Stroke
death from 22
Strongyloides 91
Strontium 106
Structural genes 433g
Substrate 433g
Sun 108–09
lip cancer 170
Sun and cancer
see *Solar radiation*
Sunscreens
and skin cancer 126
guide based on skin types, table
127
SPF described 126
table 128
Suppressor cells (T8) 395
Supraclavicular nodes 433g
Suramin
and AIDS 4055
Surgeon General
report on smoking and lung cancer
11
Surgery
aspiration biopsy 210
basic principles 209–12
biopsing principles 210
for bladder cancer 168
for bone cancers 188
for brain tumors 183
breast cancer considerations 144
cancer surgery, overview **209–12**
for central nervous system tumors
183
communication with surgeons 210
CT-guided 183
cytoreductive surgery 158, 212
for esophagus cancer 175
excisional biopsy 210
fine-needle biopsy 211
for gall bladder cancer 181
Halsted radical mastectomy 144
of the head and neck 171
incisional biopsy 210
and incurability 212
intra-arterial for oral cancer 171

Surgery *continued*
    for kidney cancer 168
    for laryngeal cancer 173
    for liver cancer 181
    lumpectomy, illustration 145
    and nutrition 272
    operating principles 212
    of the oral cavity 171
    and osteogenic sarcoma 206
    for ovarian cancer 158
    overview 208
    for pancreas cancer 179
    for penis cancer 165
    for prostate cancer 149
    for recurrence 212
    reconstructive, breast 145
    reconstructive, head and neck 171
    recovery from 212
    and sarcomas 188
    second-look operations 212
    staging 211
    for stomach cancer 177
    surgical techniques 212
    for testicular cancer 165
    for thyroid cancer 185
    types of biopsy 210
    understanding the cancer surgeon 210
    for urinary tract cancers 168
    urostomy 168
    for uterine cancer 156
    for vaginal cancer 161
    for vulvar cancer 161
Surgical oncology
    described 210
Survival
    and Auschwitz 296
Synergism 433g
Syngenic grafting 433g
Synovial sarcoma 206
Syphilis
    and cervical cancer 151
Systemic lupus erthematosis
    and multiple myeloma 201

T-cell 433g
T-cell mediated 58
T-cell growth factor 230
T-cell replacing factor (TRF) 230
T-helper cells 230
T-lymphocytes
    also see *Lymphocytes*
    and lymphoma 190
T4 (helper)
    and lymphoma 191
T4 cell
    also see *Lymphocytes*
T4-helper, illustrated 190
T8 (suppressor)
    and lymphoma 191
    also see *Lymphocytes*
    illustrated 190

Talc
    and ovarian cancer 158
Tamoxifen 145, 228
    drugs for prostate cancer
Tamoxifen citrate
    side effects 449
Tanka women 142
Tanning parlors 124
Tapeworms 91
Tar 86, 97
Taste
    changes in from cancer 272–73
Team approach to treatment 208
Technical-grade chloromethyl
    methyl ether 96
Telecobalt unit 433g
Teletherapy
    and radiation therapy 214
Telophase 40, 433g
Temin, Howard 11
Template surfacat 433g
Temple, Shirley
    see *Black, Shirley Temple*
Tendons
    cancers of 187–88
Teratomas 163
Terminal
    discussed 294
    living will 309
Terminal care
    also see *Tertiary prevention*
    discussed by Kübler-Ross 304
Terry, Luther 11
Tertiary prevention 6
    and smoking 362
Testicular cancer 163–65
    biopsy method 164
    in blacks or whites 164
    blood tests for 164
    cis-platinum 11
    and DES 163
    diagnosis 164
    drugs used in treatment 446
    early detection 164
    epidemiology 164
    an essay 153–54
    genetics 164
    geographic difference 164
    history of treatment 11
    prevention 164
    prognosis 165
    risk factors 164
    screening for 164
    seminoma or non-seminoma 163
    and sexual function 165
    summary table **120**
    survival rate trends, table 440
    symptoms 164
    theories of causation 164
    trauma and 164
    treatment 165
    type 163

underwear and 164
undescended testes 164
Testicular self-examination 164, 315
    how to **325–26**
    illustrated 325
Testis
    anatomy 163
    cancer in 163
    physiology 163
Testosterone
    and the prostate 148
Tetrachlorodibenzo-para-dioxin
    (TCDD) 97
Textile workers
    and urinary tract cancers 167
Thanatology 433g
    also see *Death and dying*
Thermography 143, 433g
Thiobendazole 230
Thiogranine
    side effects 449
Thiotepa
    side effects 449
Thomas, L. 51
Thoracotomy
    defined 134
Throat cancer **169–71**
Thrombocytopenia 198
Thromboembolism
    and smoking 88
    and the pill 88
Thymine 33, 433g
Thymine dimer 39
Thymocyte mitogenic factor (TMF) 230
Thymosin 230
    and AIDS 404
Thymus gland
    illustrated 190
    in immunity 57
    and radiation 102
Thyroid 184
Thyroid cancer 184–86
    and biopsying 185
    and radiation 104, 185
    diagnosis 185
    early detection 185
    epidemiology 185
    prevention 185
    prognosis 185
    risk factors 185
    summary table **122**
    symptoms 185
    treatment 185
    types 184
Thyroid gland
    anatomy 184
    locations 184
Thyroid scan 185
Thyroid self-examination 315
    how to **322–23**
Tilorone 230

Tissue 433g
Tissue culture 433g
Tobacco 85–89
Tobacco
    advertising 360
    and cancer 86
    and cancer deaths 86
    and carbon monoxide 86
    and cardiovascular disease 87
    and chemicals 86
    and head and neck cancers 87
    and nicotine 86
    and oral cancers 170
    and tar 86
    cancers caused, list 86
    chew 87
    costs 89
    dip 87
    revenues from 89
    smokeless 87
    snuff 87
    summary table **119–21**
Tobacco cropper's syndrome 359
Tolerance 433g
Tomograms 433g
    for the lung 134
Tongue cancer 169–71
    and smoking 87
    symptoms 170
Tonsillectomy
    and Hodgkin's disease 193
Tonsils
    and thyroid cancer 185
    radiation for 185
Tooth decay
    after radiation treatment 171
Toxic shock syndrome 91
Toxicological testing 378–79
Toxicologist 433g
Toxoplasma 23
Tracheostomy 433g
Tracheostomy tube 173
Transcription 434g
    illustrated 36
    in protein synthesis 34
Transduction 434g
Transfer factor 230
    and AIDS 404
Transfer RNA 434g
Transformation 434g
    neoplastic 65
Transfusions of blood
    and AIDS 411
Transitional cell cancer
    see *Urinary tract cancer*
Translation 434g
    illustrated 36
    in protein synthesis 35
Transmission electron microscopy
    (TEM) 376
Transplant
    and brain tumors 184

Transplantation
    spread by 19
Transrectal ultrasonography (TRUS)
    148
Transverse colon
    illustrated 288
Transverse colostomy
    illustrated 289
Trauma
    and testicular cancer 164
Treatment
    and nutrition 272
    rights of the cancer patient 240–42
    strategies, illustrated 226
    summary table **119–21**
Tribondeau, L. 101
2,4,6-Trichlorophenol 97
Trichomonas 91
    and cervical cancer 152
Trichuris 91
Trihalomethanes (TMH) 117
Triplet 434g
Trisodium phosphonoformate
    and AIDS 405
Trophoblastic tumors
    see *Placental neoplasia*
Truck drivers
    and urinary tract cancers 167
Trypanosomiasis 91
Tuberculosis 22
    in AIDS
Tuberous sclerosis
    and CNS cancer in children 203
Tuftsin 230
Tumor 434g
    benign or malignant 18
    benign or malignant, table 18
    of the bone 188
    of cartilage 188
    classifications 20
    defined 18
    growth rate 225
    see specific tumor types
    of soft-tissue 188
    solid vs hematologic 225
Tumor antigen immunoassay
    and pancreas cancer 179
Tumor-associated antigen (TAA) 230
    and lung cancer 134
Tumor board
    defined 237
    function 237
Tumor necrosis factor (TNF) 230
Tumor registry 237
Tumor resistance 225–26
Tumoricidal 434g
Tylectomy
    see *Mastectomy, partial*
Typhoid
    and gall bladder cancer 181

Uganda
    and HIV infection 392
Ulcerative colitis
    and gall bladder cancer 181
Ulcers
    and smoking 88
    and stomach cancer 177
Ultrasound 143, 434g
    for ovarian cancer 158
    for prostate cancer early detection
        148
    transrectal ultrasonography 148
Ultraviolet radiation
    history of studies 109
    list of cancers from 315
    and skin cancer **124**
    UV types 124
Uncertainty
    and AIDS 417
Understanding cancer
    a seminar 256
United Cancer Council, Inc. 453, 455
United Ostomy Association, Inc. 14,
    454
Univalent vaccine 434g
Unproven methods
    see *Quackery*
    general discussion 16
    list of scientifically unproven can-
        cer methods 246
    proponent organizations 16
Uracil 434g
Uranium 86, 117
    also see *Radon*
Urban factor 117
Ureter
    illustrated 288
Urinary tract cancer **166–68**
    also see specific site
    anatomy 166
    and coffee 167
    and cyclamates 167
    diagnosis 167
    early detection 167
    epidemiology 166
    and obesity 167
    physiology 166
    prevention 167
    prognosis 166
    risk factors 166
    and saccharine 167
    screening for 167
    and smoking 167
    symptoms 167
    treatment 166
Urination
    in prostate cancer 149
Urine
    in prostate cancer 149
Urostomy 434g
    defined
    described 168

Urostomy *continued*
  illustrated 289
U.S. Preventive Services Task Force
  336
Uterine cancer **150–56**
  also see *Cervical cancer*
  also see *Endometrial cancer*
  also see *Uterine cervix*
  also see *Uterine corpus*
  anatomy 151
  cervical **150–56**
  definition 151
  endometrial **150–56**
  and intercourse 94
Uterine-cervix cancer
  summary table **119**
  types, percentages 23
Uterine corpus
  types, percentages 23
Uterine-endometrial cancer
  summary table **119**
Uterus **150–156, 434g**
  also see *Cervical cancer*
  also see *Endometrial cancer*
  also see *Uterine cancer*
  illustrated 152–53
UV light
  general 45

Vaccines 230
Vacuole
  illustrated 29
Vaginal cancer **160–62**
  and DES 161
  diagnosis 161
  epidemiology 161
  and morning-after pill 161
  prognosis 161
  risk factors 161
  symptoms 161
  treatment 161
  types 161
Vaginal self-examination 316
  how to **326**
  illustrated 326
  rationale 326
Vaginal, vulvar cancer
  summary table **120**
Varicocele 164, 326
Vas deferens
  illustrated 326
Venereal disease
  and testicular cancer 164
Venereal warts
  and cervical cancer 152
Venezula
  and HIV infection 392
Vertical transmission 434g
Vinblastine sulfate
  for AIDS 404
  side effects 449
Vincristine sulfate

for AIDS 404
  side effects 449
Vinyl chloride 97, 118
  and brain tumors 183
  and liver cancer 181
  and lung cancer 133
Virchow, Rudolf 10
Virology 434g
Virus 434g
  defined 62
  diagram of structure 62
Virus infection of cells (oncolysates)
  230
Viruses
  and adult T-cell leukemia 67
  bacteriophages 63
  and Bittner particles 142
  and breast cancer 142
  and Burkitt's lymphoma 68
  and cancer 69–71
  and cervical cancer 70
  compared to bacteria 62
  compared to cell 62
  cytomegalovirus and AIDS 398
  discovery of 10
  DNA 63, 64
  Epstein-Barr virus and AIDS 398
  and esophageal cancer 175
  and Evan's postulates 67
  feline leukemia virus 46, 396
  first human cancer virus 12
  Gallo, Robert 12
  genes 62
  hepatitis B 69
  and herpes virus 70
  HIV 389
  HIV transmission 412
  how they infect cells 64
  HTLV-I, HTLV-II, HTLV-III 389
  HTLV (human T-cell leukemia
    virus) 12
  and human cancer 67
  and human papilloma virus 70
  illustrated 63
  immune response to a common
    cold virus, illustrated 396
  and Koch's postulates 67
  list of cancers from 315
  and liver cancer 69
  mammary tumor virus 46
  oncogenes 46
  outcomes of infection 64
  outcomes of infection, illustration
    65
  overview 61
  protein coat 62
  replication 62
  retroid viruses 63
  retroviruses 63
  retroviruses and AIDS 396
  reverse transcriptase 11
  RNA 63, 64

steps to develop vaccines for 408
  steps to infecting a cell, illustra-
    tion 64
  structure 62
  transformation 64
  types 63
  viroids 63
  and veneral wart 70
Viruses and cancer
  history of 10
  Rous, F. Peyton 10
Visualization 264
Vitamin A 349
  for leukoplakia treatment 170
  list of cancers from low intake 315
Vitamin B-12
  deficiency, and smoking 88
Vitamin C 349–51
  and home stool blood testing 329
  and stomach cancer 177
  list of cancers from low intake 315
Vitiligo 124
Vocal cord cancer
  see *Laryngeal cancer*
Voice changes
  and laryngeal cancer 173
Voice recordings
  for detection of laryngeal cancer
    173
Voice rehabilitation 173
Voicebox
  see *Larynx*
Volunteering
  American Cancer Society 317
Vomiting
  and symptoms of CNS tumor 183
Von Roentgen, Wilhelm 10, 214
Von Volkmann, Richard 10
Vulva
  anatomy 161
  illustrated 152, 153
Vulvar cancer **160–62**
  diagnosis 161
  early detection 161
  epidemiology 161
  exams for 161
  prognosis 161
  risk factors 161
  symptoms 161
  treatment 161
  types 161
Vulvar self-examination 161, 315
  how to **326**
  rationale 326

Waldeyer's ring 57
Walter, J. 105
War and cancer 105
  atomic warfare, results of 106
  late hazards of atom bombs 106
War on cancer
  see *National Cancer Act of 1971*

Warts 63
Watch dial painters 104
Water pollution 114–16
    and aquifers 118
    and cancer 374
    drinking water 117
    nitrates 118
    and PCB 118
    radioactive substances 118
    and radon 118
    trihalomethanes 117
    vinyl chloride 118
Watson, James 33, 47, 51, 71
Wegman, David H. 96
Weight
    also see *Obesity*
    ideal body weight 352
Western bolt
    and HIV antibody test 414–15
White blood cells 190
    see *Immune system, cells of*
White, Laurens P. 292, 293
Whites

5-year survival rates 440
    cancer in 381
    ovarian cancer 158
Why me?
Will to live 264, 266–70
Wilms' tumor 22, 204, 434g
    drugs used in treatment 446
    discovered during infant/child
        exam by mother 328
    epidemiology 204
    radiation treatment for 218
    survival 204
    symptoms 204
    treatment 204
Wilson, Craig 86, 358
Wofsy, Constance 420
Women's health
    vulvar/vaginal self-examination
        326
Women's Health Trial 142
Worms 91
Wynder, Ernst 82

X-ray 434g
    also see *Radiation*
    avoiding unnecessary x-rays 371–
        73
    of the breast 333–34
    in children 104
    table of doses 373
Xeromammography **333**
    also see *Mammography*
Xeroradiography 434g
Xerostomia
    and radiation therapy 171, 217
    described 171

Yamagiwa, Katsusaburo 10
Yoga 264
Yttrium 434g

Zenogenic grafting 434g
Ziegler, Daniel 26
Zinc
    and esophagus cancer 175
Zippin, Calvin 238

Bull Publishing Books of Related Interest

Bilingual Charting for Spanish-speaking Nurses and Nursing Assistants, by Georgia M. Guerrero, DSD .... $ 9.95

A Comprehensive Guide for Cancer Patients and Their Families, by Ernest H. Rosenbaum, MD and Isadora Rosenbaum $12.95

Specific sections of this book are available separately:

Cancer Patients' Guide to Social Services and Hospital Procedures .... $ 4.95

Nutrition for the Cancer Patient .... $ 7.95

Rehabilitation Exercises for the Cancer Patient .... $ 4.95

Sexuality and Cancer .... $ 2.95

The Diagnosis is Cancer: A Psychological and Legal Resource Handbook for Cancer Patients, Their Families and Helping Professionals, by Edward J. Larschan, PhD, JD and Richard J. Larschan, PhD

paper $ 9.95
cloth $17.95

Disease Prevention/Health Promotion: The Facts
by the Office of Disease Prevention and Health Promotion, U.S. Public Health Service, U.S. Department of Health and Human Services $24.95

If You Find a Lump in Your Breast, by Martha McLean .... $ 2.95

Keeping Abreast: Breast Changes that are Not Cancer, by Kerry McGinn, RN, BSN, MA .... $ 7.95

The Ostomy Book: Living Comfortably with Colostomies Ileostomies and Urostomies, by Barbara Dorr Mullen and Kerry McGinn, RN, BSN, MA $11.95

The Ostomy Book for Nurses, by Kerry McGinn, RN $11.95

Taking Charge of Your Smoking, by Joyce D. Nash, PhD $12.95

(Prices subject to change without notice)

To order copies, you can charge by phone or send check, plus $3.00 for shipping/handling, (CA residents add 6-1/2% sales tax):

Bull Publishing Company
P.O. Box 208
Palo Alto, CA 94302-0208
(415) 322-2855